FERRI'S
PATIENT TEACHING GUIDES

FERRI'S
PATIENT TEACHING GUIDES

FRED F. FERRI, M.D., F.A.C.P.

Clinical Associate Professor
Brown University School of Medicine
Chief, Division of Internal Medicine
St. Joseph's Health Services and Fatima Hospital
Providence, Rhode Island

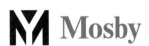 Mosby

St. Louis Baltimore Boston Carlsbad Chicago Minneapolis New York Philadelphia Portland
London Milan Sydney Tokyo Toronto

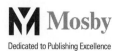

Mosby

Dedicated to Publishing Excellence

**A Times Mirror
Company**

Publisher: Susie H. Baxter
Senior Developmental Editor: Laura C. Berendson
Project Manager: Patricia Tannian
Book Design Manager: Gail Morey Hudson
Cover Design: Teresa Breckwoldt

FIRST EDITION

Copyright © 1999 by Mosby, Inc.

Mosby, Inc.
11830 Westline Industrial Drive
St. Louis, Missouri 63146

International Standard Book Number 0-8151-8397-6

98 99 00 01 02 / 9 8 7 6 5 4 3 2 1

CONTRIBUTORS

OMAR BAGASRA, M.D., PH.D.

Professor of Medicine, Thomas Jefferson University
Director, Molecular Retrovirology Laboratories
Philadelphia, Pennsylvania

Acquired Immune Deficiency Syndrome, Amebiasis, Ascariasis, Cat-scratch disease, Cellulitis, Chancroid, *Chlamydia* infection, Chickenpox, Condyloma acuminatum, Cryptococcosis, Endocarditis, Epididymitis, Epiglottitis, Fifth disease, Genital Herpes simplex, Giardiasis, Gingivitis, Gonorrhea, Granuloma inguinale, Hand-foot-and- mouth disease, Herpangina, HIV (human immunodeficiency syndrome) infection, Hookworm, Influenza, Laryngitis, Laryngotracheobronchitis (croup), Lymphangitis, Lymphogranuloma venereum, Malaria, Mastoiditis, Measles (rubeola), Mononucleosis, Mumps, Osteomyelitis, Otitis externa, Otitis media, Pharyngitis, Pinworms, Rheumatic fever, Rocky Mountain spotted fever, Rubella (German measles), Salmonellosis, Scarlet fever, Shigellosis, Sialadenitis, Sinusitis, Stevens-Johnson Syndrome, Syphilis, Tapeworm infestation, Tonsillitis, Toxic shock syndrome, Toxoplasmosis, Tracheitis, Trichinosis, Typhoid fever, Urethritis, Urinary tract infection

WILLIAM F. BINA III, M.D., M.P.H.

Associate Professor
Department of Family and Community Medicine
Mercer University School of Medicine;
Residency Director (Family Practice)
Medical Center of Central Georgia
Macon, Georgia

Furunculosis, Herpes simplex, Keloids, Marfan's syndrome, Pediculosis

JOHN MARK BOLTRI, M.D.

Associate Professor
Department of Family and Community Medicine
Mercer University School of Medicine
Macon, Georgia

Balantitis, Basal cell carcinoma, Erythema multiforme, Folliculitis, Granuloma annulare, Hyperhidrosis, Impetigo, Leukoplakia, Pityriasis rosea, Ringworm, Rosacea, Tinea capitis, Tinea corporis, Tinea cruris, Tinea pedis, Tinea unguium, Tinea versicolor, Vitiligo

MOLLY R. BURMA, R.N., M.S.N.

Department of Nursing
University of Iowa Hospitals and Clinics
Iowa City, Iowa

Costochondritis, Erythema nodosum, Fibromyalgia, Gout, Hip pain, Infectious arthritis (bacterial), Inflammatory myopathy (myositis), Juvenile rheumatoid arthritis, Low back pain, Lyme disease, Neck pain, Osteoarthritis, Polymyalgia rheumatica, Pseudogout, Psoriatic arthritis, Raynaud's phenomenon, Reiter's syndrome, Rheumatoid arthritis, Sjögren's syndrome, Systemic lupus erythematosus, Temporomandibular joint disorder, Tendinitis

CATHY C. CARTWRIGHT, R.N.C., M.S.N.

Clinical Nurse Specialist, Adjunct Faculty
Sinclair School of Nursing;
Clinical Nurse Specialist, Pediatric Neurosurgery
Childrens Hospital at University of Missouri Hospitals
    and Clinics
Columbia, Missouri

Autism, Down syndrome (trisomy 21, mongolism)

HEM ATULYA DEODHAR, M.D., M.R.C.P.

Fellow in Nephrology and Hypertension
Oregon Health Sciences University
Portland, Oregon

Acute glomerulonephritis, Acute renal failure, Pyelonephritis, Renal artery stenosis

JAMES D. DICKIE, M.D.

Mid Michigan Regional Medical Center
Midland, Michigan

Cholelithiasis

JOHN F. DONNELLY, M.D.

Associate Professor
Wright State University School of Medicine
Dayton, Ohio
Staff Physician, Greene Memorial Hospital
Xenia, Ohio
and Mercy Medical Center
Springfield, Ohio

Bullous pemphigoid, Discoid lupus erythematosus (DLE), Dermatitis herpetiformis, Pemphigus vulgaris, Psoriasis, Schleroderma (progressive systemic sclerosis)

ROBERT L. FRIERSON, M.D.

Professor of Psychiatry
University of Louisville School of Medicine;
Director, Consultation/Liaison Psychiatry
University of Louisville Affiliated Hospitals
Louisville, Kentucky

Agoraphobia and panic, Alcoholism, Anorexia nervosa, Anxiety (generalized anxiety disorder), ADHD (attention deficit hyperactivity disorder), Bipolar disorder, Bulimia nervosa, Child abuse, Major depression, Drug abuse, Elderly abuse, Encopresis, Enuresis, Erectile dysfunction, Insomnia, Obsessive compulsive disorder, Phobias, Posttraumatic stress disorder, Premature ejaculation, Schizophrenia

SCOTT R. GIBBS, M.A., M.D.

Director, Brain and NeuroSpine Center
Southeast Missouri Hospital
Cape Girardeau, Missouri

Alzheimer's disease, Amaurosis fugax, Autism, Bell's palsy, Carotid sinus syndrome, Carpal tunnel syndrome,

Cerebrovascular accident, Cervical disc disease, Cluster headache, Down syndrome (trisomy 21, mongolism), Febrile seizures, Grand mal seizure disorder, Jacksonian seizure disorder, Labyrinthitis, Lumbar disc syndromes, Meniere's disease, Meningioma, Migraine headache, Motion sickness, Multiple sclerosis, Myasthenia gravis, Narcolepsy, Parkinson's disease, Petit mal seizure disorder, Stokes-Adams attacks (Adams-Stokes-Morgagni syndrome; cardiac faints), Tension-type headache, Tourette's syndrome, Transient ischemic attack, Trigeminal neuralgia

FRED S. GIRTON, M.D.

Associate Professor
Department of Family and Community Medicine
Mercer University School of Medicine
Macon, Georgia

Acne vulgaris, Angioedema, Herpes zoster, Plantar warts, Scabies, Warts

ROBERT B. HASH, M.D.

Associate Professor
Department of Family and Community Medicine
Mercer University School of Medicine
Macon, Georgia

Animal bites, Burns, Frostbite, Heat exhaustion and heat stroke, Human bites, Hypothermia, Paronychia, Snake bites

SCOTT T. HENDERSON, M.D.

Assistant Professor of Family Practice
University of Wyoming Family Practice Residency
   Program at Cheyenne
Cheyenne, Wyoming

Achalasia, Alcoholic hepatitis, Celiac disease, Chronic hepatitis, Chronic pancreatitis, Crohn's disease, Cirrhosis, primary biliary, Cirrhosis of the liver, Diverticulitis, Diverticulosis, Dumping syndrome, Food poisoning, bacterial, Gastritis, Gastroesophageal reflux disease, Glossitis, Gilbert's Disease, Halitosis, Hepatitis A Hepatitis, alcoholic, Hepatitis B, Hepatitis C, Hepatitis, chronic, Hiatal hernia, Irritable bowel syndrome, Lactose intolerance, Pancreatitis chronic, Peptic ulcer disease, Pruritus ani, Pseudomembranous colitis, Short bowel syndrome, Stomatitis, Ulcerative Colitis, Whipple's disease

EDWARD S. HORTON, M.D.

Professor of Medicine
Harvard Medical School;
Vice President, Joslin Diabetes Center
Boston, Massachusetts

Acromegaly, Addisons Disease, Cushings Syndrome, Diabetes Insipidus, Type I Diabetes, Type II Diabetes, Hirsutism, Hyperaldosteronism, Hyperparathyroidism, Hypopituitism, Klinefelters Syndrome, Obesity, Osteoporosis, Pagets Disease, Pheochromocytoma, Prolactinoma, Syndrome or Inappropriate Anti-Diuretic Hormone Secretion (SIADH), Thyroid nodules Thyroiditis

ANDREW JAMES, R.N.

Staff Nurse II Emergency Service,
University of Missouri Hospitals and Clinics
Columbia, Missouri

Alzheimers disease, Bells palsy, Meningioma, Narcolepsy, Seizure disorder, grand mal; Seizure disorder, Jacksonian; Seizure disorder, petit mal; Trigeminal neuralgia

FRANCIS J. KELLY, M.D., M.R.C.P.I.

Fellow in Nephrology and Hypertension
Oregon Health Sciences University
Portland, Oregon

Chronic renal failure, Nephrotic syndrome, Renal calculi, Wegeners granulomatosis

JOHN W. KENNEDY, M.D.

Endocrinology and Metabolism Fellow
Harvard Medical School; Joslin Diabetes Center
Boston, Massachusetts

Acromegaly, Addisons Disease, Cushings Syndrome Diabetes Insipidus, Type I Diabetes, Type II Diabetes, Hirsutism, Hyperaldosteronism, Hyperparathyroidism, Hypopituitism, Klinefelters Syndrome, Obesity, Osteoporosis, Pagets Disease, Pheochromocytoma, Prolactinoma, Syndrome or Inappropriate Anti-Diuretic Hormone Secretion (SIADH), Thyroid nodules Thyroiditis

TODD ALAN KILE, M.D.

Chair, Division of Foot and Ankle Surgery
Mayo Clinic
Scottsdale, Arizona;
Assistant Professor of Orthopedic Surgery
Mayo Medical School
Rochester, Minnesota

Ankylosing spondylitis, Bursitis, Cervical spondylosis, Charcotjoint, Disc herniation, Frozen shoulder, Knee pain, LeggCalvePerthes Disease, Metatarsalgia, OsgoodSchlatter Disease, Osteochondritis dissecans, Rotator cuff tendinitis/tear, Tarsal tunnel syndrome, Scoliosis

JEFFREY KOVAN, D.O.

Assistant Professor
Department of Family Practice and Director of Sports
   Medicine
Michigan State University;
Staff Physician, St. Lawrence Hospital
Lansing, Michigan

Angina pectoris, Aortic regurgitation, Aortic stenosis, Atherosclerosis, Atrial fibrillation, Atrial flutter, Atrial septal defect, Bradycardia, Bundle branch block, Congestive heart failure, Dilated cardiomyopathy, Hypercholesterolemia, Hypertension, Hypertrophic cardiomyopathy, Mitral regurgitation, Mitral stenosis, Mitral valve prolapse, Multifocal atrial tachycardia, Myocarditis, Paroxysmal atrial tachycardia, Pericarditis, Premature atrial contractions, Premature ventricular contractions, Primary hyperlipoproteinemia, Restrictive cardiomyopathy, Second-degree heart block, Syncope, Tricuspid regurgitation, Tricuspid stenosis, Ventricular septal defect, Wolff-Parkinson-White syndrome, Basic description of cardiac function (Appendix I)

DELLA MAKOWER, M.D.

Assistant Professor of Medicine
Albert Einstein College of Medicine
Assistant Attending Physician,
Montefiore Medical Center
Bronx, New York

Anemia, sickle cell, Hemochromatosis, Leukemia, chronic
myelogenous, Leukemia, hairy cell, Idiopathic thrombocytopenia purpura

UMMEKALSOOM MALIK, MD

Assistant Professor of Medicine
Albert Einstein College of Medicine
Assistant Attending Physician
Montefiore Medical Center
Bronx, New York

Anemia, folate deficiency, Disseminated intravascular coagulation, Leukemia, chronic lymphocytic, Polycithemia vera

J. DOUGLAS MCDONALD, M.D.

Primary Care Sports Medicine Physician
Michigan State University
East Lansing, Michigan;
Physician, Sports and Family Medicine
Mercy Walworth Medical Center
Lake Geneva, Wisconsin

Angina pectoris, Aortic regurgitation, Aortic valvular stenosis, Atherosclerosis, Atrial fibrillation, Atrial flutter, Atrial
septal defect, Bradycardia, Bundle branch block,
Cardiomyopathy, dilated; Cardiomyopathy, hypertrophic;
Cardiomyopathy, restrictive; Congestive heart failure, Heart
block, second degree; Hypercholesterolemia,
Hyperlipoproteinemias, primary; Hypertension,Mitral regurgitation, Mitral stenosis, Mitral valve prolapse, Multifocal
atrial tachycardia, Myocarditis, Paroxysmal atrial tachycardia, Pericarditis, Premature atrial contractions, Premature
ventricular contractions, Syncope, Tricuspid regurgitation,
Tricuspid stenosis, Ventricular septal defect,
WolffParkinsonWhite syndrome, Basic Description of
Cardiac Function (Appendix I)

DIANE M. MUELLER, R.N., M.S.N., F.N.P.

Nurse Practitioner, Neurosurgery
University of Missouri Hospitals and Clinics
Columbia, Missouri

Carpal tunnel syndrome, Cervical disc disease, Lumbar disc
disease, Multiple sclerosis, Myasthenia gravis, Parkinsons
disease

YELENA NOVIK, M.D.

Assistant Professor of Medicine
Albert Einstein College of Medicine
Assistant Attending Physician
Montefiore Medical Center
Bronx, New York

Anemia, aplastic; Anemia, of chronic disease; Anemia, pernicious, Myelodysplastic syndrome, Myeloproliferative disorders, Von Willebrands disease

ERIC OLSON, M.D.

Assistant Professor of Medicine
Mayo Clinic/Mayo Medical School;
Senior Associate Consultant
Division of Pulmonary and Critical Care
Mayo Clinic Foundation
Rochester, Minnesota

Altitude sickness, Asbestosis, Atelectasis, Diffuse interstitial
pulmonary disease, Legionnaires disease, Pneumonia, bacterial; Pneumonia, mycoplasma; Pneumonia, pneumocystis
carinii; Pneumonia, viral; Sleep apnea, obstructive; Silicosis

DOUGLAS S. PARKS, M.D.

Assistant Professor of Family Practice
University of Wyoming Family Practice Residency
Program at Cheyenne
Cheyenne, Wyoming

Achilles tendon rupture, Ankle fracture, Ankle sprain,
Concussion, Epistaxis, Femoral neck fracture, Insect bites
(stings), Marine envenomation bites, Pneumothorax, Post-
concussion syndrome, Rhabdomyolysis, Spider bites

ASHOK M. PATEL, M.D.

Assistant Professor of Medicine
Mayo Clinic/Mayo Medical School;
Senior Associate Consultan,
Division of Pulmonary and Critical Care
Mayo Clinic Foundation
Rochester, Minnesota

Abscess, lung; Asthma, Bronchiectasis, Bronchitis, acute;
Chronic obstructive pulmonary disease, Cystic fibrosis,
Pertussis, Rhinitis, allergic; Sarcoidosis, Tuberculosis

PETER PETROPOULOS, M.D.

Clinical Instructor of Medicine, Brown University;
Department of Veterans Affairs
Providence, Rhode Island

Bladder neoplasms, Breast cancer, Cervical cancer, Colon
cancer, Endometrial cancer, Esophageal tumors, Hodgkin's
Disease, Kaposi's sarcoma, Lung neoplasms, primary;
Lymphoma, nonHodgkin's; Melanoma, Mesothelioma, lung;
Multiple myeloma, Ovarian Cancer,
Paget's Disease of the breast, Prostate cancer, Salivary gland
tumors, Testicular cancer, Thyroid neoplasms, Uterine malig-
nancies

KENNETH G. SAAG, M.D., M.SC.

Assistant Professor, Division of Rheumatology
Department of Internal Medicine
University of Iowa College of Medicine
Iowa City, Iowa

Costochondritis, Erythema nodosum, Fibromalgia, Gout, Hip
pain, Infectious arthritis, Inflammatory Myopathy, Juvenile
rheumatoid arthritis,
Low back pain, Lyme Disease,Neck pain, Osteoarthritis,
Polymyalgia rheumatica, Pseudogout, Psoriatic arthritis,
Raynaud's phenomenon, Reiter's Syndrome, Rheumatoid
arthritis, Sjogren's syndrome, Systematic lupus erythematosus, Tendinitis, Temporomandibular joint syndrome

CHRISTIANE SECCO, M.D.
Fellow, Albert Einstein College of Medicine
Montefiore Medical Center
Bronx, New York

Anemia, iron deficiency; Hemophilia, Lead poisoning, Priapism, Thalassemia minor

ROSLYN D. TAYLOR, M.D.
Associate Director
Department of Family and Community Medicine
  Education,
Memorial Family Practice Center
Savannah, Georgia

Erysipelas, Lichen planus, Onychomycosis, Pressure ulcer, Roseola

RICHARD TIPPERMAN, M.D.
Assistant Surgeon, Wills Eye Hospital
Allegheny University of the Health Sciences
Thomas Jefferson University
Philadelphia, Pennsylvania

Cataracts, Chalazion, Conjunctivitis, Corneal abrasion, Corneal foreign body, Glaucoma, primary angle closure

PAUL C. UTRIE, M.D.
Department of Internal Medicine
Division of Rheumatology
University of Iowa Hospitals and Clinics
Iowa City, Iowa

Costochondritis, Erythema nodosum, Fibromalgia, Gout, Hip pain, Infectious arthritis, Inflammatory Myopathy, Juvenile rheumatoid arthritis, Low back pain, Lyme Disease, Neck pain, Osteoarthritis, Polymyalgia rheumatica, Pseudogout, Psoriatic arthritis, Raynaud's phenomenon, Reiter's Syndrome, Rheumatoid arthritis, Sjogren's syndrome, Systematic lupus erythematosus, Tendinitis, Temporomandibular joint syndrome

SARAH J. VOGEL, M.D.
Albany Medical Center
Albany, New York

Amaurosis fugax, Headache, cluster; Headache, migraine, Headache, tension; Labyrinthitis, Menieres disease, Seizures, febrile; Transient ischemic attack

MAY M. WAKAMATSU, M.D.
Clinical Instructor, Harvard Medical School;
Assistant in Gynecology
Massachusetts General Hospital
Boston, Massachusetts

Breast Infection, Cervical dysplasia, Cervical polyps, Cervicitis, Contraception, Dysfunctional uterine bleeding, Dysmenorrhea, Endometriosis, Fibrocystic breast disease, Menopause, Ovarian Cysts, Vaginitis, Candida; Vaginitis, Trichomonas; Vaginosis, Bacterial;
Pelvic Inflammatory Disease (PID), Pelvic Organ Prolapse, Premenstrual Syndrome (PMS), Uterine myomas, Urinary incontinence

ROBERTA J. WEINTRAUT, M.D.
Assistant Professor of Family Practice;
Endocrinology Tutor
Mercer University School of Medicine;
Associate Director, Family Practice Residency
  Program
Medical Center of Central Georgia
Macon, Georgia

Atopic dermatitis; Contact dermatitis; Diaper dermatitis, Eczema, Graves disease, Hypothyroidism, Photodermatitis, Statis dermatitis

PREFACE

Ferris Clinical Advisor Patient Teaching Guides are designed to educate patients and their caregivers about the patients illnesses and facilitate their care. The physician may print and photocopying the handouts.

As practicing physicians we all realize the importance of patient education and the need for clear communication with our patients. The focus of each Guide is on what the patient needs to do after leaving the physicians office. In the home setting patients need to know how to speed recovery, prevent infection, administer medication, and when to contact the doctor for further assistance if certain warning signs occur.

Ferris Clinical Advisor Patient Teaching Guides are visually appealing, organized alphabetically, and written in a style that patients can easily comprehend. The format of each guide is user friendly with each topic subdivided into the following seven sections: About Your Diagnosis, Living With Your Diagnosis, Treatment, The DOs, The DONTs, When To Call Your Doctor, For More Information (Resources). Illustrations are used extensively in many topics to facilitate patient comprehension. An area for personalized instructions has also been reserved in each Guide. Additionally, several appendices provide anatomical drawings, nutritional tips, and wellness tips, especially relating to geriatric patients.

The majority of the Guides deal with diseases and disorders commonly seen by Primary Care physicians and extensively covered in Ferris Clinical Advisor, a truly state of the art medical information system for physicians.

Given the health care climate of cost containment and managed care combined with an increasingly litigious society, proper communication with patients is essential. With less time available to spend on each patient and continued need to keep patients better informed, I strongly believe that physicians and allied health professionals will find Ferris Clinical Advisor Patient Teaching Guides an essential partner in their daily practice of medicine.

Fred F. Ferri, M.D., F.A.C.P.

CONTENTS

Chlamydia infection
Cholelithiasis
Chronic obstructive pulmonary disease
Cirrhosis
Cirrhosis, primary biliary
Colon cancer
Concussion
Condyloma acuminatum
Congestive heart failure
Conjunctivitis
Contraception
Corneal abrasion
Corneal foreign body
Costochondritis
Crohn's disease
Cryptococcosis
Cushing's disease and syndrome
Cystic fibrosis
Depression, major
Dermatitis, atopic
Dermatitis, contact
Dermatitis, diaper
Dermatitis, herpetiformis
Dermatitis, stasis
Diabetes isipidus
Diabetes mellitus, type I
Diabetes mellitus, type II
Diffuse interstitial pulmonary disease
Disk herniation
Disseminated intravascular coagulation
Diverticulitis
Diverticulosis
Down syndrome (trisomy 21,
  mongolism)
Dumping syndrome
Dysfunctional uterine bleeding
Dysmenorrhea
Eczema
Ejaculation, premature
Encopresis
Endocarditis, infective
Endometrial cancer
Endometriosis
Enuresis
Epididymitis
Epiglottitis
Epistaxis
Erectile dysfunction

Erysipelas (St. Anthony's fire)
Erythema multiforme
Erythema nodosum
Esophageal tumors
Femoral neck fracture
Fibrocystic breast disease
Fibromyalgia
Fifth disease
Folliculitis
Food poisoning, bacterial
Frostbite
Frozen shoulder
Furunculosis
Gastritis
Gastroesophageal reflux disease
Giardiasis
Gilbert's disease
Gingivitis
Glaucoma, primary open angle
Glomerulonephritis, acute
Glossitis
Gonorrhea
Gout
Granuloma annulare
Granuloma inguinale
Graves'disease
Halitosis
Hand-foot-and-mouth disease
Headache, cluster
Headache, migraine
Headache, tension-type
Heart block, second-degree
Heat exhaustion and heat stroke
Hemochromatosis
Hemophilia
Hepatitis A
Hepatitis, alcoholic
Hepatitis B
Hepatitis C
Hepatitis, chronic
Herpangina
Herpes simplex
Herpes simplex, genital
Herpes zoster
Hiatal hernia
Hip pain
Hirsutism

HIV (human immunodeficiency virus) infection
Hodgkin's disease
Hookworm
Hypercholesterolemia
Hyperhidrosis
Hyperlipoproteinemia, primary
Hyperparathyroidism
Hypertension
Hypopituitarism
Hypothermia
Hypothroidism
Idiopathic thrombocytopenic purpura
Impetigo
Inflammatory myopathy (myositis)
Influenza
Insomnia
Irritable bowel syndrome
Kaposi's sarcoma
Keloids
Klinefelter's syndrome
Knee pain
Labyrinthitis
Lactose intolerance
Laryngitis
Laryngotracheobronchitis (croup)
Lead poisoning
Legg-Calvé-Perthes disease
Legionnaires' disease
Leukemia, chronic lymphocytic
Leukemia, chronic myelogenous
Leukemia, hairy cell
Leukoplakia
Lichen planus
Low back pain
Lumbar disc syndromes
Lung neoplasm, primary
Lupus erythematosus, discoid (DLE)
Lyme disease
Lymphangitis
Lymphogranuloma venereum
Lymphoma, non-Hodgkin's
Malaria
Marfan's syndrome
Mastoiditis
Measles (rubeola)
Melanoma
Meniere's disease

Meningioma
Menopause
Mesothelioma of the lung
Metatarsalgia
Mitral regurgitation
Mitral stenosis
Mitral valve prolapse
Mononucleosis
Motion sickness
Multifocal atrial tachycardia
Multiple myeloma
Multiple sclerosis
Mumps
Myasthenia gravis
Myelodysplastic syndromes
Myeloproliferative disorders
Myocarditis
Narcolepsy
Neck pain
Nephrotic syndrome
Obesity
Obsessive compulsive disorder
Onychomycosis
Osgood-Schlatter disease
Osteoarthritis
Osteochondritis dissecans
Osteomyelitis
Osteoporosis
Otitis externa
Otitis media
Ovarian cancer
Ovarian cysts
Paget's disease of the bone
Paget's disease of the breast
Pancreatitis, chronic
Parkinson's disease
Paronychia
Paroxysmal atrial tachycardia
Pediculosis
Pelvic inflammatory disease
Pelvic organ prolapse
Pemphigoid, bullous
Pemphigus vulgaris
Peptic ulcer disease
Pericarditis
Pertussis
Pharyngitis
Pheochromocytoma

Phobias
Photodermatitis
Pinworms
Pityriasis rosea
Pneumonia, bacterial
Pneumonia, *Mycoplasma*
Pheumonia, *Pneumocystis carinii*
Pneumonia, viral
Pneumothorax
Polycythemia vera
Polymyalgia rheumatica
Postconcussional syndrome
Posttraumatic stress disorder
Premature atrial contractions
Premature ventricular contractions
Premenstrual syndrome
Pressure ulcers (decubitus ulcers, bedsores)
Priapism
Prolactinoma
Prostate cancer
Pruritus ani
Pseudogout
Pseudomembranous colitis
Psoriasis
Pyelonephritis
Raynaud's phenomenon
Reiter's syndrome
Renal artery stenosis
Renal calculi
Renal failure, acute
Renal failure, chronic
Rhabdomyolyis
Rheumatic fever
Rhinitis, allergic
Ringworm
Rocky Mountain spotted fever
Rosacea
Roseola (exanthema subitum)
Rotator cuff tendinitis/tear
Rubella (German measles)
Salivary gland tumors
Salmonellosis
Sarcoidosis
Scabies
Scarlet fever
Schizophrenia
Scleroderma (progressive systemic sclerosis)
Scoliosis

Seizure disorder, grand mal
Seizure disorder, Jacksonian
Seizure disorder, petit mal
Seizures, febrile
Shigellosis
Short bowel syndrome
Sialadenitis
Silicosis
Sinusitis
Sjögren's syndrome
Sleep apnea, obstructive
Stevens-Johnson syndrome
Stokes-Adams attacks (Adams-Stokes-Morgagni syndrome; cardiac faints)
Stomatitis
Syncope
Syndrome of inappropriate antidiuretic hormone secretion (SIADH)
Syphilis
Systemic lupus erythematosus
Tapeworm infestation
Tarsal tunnel syndrome
Temporomandibular joint syndrome
Tendinitis
Testicular cancer
Thalassemia minor
Thyroid neoplasms
Thyroid nodule
Thyroiditis
Tinea capitis
Tinea corporis
Tinea cruris
Tinea pedis
Tinea unguium
Tinea versicolor
Tonsillitis
Tourette's syndrome
Toxic shock syndrome
Toxoplasmosis
Tracheitis
Transient ischemic attack
Trichinosis
Tricuspid regurgitation
Tricuspid stenosis
Trigeminal neuralgia
Tuberculosis, pulmonary
Typhoid fever
Ulcerative colitis

Urethritis
Urinary incontinence
Urinary tract infection
Uterine malignancy
Uterine myomas
Vaginitis, *Candida*
Vaginitis, *Trichomonas*
Vaginosis, bacterial
Ventricular septal defect
Vitiligo
von Willebrand's disease

Warts
Warts, plantar
Wegener's granulomatosis
Whipple's disease
Wolff-Parkinson-White syndrome

APPENDICES

FERRI'S
PATIENT TEACHING GUIDES

ABSCESS, LUNG

About Your Diagnosis

Lung abscess refers to a cavity in your lung filled with pus. Predisposing factors are stroke, excessive sleepiness, alcoholism, and poor oral hygiene. The diagnosis may be suspected from the history, although a chest x-ray and/or computed tomography (CT) scan of the chest, in addition to sputum and blood culture results are helpful. Most cases are not contagious. Successful treatment depends on the underlying cause and coexisting medical problems.

Living With Your Diagnosis

Productive cough is not always present but may be foul smelling and associated with a spiking fever, chills, and weight loss. Careful examination of the oral cavity including the teeth, the swallowing mechanism, and the heart (listening for heart murmurs) is also very useful. Complications from a lung abscess may include rupture of the abscess into the pleural space, respiratory failure and septic shock, increased shortness of breath, and chest or upper abdominal pain.

Treatment

The best treatment is a prolonged course of appropriate antibiotic therapy, initially intravenously and then orally. Postural drainage, careful monitoring for any complicating events, and occasionally surgery is necessary. With prompt and adequate treatment, most lung abscesses collapse and heal over 4–6 weeks.

The DOs

It is very important to complete the full course of antibiotic therapy as outlined by your physician. Prompt notification for any relapse in terms of fever, hemoptysis (coughing up blood), adverse medication effects, or help with smoking cessation are also important. In individuals who have problems with recurrent aspiration, changes in the diet, and consideration for feeding tube placement may be necessary. Regular performance of postural drainage especially over the affected lung segment is usually beneficial.

The DON'Ts

Don't stop your antibiotics unless advised by your doctor. Do not expect a quick recovery or complete normalization of the chest x-ray within 3–4 weeks.

When to Call Your Doctor

Notify your doctor immediately if you develop a sudden worsening in chest pain associated with shortness of breath and copious sputum production or hemoptysis. See your doctor if your symptoms persist despite completing your course of antibiotics, or if you experience significant weight loss or tiredness.

For More Information
American Lung Association
1118 Hampton Avenue
St. Louis, MO 63139
800-LUNG-USA
www.lungusa.org

ABUSE, CHILD

About Your Diagnosis

Child abuse and neglect are major sociological problems for this country. The number of alleged abuse incidents reported to state and local child protective services organizations has skyrocketed, and current statistics show that physical abuse is the leading cause of death for children younger than 1 year in the United States. As of the 1990 census figures, 160,000 children younger than 3 years were abused or neglected, representing 25% of all child abuse victims in the United States. The first year of life seems to have the highest incidence of child mistreatment in all years from birth to 18 years, and more than two third of child victims of physical abuse are younger than 6 years. Child abuse can take many forms; however, the so-called "shaken infant syndrome" is particularly disturbing and is associated with high death rates and physical injury.

Most symptoms of child abuse result in such physical conditions as bleeding into the brain, blindness, and/or injuries to the different abdominal organs, and these injuries account for most of the deaths from child abuse. Another common form of child mistreatment in infancy is the familiar syndrome of failure to thrive. As many as 30% of all cases of failure to thrive are considered to be caused by parental neglect. Because severe malnutrition in the first 6 months of life can cause permanent brain damage, failure to thrive may be associated with severe behavioral problems later in life.

It is difficult to pinpoint an exact cause or predisposing factor to child abuse. However, child abuse and child mistreatment appear to be associated with poverty, unemployment, disability of a child, psychiatric problems in the parents, substance abuse by the parents, a history of the parents being abused as a children, antisocial behavior of the parents, and whether the pregnancy was planned or not. However, none of these factors alone seems to be sufficient to predict whether a child born into this environment will be abused. In some cases, the parent-child problem may be more an example of child neglect than child abuse, and often depression or schizophrenia in the parent can lead to poor bonding and a tendency to avoid the child, thereby leaving the child susceptible to any number of consequences of child neglect. Some parents, especially young, first-time parents, may be overwhelmed by the responsibility of having to care for a child, and become frustrated. Often, parents direct their feelings of anger and frustration toward their child, using their child as a scapegoat, when in fact their anger and frustration are related to difficulties at work or difficulties in other relationships. Thus not caring for the usual needs of the child (neglect) may have different causes than deliberate mistreatment of the child (abuse). In particularly disturbing incidences of child abuse one or both parents may use the child for some form of sexual gratification. Certainly, there has been a significant rise in sexual abuse of children. However, merely witnessing the abuse of a sibling or of a mother or father by the other partner can have serious psychological consequences on a child.

Living With Your Diagnosis

Not surprisingly, studies of children who have been abused show significant problems in their emotional, social, and behavioral functioning. These children seem to have difficulty accepting emotion and tenderness, and difficulty relating in a trusting way to others. They are often unfamiliar with the concept of unconditional love. Undeserved guilt may surface because many of these children later begin to feel that they in fact were responsible for the abuse, and that if they had been quieter or less obvious, or perhaps even not born, that their parent would not be facing consequences of abuse, or the family unit would not be disintegrating. Such doubts can lead to tremendous feelings of low self-esteem among children who have been abused. Abused children also tend to exhibit anger and aggression toward their playmates and schoolmates, so social behavior is often poor. These children are certainly more likely to have major psychiatric problems such as posttraumatic stress disorder, depression, anxiety, phobias, and personality disorders, and of course, they are more likely to become abusive parents.

Treatment

Treatment of child abuse is often initiated by the reporting or suspecting of the abuse by neighbors, other family members, or medical personnel. Most emergency departments that serve children are particularly wary of children who come in frequently, especially with frequent orthopedic injuries, and who have bruises or evidence of old fractures on x-ray. In all 50 states, physicians and other medical caregivers are obligated to report suspected child abuse and can face sanctions for not doing so. In most states, there is an organization similar to a child protective agency that investigates cases of child abuse and determines whether the child should be allowed to remain in the home. If the child is removed from the home, this will often lead to placement of the child in foster care and in some cases, legal charges being made against the parents.

It is important to emphasize that in the treatment of child abuse, the primary and most important goal is the protection of the child. Obviously there is a need to evaluate and treat any medical consequences of the abuse, and to allow the child to engage in therapy for the abuse. Childhood therapy for abuse often involves the use of play therapy including puppets which provide a nonthreatening atmosphere for the child to discuss or demonstrate the abuse to the therapist by acting it out with dolls or puppets. This is especially helpful in cases of sexual abuse. If there are negative consequences, such as a parent being arrested or the child being taken from the home, often the child will blame himself for these consequences and may be reluctant to discuss the abuse.

The abusing parent also requires treatment, regardless of whether they become involved in the criminal justice system. Support groups for parents have been very helpful, and parents should be treated. In addition, many states have a program for monitoring subsequent pregnancies to assess whether it is safe for those babies to return home with the new parents.

Many adults have flashbacks to childhood physical and sexual abuse that they may have suppressed the memory of for years. Often these flashbacks are very intrusive and come at very inopportune times. It seems that childhood sexual abuse predisposes to a number of psychiatric disorders including borderline and multiple personality disorder, eating disorders, posttraumatic stress disorder, and alcohol and drug abuse. There are other peer support groups, many modeled along the lines of Adults Molested as Children (AMAC) or similar organizations.

A more desirable approach to child abuse would be preventive. Evaluating the level of support and the support network for new parents, providing parenting classes, especially for young women who are having their first child, having mother's day out days for the mothers of newborn infants, and encouraging new parents to talk about their concerns and fears about being new parents would all be helpful. Overwhelmed parents should not be ashamed or embarrassed to talk to their physicians or ministers. Of course, any episodes of abuse (even if by a family member) should be reported and investigated. Role playing between parent and child (What to Do If Approached by a Stranger, What to Do If Touched Inappropriately, etc.) can be very helpful. Unfortunately, most children are abused by someone they know. There are several commercial videos available through your local library or children's hospital. The book entitled *How to Raise a Street Smart Child* is particularly helpful.

For more information try the following Web sites:
Child Abuse Handbook Summary
http://www.fcbe.edu.on.ca/www/pubs/cah/cahsummary.htm
Sexual Abuse Information Page
http://www.cs.utk.edu/~bartley/salnfopage.htm/

In summary, the evaluation and treatment of child abuse involves both the awareness of the condition, the reporting of the condition by anyone who suspects it, and the rehabilitation of both the child and the parent.

ABUSE, DRUG

About Your Diagnosis

The abuse of prescription and illicit drugs is a major problem in this country. To understand some of the aspects of drug abuse, it is important to define the following three terms: tolerance, physical addiction, and psychological addiction.

Tolerance is present when a drug abuser needs ever-increasing amounts of the drug to achieve the same effect as before, or to avoid having withdrawal symptoms. Tolerance is a major feature of physical drug addiction. However, it is important to remember that tolerance can be lost. For instance, an individual abusing heroin who has a high tolerance to the drug decides to stop using it for a matter of months. If he then starts using the same amount he was using when he stopped, the amount could be fatal because tolerance may be lost.

Physical addiction is present when some degree of tolerance exists. An individual with physical addiction to a drug will have withdrawal symptoms when the drug is stopped. Symptoms of withdrawal include piloerection (gooseflesh), nausea, vomiting, abdominal cramps, diarrhea, a rapidly beating heart, sweating, insomnia, and strong feelings of anxiety. Withdrawal from drugs such as benzodiazepines (including Librium, Valium, and Ativan), barbiturates, and alcohol can be life-threatening. Generally, the withdrawal from drugs that are depressants is much more severe than withdrawal from drugs that are stimulants, such as phencyclidine (PCP) and cocaine.

Psychological addiction is present when an individual has a severe craving for a drug and engages in such drug-seeking behavior as forging prescriptions, faking illnesses, and even committing acts of violence to obtain the drug. Drugs causing psychological addiction often do not produce physical withdrawal when stopped. Cocaine, for instance, is extremely psychologically addicting, whereas alcohol and Valium are very strongly psychologically and physically addicting.

Living With Your Diagnosis

There is no typical drug abuser. Drug abusers can be found among housewives and businessmen, inner-city dwellers and rural inhabitants, and include individuals of all races and creeds. In the past, more men have sought treatment for drug abuse; however, that is changing. More women are being admitted to drug abuse programs, probably because of more awareness of the problem among women. There are basically five categories of drugs that are abused: depressants, stimulants, hallucinogens, inhalants, and PCP.

Depressants are drugs that make individuals feel down in the dumps and slowed down when they are used. They include alcohol, barbiturates (e.g., phenobarbital and Seconal), opiates (e.g., heroin, Dilaudid, morphine, and codeine), other pain killers (e.g., Demerol and Talwin), and drugs like meprobamate. Depressants are very strongly physically addicting, and withdrawal from these drugs can be life-threatening.

Stimulants are drugs that produce a "high" and can have the unwanted effects of causing severe insomnia, as well as a feeling of restlessness and an inability to sit still. Cocaine is a stimulant that is used in a number of forms, including the purified form, which is often smoked ("crack" cocaine). Other drugs in this group include the amphetamines, such as methamphetamine (often known as crank); caffeine; various over-the-counter stimulants, including Sinex preparations that contain a drug called phenylpropanolamine; and diet pills, including the popular FenPhen diet pill, which has recently been associated with lung and heart problems and taken off the market.

Hallucinogens are drugs that cause individuals to see things, hear things, or feel things that are not actually there, or cause individuals to misinterpret things. For instance, individuals may see intravenous tubing going into their arm and believe it is a snake, or hear leaves rustling outside and believe that someone is whispering about them. These misperceptions are called illusions. The hallucinogens were once very popular in the 1960s, and unfortunately they have made a comeback since the 1980s. They include lysergic acid (LSD), mescaline (the active ingredient of the peyote cactus), and Psilocybin, or the magic mushrooms. These drugs are very unpredictable and extremely dangerous because of behaviors individuals exhibit while using them.

Inhalants are drugs that are commonly huffed, snorted, or sniffed. Examples of inhalants include gasoline, cleaning products, anesthetics such as chloroform, nitrous oxide, and halothane, hair sprays, bug sprays, spray paints, solvents such as toluene (toluene), airplane glue, typewriter correction fluid, and kerosene. The inhalant drugs are very commonly used among teenagers and can cause severe physical damage, including kidney disease, blood disease, and a dementia or mental disorder similar to Alzheimer's. One of the major problems with these drugs, in terms of stopping the abuse, is that they are usually inexpensive, are often found in the workplace or at corner drug stores, and produce only mild physical withdrawal. However, there is strong psychological dependency or drug craving and drug-seeking behavior associated with them.

Phencyclidine (PCP) is usually considered separately from the other drugs because it has so many different features. Formerly called "angel dust," it is a drug that can produce psychosis or depression. It can cause individuals to overestimate their own strength because it does have some pain-killing properties. In addition, PCP can be stored in the body and released at another time, even without individuals using the drug again. This episode, called a "flashback," is fairly common with PCP.

One drug that we have not mentioned is marijuana. Marijuana, similar to PCP, has a number of different properties. It will often make individuals who are already depressed more depressed, and it may cause paranoia in some individuals. Many individuals consider marijuana to be a gateway drug; that is, it is often the first drug that individuals use on their way to using even stronger agents.

There are other drugs that are abused, too many to discuss in this chapter. However, two other drugs of abuse are worth mentioning: the so-called "designer drugs," which have some hallucinogenic properties; and GHB, which is a drug that has gathered notoriety as a "date-rape" drug.

Treatment

There are many different ways to treat drug abuse, but they involve one basic principle: discontinue the use of the drug. For those drugs such as the depressants that are associated with a strong physical addiction, and therefore withdrawal, the drugs should not be stopped all at once. When alcohol is the abused drug, other drugs such as Librium, Valium, and Ativan are used to slowly decrease alcohol intake in individuals who have been using alcohol for a number of years. In cases of benzodiazepine abuse, the doses of these drugs are gradually decreased. When opiates such as morphine and Dilaudid are abused, sometimes methadone is substituted and tapered for detoxifi-

cation. If you are abusing a drug, especially a depressant drug, do not try to stop the medication all at once without consulting with your doctor.

A second very important phase of treatment after detoxification is education. Most treatment programs have a very strong education component, because often individuals cannot recognize the triggers that lead to their drug abuse and cannot recognize relapse warning signs. This education is often done in peer support groups that involve other drug abusers, who can be confrontational and who are aware of some of the signs of drug abuse and denial that the counselor may not recognize. This peer support usually involves participation in some group fashioned along the lines of Alcoholics Anonymous. There are such groups for cocaine abusers (CA) and for other depressant abusers. It is strongly suggested that someone who detoxifies from drugs or alcohol go to 60 AA or NA (Narcotics Anonymous) meetings in 60 days. Patients should also obtain a sponsor, someone who has had years of clean time, and once selected, patients should call their sponsor during times when they feel they are at high risk for relapse. So a detoxification that is often medical that looks for medical complications of drug use, provides tapering of drugs if possible, education process and a peer support process are the most common stages of the treatment of drug abuse. Thus the stages of drug abuse treatment involve: (1) a medical detoxification if indicated, (2) education and maintenance of drug-free state, and (3) peer support counseling (AA, CA, or NA).

It should also be mentioned that there is a group of individuals who have what is called a "dual diagnosis"; that is, they have a psychiatric condition and drug abuse, such as major depression and alcohol abuse, or anxiety disorder and stimulant abuse, or schizophrenia and alcohol abuse. In the individual with dual diagnosis, usually the psychiatric disorder is made worse by the drug use, and the drug use is more likely because of the psychiatric disorder. Therefore if you have a dual diagnosis, it is very important that you are treated for both conditions, that you stay on your medication prescribed for your psychiatric disorder, and that you follow the 12-step recovery program for substance abuse. There are some AA-type groups called "double trouble" groups where all the members also have psychiatric disorders. If you have a dual diagnosis, you might choose a sponsor who also has a dual diagnosis, who will be able to understand your need for psychiatric care and recovery. In some AA or NA groups, there is a very strong bias against medication, so you may have to look around to find a group in which you feel comfortable. It is very important to participate in a recovery program and stay on medication if you have a dual diagnosis.

The DOs

It is very important for the individual who has been detoxified from drugs and is in a recovery program to follow some simple common-sense steps.

- You should inform your doctor or any emergency room physician that you are a recovering drug abuser, so they will not give you medication that might jeopardize your sobriety.
- You should remember that you will probably have strong urges during your sobriety to see whether you can use drugs again or use them in a social setting. These are signs of denial and relapse; if you experience them, you should definitely contact your sponsor. It probably is more common to have these kind of symptoms after anniversaries, especially the first year anniversary of sobriety.
- During your recovery, such basic things as eating well, getting plenty of fluids, getting plenty of rest, exercising moderately, and reducing stress will all play a major role in your attempts to continue your sobriety.

The DON'Ts

You should not see those friends and relatives who still abuse drugs or remind you of when you were abusing drugs. Your new community should revolve around your sponsor and your AA or Narcotics Anonymous (NA) members.

When to Call Your Doctor

You should contact your counselor or sponsor for any relapse warning sign. You should contact your physician if you notice any physical consequences of your drug use or of withdrawal, such as seizures, psychosis, or suicidal thoughts. You should also notify your doctor before you take any medications, including over-the-counter drugs, because many of these agents have properties similar to drugs of abuse.

For More Information

Contact your local crisis center hot line, the Salvation Army treatment program, or local AA/NA/CA directories. The following online sites may also be helpful:

Web of Addictions @:
http://www.well.com/www/woa
National Clearinghouse of Alcohol and Drug Information @:
http://www.health.drg
Habit Smart @:
http://www.cts.com/~habtsmrt
Alcoholics Anonymous Information @:
http://www.csic.com/aa
The Big Book @:
http://www.recovery
org/aa/bigbook/ww/index.htm/
Cocaine Anonymous @:
http://www.ca.org
Narcotics Anonymous @:
http://www.wsoinc.com
You can even attend a live AA meeting online at http://www.cr/.com/~pac/aa.

ABUSE, ELDERLY

About Your Diagnosis

Elderly abuse has become increasingly common in the last 20 years. In the United States alone, about 4% of individuals older than 65 years (approximately 1 million individuals) experience abuse or neglect. There are four types of mistreatment of the elderly: physical abuse, physical neglect, psychological abuse, and material abuse. Physical abuse consists of assaults, rough handling, burns, sexual abuse, and unreasonable confinement. Physical neglect often includes dehydration, malnutrition, poor hygiene, allowing the wearing of inappropriate or soiled clothing, improper giving of medication, and failure to obtain medical care for the elderly individual. Psychologic abuse involves verbal or emotional abuse, threats, and isolation/confinement. Finally, the elderly may experience material abuse, such as the withholding of finances, misuse of their funds or outright theft, and withholding the means of daily living.

Elderly victims of abuse are usually (1) older than 75 years, (2) women, (3) white, and (4) widowed. In addition there are other characteristics of elderly individuals who are abused. They have behavioral problems, are incontinent, display shouting (especially nighttime shouting), exhibit paranoia, have many physical complaints, and are fairly socially isolated so that abuse is less likely to be discovered. Those elderly individuals with emotional and/or physical problems, and those who are totally dependent on a caregiver are more likely to be abused.

The abusers of the elderly are usually (more than 60% of the time) married to them. In about a quarter of cases, the abuser is an adult child living in the home, who is dependent on the older individual. Elderly abuse occurs in all races and economic classes.

The assessment of elderly abuse should first involve a suspicion that it is happening. Elderly abuse should be suspected in those individuals who have frequent falls and orthopedic injuries, who seem to have a lot of problems with their medication, and who seem to be losing weight without explanation but who gain weight while hospitalized. Unexplained incontinence and body odor may be signs of elderly neglect.

Treatment

The treatment of elderly victims of abuse involve treating whatever medical problems may be the result of the abuse. It is often necessary to contact a reporting agency such as Adult Protective Services. Depending on the nature of the abuse, immediate hospitalization for urgent medical care may be indicated. Treatment should also involve providing support for the abuser and reducing the level of stress in the environment. In some cases, the filing of legal charges and the removal of the elderly individual from the home may be needed.

Like children, the elderly are susceptible to abuse because they are often more vulnerable and dependent. Prevention of abuse of the elderly requires a heightened sense of awareness that it exists, sharing the responsibilities for caring for an elderly parent among different family members, so no one individual is overwhelmed, promptly treating any medical or psychiatric problems in the elderly, and increasing social outlets for elderly patients. It is essential that all of us check on the elderly in our neighborhoods, families, and churches, to prevent mistreatment of our older citizens.

ACHALASIA

About Your Diagnosis

Achalasia is a disorder of the esophagus, the tube that connects the mouth and stomach. With this disease, the esophagus has a decreased ability to move liquid and solids down to the stomach. This movement is known as peristalsis. Also the lower esophageal sphincter (the muscle between the esophagus and stomach) does not relax in response to swallowing. The causes of this disorder include damage to the nerves to the esophagus, parasitic infections, and hereditary factors. Achalasia may occur at any age but is more common as you grow older. The incidence of achalasia is 2 cases per 10,000 individuals.

Achalasia is detected by a barium swallow x-ray. On x-ray there is a narrowing of the lower portion of the esophagus and widening of the upper portion. A chest x-ray may be useful if it shows the esophagus is enlarged with air or fluid. Pressure measurements (manometry) may be done to prove the lack peristalsis and the increased pressure at the lower esophageal sphincter. Endoscopy, using a small light tube with a tiny video camera on the end, can be used to confirm a tight sphincter.

There is no cure for achalasia, but treatment can improve the symptoms in 60% to 85% of cases and help prevent complications.

Living With Your Diagnosis

The main symptom of achalasia is difficulty swallowing. Typically, problems with swallowing liquids occur first. It can progress to problems swallowing solid foods. When this occurs weight loss is not uncommon. Chest pain and pain on swallowing are not typical but can occur. Heartburn and belching are rare. In advanced cases, halitosis or bad breath can occur. Rarely does vomiting occur, but when it does it is caused by the overflow of food in the esophagus. Symptoms associated with the respiratory system such as coughing and wheezing can also occur.

Without treatment complications can arise. These include perforation (tearing) of the esophagus and regurgitation of acid or food from the stomach into the esophagus (gastroesophageal reflux disease [GERD]). Another complication is aspiration pneumonia. It can occur if the stomach contents are aspirated into the lungs. About 5% of patients with achalasia have a chance of developing esophageal cancer.

Treatment

The goal of treatment is to reduce the pressure at the lower esophageal sphincter. This is done by dilating the sphincter with special weighted instruments or balloons that are inflated to dilate the sphincter. Even after dilation the esophagus will not have normal movement. The procedure may have to be repeated if symptoms reoccur. A rare complication of this procedure is esophageal perforation.

Medications such as long-acting nitrates or calcium channel blockers can also be used to lower the pressure at the lower esophageal sphincter. The medications usually are used in individuals who are unable to tolerate the dilation procedure.

Surgery to decrease the pressure in the lower sphincter (called an esophagomyotomy) may be indicated if other treatments fail.

The DOs

- Seek medical advice.
- Eat and drink in an upright position.
- Eat and chew slowly.

The DON'Ts

- Avoid eating and drinking in a lying position.
- Avoid hot or cold liquids because they may make the condition worse.

When to Call Your Doctor

- If you have persistent difficulty swallowing.
- If painful swallowing develops.
- If symptoms persist despite treatment for achalasia.
- If you are vomiting blood or other new symptoms develop.

For More Information
National Digestive Diseases Information Clearinghouse
2 Information Way
Bethesda, MD 20892-3570
www.niddk.nih.gov
nddic@aerie.com

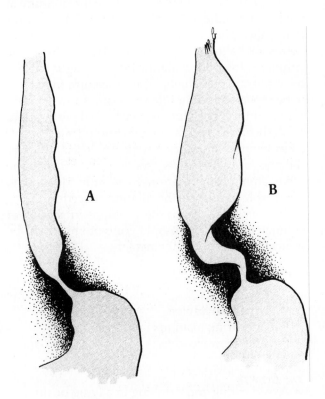

Esophageal achalasia **A,** Early stage showing narrowing of lower esophagus. **B,** Advanced stage showing dilated middle esophagus.(From Phipps WJ, Cassmeyer VL, Sands JK, et al: *Medical-Surgical Nursing: Concepts and Clinical Practice,* vol 5. St. Louis, Mosby–Year Book, 1994. Courtesy of Price SA, Wilson LM: *Pathophysiology: Clinical Concepts of Disease Processes,* 4th ed. St. Louis, Mosby, 1992. Used by permission.)

ACHILLES TENDON RUPTURE

About Your Diagnosis

The Achilles tendon is the tendon that connects your calf muscles to your heel. You use it for jumping and standing on tiptoe. You can rupture or tear it either partially or completely when jumping, by forcefully bending the foot toward the shin, or by receiving a direct blow. Men aged 40–50 years who are occasional athletes are the most common victims, but it can occur at any age. History and a physical examination will usually identify the injury. Sometimes it is treated with casting, but it usually requires surgery for repair. Recovery is slow and may take up to 6 months, but is usually complete.

Living With Your Diagnosis

The most common symptom of an Achilles tendon tear is stabbing pain at the lower calf at the time of injury. Frequently, you will not be able to walk without pain, especially when you try to push off of the toe. Swelling is seen at the site of injury. The calf muscles may appear bunched up. You may be unable to stand on tiptoe on the injured foot.

Treatment

The most common treatment for a complete Achilles tear is surgery. After surgery, the foot is immobilized with a cast that keeps the toe pointed down somewhat. This is changed in about 3 weeks to a smaller cast that holds the foot at more of a 90-degree angle. This is removed in about 4 more weeks, and any wires put in to hold the tendon together until healed are taken out at that time. Your doctor will probably advise a heel lift or high-heeled shoe for another couple of months after that. If it is possible to get the ends of the tendon back together without surgery, your doctor may recommend casting for 10–12 weeks, with cast changes at 6 weeks and around 8–9 weeks. You will be placed in a heel lift for around 3 months after removal of the last cast. In any case, with exercise and physical therapy, most individuals will have a full recovery.

The DOs

You should take pain medicines as prescribed. You should protect your cast because it is crucial to protect the tendon until it has a chance to heal, and that will take time. After the cast removal, you should follow instructions for physical therapy and exercise to recover muscle strength and range of motion at the ankle. Proper conditioning is important to prevent reinjury of the tendon. If you have a partial tear of the tendon, it is essential to follow your rehabilitation prescription to the letter. There is a significant risk of complete rupture if the tendon is stressed too much before it can heal.

The DON'Ts

You should avoid cortisone or steroid injections around the Achilles tendon because the injections are a significant risk factor for Achilles tendon rupture. If you have a rupture, you should not remove or damage your cast. If you tear the repair loose, you start over again in your course of treatment, and this will significantly prolong your time to complete healing. You should not do anything that will cause excessive force on the tendon until healing is complete because of the risk of reinjury. For this reason, you should follow your physical therapy instructions to the letter until released to full activity.

When to Call Your Doctor

You should call your doctor if you damage your cast. If you have had an injury repaired, you should call your doctor if you experience a reinjury. You should also call if you have increasing symptoms of pain in the calf or are unable to raise onto tiptoe or walk. These may be signs of reinjury, as may increased swelling at the site of injury.

For More Information
Description of the injury and surgery
http://www.medmedia.com/05/243.htm

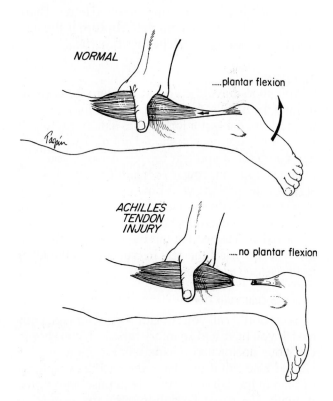

The Thompson test or "squeeze" test for complete rupture of the Achilles tendon. With an intact or partially torn tendon, squeezing the calf muscles produces passive plantar flexion of the ankle. With loss of continuity of the Achilles tendon, this maneuver fails to produce ankle motion. (From Burke JH, Boyd RJ, McCade CJ: *Trauma Management—Early Management of Visceral, Nervous System, and Musculoskeletal Injuries*, vol 1. St. Louis, Mosby–Year Book, 1988. Used by permission.)

ACNE VULGARIS

About Your Diagnosis

Acne is one of the most common problems of adolescence. The unsightly pimples and blemishes of acne can result in embarrassment, anxiety, social difficulties, and eroded self-confidence far beyond the minor health risk of the disease.

The skin disease of acne commonly occurs in adolescence. The peak for acne activity is in the mid teens. During this time the skin oil (sebaceous) glands begin to become more active and produce more oil. This increased oil is noted as oily skin, but in some individuals (more than 18 million in the United States) this oil will be blocked. The blockage occurs at the skin pore openings. The pores are blocked because of sticky cells, bacteria, oil, and other materials. When the oil cannot escape through the normal skin pore, it backs up and forms a whitehead; if this is opened and exposed to the air, it becomes a blackhead. If the backed-up oil leaks into the surrounding skin, inflammation and infection occur, which will cause pimples and cysts. In other words, ACNE.

Acne can occur in both girls and boys, but boys usually have more oily skin and for that reason often have worse acne. Heredity plays a part as well; if your parents had bad acne, you may too. Foods do not seem to affect acne, and there are no known foods that make acne worse. But if you note a certain food that makes your acne worse, try to avoid it. Stress has been found to be the only consistent cause of worsening acne. For this reason, acne often gets worse before exams, before big dates, or when students begin college.

Living With Your Diagnosis

Acne is usually found on the face, shoulders, and back. The rash is made of small bumps with whitish or black tops. Squeezing or expressing these bumps is NOT helpful and can lead to infection and scarring. In severe acne, large and deep cysts may form, which can result in significant scarring if not properly treated.

Acne is not an infection, although normal bacteria on the skin are part of the problem. For this reason, acne cannot be given or caught. For this same reason, antibiotics will not cure acne, although they do often help calm it down. Most individuals will outgrow acne by their mid 20s, but in some cases it continues. In severe cases after active acne has stopped, some small, depressed, or lumpy scars may be left. If scarring occurs, special treatment may be required, often involving surgical procedures.

Treatment

There are many ways to treat acne. No matter what treatment is used, it will take 8–10 weeks before you notice improvement in your skin. In some case the acne may actually get worse for a few weeks before improving. Nonmedical treatment consists of a good diet, regular exercise, daily skin hygiene with a medicated acne soap, and gentle washing (scrubbing can actually make acne worse). Salicylic acid compounds and cleansing soaps may be beneficial in washing the acne-prone areas. Oil-based makeup, suntan oil, and oils of any kind should be avoided. Stress and strong emotions can cause a flare of your acne, and if possible should be avoided.

The first medications used for treating acne are those applied to the skin. These are usually topical antibiotics and comedolytics (peeling agents). Antibiotics that are prescribed include benzoyl peroxide, erythromycin, clindamycin, and meclocycline.

Benzoyl peroxide has both comedolytic and antibiotic properties. It can be purchased without prescription in several strengths (always start at the lowest concentration). It must be used according to directions. It can be very irritating to the skin and should be stopped if the skin becomes sore. You must thoroughly and gently wash and dry your face before applying the medication to the skin. Apply the proper amount over the entire area of skin that has acne. Don't apply too much. Apply at bedtime and wash off in the morning. If it fails to work after 8–10 weeks or if your acne significantly worsens, see your doctor.

Oral medication or pills such as antibiotics, peeling agents (tretinoin, Retin-A, or isotretinoin), or hormones require a doctor's prescription and supervision. Antibiotics can lead to diarrhea, upset stomach, allergic reactions, and in women, yeast infections. Hormone treatment is helpful as a means to decrease oil production, but requires close doctor supervision. Isotretinoin absolutely cannot be used in patients who are pregnant or those who may become pregnant.

The DOs

- Eat regularly, exercise regularly, and wash oily skin gently everyday with medicated acne soap and water.
- Use cosmetics, suntan lotions, and shampoos that are oil free.
- Start treatment with the lowest strength lotion of benzoyl peroxide or over-the-counter topical medication.
- Be patient; almost everyone grows out of acne.

The DON'Ts

- Don't alter eating habits, i.e., don't avoid chocolate, french fries, unless you notice certain foods make your acne worse.
- Don't pinch, squeeze, express, or pick your pimples. This can lead to infection and scarring.
- Don't rub or massage acne, and avoid chin straps, shoulder pads, straps, and spandex garments that rub the skin where acne is present.
- Don't sunbathe; this can actually make some cases of acne worse. Besides, sun exposure is *dangerous*.
- Don't expect improvement for at least 8–10 weeks.
- Don't use over-the-counter medication while taking prescription medication unless your doctor knows.
- Don't hesitate to ask your doctor about acne and to tell him how you feel about it.

When to Call Your Doctor

- If your acne is worsening despite treatment.
- If you are having emotional problems because of your acne.
- If you have significant scarring.

For More Information
American Academy of Dermatology
930 N. Meachum Road
Schaumburg, IL 60173
847-330-0230

ACQUIRED IMMUNODEFICIENCY SYNDROME (AIDS)

About Your Diagnosis

Acquired immunodeficiency syndrome is a failure of the body's immune system. It leaves the body with an inability to fight infection or to suppress the growth of abnormal cells, such as cancer. The disease affects the white blood cells and the cells of the bone marrow, liver, spleen and lymph glands. As of the end of 1996, an estimated 22.6 million individuals worldwide were living with AIDS.

Acquired immunodeficiency syndrome is caused by the human immunodeficiency virus (HIV). The virus can be transmitted from an infected mother to her unborn child; through sexual intercourse; through the use of contaminated needles by intravenous drug users; and from a transfusion of blood or blood products from an infected individual. It is not spread by casual contact. There is no cure, but new medications can relieve and control the symptoms.

Living With Your Diagnosis

Signs and symptoms of the disease include fever, unexplained weight loss, fatigue, chronic respiratory and skin infections, swollen lymph glands, diarrhea, night sweats, headaches, and muscle weakness. As the disease progresses, it leaves the body more prone to other infections such as pneumonia, meningitis, and cancer.

Treatment

Current treatment includes a strict regimen of medications. Combinations of antiviral agents and protease inhibitors are showing great promise. Common side effects of the drugs are anemia, loss of appetite, nausea and vomiting, headache, and insomnia. Antibiotics may be needed if other infections are present.

The DOs

- Take your medications as directed. Doses must not be skipped.
- Follow a well-balanced diet to maintain a stable body weight. Loss of appetite is common, as is nausea from the disease or the medication, so it is best to eat small, frequent meals and to avoid fried and acidic foods. Most individuals can tolerate the "BRAT" diet when nauseated—bananas, rice, applesauce, and toast.
- Participate in your treatment and care decisions.
- Normal exercise and activity are unrestricted depending on the patient's tolerance. Do try to schedule rest periods as needed.
- Contact local social agencies about AIDS support groups.
- Practice infection control. Good hand washing is an essential first step in preventing other infections.
- Avoid others with infections such as the "flu."

The DON'Ts

- Skip or stop your medications. If you cannot tolerate the medications, notify your doctor.
- Have unprotected sexual contact with others.
- Share needles or donate blood.
- Get pregnant, because there is a possibility that the infant will be infected with the virus.

When to Call Your Doctor

- If you have shortness of breath.
- If pain or new skin lesions develop.
- If a new cough develops.
- If visual changes occur.
- If you have increased fatigue or weakness.
- If your temperature is greater than 101°F.
- If you have difficulty staying awake or are confused.

For More Information

The following resources are available nationally. Check your local phone book for support groups in your area.
The CDC National AIDS Hotline
800-342-AIDS
800-344-SIDA (Spanish)
800-AIDS TTY (Hearing impaired)
The National Association of Individuals with AIDS
1-202-898-0414
AIDS Treatment News
800-873-2812
National Native American AIDS Prevention Center
2188 Lake Shore Avenue Suite A
Oakland, CA 94686
Indian AIDS Hotline
800-283-AIDS
National Pediatric HIV Resource Center
15 South 9th Street
Newark, NJ 07107
800-362-0071
Internet Sites
www.healthfinder.gov
www.healthanswers.com
www.teleport.com/~celinec/aids.shtml

ACROMEGALY

About Your Diagnosis

Acromegaly is a disease caused by excess growth hormone (GH). Growth hormone levels are tightly regulated by the body to allow for normal growth and development. Growth hormone–releasing hormone (GHRH) is secreted from the hypothalamus in the brain, causing the pituitary to secrete GH. Growth hormone circulates in the blood and causes the liver to secrete insulin-like growth factor-1 (IGF-1). Insulin-like growth factor-1 acts on the bones and body tissues to promote growth and development. In most individuals, GH is decreased by IGF-1 and a hormone called somatostatin. In acromegaly, there is abnormal secretion of GH from a tumor, usually located in the pituitary. The tumor does not decrease GH secretion in response to IGF-1 or somatostatin, leading to increased GH levels over time. Occasionally, tumors elsewhere in the body may produce extra GHRH, which causes the pituitary to secondarily overproduce GH.

There are approximately 750 new cases of acromegaly each year in the United States. However, 10–20 times as many individuals are currently living with the disease.

After a complete medical history and physical examination, acromegaly is detected by measuring levels of GH and IGF-1 in the blood. Levels of IGF-1 are more easily measured because they are stable throughout the day. Insulin-like growth factor-1 levels may be falsely elevated during pregnancy, whereas IGF-1 levels decrease in older individuals and individuals with diabetes. Because GH levels fluctuate widely during the day, GH is best measured 1 hour after drinking a sweet liquid during an oral glucose tolerance test (OGTT). Acromegaly is confirmed by an elevated GH level. Pituitary magnetic resonance imaging (MRI) is then used to locate the lesion. If the pituitary MRI is normal, a GHRH level is measured. An elevated GHRH suggests a tumor elsewhere in the body is causing acromegaly.

Most individuals can expect significant relief of their symptoms once the diagnosis is established and the tumor is surgically removed. Some tumors may not be completely resectable. Symptomatic relief may still be obtained through a combination of surgery, radiation therapy, and medications.

Living With Your Diagnosis

Signs and symptoms include an increase in the size of hands and feet (gloves, rings, and shoes are too tight), headaches, blurry vision, high blood pressure, joint pains, carpal tunnel syndrome (numbness of the fingers in the hand), high blood sugars, changes in a woman's menstrual cycle, or male impotence. There may be a change in facial features (more prominent forehead, jaw, lips, tongue, and increased space between teeth), deepening of the voice, or increased snoring.

Acromegaly may cause hypertension, diabetes, arthritis, carpal tunnel syndrome, heart disease, and sleep apnea.

Treatment

The best treatment is transsphenoidal surgery to remove the pituitary tumor. The operation is performed through the nose or above the lip. No scar is noticed on the skin. Cure rates of 60% or greater are achieved by the most experienced surgeons. Transsphenoidal surgery may be complicated by infections of the cerebrospinal fluid, leakage of cerebrospinal fluid into the mouth, or damage to the pituitary.

Medications are also effective for acromegaly. Bromocriptine is the most commonly used medicine. It should be taken at bedtime with food and started at a very low dose to minimize side effects such as nausea, lightheadedness, and nasal congestion. Approximately 50% of those individuals not cured by surgery will have normal GH and IGF-1 levels with bromocriptine. Octreotide, a somatostatin analogue, may be used for the remaining patients. This medicine must be given via subcutaneous injection every 8 hours. Octreotide may cause nausea, diarrhea, gallstone formation, or diabetes.

Finally, radiation therapy may be used to control acromegaly. This is best used for patients who are not candidates for surgery or who are not cured by surgery alone. Approximately 50% of patients will have normal GH and IGF-1 levels within 2–5 years of therapy. Visual loss may occur if the optic nerves are damaged from the radiation.

The DOs

- Initially take bromocriptine at bedtime with food.
- Start with a low dose of bromocriptine and increase the dose slowly (over several weeks).
- Follow-up with your doctor regularly. Tumors may recur.

- Have your blood pressure, blood sugars, and heart examined regularly for possible complications from acromegaly.

The DON'Ts
- Don't expect immediate relief of all your symptoms.
- Don't be afraid to try a combination of treatments.
- Don't eat before your OGTT. This will invalidate the test.
- Don't forget to have your eyes examined.

When to Call Your Doctor
- Your vision changes.
- You have worsening headaches.
- You notice new nerve pains or numbness anywhere in your body.
- You have chest pain or pressure.
- You have side effects from your medication including nausea, dizziness, or lightheadedness.

For More Information
Pituitary Tumor Network Association   16350 Ventura
Boulevard #231   Encino, CA 91436
805-499-9973
National Institute of Diabetes and Digestive and Kidney Diseases
http://www.niddk.nih.gov/acromegaly

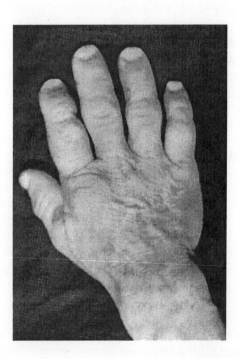

Hand with characteristics of acromegaly. (From LaFleur-Brooks ML: *Exploring Medical Language—A Student Directed Approach.* vol 3. St. Louis, Mosby–Year Book, 1993. Used by permission.)

ADDISON'S DISEASE

About Your Diagnosis

Addison's disease occurs when the two small glands sitting atop the kidneys, called the adrenal glands, fail to produce enough cortisol. Cortisol is a hormone that circulates in the bloodstream and is important for maintaining normal blood pressure and metabolism. Cortisol levels are regulated by a hormone secreted from the pituitary gland in the head called adrenocorticotropic hormone (ACTH).

There are three main reasons for low cortisol levels: adrenal failure (Addison's disease), pituitary failure (low ACTH), or suppression of the normal response caused by medications. Most commonly, adrenal failure is caused by destruction of the adrenal cortex, or outer shell, by the body's own immune system. Doctors are not sure why this occurs. Other causes include infections that spread to the bloodstream, including tuberculosis or fungus infections. Cancer that has spread to the adrenal glands may also cause Addison's disease. Pituitary failure may result from local tumor growth and compression, or from pituitary surgery. Medications such as oral steroids taken for asthma, bronchitis, or arthritis may cause a temporary shutting off of normal cortisol response, especially if doses are rapidly withdrawn.

Addison's disease is relatively rare, affecting only 1 of every 100,000 individuals. Addison's disease is best detected by a complete medical history and physical examination, followed by an ACTH stimulation test. This test involves injection of ACTH into the muscle, with the measurement of blood cortisol before the test and 60 minutes later. In addition, ACTH hormone levels and aldosterone levels may be drawn. The diagnosis is established with a subnormal cortisol response to the administered ACTH. Elevated ACTH levels and suppressed aldosterone levels confirm the diagnosis of Addison's disease.

There is no cure for Addison's disease; however, it is treatable with oral medicines.

Living With Your Diagnosis

Patient's typically complain of tiredness, weakness, decreased appetite, depression, or weight loss. Some may have nausea, vomiting, and diarrhea. The skin and mucous membranes may become hyperpigmented. This is especially notable on the creases of the palm. Other patients may have no symptoms.

Addison's disease may cause low blood pressure, especially during times of stress or upon standing. This can lead to dizziness and fainting. Addisonian crisis is a medical emergency manifested by cardiovascular collapse and associated with back pain, severe nausea, vomiting, and diarrhea. This may occur suddenly in response to severe stress, trauma, or illness.

Treatment

Treatment of acute Addisonian crisis involves intravenous fluids and glucose plus intravenous steroids such as dexamethasone. Chronic treatment involves oral glucocorticoid replacement with hydrocortisone. Fludrocortisone is also available for patients with low aldosterone levels. In addition, a high-salt diet is often helpful.

Overtreatment with hydrocortisone could lead to the Cushing's syndrome, which involves weight gain and change in body habitus caused by extra steroids circulating in the blood. High blood pressure or diabetes may result from excess hormone replacement. Undertreatment leaves patients feeling weak and tired.

The DOs

- Carry injectable cortisol (Solucortef) for emergency purposes and have someone in your family learn to administer this medicine for you in case you are too ill to give yourself medicine.
- Get a Medic Alert bracelet which states that you have Addison's disease and require cortisol in emergencies.
- Increase your hydrocortisone dose if you notice a fever or if you have decreased oral intake caused by mild gastrointestinal illness.
- Call your doctor whenever you feel poorly.

The DON'Ts

- Don't skip doses of your medicine, especially if you are feeling sick.
- Don't forget to take your medicine, and make sure you don't run out of medicine.
- Don't be afraid to slowly decrease your medicine if your doctor recommends a lower dose. After an initial adjustment period, you will continue to feel well and will avoid complications from overtreatment such as weight gain, diabetes, and high blood pressure.

When to Call Your Doctor

- You are having nausea and vomiting or a fever.
- You have elective surgery scheduled; the dose of your medicines needs to be adjusted.
  - You feel weak and tired and have noticed weight loss.
- You or your family members do not know how to inject cortisol in an emergency.

For More Information

National Adrenal Disease Foundation   505 Northern Boulevard Suite 200   Great Neck, NY 11021 516-487-4992.
National Institute of Diabetes and Digestive and Kidney Diseases http://www.niddk.nih.gov/AD
Medic Alert Foundation International   2323 Colorado Turlock, CA 95391   209-668-3333.

ADHD (ATTENTION DEFICIT HYPERACTIVITY DISORDER)

About Your Diagnosis

Attention deficit disorder (ADD) in children is often considered in conjunction with other disruptive behavior disorders, including conduct disorder and oppositional defiant disorder. It is only recently that we have begun to pay more attention to ADD in adults. To diagnose ADD, the child must demonstrate either signs of *inattention* (ADD) or signs of *hyperactivity* (ADHD). Signs of inattention include:

1. Failing to pay attention to details, or making careless mistakes in schoolwork or other activities.
2. Difficulty sustaining attention in either task or play activities.
3. Not listening when spoken to directly.
4. Not following through all instructions, and failing to finish schoolwork, chores, or duties in the workplace.
5. Difficulty organizing tasks and activities.
6. Avoiding, disliking, or being reluctant to start tasks that require sustained mental effort.
7. Losing things necessary for tasks or activities.
8. Being easily distracted by other stimuli that have nothing to do with the task at hand.
9. Forgetfulness in daily activities.

Of course, these behaviors are fairly common, even in normal children. Therefore six or more of these eight criteria must be present for at least 6 months to a degree that is interfering with a child's daily function and is inappropriate for the child's anticipated level of development, for the diagnosis of ADD to be made.

In addition to or instead of signs of inattention, the child often shows signs of *hyperactivity* as indicated by:

1. Fidgeting with hands or feet or squirming in the seat.
2. Leaving a seat in the classroom or in other situations in which remaining seated is expected.
3. Running about or climbing excessively in situations in which that is inappropriate.
4. Difficulty playing or engaging in leisure activity quietly.
5. Being on the go or active as if driven by some kind of motor.
6. Talking excessively.
7. Impulsively blurting out answers before questions have even been asked or completed.

8. Difficulty waiting their turn.
9. Interrupting or intruding on others.

In addition, for the diagnosis of ADHA to be made six or more of these signs of hyperactivity must persist for 6 months to a degree that is interfering with the child's development and is inappropriate for the child's stage of development. ADD accompanied by hyperactivity is defined as ADHD.

Living With Your Diagnosis

ADD is identified as a persistent, severe pattern of inattention or hyperactivity (ADHD)/impulsivity symptoms as compared with the behavior of other children at the same developmental level. The onset of these symptoms must occur before 7 years of age, and the symptoms must be present in more than one setting; for instance, at school and at home. Of course, other conditions such as anxiety disorders might explain these symptoms.

Between 2% and 7% of all children have ADD, and it seems that in schoolage children, its prevalence is higher in boys. By adolescence, the prevalence of ADD has narrowed considerably between boys and girls.

It seems that ADD does run in families, because children of parents with ADD have an increased risk of developing the disorder, compared with that of children whose parents are unaffected. Some environmental factors also may play a role in the progression of ADD, including growing up in a very chaotic, crowded environment, growing up in a lower socioeconomic status home, and growing up in a family where the entire family unit, especially parents, is not intact. Also, childhood neglect and child abuse may predispose to its development.

Often, the early behavior associated with ADD and ADHD is seen in very young children. Some studies suggest that children as young as 1-1/2 years are brought to physicians because parents are concerned that their children move too much during sleep. At about 3 years of age, however, the symptoms described by parents usually include difficulty playing quietly and excessive climbing and running. Usually parents notice the hyperactivity (ADHD) more than the attention problems (ADD, alone), probably because inattention is often not noticed until a child begins school and grades suffer because of it. Although hyperactivity, impulsivity, and attention problems decline through adolescence, in some individuals they persist well into adulthood. In some populations of adolescents, it has been noted that those with ADD and ADHD have a higher incidence of delinquency, truancy, and substance abuse during adolescence. This pattern of antisocial behavior may also continue through adulthood.

Often, other family members, neighbors, or teachers encourage the parents to have their child evaluated for ADD and especially ADHD. Many of these ADHD children are typically described as very active or just "normal boys"; however, looking back, many parents point out that their child's behavior was not normal.

In assessing a child for ADHD, other psychiatric and medical conditions that might be causing hyperactivity must be looked for, as well as family events that the child may be reacting to. The most common way of diagnosing this disorder is through the use of rating scales. Usually the rating scales are completed by teachers and parents because often the child does not display the hyperactivity in the psychiatrist's presence. Although the parents may be more aware of the child's behavior at home, teachers are often more aware of different problems in attention because of the more structured nature of the classroom. One of the more common scales used to diagnose ADHD is the Conner's teacher rating scale, which is used for children from 3 to 17 years of age. The Utah rating scale, also commonly used to diagnose ADD and ADHD, describes certain behaviors. The parents or teachers have to determine how often these behaviors occur and rate the frequency of their occurrence as follows: "not at all," "seldom," "often," or "frequent." A different number of points is given for each category, and the points are then added. If the child's behavior score falls outside the norms, then the diagnosis of ADHD or ADD is suspected. In addition to the rating scales, interviewing the child with suspected ADHD and the child's parents is essential. Finally, there is a role for observing the child and commenting on those observations as part of the diagnosis. Therefore the diagnoses of ADD and ADHD are generally made by considering a combination of factors, including the interviews, the rating scales, and observation. Presently, no specific laboratory tests are available that can help in the diagnosis of these disorders.

Treatment
The most effective treatment of ADD and ADHD is a combination of psychosocial and drug therapy.

The drugs most commonly used are the so-called psychostimulants, which seem to have an opposite effect on children with this disorder. Instead of over-stimulating these children, these drugs help them feel calmer, more relaxed, more focused, and less scattered in their thinking. Drugs used to treat this condition include methylphenidate (Ritalin), dextroamphetamine, and pemoline (Cylert). Ritalin is the most commonly prescribed drug in this country for treating ADD and ADHD and accounts for more than 90% of all stimulant use in the United States. Because of their tendency to improve attention, the stimulants used in children with ADD and ADHD often lead to an improvement in their school function. Ritalin is often used because it is less likely to cause side effects than some of the other drugs. Ritalin can cause insomnia and appetite suppression, and so the drug is usually given in the morning. The typical dose is 5 mg to start, and is increased by 5 mg until the desired effect is achieved. If the drug is given three times a day, the last dose of the day is usually one half the morning or noon dose. The recommended maximum dose is 60 mg, although in some cases, higher doses have been used successfully. If dextroamphetamine is to be used, it should only be used after failure of a trial of Ritalin. Dextroamphetamine is more potent, so the dose is lower than that which would be used for Ritalin to treat ADHD. Antidepressants have also been used, especially imipramine and desipramine. They do, of course, have side effects that include rapid heart rate, a drop in blood pressure when standing, and some blurry vision. Generally these problems are not sufficient to discontinue the medication if it is working. It is important to point out that there have been rare reports of sudden death in infants who were taking desipramine. The serotonin drugs, such as Prozac, are currently under investigation for the treatment of this disorder, and a drug used to treat high blood pressure, clonidine, has also been used successfully. However, the hallmark of treatment with medication for ADHD remains the psychostimulants and preferably Ritalin.

In adults with ADHD and ADD (formerly known as residual ADD), there is often a history of failed relationships, problems at work and frequently changing jobs, many activities started but never completed, and occasionally alcohol and drug abuse. Many of these patients as adults have been in different psychiatric facilities where they may have been misdiagnosed as having either anxiety disorders or manic depressive disorder. The use of psychostimulants in this population is often very effective in helping patients return to functioning fairly normally. One major concern is the use of psychostimulants in populations that have had a history of substance abuse, particularly stimulant abuse involving cocaine, PCP, or the amphetamines. Ritalin and dextroamphetamine should not be used in this population. Instead, those individuals with substance abuse and ADHD or ADD should be treated primarily with the more stimulating antidepressants such as desipramine, imipramine, and fluoxetine (Prozac). Some reports indicate that patients with ADD and a history of drug abuse have been treated successfully with Cylert, which may have a less addictive potential than dextroamphetamine and Ritalin.

Having a child with ADD or ADHD can be extremely distressing for parents, often stretching their patience to the limit. These children can be extremely irritable and aggressive, and parents have to keep a close watch on them. Therefore, support for the parents is essential.

In adults, the ADD may coexist with depression, and some studies have reported successful treatment of major depression in ADD with a combination of Ritalin and either imipramine or Prozac. Some studies have shown that growth retardation can occur with dextroamphetamine and other agents besides Ritalin, but this has not been well documented. Of course, the traditional side effects of antidepressant drugs such as desipramine include dry mouth and blurry vision, and Prozac can cause nausea, upset stomach, and, in adults, sexual dysfunction. In higher dosages, the psychostimulants can increase the occurrence of cardiac arrhythmias and potentially cause seizures. Although it is important to remember that not all active children have ADHD, parents should not hesitate to have their children evaluated if their behavior seems to be different in terms of their level of activity, compared with the activity level of siblings or neighbors' children. The use of the medications mentioned above can give a child a sense of accomplishment and increase self-esteem that is often lacking in individuals who have this disorder.

The DOs

If irritability is a problem, adults with ADD should consider support groups for anger control. Patients with ADD should engage in a regular exercise program and try to maintain some structure and routine in their lives.

The DON'Ts

Individuals with ADD should not attempt to self-medicate hyperactivity with drugs or alcohol, or use excessive amounts of caffeine or sugar. They should prioritize activities and not begin several tasks at one time. Also, doses of Ritalin or amphetamine should only be increased by a physician. These drugs do have addictive potential.

When to Call Your Doctor

You should call your doctor if you notice any side effects of medication, including muscle twitching, nausea, rapid heartbeat, or confusion. Depression, aggressive behavior and/or psychosis should also be reported. You should also contact your physician if you feel the need for a mental health referral or a support group to help you deal with your child's condition.

For More Information

Contact your pediatrician or crisis center hotline. You can also obtain information about ADD and ADHD over the Internet at the following sites:
ADD Archive
http://www.seas.upenn.edu/~mengwong/add
ADD Checklist
http://www-leland.stanford.edu/group/dss/disability/add/adult.checklist.htm
Children and Adults with ADD
http://turnpike.net/metro/B/bernstp/chadd544.htm
Facts About Ritalin
http://services.bunyip.com:2331/medica/c/pharmacy/ritalin.htm/

AGORAPHOBIA AND PANIC

About Your Diagnosis

Agoraphobia is a condition very closely related to panic. Agoraphobia is the fear of wide open spaces and also usually involves the fear of being in locations such as shopping centers, stadiums, or arenas, where you might feel that there is no escape. Many patients with agoraphobia tend to stay in their homes for long periods, often finding someone to bring them food and do their shopping. If they do go out, patients with agoraphobia tend to do much better if they go to a familiar place, go to a location at times when it is not excessively busy, or take a trusted companion with them when they leave the house.

Living With Your Diagnosis

In panic disorder with agoraphobia, the patient has unexplained panic attacks. It is important to remember that nothing has to happen to cause a panic episode. It can come "out of the blue" for no apparent reason. Usually the panic episode, whether associated with agoraphobia or not, involves many physical findings. These include tightness and pain in the chest; rapid, shallow breathing; shortness of breath; and a pounding, rapidly beating heart. Many patients have described the feeling that "their heart will come out of their chest" because it is beating so hard and fast. In addition, patients usually have diffuse sweating and a feeling that something bad is about to happen which cannot be prevented. When they experience these episodes, many patients feel they are dying and often go to the emergency room, believing they are having a heart attack.

Panic disorder with agoraphobia is more common in women, and usually begins in the late teenage years or in early adulthood. Although subsequent episodes do not involve a stimulus, the initial episode often occurs within 3–6 months after a significant life event, such as a death, a move, an engagement, a marriage, or a change in job status. Agoraphobia is actually a form of fear related to panic disorder, and it can lead the patient to become house bound and debilitated. The presence of agoraphobia makes panic disorder even more serious; patients will often avoid situations that they feel might cause increased anxiety, or areas where they might feel trapped and unable to escape. Typical agoraphobic situations include being alone, traveling far from home, using public transportation, going over bridges or through tunnels, or being in crowded places or restaurants, department stores, malls, theaters, churches, or other public places, especially if the individual perceives that escape may be difficult. Ultimately, patients with agoraphobia are often socially isolated, have difficulty initiating new relationships, and have a significant problem with self-esteem and self-confidence.

Treatment

The treatment of panic disorder with agoraphobia initially involves education. There are many different types of treatment, but the immediate goal is to decrease the subjective feelings of panic and to improve the patient's quality of life. For treatment to be successful, it is very important that patients have a trusting relationship with their doctor.

Medications are very effective in the treatment of panic disorder with agoraphobia. Although many medications can be used for this condition, it seems that the benzodiazepines, especially alprazolam (Xanax) and lorazepam (Ativan), are very effective. Other drugs that have been used effectively include serotonin drugs, such as paroxetine (Paxil), fluoxetine (Prozac), and sertraline (Zoloft). The use of benzodiazepines, the so-called minor tranquilizers, may not be possible if the patient has significant liver or lung disease, or if there is a history of alcohol abuse or abuse of similar medications. Imipramine, a tricyclic antidepressant, has also been used to treat panic. Medications commonly prescribed for panic disorder have some side effects, including jitteriness; fast heartbeat; insomnia; some gastrointestinal distress, (especially nausea, vomiting, and diarrhea) and a decrease in sexual interest and function. You should also be aware that most of these medications, especially the antidepressants, do not produce immediate resolution of the panic disorder; it usually takes about 2–3 weeks before improvement is seen. You may get more immediate benefit from a drug such as alprazolam (Xanax); however, its major disadvantage is the potential for physical addiction, as well as the occurrence of withdrawal symptoms when it is discontinued after long periods of use. Occasionally your doctor may combine an antidepressant and an antianxiety drug to treat your panic disorder. Another drug called BuSpar has been used in some cases to treat panic, but it is probably less effective than the benzodiazepines, the tricyclic antidepressants, or the other antidepressants. The advantage of BuSpar is that it is not physically addicting. In addition to treatment with medication, psychosocial treatment is very effective and is often used in conjunction with medication. Psychosocial treatment involves gradually exposing the patient to the feared situation; teaching relaxation training, deep breathing exercises, and meditation; and helping the patient to overcome thought processes that might be contributing to the panic and agoraphobia. Of course, psychosocial treatment by itself has no side effects. Psychosocial treatment usually involves about 12 sessions and has been found to provide full panic relief in the majority of the patients.

The DOs

Avoid medications that might produce or increase anxiety, including those that contain large amounts of caffeine or sugar. Drugs such as cocaine, phencyclidine (PCP), and amphetamines should also be avoided. Limit your intake of coffee or tea, especially during the evening hours. Exercise might be of some benefit in panic because it provides an outlet for the overwhelming anxiety some patients have.

The DON'Ts

You should not take any medications that are not prescribed by your doctor. You should not use prescribed addictive medications more frequently or in higher dosages than your doctor recommends.

When to Call Your Doctor

You should call your physician if the medication he has prescribed is not working; if you experience overwhelming episodes of pain, anxiety, or an increase in agoraphobia; or if you are thinking about suicide. It is important to remember that although panic is a very disabling condition, especially if associated with agoraphobia, and can lead to a patient becoming a virtual recluse in his own home, this condition is treatable.

For More Information

It is important to contact your family physician or a local mental health center if you find you have some of the symptoms of agoraphobia. In addition, crisis center lines are available in most states, and they can also help you if you need more information about panic disorder and agoraphobia. On the Internet, check out Web sites for attacking anxiety @:
http://www.sover.net/schwcof
Treatment of Panic Disorder @:
http://text.nlm.nih.gov/nih/cdc/www/85txt.htm

ALCOHOLISM

About Your Diagnosis

The term "alcoholic" has been used to describe any number of patterns of alcohol abuse. However, it is important to distinguish two separate groups of individuals who use alcohol excessively. The first group includes those individuals who drink regularly on a chronic basis and who experience withdrawal signs when the alcohol is discontinued abruptly. These individuals obviously suffer from serious social and occupational consequences of their drinking behavior and are truly physiologically addicted to alcohol. The term alcoholic is often used to describe that population. A less talked about but probably larger group of individuals are those who experience problems with their drinking, but who may not be physically dependent on alcohol. They may drink sporadically, but when they do drink, they may have legal, marital, and occupational consequences that stem from alcohol use. These individuals are generally referred to as "problem drinkers." Therefore some authors prefer to talk about two worlds of alcohol problems: the first is characterized by heavy drinking and the immediate problems of intoxication; the second is characterized by severe dependence, continuous drinking, and the consequences of long-term drinking. It may be that these two populations need a different treatment approach if we are to be successful.

Alcohol is one of the most widely used drugs in the world. Its consumption is very high in the United States, and various studies have suggested that there are between 9 and 15 million alcoholics in this country. Because the drug is so popular, there has grown up a complete industry associated with alcohol abuse, and along with nicotine, alcohol is one of the most commonly abused drugs in the United States.

In the United States, alcohol abusers are more likely to be men. Studies suggest that only a third of men describe themselves as abstainers from alcohol, whereas about 50% of women do so. Certainly, men are more likely to go to treatment centers for alcohol abuse. Black and Hispanic populations are more likely to abstain from alcohol than are whites, and about two thirds of black and Hispanic women describe themselves as abstaining.

Living With Your Diagnosis

There are obviously a number of consequences of drinking, and these include a variety of social, legal, and medical problems. Alcohol-related deaths account for about 5% to 7% of all deaths, ranking it as one of the four most common causes of death in the United States. The health hazards of alcohol abuse are well known and primarily involve diseases of the liver, such as cirrhosis and hepatitis; ulcer disease, including esophagitis; heart disease, including cardiomyopathy and congestive failure; and mental disorders, such as Wernicke-Korsakoff and alcohol dementia and delirium tremens (DTs) or alcohol withdrawal delirium.

Alcohol abuse appears to run in families, especially on the father's side. Because of this, the children of alcoholic fathers should be counseled never to drink even socially, because their potential for becoming alcohol abusers is much greater than that of the average individual. In fact, there is a sevenfold risk of alcoholism in first-degree relatives of alcohol-dependent individuals, and the greatest risk is for male relatives of alcohol-dependent men. There are, however, other environmental and social factors that also play a role in the development of alcoholism.

To diagnose alcohol dependence, there must be a pattern of drinking that causes problems, and evidence of tolerance and withdrawal. Withdrawal is a typical pattern of symptoms related to the abrupt discontinuation of alcohol. Alcohol dependence is characterized by the consumption of alcohol in larger amounts or over a longer period than the individual intended; by a persistent desire to cut down or control drinking (going on the wagon); by a great deal of time spent either drinking or recovering from drinking; by the reduction or relinquishing of important social, occupational, or recreational activities because of drinking; and by the continuation of drinking despite the individual's knowledge of having a persistent physical or psychological problem that is most likely secondary to alcohol abuse. If these criteria are met, the diagnosis of alcohol dependence is made. Alcohol abuse, on the other hand, only requires a recurrent drinking that results in a failure to fulfill a major role obligation like school or work, recurrent drinking in situations in which it is physically hazardous, recurrent alcohol-related legal problems, and continued drinking despite having persistent or recurrent social or interpersonal problems that are caused by drinking.

The diagnosis of alcoholism is usually made on the basis of the history. In addition, there are different tests that are given to screen for alcohol abuse. Examples of these tests are the Michigan Alcohol Screening Test (MAST) and CAGE questions. The CAGE survey measures repeated efforts to cut down ((C) amount of alcohol consumed, annoyance (A) when others comment on your drinking, feeling guilty (G) about drinking and trying to hide it and needing alcohol as an "eye opener" (E) to get started in the morning. Of course, the first thing that should be done when diagnosing alcohol abuse is creating a setting where the individual can become abstinent and then, in that setting, performing a complete examination to identify any health problems caused by alcohol abuse. After that, the alcoholic will probably need detoxification. This is accomplished using a variety of drugs, including vitamins such as thiamine and folic acid, and the benzodiazepines such as Librium, Valium, and Ativan for slowly tapering the individual off the alcohol. Discontinuing large amounts of alcohol after a persistent pattern of drinking can be dangerous and can produce delirium tremens (DTs), and seizures which can be fatal. Health problems during this period that should be screened for include the consequences of malnutrition such as muscle wasting, the presence of infectious diseases (alcohol lowers the individual's ability to fight off infections), hepatitis, pancreatitis, gastritis, and head trauma (secondary to fights and other behavior exhibited while drinking), and signs of alcohol-related mental disorders, especially brain damage from alcohol.

Women drinkers tend to begin heavy drinking much later than men do, and tend to exhibit the consequences of heavy drinking much faster, so they may exhibit the medical complications of drinking at an earlier age than men do. The concept of telescoping has been used to describe the course of symptom progression in women who, despite beginning heavy drinking later than men, begin to experience alcohol-related problems and seek treatment sooner than men do. Also, compared with men, women with alcohol abuse are more likely to drink alone, and are at greater risk for using other drugs in addition to alcohol. Both of these tendencies may partly explain why women seek treatment sooner than men do for alcohol abuse.

Although it is beyond the scope of this chapter, we should mention that perhaps even mild alcohol use during pregnancy can lead to serious consequences, namely, the fetal alcohol syndrome. In the United States, this birth defect has an incidence of between 1 case per 1,000 and 1 case per 300 live births and can lead to serious physical deformities and mental retardation. We should also mention the elderly, because this is a population that has been often overlooked when examining alcohol abuse. Certainly elderly patients who complain of frequent falls or exhibit frequent hip injuries should be evaluated for alcohol dependence and abuse. Older alcoholics, not unexpectantly, have far more medical problems and have more inpatient medical days than do the elderly who do not drink. In addition, there is much more likelihood of a drug-alcohol interaction occurring because many of these elderly patients are taking medications, some of which are sedating and can interact in an additive way with the alcohol. Many times the elderly attempt to self-medicate depression and loneliness with alcohol.

Treatment

The treatment of alcohol abuse most often involves adherence to a 12-step recovery plan. The initial objective is abstinence, followed by education, detoxification, and peer support group treatment. The hallmark of the 12-step program is that alcoholism is a disease which cannot be cured merely by willpower, and that individuals, in fact, are powerless over their drinking. This is the first of 12 steps. While in the recovery program with Alcoholics Anonymous (AA), individuals attend a number of meetings where they are surrounded by other people who abuse alcohol, and they are charged with obtaining a sponsor who has a significant degree of sobriety and whom the individuals feel will have a compatible personality. The goals of alcohol treatment are:

1. Stabilize the acute medical condition, including withdrawal.
2. Increase motivation for recovery.
3. Initiate treatment for chronic medical and psychiatric conditions, especially in those individuals who may have a dual diagnosis.
4. Assist the patient in locating suitable housing. This very often requires transfer to a so-called halfway house as a transitional move before going home.
5. Enlist social support for recovery such as intro-

ducing the patient to 12-step programs and AA, and getting the family involved in support groups for families of alcohol abusers.

6. Teach the patient coping skills to use instead of drinking, and work on changing old habits, such as drinking with friends and going to places where alcohol use was formerly a major order of business.
7. Improve occupational function.
8. Promote maintenance of recovery through ongoing participation in AA, gradually involving more leadership roles.

These are the goals of alcohol treatment. It should be pointed out, however, that there is a very high rate of relapse for alcoholics. It is very important that alcoholics who relapse not get totally down on themselves. They must accept that relapse is part of the disease and work toward maintaining an abstinence state again. For depressed individuals alcohol is an additional depressant which will make an existing sadness much more intense. Alcohol should not be used as a treatment for depression.

There are several medications that are used during alcoholism treatment. The benzodiazepines, clonidine, and vitamins are used during the immediate withdrawal phase of alcohol abuse. Occasionally, long-term drugs are used, such as naltrexone and disulfiram (Antabuse). Naltrexone significantly decreases the craving for alcohol after someone is detoxified, whereas Antabuse interacts with any alcohol that the individual may have taken to produce serious physical symptoms, including chest discomfort and shortness of breath. In this way, Antabuse serves as a deterrent to drinking. Antabuse can also be used in particularly vulnerable times, such as anniversaries of deaths, during premenstrual syndrome (PMS), or at the anniversary date of sobriety when chances for relapse are high.

The DOs

Avoid medication during drinking binges, and of course, never drink and drive. It is also important to find other friends and become part of a community.

The DON'Ts

Don't drink. Do not see those friends who drink. Alcohol abusers should also not have any alcohol in the house. Anyone who cares for the abuser will understand that.

When to Call Your Doctor

Call your doctor if you are having any significant medical consequences of alcohol abuse, including nausea, persistent vomiting, constant diarrhea, heartburn or tightness in your chest, blood in the stools, especially dark red blood, and vomiting blood. These are all life-threatening conditions that should be reported to your physician. In addition, because alcohol is a depressant, suicidal thoughts and suicidal behavior are very common among alcohol abusers, so you should discuss with your doctor any suicidal thoughts you may be having. Most important, do not lie to your doctor when he asks about alcohol abuse and if he does not bring it up, you should.

For More Information

The best place to get additional information about alcoholism is at your local AA central office. In addition, most mental health centers also can be of some assistance, or you can check out the following Internet Web sites:
National Association of Children of Alcoholics
http://www.health.org/nacoa
Information about AA   http://www.moscow.com/Resources/Selfhelp/AA
Listings for your local AA chapters can be found @ http://www.casti.com/aa

ALDOSTERONISM

About Your Diagnosis

Aldosteronism is a syndrome of high blood pressure and low blood potassium levels caused by an excess of the natural mineralocorticoid called aldosterone.

Aldosterone is a hormone normally produced by two small glands sitting atop the kidneys called the adrenal glands. There are two main types of aldosteronism, primary and secondary. Primary aldosteronism means that the extra aldosterone being produced arises from the adrenal gland. This is usually caused by a tumor of a single adrenal gland that overproduces aldosterone. This is also known as Conn's syndrome. More than 95% of the cases of Conn's syndrome are benign. Rarely, however, these tumors may be malignant. Primary aldosteronism may also be caused by a condition known as bilateral adrenal hyperplasia in which both adrenal glands are overproducing aldosterone. Researchers do not know the reason why this disorder occurs.

Secondary aldosteronism may be caused by a variety of conditions outside of the adrenal gland, such as congestive heart failure, liver failure, kidney disease, and dehydration, or caused by certain medicines such as diuretics or fludrocortisone. Aldosteronism is relatively uncommon but still accounts for about 0.5% of cases of hypertension in the United States.

Aldosteronism is suspected in patients with high blood pressure and low blood potassium levels, because aldosterone's normal function is to increase sodium and fluid in the bloodstream and to increase potassium excretion in the kidney. Elevated aldosterone levels can be measured in the blood or urine. A special blood test called plasma renin activity (PRA) is measured to distinguish between primary aldosteronism (low PRA) and secondary aldosteronism (high PRA). If primary aldosteronism is diagnosed, special testing by an endocrinologist is then needed to distinguish an adenoma from bilateral hyperplasia. Once all the biochemical testing is completed, a computed tomography (CT) scan of the abdomen may be performed to confirm the location of the disease. Sometimes other special radiologic techniques are needed as well.

Aldosteronism is curable by surgery if the cause is a single adenoma. Bilateral adrenal hyperplasia is not curable without removing both adrenal glands. This may cause more side effects than the patient was experiencing with aldosteronism. Therefore, these patients are treated with medication whenever possible. Secondary causes of aldosteronism are treated by treating whatever condition is leading to the elevated aldosterone levels.

Living With Your Diagnosis

High blood pressure, weakness, cramping, nausea, constipation, muscle spasm, and frequent urination may occur. Some patients may have no symptoms.

Untreated aldosteronism can lead to uncontrolled hypertension, which over time can be a risk factor for stroke or heart disease. Rarely, patients with a very low potassium level may be susceptible to arrhythmias, especially if they are taking the drug digitalis at the same time. Left untreated, very low potassium levels can lead to paralysis and even death caused by respiratory failure.

Treatment

Bilateral adrenal hyperplasia is treated with spironolactone, a medication in the class of drugs known as potassium-sparing diuretics. This helps to maintain the blood potassium level in the normal range. Side effects from this medicine include gynecomastia (male breast development), impotence, and feelings of being tired, lethargic, and drowsy. Treatment for Conn's syndrome involves surgical removal of the tumor. This can be complicated by bleeding, infection, low blood pressure, and high potassium levels after surgery. By pretreating with spironolactone before surgery, blood pressure and potassium levels are generally more stable. Secondary aldosteronism is treated by treating the underlying cause.

The DOs

- Add 1/4 teaspoon of salt to each meal or take salt tablets as prescribed by your doctor for the special endocrine tests required to diagnose aldosteronism.
- Tell your doctor if you have a history of congestive heart failure before beginning this high-salt diet.
- Take spironolactone preoperatively to minimize the low blood pressure and high potassium levels that can sometimes occur postoperatively.
- Find an experienced surgeon to remove the tumor.

The DON'Ts

- Don't obtain radiology studies until your doctor knows whether you have a primary aldosteronoma, bilateral hyperplasia, or secondary aldosteronism. This will prevent unnecessary procedures.
- Don't let your potassium level fall below normal, especially if you are taking digitalis. This can predispose you to cardiac arrhythmias.

When to Call Your Doctor

- You have male breast development or impotence, nausea, drowsiness, or lethargy while taking spironolactone.
- You have excess cramps or palpitations. Your potassium level may be dangerously low.
- You feel extremely weak and tired or dizzy when you stand up. You may need extra hormone replacement postoperatively.

For More Information

National Adrenal Disease Foundation
505 Northern Boulevard, Suite 200
Great Neck, NY 11021
516-487-4992
The Endocrine Society
435 East West Highway, Suite 500
Bethesda, MD 20814-4410
1-888-ENDOCRINE

ALTITUDE SICKNESS

About Your Diagnosis

High altitudes are low oxygen environments. As you go up, an adequate oxygen supply is maintained by various compensations such as increases in breathing rate and heart rate. High altitude causes fluid shifts that may lead to swelling of the hands, face, and feet. Rapid exposure to altitudes of 7,000–8,000 feet or more (for comparison, most Colorado ski resorts are near 9,000 feet) may overwhelm your body's ability to adapt, potentially leading to such altitude illnesses as acute mountain sickness, high-altitude pulmonary edema, and high-altitude cerebral edema.

Living With Your Diagnosis

Acute mountain sickness (AMS) is characterized by headache, nausea, vomiting, shortness of breath, difficulty sleeping, dizziness, and malaise, which typically occur 6–48 hours after ascent. Symptoms may be mistaken for alcohol hangover, exhaustion, or infection. Acute mountain sickness is the most common altituderelated illness; 25% of individuals may be affected at 7,000 feet and as many as 50% at 15,000 feet. Men and women are equally susceptible, yet younger adults may be more vulnerable. Acute mountain sickness is also more common in individuals with underlying lung problems, previous history of AMS, and those who usually live at sea level.

High-altitude pulmonary edema refers to the abnormal accumulation of fluid in the lungs at altitudes higher than 8,000 feet. This is a life-threatening condition that often strikes young, fit climbers who have made previous trips to high altitudes without problems. Symptoms usually develop within 2–4 days and begin with decreased exercise performance. Symptoms of AMS may also be present. Later symptoms may include cough, chest congestion, shortness of breath at rest, decreased level of alertness, and incoordination.

High-altitude cerebral edema is an illness caused by brain swelling. Severe headache, walking problems, and mental dysfunction (hallucinations, reduced responsiveness, and even coma) are the characteristic symptoms. This is a life-threatening condition and frequently occurs together with high-altitude pulmonary edema.

Treatment

Treatment of altitude-related conditions depends on the severity of the illness and the environment. Symptoms of AMS usually spontaneously resolve in as little as 1–3 days. Some minor symptoms, such as headache, can be treated with acetaminophen or aspirin. More significant symptoms can be relieved with descent or drugs such as acetazolamide, which stimulates breathing and helps prevent fluid retention.

For high-altitude pulmonary edema, rest and supplemental oxygen are usually the initial treatments. For severe illness or when oxygen is not available, decent is mandatory.

Immediate decent and oxygen therapy are recommended for high- altitude cerebral edema to help prevent serious neurologic damage or death. Dexamethasone, a steroid, is often used to help prevent or reduce brain swelling.

The DOs

The most effective preventive measure for altitude-related illness is a gradual ascent allowing for 2–4 days of acclimation at altitudes of 6,000–8,000 feet before ascending to higher elevations.

Discuss with your health care provider the need for drug therapy to help prevent altitude-related illness. Acetazolamide is often used to prevent altitude-related symptoms. It is usually started 1–2 days before ascent and continued for 2 or more days at high altitude. The most common side effects are nausea and numbness/tingling of the lips, fingers, and toes. Acetazolamide preventive therapy is usually reserved for those known to be at risk for AMS or for those who must reach altitude very quickly.

The DON'Ts

- Avoid alcohol and sleeping pills at high altitude because they may worsen both sleep quality and AMS symptoms.
- Avoid overexertion when initially arriving at high altitude. Unfortunately, exercise before traveling to high altitude does not help prevent altitude-related illnesses.
- Avoid acetazolamide if you are allergic to sulfa drugs.
- Avoid reexposure to high altitude if you have had previous problems with high-altitude pulmonary edema or high-altitude cerebral edema.

When to Call Your Doctor

Altitude-related illness may occur in an area where contact with a doctor is not possible. The development of neurologic or respiratory problems should be taken very seriously and should initiate as safe and quick of a descent as possible.

For More Information
Medical Letter 34:84–86, 1992.

ALZHEIMER'S DISEASE (SENILE DEMENTIA)

About Your Diagnosis

Alzheimer's disease is a degenerative brain process causing dementia in older individuals. It usually presents as a progressive loss of mental function disrupting the way the brain normally works, affecting memory, thinking ability, and language. The cause remains unknown. An estimated 5% to 10% of individuals older than 65 years have some form of dementia, and Alzheimer's accounts for at least half of these. The diagnosis of Alzheimer's is made by excluding other known causes of dementia. At this time there is no cure.

Living With Your Diagnosis

A rapidly progressive form begins in adults aged 36–45 years, with a more gradual form occurring in adults 65–70 years of age. Seventy-five percent of all cases of Alzheimer's dementia are inherited. Early signs and symptoms include forgetfulness of recent events, increasing difficulty with everyday tasks, and personality changes. The disease is progressive and may develop into an inability to take care of oneself and failure to recognize familiar individuals.

Patients with Alzheimer's dementia have difficulty adapting to changing living environments. It is important to establish more than one caregiver. Try not to change their caregivers nor their place of residence any more than absolutely necessary. To assist their failing memory, it is helpful to print information (in large type) that they often forget and make it available in several places in their living quarters. It is also advisable to have them fitted with a medical alert bracelet or a tag that lists their address in the event that they wander and become lost. Many of these patients are unsteady on their feet and are prone to falling. Some may benefit from using a walker or being in living quarters fitted with handrails.

Treatment

Presently, no cure exists; however, there are some medications that may help to manage the patients' behavior and improve their level of function. Reversible cholinesterase inhibitors are sometimes used to inhibit the normal breakdown of neurotransmitters (chemical messengers sent from one brain cell to another). These inhibitors may effectively improve some patients' level of function. Other medications may be used to control their anger and agitation.

The DOs

- Simple reminders can help with memory.
- Create pleasant distractions if the patient is upset or angry.
- Make the living quarters safe (handrails, door locks to prevent the patient from wandering and becoming lost).
- Join an Alzheimer's support group.
- It is likely that nursing home care will eventually become necessary.
- Allow the patient to remain as active and independent as possible. Use supervision as necessary.
- Have the patient wear an identification band.
- If the patient is living with family members, arrange for respite periods for the primary caregiver.

The DON'Ts

- If someone you know has signs and symptoms of dementia, do not assume that this is Alzheimer's dementia. There are many causes for mental changes that are reversible or treatable. Consult your physician.
- Don't change the patient's living environments any more than absolutely necessary.

When to Call Your Doctor

- If you see a sudden marked worsening of symptoms.
- If the patient has any new health problems.
- If the patient has any problems associated with medications.

For More Information

Alzheimer's Association
919 N. Michigan Ave.
Suite 1000
Chicago IL 60611-1676
800-272-3900
312-335-8700
Alzheimer's Disease Education and Referral Center
P.O. Box 8250
Silver Spring, MD 20907-8250
800-438-4380
e-mail: adear@alzheimers.org
The Alzheimer's Foundation (AF)
8177 South Harvard
M/C-114
Tulsa, OK 74137
918-481-6031
World Wide Web
http://www.alz.org
http://www.rxmed.com/illnesses/alzheimer's disease.html
http://www.alzheimers.org/adear

AMAUROSIS FUGAX (TRANSIENT MONOCULAR BLINDNESS)

About Your Diagnosis

Amaurosis fugax is a short-lived episode of blindness in one eye (monocular). This symptom usually develops suddenly, and many individuals describe the event as "it was as if a shade or curtain came over my eye." It is caused by a blockage or low blood flow within the main blood vessel supplying the eye. Blockages are usually due to a blood clot or plaque (small piece of cholesterol) that breaks off from a larger artery and travels upward to the brain or eye, becoming lodged in the main artery supplying the eye. Low blood flow to the eye may also result from a critical narrowing of one of the main blood vessels supplying blood to the brain and eye. The monocular blindness of amaurosis fugax is generally brief, but in rare cases it may be prolonged or permanent.

Living With Your Diagnosis

An episode of amaurosis fugax is often frightening. Although the visual loss most often gradually resolves, one should seek medical attention right away because this is often one of the warning signs of a stroke.

Treatment

The treatment of amaurosis fugax depends upon identifying the source of the blood clots or cholesterol that have caused low blood flow or blocked the main artery to the eye. Blood clots may come from arteries inside the head, arteries in the neck, or from the heart. Several different tests may need to be done to find the source. These tests may include an ultrasound of the carotid arteries in the neck, a study of the electrical system of the heart, a magnetic resonance angiography (MRA) scan of the blood vessels in the head and neck, an echocardiogram of the heart, or an angiogram (dye imaging of the blood vessels). If these studies reveal the source of the problem, medication and/or surgery may be necessary.

The DOs

- If you are a diabetic, maintain especially good control of your blood sugar.
- If you use tobacco, immediately begin a program to quit smoking. Ask your physician for help.

The DON'Ts

- DO NOT DRIVE. A sudden loss of vision in one eye could put you and others in danger.
- Don't use tobacco because it promotes vascular disease.
- Don't ignore any of the above signs or symptoms because they may be an early warning sign of a major stroke.

When to Call Your Doctor

- If you have an unusually severe headache.
- If you have another episode of vision loss, call immediately.
- If you have signs or symptoms of a transient ischemic attack (TIA), call immediately. The following are some of the more common symptoms of a TIA:

  Weakness or numbness on one side of the face or body (face, arm, leg).

  Changes in vision.

  Confusion.

  Dizziness.

  Blindness.

  Double vision.

  Slurred speech, inability to talk, or difficulty swallowing.

  Loss of coordination or balance.

For More Information
World Wide Web
http://www.ninds.nih.gov
National Institute of Neurological Disorders and Stroke (NINDS)
9000 Rockville Pike
Building 31, Room 8A16
Bethesda, MD 20892
Phone: 301-496-5751
Fax: 301-402-2186

AMEBIASIS (AMEBIC DYSENTERY)

About Your Diagnosis

Amebiasis is an infection of the large intestine and sometimes the liver, caused by a parasite. It is common in subtropical locations, especially in crowded or unsanitary living conditions. The common sources of the infection are contaminated food, polluted water, or faulty plumbing. It is spread by flies or other insects and by direct contact with hands or food contaminated with feces. It is curable with treatment but may last 3 weeks. In some cases there may be no symptoms, but you can still be a carrier of the disease.

Living With Your Diagnosis

The most common symptom is diarrhea. It may be foul smelling and may be streaked with mucus or blood. Gas and abdominal cramping along with fever are common. If the liver is involved, there may be tenderness in the upper right side of the abdomen and yellowing of the skin.

Treatment

Medications to kill the parasite will be prescribed by your doctor. You must take them as directed. Side effects of the medication may include nausea, headache, dry mouth or a metallic taste, and darkening of the urine. Alcohol must not be consumed while taking these medications. Bed rest during the acute stage is needed. Normal activities should be resumed gradually after the fever is gone and the diarrhea improves. Fluids must be increased to prevent dehydration. If solid foods are not tolerated, a liquid diet of broths, juices, and ice cream can be taken until the appetite improves, with gradual progression to a normal diet.

The DOs

- Take the medication as prescribed.
- Rest in bed until the fever subsides and the diarrhea decreases.
- Increase fluids to prevent dehydration.
- Wash hands frequently, always before eating.
- Drink bottled water if traveling in developing countries.

The DON'Ts

- Don't drink alcohol when taking the medication prescribed for this disease.
- Don't drink water or use ice if in a country where the water may be contaminated.
- Don't eat raw vegetables, unpeeled fruit, raw fish, or shellfish in questionable areas.

When to Call Your Doctor

- You experience severe abdominal cramping for longer than 24 hours.
- Diarrhea increases or there is an increase in blood in the stools.
- Pain occurs in the right upper side of the abdomen.
- Yellowing of the skin occurs.
- A rash develops.
- Vomiting starts.
- You cannot tolerate fluids or the medications prescribed.

For More Information:
The National Institute of Allergy and Infectious Diseases of the NIH
Office of Communications
9000 Rockville Pike
Bethesda, MD 20892
301-496-5717
Internet Sites
www.healthfinder.gov (Choose SEARCH to search by topic)
www. healthanswers.com

ANEMIA, APLASTIC

About Your Diagnosis

Aplastic anemia is failure of the bone marrow to produce blood cells. It results in decrease in all types of blood cellsred blood cells, white blood cells, and platelets.

The cause of most cases (65%) of aplastic anemia is unknown. The incidence averages five to ten new cases per million persons per year. Exposure to chemicals such as benzene, insecticides (DDT), and explosives (TNT) is associated with some cases of the disease. Ionizing radiation also may cause aplastic anemia. Several medications, such as chloramphenicol (an antibiotic) and gold salts (therapy for rheumatoid arthritis), and some viral infections, such as hepatitis, can lead to the development of aplastic anemia. An immune system defect may cause suppression of bone marrow production.

A patient with aplastic anemia has signs of low blood counts. Evaluation of a blood smear and bone marrow test are necessary to make the diagnosis. The only curative treatment is allogeneic bone marrow transplantation. Several medications can produce remissions of the disease, but the remissions are temporary.

Living With Your Diagnosis

Severe aplastic anemia is a life-threatening disease. A low platelet count leads to bleeding and bruising and a low red blood cell count to anemia. A low white blood cell count predisposes the patient to infections.

Anemia can manifest itself as weakness, fatigue, and decreased tolerance of exercise. It can cause chest pain, dizziness, and shortness of breath. Lowering of the white blood cell count (leukopenia) decreases resistance to infection. Patients have recurrent infections, such as pneumonia, sinusitis, and skin infections. A low platelet count can cause prolonged bleeding from the vagina or nose, bleeding into internal organs, and easy, frequently spontaneous bruising.

Treatment

Rapid diagnosis and initiation of therapy are necessary. Bone marrow transplantation from a family member or sometimes a matched, unrelated donor can bring a cure. Bone marrow transplantation can be performed, however, only on young patients.

Only one fourth to one third of patients with aplastic anemia can undergo transplantation. For young patients with a suitable related donor, bone marrow transplantation is the treatment of choice. A compatible unrelated donor may be found through the National Marrow Donor Program and International Bone Marrow Registry. Blood transfusions should be limited before transplantation.

Bone marrow transplantation involves high doses of chemotherapy and infusion of bone marrow cells from a donor followed by a long course of immunosuppressive medications. A combination of immunosuppressive medications, such as cyclosporine, antilymphocyte globulin, and prednisone, produces remissions for as many as 70% of patients who cannot undergo a transplant. Treatment with immunosuppressive agents should be carefully monitored. The use of male hormones (androgens) can lead to improvement of symptoms for some patients. Supportive care with red blood cell and platelet transfusions is essential for all patients.

Allogeneic bone marrow transplantation is an intensive and toxic treatment. The procedure carries risk for infection and toxic effects of chemotherapy on the liver, lungs, and brain. These effects can be fatal for a small proportion of patients. Prolonged use of immunosuppressive drugs decreases resistance to some types of infections. Steroids, such as prednisone, can increase blood glucose level, elevate blood pressure, and cause stomach distress, loss of calcium and other salts, fluid retention, and weight gain. Infusion of antilymphocyte globulin can produce serum sickness. Androgenic hormones can cause liver damage, menstrual irregularities, and unwanted hair growth.

The bone marrow cells of the donor can attack the body and produce a serious complication called *graft-versus-host disease*. A skin rash, diarrhea, liver dysfunction can develop. Continuous use of immunosuppression can prevent and manage graft-versus-host disease. Failure of the transplanted marrow to grow and function (graft failure) is another complication of bone marrow transplantation. Acute leukemia (myelodysplastic syndrome) can develop years after transplantation, but this is rare. However, among some patients acute leukemia may develop even without treatment.

Medications that protect the stomach may be necessary for patients who take steroids. Specific prophylactic antibiotics are administered. Frequent blood tests are used to monitor blood glucose, electrolytes, blood counts, and liver function tests.

The DOs
- Take your medications as prescribed.
- Report for laboratory tests as directed.
- Eat a special protective diet as recommended if you have a low white blood cell count, to limit bacterial contamination.
- Use medical alert identification.
- Undergo re-vaccination if you undergo bone marrow transplantation.

The DON'Ts
- Avoid crowds and contacts with people with obvious infections.
- Do not take aspirin and aspirin-like medications; they can increase the bleeding.
- Inform household members that they should not be vaccinated with live vaccines, such as live polio vaccine.
- Avoid eating fresh leafy vegetables, fruit, cheese, and yogurt.
- Limit interactive sports and strenuous exercise.

When to Call Your Doctor
- If you have a fever, bleeding, chest pain, or dizziness. Prompt treatment is necessary.

For More Information
Leukemia Society of America
600 Third Ave.
New York, NY 10016
800-955-4LSA
Oncolink: Bone Marrow Transplantation
http://www.oncolink.upenn.edu/specialty/chemo/bmt/
Blood & Marrow Transplant Newsletter
http://nysernet.org/bcic/bmt/bmt.news.html

ANEMIA, OF CHRONIC DISEASE

About Your Diagnosis

Anemia of chronic disease is anemia, or a decreased hemoglobin level, that accompanies a chronic disease. Any type of chronic disease of more than 1 or 2 months duration can cause anemia. Inflammatory, infectious, or malignant conditions can cause anemia. Anemia of chronic disease is associated most frequently with rheumatoid arthritis, tuberculosis, acquired immune deficiency syndrome (AIDS), endocarditis, lung abscess, chronic osteomyelitis, malignant tumors, and lymphoma.

The mechanism of anemia of chronic disease is not fully understood. The immune disturbance of chronic inflammation causes decreased production of a growth factor for red blood cells. An impaired incorporation of iron into the red blood cells occurs. The life span of the red blood cells shortens. Anemia of chronic disease is common; the only type of anemia that is more common is iron deficiency anemia.

Microscopic examination of the blood provides the basis for the diagnosis. Special blood tests used to measure the content of iron (ferritin, serum iron, iron-binding capacity) help confirm the diagnosis. A bone marrow examination frequently is necessary to rule out deficiency in iron and other conditions that lead to anemia.

Successful management of underlying disease results in marked in the anemia. Special treatments can improve the anemia and its symptoms.

Living With Your Diagnosis

Anemia of chronic disease is usually moderate and rarely causes symptoms. If left unrecognized, the anemia worsens. This manifests as easy fatiguability and decreased tolerance of exercise. Patients with underlying cardiovascular and pulmonary diseases are at particular risk. Combinations of these diseases with anemia deserve special attention. Severe anemia can cause chest pain, shortness of breath, and palpitations.

Treatment

The main treatment is control and correction of the underlying disease. This is likely to improve the anemia and its signs. Patients with symptomatic anemia related to diseases that cannot be managed effectively, can benefit from treatment with erythropoietin (eg, Epogen, Procrit). This is a growth factor for red blood cells that is produced by means of special technology. It stimulates the red blood cells to grow and develop normally. An increase in hemoglobin can be observed during 3 to 4 weeks of treatment. Patients who respond to erythropoietin continue long-term therapy. Blood transfusions may be necessary for patients with severe anemia.

Erythropoietin treatment is prescribed and monitored by a physician. Patients receive erythropoietin as an injection under the skin three times a week. Follow-up blood tests are performed to determine whether there is a response. Continuous use of erythropoietin may be necessary. Erythropoietin therapy is usually well tolerated. Erythropoietin can cause elevations in blood pressure, but this is rare. Patients with preexisting seizure disorders should be monitored for seizures.

The DOs

- Follow treatment recommendations for the underlying condition.
- Discuss with a physician any new medications and their effects on anemia.
- Eat a well-balanced diet rich in iron and folic acid to maintain production of red blood cells.
- Participate in nonstrenuous exercise if you have mild or moderate anemia.
- Use medical alert identification if you have severe anemia.

The DON'Ts

- Do not take iron-containing vitamins. Iron overload can develop.
- Avoid strenuous exercise.

When to Call Your Doctor

- If you experience chest pain, palpitations, dizziness, or shortness of breath. These are symptoms of severe anemia.

For More Information
National Heart, Lung, and Blood Institute Information Center, P.O. Box 30105
Bethesda MD 20824-0105
301-251-1222
MedWeb Hematology: http://www.gen.emory.edu/medweb.hematology.html
MedMark Hematology: http://medmark.bit.co.kr/hematol.html

ANEMIA, FOLATE DEFICIENCY

About Your Diagnosis

The term *folate deficiency anemia* means that low blood counts are caused by a deficiency of folic acid in the body. It is also called *megaloblastic anemia* because the blood cells become larger in this anemia. Folic acid is a vitamin needed by the body for making DNA (deoxyribonucleic acid), which is the basic genetic material in all cells. Megaloblastic anemia also can result from lack of vitamin B_{12}. The factors that lead to folic acid deficiency are dietary deficiency, defective absorption of ingested folate, increased need for folate, and inability of the body to use available folate.

The main cause of folate deficiency is a folate-poor diet. This commonly occurs among elderly persons, poor persons, and persons with alcoholism. Patients undergoing hemodialysis or hyperalimentation also can have folate deficiency. Malabsorption of folate commonly occurs in diseases of the small intestine, such as tropical sprue, nontropical sprue, regional enteritis, leukemic or lymphomatous infiltration of the small intestine, Whipple's disease, scleroderma, amyloidosis, and diabetes mellitus.

Folate deficiency is most common among women who have given birth multiple times. Folate needs increase five- to tenfold during pregnancy because of transfer of folate to the growing fetus. Poor diet, infection, and coexisting hemolytic anemia also may contribute to folate deficiency.

Folate deficiency also occurs in conditions such as hemolytic anemia, and exfoliative dermatitis because of increased folate requirements. Patients taking antiepileptic drugs can have folate deficiency anemia.

The incidence of folate deficiency varies in different parts of the world. This disorder is not hereditary. It is always caused by deficiency of folic acid in the body. It cannot be transmitted from one person to another.

The serum folate level is the single most useful laboratory test in the diagnosis of this disorder. Other blood tests reveal abnormalities suggestive of folic acid deficiency anemia.

This is a manageable disorder. Folic acid supplementation is the mainstay of treatment.

Living With Your Diagnosis

Fatigue, palpitation, progressive loss of appetite, shortness of breath, lightheadedness, and mental depression are the principal symptoms of folate deficiency anemia. Inflammation of the tongue and gums, vomiting, and diarrhea occur frequently. There are no neurologic findings in this type of megaloblastic anemia.

A complete blood cell count reveals a low hemoglobin level. The red blood cells look larger than normal on a blood smear. The peripheral white blood cells are hypersegmented.

The serum folate level is the single most useful laboratory test in the diagnosis of folate deficiency anemia. Red blood cell folate concentration does not fall into subnormal range until all of the body stores have become depleted. Red blood cell folate levels are low among more than half of patients with vitamin B_{12} deficiency anemia; therefore it cannot be used to differentiate folate deficiency and vitamin B_{12} deficiency anemia.

Treatment

It is easy to manage folate deficiency anemia. Blood counts start improving in 2 to 3 weeks after treatment begins. Once the diagnosis is made, every attempt should be made to find and manage the problem causing anemia. Folate is usually given orally 1 to 5 milligrams daily, although 1 milligram is usually enough. At this dose, the anemia is corrected even among patients with malabsorption. Pregnant women should take a 1 milligram folate supplement daily. Patients start feeling better after taking folic acid for a few weeks. There are no side effects of the treatment.

Megaloblastic anemia can be caused by vitamin B_{12} deficiency, and therapeutic doses of folic acid partly correct the hematologic abnormalities in vitamin B_{12} deficiency. However, the neurologic symptoms can progress with disastrous results. Therefore, it is important to have both folate and vitamin B_{12} measured early in the evaluation of megaloblastic anemia.

The DOs

- Take folic acid supplements as prescribed.
- Eat a healthful diet that includes foods high in folate, such as green leafy vegetables, meat, and cereals.
- If you are pregnant, take a daily folic acid supplement in addition to your multivitamin. Folate

deficiency can cause several congenital fetal abnormalities.

- Increase your physical activity gradually. There are no restrictions for exercise as long as you do not feel tired.
- Talk to your physician about taking a folate supplement if you are taking any of the following medications: phenytoin (eg, Dilantin), antibiotics, chemotherapeutic agents, or oral contraceptives.

The DON'Ts
- Do not use medications more frequently than recommended.
- Refrain from drinking alcoholic beverages, because they can aggravate anemia.
- Avoid foods such as pastry and soft drinks because they tend to displace more nutritious foods.
- Do not overcook your food, because excessive cooking can destroy folic acid.
- Avoid physical exertion to the point of fatigue.

When to Call Your Doctor
- If you experience numbness, problems with balance, or any visual disturbances during treatment.

For More Information
Med Web Hematology: http://www.gen.emory.edu/medweb.hematology.html
MedMark Hematology: http://medmark.bit.co.kr/ hemato,html
National Heart, Lung, and Blood Institute Information Center
P.O. Box 30105
Bethesda MD 20824-0105
301-51-1222

ANEMIA, IRON DEFICIENCY

About Your Diagnosis

Iron deficiency anemia occurs when your body does not have enough iron to produce red blood cells. Iron is an essential component of red blood cells. Most of your iron comes from food, but you may lose iron if you lose a large amount of blood. In developing countries, inadequate nutrition is the principal cause of iron deficiency anemia. In Europe and United States, chronic blood loss is more frequently responsible for the iron deficiency.

The body has many ways of conserving iron. When red blood cells are destroyed, the iron inside them is reused in the production of new red blood cells. However, there is a daily iron loss that should be replenished with nutrition. Foods that have a high amount of iron are animal products such as meat, milk, and eggs. Vegetables such as spinach and broccoli have a large amount of iron, but the intestine is not able to absorb it.

Patients at risk for iron deficiency anemia are strict vegetarians (those who do not consume any animal products) and who eat an inadequate diet and at the same time require large amounts of iron, such as pregnant or lactating women or women with heavy menstrual losses. Also at risk are patients with chronic blood losses due to conditions such as gastric ulcers or intestinal tumors. Many times the first sign of a malignant intestinal tumor is iron deficiency anemia.

Living With Your Diagnosis

You may feel fatigued or unable to perform your normal daily activities. In severe cases, you may have shortness of breath, palpitations, and even chest pain. If you have an iron deficiency for a long period of time, other symptoms such as sore mouth, difficulty swallowing, or a tendency for your nails to soften and curl, sometimes taking the shape of a spoon, may occur.

A simple blood test is the most common method of diagnosis. The blood is examined with a microscope, and the red blood cells show a characteristic shape. Sometimes the diagnosis is not clear, and a bone marrow examination is necessary. This is performed at the doctor's office under local anesthesia, and the results usually are available in 2 to 3 days.

Determination of the cause of iron loss is essential to the diagnosis of iron deficiency anemia. Because the cause is most often chronic blood loss, signs of abnormal bleeding are sought.

The tenuous nature of iron balance among infants, adolescents, and pregnant women make evaluation unnecessary in most instances of iron deficiency anemia. A trial with iron supplementation is usually sufficient. However, any abnormality among men or postmenopausal women necessitates prompt investigation.

Treatment

The immediate treatment of patients with iron deficiency anemia depends on the severity of the condition. In the worse cases, blood transfusion may be necessary. All other cases can be managed with an iron tablet taken three to four times a day. A typical regimen is one tablet after each meal and at bedtime. As many as 25% of patients have some nausea and upper abdominal pain; diarrhea and constipation may occur. If that is the case, a physician should be told, and the dose of iron will be reduced. After any surgical procedure, especially a gastric operation, the body absorbs less iron than normal. In that case a liquid iron preparation is usually prescribed.

The DOs

- Undergo a screening blood test if you are at risk for iron deficiency anemia.
- Participate in your prenatal care, and take your prenatal vitamins. Continue to take your prenatal vitamins if you are lactating.
- Eat a well-balanced diet to maintain your iron balance.

The DON'Ts

- Avoid overexertion.

When to Call Your Doctor

- If you experience severe fatigue, dizziness, chest pain, or shortness of breath.
- If you have bleeding or if chronic bleeding increases.
- If you have abdominal pain from their iron supplement pill. This is a side effect of some formulations of iron and can usually resolves or improves with lowering of the dose or changing to a different iron formulation.

For More Information
MedWeb   Hematology: http://www.gen.emory.edu/

medweb.hematology.html
MedMark Hematology: http://medmark.bit.co.kr/hematol.html
National Heart, Lung, and Blood Institute Information Center
P.O. Box 30105
Bethesda, MD 20824-0105
301-251-1222

ANEMIA, PERNICIOUS

About Your Diagnosis

Pernicious anemia is deficiency of red blood cells and hemoglobin that results from a deficiency or abnormal absorption of cobalamin (vitamin B_{12}). This vitamin is essential for normal growth and development of red blood cells, other blood cells, and cells of the nervous system. Insufficient intake of vitamin B_{12} rarely causes anemia. Most frequently absence of a specific protein, intrinsic factor, necessary for absorption of vitamin B_{12} causes pernicious anemia. This occurs when the immune system attacks the cells of the stomach lining and prevents them from producing intrinsic factor. Other mechanisms include absence of the stomach or small intestine after an operation, tapeworm infestation, or tropical sprue.

Pernicious anemia is rare. Both sexes are affected equally. This form of anemia rarely occurs before 30 years of age. It is more common among persons of northern European descent.

The diagnosis of pernicious is made by means of microscopic examination of the blood and measurement of vitamin B_{12} and the products of its breakdown in the blood. Special tests may be needed to observe abnormal absorption of the vitamin (Schilling test) and document the presence of specific antibodies.

Supplementation of vitamin B_{12} leads to full correction of anemia. Patients with deficient absorption of the vitamin need long-term supplementation.

Living With Your Diagnosis

Anemia becomes apparent as fatigue and poor exercise tolerance. In severe cases anemia can cause chest pain, shortness of breath, and a rapid heart beat. Patients with pernicious anemia, however, almost never need blood transfusions. Deficiency of vitamin B_{12} can produce decreased sensation and numbness in the feet and hands. Severe deficiency can cause severe neurologic deficits, such as confusion and disorientation, but this is rare.

Treatment

Therapy for pernicious anemia is administration of vitamin B_{12} as injections under the skin or into the muscle. Initial treatment involves daily injections followed by weekly and eventually monthly injections. Improvement in the sense of well-being occurs in a matter of days. It takes 4 to 8 weeks to demonstrate an increase in hemoglobin concentration. Treatment is lifelong. Patients with insufficient intake can take oral vitamin B_{12}. There are no known side effects or complications of taking vitamin B_{12}. Vitamin B_{12} is also available as a gel solution for intranasal administration (Nascobal), which is administered via a metered dose nasal inhaler once weekly in place of monthly injections. Intranasal administration for maintenance therapy of pernicious anemia should be used only after the initial deficiency has been corrected with vitamin B_{12} injections. Medical supervision is necessary for the initial treatment with vitamin B_{12}, because lowering of blood potassium level may occur. A simple blood test can determine this. Potassium taken as a pill corrects this temporary problem.

The DOs

- Continue treatment on a monthly basis (if injections are used), even if the anemia is corrected. Discontinuation of treatment leads to recurrence of anemia and all the symptoms.
- Follow the schedule of vitamin B_{12} injections recommended by your physician.
- Discuss a supplementation schedule with your physician if you are pregnant.
- Eat a well-balanced diet, rich in folic acid (another vitamin important for the blood cells) and other essential nutrients.
- Supplement your diet with oral vitamins if you eat a special diet, such as a vegetarian, especially vegan, diet.

The DON'Ts

- Avoid exercise until the anemia is corrected.

When to Call Your Doctor

- If you experience any signs of severe anemia, such as chest pain, palpitations, or shortness of breath.

For More Information
National Heart, Lung, and Blood Institute Information Center P.O. Box 30105
Bethesda, MD 20825-0105
301-251-1222
MedWeb Hematology: http://www.gem.emory.edu/medweb.hematology.html
MedMark Hematology: http://medmark.bit.co.kr/hematol.html

ANEMIA, SICKLE CELL

About Your Diagnosis

Sickle cell anemia is a genetic disease in which the red blood cells contain an abnormal hemoglobin known as *hemoglobin S* (Hb S). Hemoglobin is the material in red blood cells that carries oxygen from the lungs to the rest of the body. The abnormal hemoglobin has a tendency to aggregate, especially in parts of the body where oxygen content is low. This aggregation causes the red blood cells to form a sickle shape, which gives the disease its name.

Sickle cell anemia is caused by a mutation in the DNA (deoxyribonucleic acid) that codes for beta-globin, one of the proteins that makes up hemoglobin. More than 50,000 persons in the United States have sickle cell anemia. The disease is most common among African-Americans, but is also seen among persons of Mediterranean, Caribbean, South and Central American, Arabian, and East Indian ancestry.

Sickle cell anemia is a hereditary disease. Patients inherit the abnormal gene from both their mother and their father; therefore their bodies can make only Hb S. The parents of patients with sickle cell anemia may have either sickle cell disease or sickle cell trait. Persons with sickle cell trait have one sickle cell gene and one normal beta-globin gene. They can make both Hb S and normal hemoglobin (Hb A). Persons with sickle cell trait are healthy but can have children with sickle cell anemia.

Sickle cell anemia is diagnosed by means of a blood test to determine that the red blood cells form a sickle shape. The blood test is followed by a more detailed examination of the blood to determine the presence of Hb S, Hb A, or any other abnormal hemoglobin.

A few patients with sickle cell disease have been cured with bone marrow transplantation from a brother or sister. However, this treatment remains highly experimental.

Living With Your Diagnosis

Sickle cell anemia is characterized by acute episodes of illness, known as *crises*. The most common type of crisis is a vasoocclusive or painful crisis; it is believed to be caused by blockage of blood vessels by sickled red blood cells. Patients experience severe pain, usually in the bones, and may have a fever. Symptoms usually last several days but may persist for more than a week.

Sickle cell anemia can affect every organ of the body, leading to complications such as kidney disease, eye disease, chronic hip or shoulder pain, heart disease, and leg ulcers. Sickling of red blood cells in the blood vessels of the brain may lead to strokes. Men with sickle cell anemia may have priapism, a persistent, unwanted erection. Sickling in the spleen causes the organ to become inactive, making patients with sickle cell anemia prone to infections. Some of the more common infections are osteomyelitis (bone infection) and pneumonia.

Patients with sickle cell anemia may have a serious lung disorder known as *acute chest syndrome*. This syndrome is believed to be caused by a combination of sickling in the blood vessels of the lung and ribs and pneumonia. Patients with sickle cell anemia also may experience a type of crisis known as *aplastic crisis*, in which the bone marrow temporarily stops making red blood cells. This type of crisis is usually associated with an infection (especially with the organism parvovirus B19) and can lead to severe anemia.

It is safe for patients with sickle cell anemia to travel in pressurized aircraft. However, travel in nonpressurized aircraft at high altitudes may trigger a crisis.

Treatment

Treatment of sickle cell crisis involves controlling the pain. Mild crises can be managed with oral medications, which may or may not be narcotics. More severe pain crises may necessitate use of narcotics administered by means of intramuscular or intravenous injection. Fluids are given to prevent dehydration. Severe complications of sickle cell disease, such as stroke or acute chest syndrome, may be managed by means of exchange transfusion, which involves removing the patient's abnormal red blood cells and replacing them with normal red blood cells.

Hydroxyurea is a chemotherapeutic drug that appears to decrease the frequency of pain crises among patients with sickle cell anemia. Some patients with severe symptoms of sickle cell anemia may be treated with this drug.

Narcotic pain medications can cause drowsiness and constipation. Aspirin and nonsteroidal anti-inflammatory drugs (NSAIDs), such as ibuprofen, can cause stomach pain and platelet abnormalities (platelets are blood cells that help form clots). Hydroxyurea can cause a decrease in all blood cell counts: red blood cells, white blood cells, and platelets. A low red blood cell count (anemia) can cause fatigue and shortness of breath. A low white blood cell count (neutropenia) can increase susceptibility to infection. A low platelet count (thrombocytopenia) can lead to easy bruising or bleeding.

Use of narcotics can lead to physical dependence and symptoms of withdrawal if the drug is stopped too quickly. However, true addiction (a psychological need for the drug) is rare. Overuse of aspirin or NSAIDs can cause stomach ulcers and kidney disease. Overuse of acetaminophen (eg, Tylenol) may produce liver damage. Hydroxyurea can cause fetal abnormalities; therefore patients should not become pregnant or father a child while taking it.

Children with sickle cell anemia generally receive prophylactic penicillin to prevent bacterial infection. Many sickle cell crises may be managed at home with oral pain medications, hydration, and rest.

The DOs
- Take a daily folate supplement.
- Drink plenty of fluids to avoid dehydration, especially if you begin to have a painful crisis.
- Eat a healthy diet that contains green, leafy vegetables, which are high in folate.
- Participate in mild to moderate exercise as tolerated but be careful to rest if you feel tired and drink fluids after exertion.
- Dress warmly and avoid exposure to cold if possible; cold temperatures may trigger a crisis.
- Inform the surgeon or dentist that you have sickle cell anemia if you are undergoing elective surgical or dental procedures.
- Consider genetic counseling to determine your risk for having an affected child.
- Undergo prenatal care with both your obstetrician and your primary care physician. Although you may have a more complicated pregnancy than women without sickle cell disease, your likelihood of delivering a healthy baby is excellent.

The DON'Ts
- Do not overuse pain medications.
- Avoid excessive consumption of alcohol.
- Avoid overexertion.
- Avoid swimming in cold water, which may trigger a crisis.

When to Call Your Doctor
- If you have a fever, shortness of breath, severe abdominal pain, priapism, neurologic symptoms (such as weakness on one side of your body or difficulty speaking), or a painful crisis that does not respond to management at home.

For More Information
National Heart, Lung, and Blood Institute Information Center
P.O. Box 30105
Bethesda, MD 20824-0105
301-251-1222
MedMark Hematology: http://medmark,bit.co.kr/hematol.html
Sickle Cell Disease Association of America, Inc.
200 Corporate Point, #495
Culver City, CA 90230-7633
Operation Sickle Cell, Inc.
2409 Murchison Road
Fayetteville, NC 28301
910-488-6118
http://www.uncfsu.edu/osc/
Joint Center for Sickle Cell and Thalassemic Disorders
http://cancer.mgh.harvard.edu/medOnc/sickle.htm

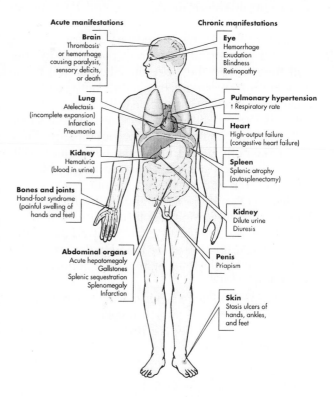

Clinical manifestations of sickle cell disease. (From Lewis SM, Collier IC, Heitkemper MM: *Medical-Surgical Nursing: Assessment and Management of Clinical Problem*, vol. 4. St. Louis, Mosby–Year Book, 1995. Used by permission.)

ANGINA PECTORIS

About Your Diagnosis

Angina pectoris is heart-related pain. Pain may be felt in the chest or the upper arms or jaw. It occurs when the heart has an inadequate oxygen supply in the blood. Any condition that causes the heart to increase work increases its need for oxygen. If blood flow to the heart is decreased because of coronary artery disease from atherosclerosis (scarring and fatty deposits in the blood vessels) or from vessel spasm (contracting closed), angina may result.

The coronary arteries are the vessels that supply blood to the heart muscle. Abnormal heart valves may decrease blood flow through the heart and to the coronary vessels. Abnormal heart rhythm (arrhythmias) may keep the heart from moving blood effectively. If the heart must work harder because of exercise, stress, or illness and blood flow does not meet demands, angina may result. A decrease in the number of oxygen-carrying cells (red blood cells) in the blood (anemia) makes it difficult for the heart to deliver oxygen. Damage to the heart muscle from disease or heart attack (myocardial infarction, which means a portion of the heart muscle dies because it does not have enough blood) causes the heart to pump less effectively. Angina pectoris may be a sign of more serious heart problems and requires immediate attention from a physician. The following persons are at risk for heart disease:

Men
Women after menopause who are not taking estrogen replacements
Persons older than 55 years
Persons with a family history of heart disease
Persons who smoke
Persons who are overweight
Persons with diabetes
Persons with hypertension (high blood pressure)
Persons with high cholesterol levels
Sedentary persons (those who do not exercise regularly)
Persons who eat diets high in fat and cholesterol

Living With Your Diagnosis

Angina is described in several ways. Some patients describe a smothering or crushing pain as if someone is sitting on their chest. The pain may be dull or sharp and may last several minutes or just a moment. The pain may be in the center of your chest or in your back, shoulder, or jaw. It may feel like heartburn. It may be accompanied by sweating, dizziness, or shortness of breath (fig 1). If pain occurs with exercise or increased work for the heart, rest may help. Pain that occurs at rest is called *unstable angina*.

Exercise can improve some patients' symptoms and their ability to work. Aerobic exercise such as swimming, bicycling, and walking or jogging is the best form of exercise for patients with heart disease who can tolerate exercise. Before an exercise program is begun, an exercise test must be conducted. A physician's clearance is necessary for strenuous activity.

It is normal to have concerns about the effects on your heart of having sexual relations. Most people with heart disease or angina may engage in sexual activity safely with the same risk as those for moderate exercise. If you are concerned, speak to your doctor.

Treatment

The diagnosis of angina pectoris is made by a physician on the basis of the symptoms and examination findings. Tests may be performed to evaluate the heart. These may include electrocardiograms (ECGs), treadmill or exercise tests, or catheterization (checking the blood flow at the heart by means of inserting a device through a vein to the heart). Severe cases of angina pectoris may necessitate angioplasty (opening clogged blood vessels with a balloon-like device) or coronary artery bypass grafting. Laboratory tests may be performed to monitor for evidence of heart damage or other conditions, such as anemia, diabetes, hyperthyroidism, or high blood cholesterol levels.

Chest pain is controlled with attempts to improve the blood flow to the working heart muscle or to decrease the work of the heart. Resting or decreasing activity is the first treatment you should try. Some patients can improve the blood flow to their hearts with nitrates such as nitroglycerin (a small pill placed under the tongue). Hypertension (high blood pressure) makes the heart work harder, so antihypertensive medicines such as beta-blockers or calcium channel blockers may be given. There are many different types of these medications, so a physician should review the side effects with you. Arrhythmias may be treated with antiarrhythmic medicines. High blood cholesterol should be treated.

Underlying medical conditions that may be contributing to the angina or heart disease require careful management. Control of diabetes and hypertension is extremely important. Monitoring thyroid disease and high blood cholesterol are important. Anyone with angina or heart disease should take aspirin daily unless otherwise directed by a physician.

The DOs
- Stop smoking.
- Lose weight if you are overweight.
- Reduce calories in your diet. Include reduced-fat and low-cholesterol items in your diet.
- Take your medications as directed.

The DON'Ts
- Do not forget to take your medications as scheduled. Do not ignore your symptoms. If they do not improve, you may need medical attention immediately.

When to Call Your Doctor
- If you have worsening chest, arm, or jaw pain not controlled with your usual medicines or resting.
- If you have taken your nitroglycerin three times without relief. Call 911 or get to an emergency facility as soon as possible.
- If you have new or worsening cardiac symptoms such as shortness of breath, sweating, or feeling faint that are not controlled with your medication. Seek immediate medical care.

For More Information
Living with Angina is a booklet available from the American Heart Association that is very helpful for persons with this condition. Call 1-800-242-8721 and ask for the literature department.

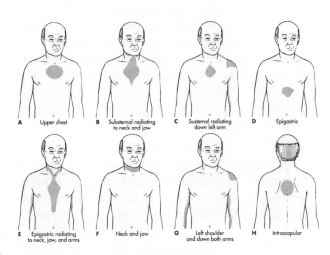

Location of chest pain during angina or myocardial infarction. **A,** upper chest. **B,** substernal area with radiation to neck and jaw. **C,** substernal area with radiation down left arm. D, epigastric area. E, epigastric area with radiation to neck, jaw, and arms. F, neck and jaw. G, left shoulder and down both arms. H, intrascapular area. (From Lewis SM, Collier IC, Heitkemper MM: *Medical-Surgical Nursing: Assessment and Management of Clinical Problem*, vol. 4. St. Louis, Mosby–Year Book, 1995. Used by permission.)

ANGIOEDEMA

About Your Diagnosis

Angioedema is almost identical to the common skin condition of urticaria or hives. In hives, raised, red, itchy, irregular bumps appear on your skin, whereas in angioedema the same thing is happening but deeper in the skin. You cannot see the raised, red bumps, but you can feel a firm swelling pushing up your normal skin. Instead of angioedema being itchy, it may be tender or painful.

Angioedema can occur anywhere on the body, but it more commonly involves the eyelids, lips, tongue, and external genitalia. It can also occur inside the body. In the intestines it can cause abdominal pain, and in the airways it can cause difficulty in breathing, which can be fatal. Fortunately the most common occurrence of angioedema is on the outside of our body, and although uncomfortable it is not dangerous.

Anyone can get angioedema. About 15% to 20% of all individuals will have at least one episode of hives or angioedema in their lifetime.

The swelling of angioedema is usually present for only a day or two at any one spot. However, it often will move from one location to another and last for several days. Sometimes it can become chronic.

Angioedema is an allergic reaction that somehow has come into your body. It is not an infection, although infections can cause an attack of angioedema. It is not contagious, although certain types are hereditary, and you should check to see whether other family members have had a similar problem. The usual causes of angioedema are a new drug, a new food, a new perfume, etc. You may even have taken that drug or food in the past without problem, but now you have developed an allergy to it.

Although no cure exists for angioedema, it can be treated and the symptoms controlled. The main treatment is to prevent recurrences.

Living With Your Diagnosis

The diagnosis of angioedema is made by the typical appearance of the swollen skin and its tendency to come and go. There are some blood tests that can be done, but they are not always helpful and do not affect treatment. A family history of angioedema is very important; therefore family members should be asked about any episodes of angioedema they have had, and you should tell your doctor about these.

The typical rash of angioedema is puffy or swollen skin that is firm and may be painful. The rash can occur anywhere but usually involves the eyelids, lips, genitalia, tongue, hands, and/or feet. The swelling can occur inside the body as well. You must contact your doctor immediately if you are having any trouble breathing or are wheezing, or are having abdominal pain. Angioedema often resolves in a day or two to a week, but in some cases it can persist and may require long-term treatment. Chronic angioedema, although uncomfortable and irritating, usually will not progress to a more serious disease.

Treatment

The primary treatment for angioedema is removal of whatever is causing the allergy. Unfortunately the exact cause of the angioedema is often not known, and even if it is (e.g., pollen), it may be impossible to remove it. Therefore the main treatment of active angioedema is to control the symptoms.

Application of cold compresses may provide local comfort. Lotions and creams are usually not helpful because they don't penetrate deep enough under the skin to reach the angioedema.

Oral antihistamines work well but must be taken in adequate amounts on a regular basis. Failure to take antihistamines regularly may result in the angioedema coming back. Antihistamines are well known for their tendency to make individuals drowsy, as well as to cause other side effects such as dry mouth. Newer antihistamines have fewer side effects. If antihistamines are not controlling your symptoms, see your doctor. Your doctor can prescribe stronger medications such as steroids.

The best treatment is always prevention. You should carefully examine potential causes for your angioedema. Note if you ate a new food, wore new clothes, took a new drug, wore a new perfume, were exposed to a new smell, or have a new job. Anything that you can think of which might have caused your angioedema is helpful. Sometimes your doctor may need to perform tests to find out what the allergic problem is. If you know what triggers your angioedema, the best treatment is to avoid that trigger.

The DOs

- Do seek medical aid immediately if you are having trouble breathing or are having chest pain.
- Do use cold compresses on the swollen areas.
- Do take antihistamines in proper doses for the swelling.
- Do note immediately any possible causes for your angioedema (new food, drug, soap, perfume, etc.).
- Do remove or stop any possible cause of the swelling, such as new food, new soap, or new perfume. Ask your doctor about any drugs you are taking.

The Don'ts

- Don't use heat on the swelling
- Don't use creams, ointments, or lotions.

When to Call Your Doctor

If you are having trouble breathing, having chest pain, or having abdominal pain, contact you doctor immediately.

- If your angioedema is not responding to antihistamine therapy after 2 or 3 days of continuous treatment.
- If you are having recurrent attacks of angioedema.

For More Information
American Academy of Dermatology
930 N. Meachum Road
Schaumburg, IL 60173
847-330-0230

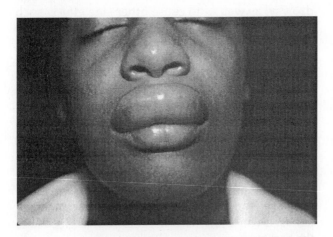

Angioedema of the upper lip, with severe swelling of deeper tissues. (Courtesy of Beverly Sanders, M.D. From Goldstein BG, Goldstein AO: *Practical Dermatology,* vol 1. St. Louis, Mosby–Year Book, 1992. Used by permission.)

ANKLE FRACTURE

About Your Diagnosis

An ankle fracture is a break of any of the bones of the ankle joint. Causes include a blow to the ankle, a fall landing on the feet, or most commonly a twisting injury to the ankle. A physical examination and usually an x-ray will diagnose the injury. Most of the time an ankle fracture will heal, but it is possible to have some long-term pain and disability depending on the circumstances of the injury.

Living With Your Diagnosis

The symptoms of an ankle fracture are pain in the ankle, particularly when bearing weight or moving the ankle. The signs include swelling, bruising, and possibly deformity of the joint. Depending on the severity, an ankle fracture may not be more than a severe sprain in which the ligament has pulled its attachment off the bone. On the other hand, a fracture can result in a major disruption of the joint. This may include a dislocation of the ankle.

Treatment

Treatment will depend on the severity and location of the fracture. It can range from treatment similar to a sprain with rest, ice, compression, and bracing for protected mobility, to surgery with placement of screws and plates to hold the bones together while they heal. A cast or a removable splint that will hold the bones in a stable position until they heal is the most common treatment. This will take 4–6 weeks in most cases. If a cast is used, there will be some weakness of the lower leg muscles after removal. This is probably the most common side effect and will resolve with physical therapy. Potential complications include failure of the fracture to heal (called a nonunion). Other complications include restriction of blood flow to the foot or toes if the cast is too tight or if there is swelling in the cast. Infection or bleeding related to surgery can also occur.

The DOs

You should take medications for pain control as prescribed. A diet containing adequate supplies of calcium will help with bone healing. You should keep your foot elevated for the first few days to minimize swelling. You may have crutches to use for walking. You should apply cold to your ankle the first day or so to minimize swelling. You will probably not receive any exercises to do until removal of the cast. Following those exercises or participating in physical therapy will shorten your recovery.

The DON'Ts

You should minimize swelling in your ankle. You should avoid spending too much time on your feet or with your foot hanging down in that this will increase swelling. You should not place heat on the ankle for the same reason. Swelling may result in restriction of circulation to the foot. You should not get a plaster cast wet; even a fiberglass cast takes a long time to dry if it gets wet, so you should try to keep it dry. You should not stick objects such as coat hangers, pencils, or knitting needles down the cast to scratch itching places. If you break the skin, you may get an infection. Although a cast is designed to protect the ankle, it is not indestructible. You should try to avoid damaging the cast because that will make it less effective. Do not remove your cast too soon. This may result in reinjury that will significantly prolong the time to recovery. Do not remove your plastic or metal splint unless instructed to. It cannot keep your bones in position for healing unless it is in place.

When to Call Your Doctor

You should call your doctor if you notice any numbness, tingling, coldness, or duskiness of your toes. This could indicate that the cast is too tight or that there has been swelling of the ankle, resulting in restriction of circulation to your foot. You should call if you have damaged your splint or cast so that it is loose, or is allowing your ankle to move more than it should. If you had surgery, you need to call if fever develops, or if redness, swelling, or pus are present at the incision; these signs suggest that an infection is present. You should contact your doctor if you have increasing pain or are unable to use your ankle at some time after surgery, because this could be an indication that plates or screws have broken or shifted.

For More Information
Description of the injury, x-rays, and surgical treatment
http://www.medmedia.com/00a1/29.htm

ANKLE SPRAIN

About Your Diagnosis

Ankle sprains are the result of stretching, or partially or completely tearing one or several of the ligaments that hold the ankle joint together. Ankle sprains occur when the ankle joint is forced to bend further than normal. The most common type of sprain occurs when the foot is turned inward and the full weight comes down on the ankle. This causes a sprain on the outside of the ankle. Almost everyone has a sprain sometime in their life. Almost all resolve completely without further problems.

Living With Your Diagnosis

The symptoms of a sprain include a popping or tearing sensation at the time of injury. This results in pain whenever the ankle bears weight. Usually there is fairly quick swelling at the site of injury. Bruising will often develop during the next 24 hours.

Treatment

Treatment will help prevent swelling, protect the joint until it heals, and prevent unnecessary muscle weakness. Treatment also helps remove any swelling, enabling you to get moving again as quickly as possible. The initial treatment helps to prevent swelling and consists of four components. First, apply ice to the injury immediately because the swelling can start in a few minutes. The less swelling you have, the quicker you will be back to normal activity. Second, rest the joint for 1 or 2 days. This may include using crutches to rest the ankle if you have to be up and around during the first day or two. Third, compress the injured area with a compression wrap or air splint. Fourth, elevate the ankle above the level of the hip. You can remember these treatment components with the acronym RICE (*R*est, *I*ce, *C*ompression, and *E*levation).

The next treatment is protected motion that allows the ankle to move without moving too far and further injuring the joint. This may be as simple as using a compression wrap or a splint or brace. Your doctor may prescribe physical therapy. This will keep muscles from weakening and help remove any swelling that has taken place. Sometimes your doctor may suggest heat or alternating cold and heat to try to remove swelling that is present. Do not ever use heat before 72 hours after the injury because it will nearly always cause more swelling that will slow recovery. Lastly, your doctor may recommend exercises or physical therapy after you have recovered to try to prevent future injuries. Severe injuries may require casting of the foot or even surgery. This is usually necessary when the ligaments are completely torn or if there are multiple ligaments injured.

The DOs

You should take any medicines prescribed by your doctor. Prescription pain medicines may be used for severe sprains. Over-the-counter medications may be used for less severe sprains. You should follow your instructions for RICE immediately after your injury. Your doctor may prescribe physical therapy. Use your crutches as directed. If you are an athlete, your trainer may be able to help speed your recovery. After you have recovered, you may want to consider exercises to increase the strength of the lower leg muscles. There are also exercises that may improve "proprioception" (the ability to recognize the position of your foot without looking at it). Both types of exercises may help prevent future injury.

The DON'Ts

You should avoid activities that will increase swelling because this will slow your return to complete activity. Therefore, early application of heat, excessive activity, standing, or sitting with the ankle hanging should be avoided. If you keep a shoe on or apply a splint, brace, or compression wrap, you should watch for signs that it is getting too tight and cutting off circulation to the toes. Symptoms would include numbness or tingling in the foot or toes, blueness or duskiness of the toes, or coldness in the toes. If any of these occurs, loosen whatever is tight or contact your doctor. Although it is desirable to keep the joint moving, you must avoid a second injury before the first one heals.

When to Call Your Doctor

You should call if swelling is increasing or if you notice any of the above symptoms of decreased circulation to the foot. You should call if you are not noticing significant improvement within 7–10 days after the sprain. You should call if there is any popping, catching, or giving way of the ankle after the swelling has gone away. These may be signs of a more severe injury than was originally apparent.

For More Information
Description of the injury, the ligaments involved, and treatments
for severe sprains
http://www.medmedia.com/00a1/25.htm

ANKYLOSING SPONDYLITIS

About Your Diagnosis

Ankylosing spondylitis is a form of arthritis that primarily affects the entire spine, although it may involve the hips and shoulders. It usually affects young men, and there seems to be a genetic link. Back pain is the most common symptom, and it may be quite difficult to make the correct diagnosis in the early stages of the condition. Most of the usual blood tests for arthritis are normal. In the later stages of the condition, radiographic (x-ray) findings can be quite dramatic, showing complete fusion of the spine. This may cause the patient to walk in a stooped posture. Ankylosing spondylitis can have features such as eye irritation, heart problems, and spinal cord compression. A decreased ability to expand the chest can be another early finding.

Living With Your Diagnosis

Ankylosing spondylitis is a gradually progressive disease, and it can result in serious impairments. Precautions include sleeping without pillows to prevent the neck from fusing in an abnormally flexed position. If this happens, it becomes difficult to see straight ahead when walking or driving. Physical therapy, including water therapy, is combined with use of medications such as aspirin and anti-inflammatory drugs to minimize deformity and pain.

Treatment

Nonsurgical treatment is geared toward preventing fusion in undesirable positions. Physical therapy is important but possibly not cost effective. Analgesics and anti-inflammatory drugs can be effective in managing the pain. Surgical treatment involves cutting the bones in the spine to realign the body into a functional position. This is a complex surgical procedure with considerable risk, and patient and surgeon should choose this option with care. The hips are sometimes involved, and replacement arthroplasty may be needed.

The DOs

- Maintain as much motion as possible to prevent fusion in an awkward position.
- Perform regular non-weight-bearing exercise.

The DON'Ts

- Do not spend long periods in a poor posture, particularly with the head hanging forward.

When To Call Your Doctor

- If you fall and notice a sudden change in the alignment of your neck or back, whether or not you are feeling pain.

For More Information
http://www.spondylitis.org/symptoms.htm
http://www.medmedia.com/oa4/46.htm

ANOREXIA NERVOSA

About Your Diagnosis

Anorexia nervosa is a form of eating disorder. It is a condition that can have life-threatening consequences if not properly treated. In this condition, there is a refusal on the part of patients to maintain body weight at or above what is normal for their age and height. In addition, individuals with anorexia nervosa also have an intense fear of gaining weight or becoming fat, even though they are generally underweight. When asked about their ideal weight, patients with anorexia nervosa will never be able to give a number because they will always believe they should be thinner than they actually are. Individuals who have anorexia nervosa also seem to have an abnormal perception of how their body looks, despite normal weight for their height. There also is a strong denial about the serious physical consequences of low body weight and rapid weight loss. In women who have already had their first menstrual period, there is generally an absence of menstrual cycles secondary to malnutrition and starvation. To make a diagnosis, there needs to be at least three consecutive menstrual cycles missing. This loss of menstruation in someone who has already begun to have periods is called secondary amenorrhea. The individual with anorexia nervosa may have periods of binge eating behavior, but this is usually followed fairly rapidly by some sort of activity to eliminate the food (purging).

Although anorexia nervosa is often depicted in the media, it is actually a fairly rare illness. The groups at highest risk for this condition are adolescent girls and young women, but even there, it affects only about 0.5% of that population. It is true, however, that the occurrence of anorexia nervosa has increased significantly during the last 50 years, mainly related to societal attitudes about weight loss and acceptable physical appearance.

Anorexia nervosa is basically a condition that affects women, much more commonly than men in a ratio of 10:1 or even 20:1. It is more common in higher socioeconomic classes. Some occupations such as modeling, ballet dancing, figure skating, and being a jockey appear to confer a much higher risk for the development of anorexia nervosa, probably because of the emphasis in these occupations on thinness.

Living With Your Diagnosis

Anorexia nervosa seems to develop more rapidly in environments in which food is readily available, but in which being thin is to perceived to be desirable. We really do not know what causes anorexia nervosa, but some other risk factors are associated with the disease. There may be a genetic component; that is, it may be passed on from parents to children. The mothers of patients with anorexia nervosa are often described as overprotective, intrusive, orderly, and very much concerned with perfection. They are also described as being fearful of separation. On the other hand, fathers of patients with anorexia nervosa are often described as withdrawn, passive, very emotionally distant, moody, workaholics and in general fairly ineffective and absent. Undoubtedly the American fascination with thinness increases the risk for anorexia nervosa in this population. It is much more common among Caucasian women than among African-American or Hispanic women.

In looking at the childhood of women who later become anorexic, they were often very compliant children. They did not go through the usual acting out and difficult stages that occur around 2 years of age, the so-called terrible twos. When they approached adolescence, they began to develop the eating disorder, which served as a very powerful tool to disrupt the family and became their first rebellious act against their parent's wishes. In addition, there may also be some concern among pubertal women revolving around their budding sexuality. They may have concerns about heterosexual contact, and some fear of menstruation and the possibility of pregnancy. The development of anorexia nervosa with its secondary amenorrhea delays the onset of sexual maturity, leading to decreased anxiety about sexual issues among these patients.

As might be expected, there are many medical problems associated with anorexia nervosa. These include abnormalities of the skin, cardiovascular problems such as low blood pressure, slow heart rate, and abnormal heart rhythms, anemia, inability to fight infection, abnormal blood chemistry (such as low potassium, sodium, albumen, and total protein), dehydration, constipation, low thyroid hormone levels, and osteoporosis or bone disease. In assessing a patient with suspected anorexia nervosa, it is very important to obtain a weight history, including the individual's highest and lowest weights and the weight that she would like to be now. It is also important to take a dietary history and have the patient describe a typical day in terms of food intake and any food restrictions. Many times anorexic patients will engage in elaborate behavior to purge themselves of food they have eaten. This includes self-induced vomiting, which may cause dental caries and cavities, excessive exercise, abuse and misuse of laxatives and enemas, and use of diet pills and water pills. Abuse of syrup of Ipecac to induce vomiting is also fairly common. In the initial assessment, there may be a strong sense of denial on the part of the patient about the anorexia nervosa. A complete physical examination and laboratory testing should be done to rule out some of the physical problems mentioned earlier, and a decision should be made as to whether to treat the patient as an outpatient or to admit the patient to the hospital.

Treatment

The first goal of treatment for the patient with anorexia nervosa is to engage the patient and her family. Frequently there are strong feelings of guilt, and these must be addressed. The patient will often minimize problems and suggest that the concerns of the family are simply an overreaction. A second goal of treatment is to assess and address the patient's active medical problems. Depending on the severity of the illness, this may require hospitalization. Treatment usually involves psychotherapy, and occasionally medication if there is a depressive or anxious component. It should be remembered, however, that medications that cause a rapid weight gain, such as antidepressants like Elavil and Sinequan, should be avoided because the patient will rebel against any rapid weight gain. The patient is usually weighed once a week, and a gain in body weight of about 2–3 pounds a week is expected.

Many programs use negative and positive feedback, allowing patients to do things that they enjoy if they gain the weight or preventing them from doing so if they do not. It is important during this phase to provide patients with significant emotional support and reassurance, to address their fears about gaining weight, to educate these patients about the dangers of semistarvation, and to reassure them that they will not be allowed to gain "too much weight." In most treatment units that are experienced in treating anorexia nervosa, invasive techniques such as nasogastric feeding or intravenous feeding are rarely needed and are only used

for life-threatening circumstances. Unfortunately, a large percentage of patients with anorexia nervosa remain chronically ill. About 30% to 50% of patients successfully treated in the hospital require hospitalization again within 1 year of discharge, so outpatient programs after hospitalization are essential. There are, of course, side effects from medications used to treat anorexia nervosa. For example, some of the tricyclic antidepressants used to treat depression in anorexia can cause weight gain, drowsiness, blurred vision, constipation, and a fast heartbeat. There remains a significant mortality rate (death rate) associated with this condition.

The DOs

If you have anorexia nervosa, it is very important to follow your doctor's recommendations to avoid binging behavior, and to talk to a nutritionist about a safe diet. When shopping, you should buy clothes that fit, not clothes that you have to lose weight to get into.

The DON'Ts

If you have anorexia nervosa, you should not weigh yourself daily; you should avoid use of drugs, diet pills, and caffeine designed to promote weight loss; you should not use laxatives unless instructed to do so by your physician; and you should not engage in activities/occupations (modeling, ballet dancer, being a jockey) where emphasis is placed on weight loss. You should shop for food judiciously and avoid eating alone, if possible.

When to Call Your Doctor

You should report any unusual problems to your physician such as unusual thoughts, paranoia or hallucinations, significant depression, and any suicidal thoughts. Also, if you have done well for some time, notify your doctor if your urge to binge and purge begins to increase. Also, it is very important to minimize stress in your family, so some sort of family therapy is often helpful.

For More Information

In most cities, there are many support groups for patients with anorexia nervosa and their families. You can find out about them by calling your crisis center hot line or the psychiatric department at your local medical school.
Online Web sites of interest include:
Anorexia and Bulimia
http://umt.umt.edu:700/o/general/anorexia.txt
Eating Disorder Resources on the Internet:
http://www.stud.unit.no/studorg/ikstrh/ed/ed.hmt/

ANXIETY (GENERALIZED ANXIETY DISORDER)

About Your Diagnosis

Generalized anxiety disorder (GAD), one of many different anxiety disorders, is characterized by excessive anxiety and worry about a number of events and activities, such as work or school performance. In GAD, anxiety and worry occur on most days and have been present for at least 6 months. In addition to the anxiety, individuals find it very difficult to control their worrying even when reassured by others. In GAD, anxiety and worry are associated with specific symptoms, including restlessness or feeling keyed up, uptight, or on edge; being easily fatigued or feeling "drained": having difficulty concentrating or feeling that one's mind has gone blank; irritability out of proportion to whatever may have caused it; and feeling angry for no apparent reason. Muscle tension or tightness occurs, as well as sleep disturbances, especially difficulty falling or staying asleep or having a very restless, unsatisfying sleep. For GAD to be diagnosed, the intensity of anxiety has to cause some impairment in the individual's ability to function either on the job or in social relationships. The anxiety may also cause physical symptoms including shortness of breath, chest tightness, rapid and pounding heartbeat, sweating, a sensation of choking, and abdominal distress.

Some forms of anxiety besides GAD include *panic attacks,* in which the physical symptoms just mentioned occur "out of the blue" for no apparent reason, last for a very brief period, and then resolve. The individual with panic attacks may not, in fact, be anxious most of the day and may be relatively calm between the episodes of panic.

Agoraphobia, another form of anxiety, is a fear of being out in open spaces alone, where one might feel trapped and unable to get home. Agoraphobia often occurs in conjunction with panic and sometimes leads individuals to become virtual prisoners in their own homes.

Phobias are a type of anxiety involving fears of specific objects, places, or behaviors. Examples of phobias include fear of urinating in public restrooms, fear of using public transportation, or specific fears such as fear of heights (acrophobia), fear of foreigners (xenophobia), and fear of closed-in places (claustrophobia).

Other forms of anxiety include the obsessive-compulsive disorder, the posttraumatic stress disorder, and the acute stress disorder, as well as the anxiety caused by legal drugs such as caffeine, the anxiety caused by drugs of abuse such as amphetamines or cocaine, and the anxiety caused by medical conditions and medications, such as those used to treat asthma (steroids, aminophylline). In general, anxiety is a state of fear or worry that (1) may or may not have a cause, (2) the individual cannot control, and (3) that significantly compromises the individual's ability to function normally.

It should be pointed out that worry and anxiety are normal feelings; however, it is all a matter of degree. Sometimes anxiety can allow us to make plans and provisions for the future and can, in fact, be beneficial. Such beneficial anxiety is called anticipation.

Living With Your Diagnosis

Generalized anxiety disorder is fairly common, affecting up to 10% of individuals at any particular point in time. Its childhood equivalent, the so-called overanxious anxiety disorder of children is also fairly common. Studies of families suggest that anxiety can be transmitted to children genetically, especially in conditions such as panic disorder. The matters about which anxious patients can worry are endless. They are likely to report worry over minor matters, and they are often anxious for at least half the day during an average day. In children and adolescents, the worries will center around the quality of their school performance or some aspect of their social functioning in school. They may also be concerned with their own physical or mental imperfections as they see them, and such anxious adolescents will require constant reassurance. There are some medical conditions that have a high correlation with anxiety. These include such conditions as ulcerative colitis, Crohn's disease, asthma, hypertension, heart disease, ulcer disease, reflux esophagitis, and headaches. During evaluation, anxious patients often have rapid or pressured speech and often shift from one subject to another without any apparent connection. These patients may be extremely restless, shifting about in their chair or tapping their fingers or toes, ringing their hands, putting their head in their hands, and often even getting up and walking across the room. Patients will use such phrases as "I feel like I'm going to jump out of my skin," "My whole body's on fire," "I think

I'm going to have a heart attack," or similar comments.

In the treatment of anxiety, it is very important to determine whether some medical condition or substance abuse is causing the anxiety. Common drugs that can produce anxiety include theophylline, any medications with caffeine, steroids, many antihypertensives including Aldomet, stimulating antidepressants such as Prozac, inhalers used for breathing problems such as Breathine and Vanceril, thyroid medication, and diet pills. Many over-the-counter medications such as some antihistamines, some cough and cold preparations, and diet pills that contain caffeine can also cause anxiety, and dietary intake of excessive amounts of caffeine and sugar can make any anxiety syndrome worse. Once a medication or a medical condition has been eliminated as a cause of anxiety, then an adequate history should be obtained for substance abuse to eliminate the possibility that the individual may be using some kind of psychostimulant that might be producing anxiety. Attention should also be directed toward uncovering any precipitants in the individual's home environment or any major stressors that might be contributing to the anxiety.

Treatment

The treatment of anxiety involves both behavioral techniques and medication. One behavioral technique used is biofeedback, wherein patients are hooked to a machine and learn to decrease their muscle tone or control their brain waves by regulating their breathing. Other behavioral techniques include progressive muscle relaxation, which is often done to a prerecorded tape; imagery, where individuals imagine that they are in some pleasant setting; meditation; and hypnosis. Behavioral techniques have been very effective in treating anxiety and are the commonly used methods in those patients who prefer not to take medication.

If you have been prescribed a medication for anxiety, it is most likely one of the minor tranquilizers of the benzodiazepine class. This would include such drugs as alprazolam (Xanax), lorazepam (Ativan), or diazepam (Valium). Although these drugs are very effective for the rapid relief of anxiety, they do have side effects. They typically slow down breathing and therefore may not be the best drugs to use in someone who has asthma, bronchitis, or emphysema. They also are broken down by the liver, so they may be bad choices in someone

who has severe liver disease, such as cirrhosis or hepatitis. Finally, these drugs can be habit forming; that is, they cannot be discontinued without being tapered for fear of withdrawal signs and symptoms. Those individuals who have a history of substance abuse, particularly abuse of depressant drugs, such as alcohol, barbiturates, or benzodiazepines should not be prescribed these drugs. Because the duration of action of some of the benzodiazepines, such as Xanax and Ativan, is fairly short, they may have to be given three or four times a day. Also, the benzodiazepines may produce a significant degree of sedation, which can impair driving and the ability to operate certain machinery.

Another group of drugs that are used to treat anxiety are the antidepressants. The tricyclic antidepressant drugs, such as imipramine, have been very effective for years in treating anxiety disorders. The major drawback of these medications is that they are not effective as quickly as the benzodiazepines. It may take 10 days to 2 weeks before the beneficial effects of imipramine and other tricyclic antidepressants are seen. They also may initially increase anxiety before relieving it, and they have side effects such as weight gain, sexual dysfunction, dry mouth, constipation, and blurry vision. The advantages of the tricyclic antidepressants are two-fold: (1) they can be given once daily, and (2) they may be more effective than the benzodiazepines when depression is associated with the anxiety, as it often is.

Other antidepressants used to treat anxiety are the selective serotonin reuptake inhibitors (SSRIs). In particular, paroxetine (Paxil) seems to have significant antianxiety effects. It can be given once daily, usually in the evening, and may improve sleep. It has few side effects, except for diarrhea, constipation, and some sexual side effects. Paxil is similar to imipramine in that its therapeutic onset is delayed; it may take 2–3 weeks before the beneficial effects are seen. In addition, you may have to avoid using Paxil if you are taking certain other medications because of its interaction with them.

Buspirone (BuSpar) is also used for anxiety. It is the only drug approved for anxiety that is not potentially physically addicting, so it is often substituted for the benzodiazepines. The advantages of using BuSpar are that it is less likely to cause sedation and that there is no withdrawal on discontinuing it. Side effects of Buspar may include gastrointestinal distress and headaches.

Finally, the beta-blocker, propranolol (Inderal) is often used for treating some of the effects of anxiety and is particularly effective for treating the runaway heartbeat and sense of heart pounding that many anxious patients feel. Because Inderal is also used to treat high blood pressure, individuals with low blood pressure should not take it. It can also sometimes make individuals feel very tired, and should not be used in patients who have severe lung disease.

Anxiety disorders can cause significant suffering and worry for patients. However, these are treatable conditions.

The DOs

If you have an anxiety disorder diagnosed, it is very important to minimize your level of stress; to have some activity that you enjoy doing such as reading, writing, or knitting; to participate in a regular exercise program; and to watch your diet. If you are taking antianxiety medications, you should be very careful when driving or operating dangerous machinery.

The DON'Ts

Do not use products containing caffeine, and decrease your sugar intake as much as possible. In addition, remember that most prescribed medications for anxiety have some sedating effects; therefore you should avoid drinking alcohol.

When to Call Your Doctor

You should call your doctor if the nature of your anxiety changes, if you notice any side effects from your medications, or if your anxieties are accompanied by depression and suicidal ideation or thoughts.

For More Information

For more information on anxiety, please contact your local mental health center or your local community hotline. There are various support groups in most communities for specific anxiety disorders such as panic, obsessive-compulsive disorder, and posttraumatic stress disorder. On the Internet, check out the following Web sites:
http://www.soven.net/~schwcof
http://www.cts.com/~health
National Panic/Anxiety Disorder Newsletter @
http://spiderweb.com/npadnews

AORTIC REGURGITATION

About Your Diagnosis

The aorta is the large artery that leaves the heart from the left ventricle. The aortic valve is between the left ventricle and the aorta. Aortic regurgitation (also called *aortic insufficiency*) is the leaking of blood from the aorta back through the aortic valve into the left ventricle when the ventricle is contracting. This causes the left ventricle to swell over time to compensate for the extra blood in it. Left heart failure may occur after many years if this should happen. If the valve regurgitation is more severe, it may cause failure sooner. Because the valve is not functioning normally, the blood flowing through creates a turbulence called a *heart murmur*.

Aortic regurgitation is caused by a defect in the aortic valve. This may be caused by infections such as rheumatic fever (usually from streptococcal infections earlier in life) or endocarditis (a bacterial infection in the heart). Aortic regurgitation also may be caused by enlargement of the base of the aorta from injury or a genetic condition. It is detected by means of listening to the heart with a stethoscope and hearing a specific type of murmur in a specific area. If the patient already has symptoms of heart failure, the signs are found during an examination or on a chest radiograph (x-ray). An echocardiogram (ultrasound examination of the heart) is performed to give a better view of the valve.

Living With Your Diagnosis

Most patients with aortic regurgitation have no symptoms. The symptoms that do occur are those of heart failure, such as fatigue, difficulty breathing, especially when lying down, coughing, or shortness of breath. Some patients feel chest pain or pain in the upper middle back.

Abnormally functioning valves are often targets for infection. If you have aortic valve problems, you should take antibiotics as prescribed before and after dental or surgical procedures. If you have no symptoms, no changes in lifestyle or treatment are needed. Smoking and obesity strain the heart. Lose weight and stop smoking to lessen the workload of the heart. If you have no symptoms, you can exercise.

Treatment

If symptoms exist, the therapy is similar to that for heart failure. This means weight loss, stopping smoking, restricting salt and excess fluid in the diet, and rest. Medications may be needed. Once symptoms of aortic regurgitation occur, aortic valve replacement may be necessary.

The DOs

- Exercise regularly.
- Lose extra body weight.
- Take antibiotics (if prescribed) before and after dental or surgical procedures.

The DON'Ts

- Do not be concerned if you have no symptoms.
- Do not delay treatment if you do have symptoms.

When to Call Your Doctor

- If symptoms develop such as shortness of breath, chest or upper back pain, palpitations or rapid heartbeat, or fainting.

For More Information

The American Heart Association has information on heart murmurs and heart valve defects. Call 1-800-242-8721 and ask for the literature department.

AORTIC VALVULAR STENOSIS

About Your Diagnosis

Aortic stenosis is narrowing in the aortic valve, where blood leaves the left ventricle and enters the aorta. This narrowing causes the left ventricle to do more work. Like other muscles in the body forced to work hard, the ventricle thickens to generate more force. The abnormality in the valve may have several causes. Among young persons, it is usually from congenital abnormalities (those present at birth). Some persons are born with damaged valves or have a two-sided (bicuspid) aortic valve instead of a normal, three-sided valve.

Aortic stenosis may occur among 1% to 2% of the population. Rheumatic fever from streptococcal infections early in life or heart disease such as cardiomyopathy may damage the valve and affect normal or damaged valves later in life. The most common cause is calcium and cholesterol deposits on the valve that occur as we age. Aortic stenosis is about three times more common among men than among women.

Living With Your Diagnosis

Most persons with aortic stenosis have no symptoms early. If the valve narrows enough to create flow problems, you may have fatigue, fainting, chest pain, or symptoms of left heart failure, such as shortness of breath. As the left ventricle thickens, that side of the heart enlarges. A chest radiograph (x-ray) shows this abnormality. Your doctor hears a heart murmur in a specific area over the heart. A murmur is a sound made by the flow through an abnormal valve. An echocardiogram (ultrasound examination of the heart) is obtained to confirm the diagnosis and check the severity of the stenosis.

If you have no symptoms, the condition merely is checked each year. Because abnormal valves may be the target of some bacterial infections, you should take antibiotics as prescribed before and after dental or surgical procedures. If the stenosis is mild, you may exercise moderately without many difficulties.

If the stenosis is moderate or severe or there are symptoms, you need to limit your exertion because overexertion can worsen symptoms quickly. You may need medications to help control the symptoms of heart failure or arrhythmias that may occur. An operation to replace the valve may be necessary.

Treatment

The best treatment is to take all medications prescribed and to closely monitor for changes in symptoms. Antibiotics are necessary before and after dental or surgical procedures. Diuretics reduce the excess fluid in the blood. Taking diuretics may cause dehydration or electrolyte problems. Vasodilator medicines such as nitrates reduce the workload of the heart. These drugs may cause headaches or symptoms of low blood pressure such as fainting or lightheadedness. Digitalis (digoxin) used for heart failure helps the heart contract better. The level of this drug in the blood must be measured periodically with a laboratory test.

The DOs
- Take your medications as directed.
- Stop smoking.
- Start a salt-restricted diet and lose weight if you have congestive heart failure.

The DON'Ts
- Do not neglect worsening symptoms.
- Do not forget to take your antibiotics before and after dental or surgical procedures.

When to Call Your Doctor
- If easy exercise is becoming difficult. Rest until evaluated by your doctor.
- If symptoms of heart failure or heart disease occur, such as chest pain, shortness of breath, palpitations or rapid heartbeat, or fainting.

For More Information
The American Heart Association has information on heart murmurs and heart valve defects. Call 1-800-242-8721 and ask for the literature department.

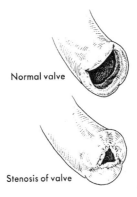

Aortic stenosis. (From LaFleur-Brooks ML: *Exploring Medical Language—A Student Directed Approach.* vol 3. St. Louis, Mosby–Year Book, 1993. Used by permission.)

ARTHRITIS, INFECTIOUS (BACTERIAL)

About Your Diagnosis

Infectious arthritis (sometimes called septic arthritis) is an infection inside of a joint. It is usually caused by bacteria. Normally, the inside of joints are free of germs (sterile). When bacteria get into the sterile joint they cause inflammation, resulting in pain and swelling. Usually only one joint becomes infected at a time such as the knee, hip, wrist, shoulder, elbow or ankle.

Anyone can develop a joint infection, but it is most common in young children and older adults. There are several reasons why joint infections develop in individuals. Most of the time it is because of abnormal changes in the joint from other forms of arthritis, a poorly working immune system (possibly caused by certain medicines or other conditions such as diabetes or kidney disease), or an artificial joint (joint replacement).

Joint infections are diagnosed by removing the infected fluid from the joint with a needle and testing it in the laboratory. With antibiotic treatment and drainage of the infected fluid from the joint, the infection can usually be cured.

Living With Your Diagnosis

Infected joints swell quickly and are very painful and difficult to bend. They cause high fevers, chills, shakes, muscle aches, and fatigue. Depending on the joint involved, individuals with joint infections may not be able to walk or use their arms. Patients usually receive initial intravenous (IV) antibiotic treatment in the hospital before continuing treatment at home. After treatment is started the symptoms slowly improve over the next 1–2 weeks. However, even after the infection is treated joint pain may persist. In addition to antibiotic treatment, it is necessary to receive physical therapy to help maintain motion in the joint. This requires dedication to performing the exercises on a regular basis. Because of possible permanent damage from the infection, some individuals never recover full motion in the affected joint even with the therapy.

Treatment

Joint infections require three stages of therapy: antibiotics, drainage of the joint, and therapy to restore normal motion in the joint.

Antibiotics are usually given through a vein for the first 2 weeks and then by mouth for an additional 2–4 weeks. Sometimes longer treatment is needed. The most common side effects from antibiotics are allergic reactions, rashes, and diarrhea. Women sometimes have yeast infections develop while taking antibiotics.

During the first week of treatment the infected joint fluid must be drained regularly. This is performed in one of two ways depending on the affected joint. Most joints can be drained by sticking a needle into the joint and drawing the fluid off usually once a day. Other joints are more difficult to drain this way and instead require drainage by an operation.

After the first few days of treatment, individuals with joint infections should begin therapy to restore normal motion in the joint. Therapists teach and assist with this part of the treatment. Therapy should continue until after the pain is gone and the joint is working normally again.

The DOs

- Take your medicines as prescribed.
- Ask your doctor which over-the-counter medications you may take with your prescription medications.
- Perform exercises to maintain joint motion and preserve strength.

The DON'Ts

- Don't wait to see whether side effects from medications will go away.
- Don't continue an exercise program that causes pain. If pain after exercise continues, it usually means the exercise program needs to be modified specifically for you.

When to Call Your Doctor

- If you have any medication side effects.
- If the medication and treatments are not decreasing the pain.
- If a new fever, chills, or worsening pain or swelling develop.
- If you believe you need a referral to a physical or occupational therapist.

For More Information

Contact the Arthritis Foundation in your area. If you do not know its location, you may call the national office at 800-283-7800 or access the information on the Internet at www.arthritis.org.

ARTHRITIS, JUVENILE RHEUMATOID

About Your Diagnosis

Juvenile rheumatoid arthritis (JRA) refers to a form of arthritis occurring in children that is different from adult rheumatoid arthritis. Juvenile rheumatoid arthritis will develop in 1 of every 1,000 children. The arthritis is caused by inflammation (changes in the immune system) in the joint that can cause stiffness, warmth, swelling, and pain. Although there is no cure for this type of arthritis, there are many very good treatments, and a substantial number of children will have a complete remission of their condition. There are three types of JRA, and these can be associated with different types of problems.

Pauciarticular JRA affects only a few joints (usually less than four joints) and occurs in half of the children with JRA. This type most commonly starts in the preschool years and is more likely to occur in girls. Knees, elbows, and ankles are usual spots for the arthritis to occur. Inflammation in the eyes develops in about half of children with pauciarticular JRA. The eye disease can develop at any point during the course of JRA; thus all children with JRA must be seen by an eye doctor regularly. The inflammation is usually detected by the eye doctor by examining the eyes with a special light (called a slit lamp). Untreated, the eye inflammation can lead to vision loss and scarring, so it is important to continue regular eye examinations.

Polyarticular JRA affects many joints and occurs in about 40% of children who have JRA. Often the arthritis involves the small joints of the hands and fingers. Joints commonly affected include the neck, knees, ankles, feet, wrists, and hands. Again, girls are more likely to develop this condition. Some children have a positive blood test called a rheumatoid factor, and their arthritis can be very similar to adult rheumatoid arthritis. Children with polyarticular JRA can also have eye inflammation develop, but this does not occur as often as in the children with pauciarticular JRA.

Systemic JRA occurs in about 10% of children with JRA, with boys and girls both affected equally. Often this condition starts with fever, rash, changes in the blood cells, and joint pain. The inflammation of the joints may not develop for many weeks to months, so this type of JRA can be very hard to diagnose at first. Rarely, systemic JRA can involve the heart, lymph nodes, liver, and lungs.

Approximately 70,000 children in the United States have some form of JRA. Although certain hereditary and environmental factors may increase an individual's risk of developing JRA, the exact cause is unknown. Juvenile rheumatoid arthritis is not an infectious illness. In other words, you cannot "catch" it from another individual.

To diagnose JRA in a child, a physician obtains a medical history, performs an examination of the joints, and orders laboratory tests and possibly x-rays of the joints. Laboratory tests may include an erythrocyte sedimentation rate (ESR), which measures inflammation in the body, a complete blood cell count (CBC), a rheumatoid factor (RF), and an antinuclear antibody (ANA). The RF and ANA are specific proteins found in the blood and may aid a physician in the diagnosis of JRA. However, there is no single blood test that will prove or disprove whether a child has JRA.

Juvenile rheumatoid arthritis is a chronic disease that may last for many months or years. However, about 75% of children eventually outgrow this disease. Although there is no cure for JRA, earlier detection, improved medications, and comprehensive treatment greatly improve the chances for a full and active life.

Living With Your Diagnosis

Juvenile rheumatoid arthritis causes joint pain and stiffness that can affect a child's ability to do daily activities. Stiffness and discomfort are usually worse in the morning, then get better toward the end of the day. The child may hold the affected joint close to the body because of the pain. Arthritis affecting the hands and wrists can affect the ability to write, dress, and carry items. Arthritis affecting the hips, knees, or feet can decrease the ability to walk, play, or stand. If arthritis affects the neck, it can decrease the ability to look around. A child may not want to participate in play activities because of the pain and fatigue. The pain of JRA may also keep the child awake at night, which may increase the fatigue.

Treatment

The best way to manage JRA is through a combination of medication, therapies, exercise, education, and "pacing" of activities to prevent fatigue. Treatment should be from a physician experienced in the treatment of arthritis. Medications help to decrease the inflammation that causes pain and swelling. Nonsteroidal anti-inflammatory drugs (NSAIDs) are often the first line of therapy. Possible side effects of NSAIDs include stomach upset, ulcers, diarrhea, constipation, headache, dizziness, difficulty hearing, and a rash. If these medications do not adequately control the pain, a physician may prescribe "disease modifying" medications that often are effective in slowing the progresssion of the disease. These medications include gold shots, hydroxychloroquine, and methotrexate. Gold shots and methotrexate may affect the blood, liver, or kidneys and possibly cause a rash. Hydroxychloroquine may affect the eyes and cause a rash. Prednisone, a potent anti-inflammatory drug, is used if the disease cannot be managed by other medications or if the child has serious systemic JRA. Prednisone may cause acne, high blood sugar, increased blood pressure, difficulty sleeping, and weight gain. When used for a long time, prednisone may also slow down a child's growth rate and cause thinning of the bones. The eye disease is treated with prednisone eye drops, and if severe, may require more potent oral medications.

Learning about JRA is essential because your child may have the disease for a long time, and careful management is important to prevent problems. Exercise is important to maintain joint movement and muscle strength. Pacing activities helps manage fatigue. The use of splints can help in resting painful, swollen joints.

The DOs
- Have your child take medications as prescribed.
- Call the doctor if your child experiences any side effects from medications. Learn as much as you can about this condition and its treatments.
- Encourage your child to exercise.
- Encourage your child to participate in the same activities other children of that age are participating in; however, your child should alternate periods of activity with rest.
- Speak to your child's teachers and school nurse. Ask them what services are available in the school system to help your child manage pain and fatigue.

The DON'Ts
- Wait and see whether a medication side effect will go away. Always call your doctor if you have any questions.

- Give up. If one medication doesn't work for your child, discuss this with your physician until you find a medicine that helps decrease the pain and stiffness.
- Have your child continue with an exercise program that continues to cause increased pain. This may mean that the program needs to be modified.
- Forget to have regular eye examinations. Children with JRA can have eye inflammation develop. Also, some of the drugs used to treat JRA can cause side effects in the eyes.

When to Call Your Doctor
- Your child has any side effects listed above from any of the medications.
- The medication is not helping the joint pain, stiffness, swelling, or fatigue.
- Your child needs a referral to a physical or occupational therapist for exercise, joint protection, or splinting.

For More Information
Contact the Arthritis Foundation in your area. If you do not know the location of the Arthritis Foundation, you may call the national office at 1-800-283-7800 or access the information on the Internet at www.arthritis.org. Children with JRA will benefit from contact with other children, and the Internet can be a good way to find a pen pal. Many cities have support groups for children with JRA and their parents.

ARTHRITIS, PSORIATIC

About Your Diagnosis

Psoriatic arthritis causes inflammation leading to pain, swelling, and warmth of certain joints and a rash. The joints most frequently affected are the fingers, neck and lower back. Although the psoriasis rash usually occurs before the joint pain, some individuals are unaware of this rash. Psoriasis may affect the nails, scalp, umbilicus (belly button), and genital areas. Fatigue may also occur in this disease. Less commonly, psoriatic arthritis may also cause inflammation of the eyes, nails, and heart.

Although certain hereditary and environmental factors may increase an individual's risk of developing psoriatic arthritis, the exact cause of this disease is unknown. Psoriatic arthritis is not an infectious illness. In other words you cannot "catch" it from another individual.

Psoriatic arthritis usually begins between the ages of 30 and 50 years. It occurs equally between men and women. To diagnose psoriatic arthritis, a physician obtains a medical history, performs an examination of the joints, skin, and nails, and orders laboratory tests and possibly x-rays of the joints, neck, and lower back. Laboratory tests may include an erythrocyte sedimentation rate (ESR), which measures inflammation in the body, and a complete blood cell count (CBC).

Living With Your Diagnosis

The joints most frequently affected are the fingers, neck, and low back. Psoriatic arthritis of the fingers can decrease your ability to write, open jars, and lift and carry items. If the back is affected, it can decrease your ability to bend or stand. If the neck is affected, it may affect your ability to look around. For some individuals, the rash of psoriasis causes embarrassment in social situations. There is no cure for psoriatic arthritis. However, with earlier detection, improved medications, and comprehensive treatment, individuals with psoriatic arthritis can lead a full life.

Treatment

The best way to manage psoriatic arthritis is through a combination of medications, therapies, exercise, and education. Medications help to decrease the inflammation that causes pain and swelling. Nonsteroidal anti-inflammatory drugs (NSAIDs) are of-

ten the first line of therapy. Potential side effects of NSAIDs include stomach upset, diarrhea, constipation, ulcers, headache, dizziness, difficulty hearing, and a rash. If these medications do not adequately control the pain and swelling, a physician may prescribe "disease modifying" medications that may slow down the disease process. These medications include hydroxychloroquine, sulfasalazine, and methotrexate. Hydroxychloroquine may cause nausea, diarrhea, and a rash, and rarely affect the eyes. Sulfasalazine and methotrexate may affect the blood and liver, and may cause a rash. A dermatologist (skin doctor) may prescribe medications to manage the psoriasis.

Learning about your arthritis is essential because you may have psoriatic arthritis for the rest of your life. Exercise is important to maintain joint movement and muscle strength. Alternating periods of rest and activity helps to manage fatigue.

The DOs

- Take your medication as prescribed.
- Call your doctor if you are experiencing side effects from medications.
- Ask you doctor what over-the counter pain medications and skin products you may take with the prescription medications.
- Exercise, because this can help maintain joint range of motion and muscle strength.

The DON'Ts

- Wait and see if a medication side effect will go away. Always call your doctor if you have any questions.
- Give up. If one medication does not work for you, discuss this with your physician until you find a medicine that helps decrease joint pain, stiffness, and the skin disorder.
- Go on a specific diet without the consent of your physician.
- Continue an exercise program that causes pain. If pain after exercise continues, it usually means the exercise needs to be modified specifically for you.

When to Call Your Doctor

- You experience any of the side effects listed above from any of the medications.
- The medication is not helping the joint pain, stiffness, or swelling, or the skin disorder.
- You need a referral to a physical or occupational therapist for exercise or joint protection.

For More Information

Contact the Arthritis Foundation in your area. If you do not know the location of the Arthritis Foundation, you may call the national office at 1-800-283-7800 or access information on the Internet at www.arthritis.org. The National Psoriasis Foundation may be reached at 503-297-1545.

ARTHRITIS, RHEUMATOID

About Your Diagnosis

Rheumatoid arthritis (RA) causes inflammation leading to pain, stiffness, and swelling in joints. The joints most frequently affected are the hands, wrists, feet, and knees. Fatigue can also be severe in RA. Less commonly, RA can cause inflammation in other parts of the body including the lungs, eyes, heart, blood vessels, skin, and nerves. Rheumatoid arthritis used to be called "crippling" arthritis because of the potential joint damage. Now, because of better treatment, less joint damage may occur.

Although certain hereditary and environmental factors may increase an individual's risk of developing RA, the exact cause of RA is unknown. Rheumatoid arthritis is not an infectious illness. In other words, you cannot "catch" it from another individual.

Rheumatoid arthritis affects 1% to 5% of the adult population throughout the world. It occurs two to three times more frequently in women than in men, and occurs more commonly during a women's childbearing years. To diagnose RA, a physician obtains a medical history, performs an examination of the joints, and orders laboratory tests and possibly x-rays of the joints. Laboratory tests may include an erythrocyte sedimentation rate (ESR), which measures inflammation in the body, a complete blood cell count (CBC), and a test called a rheumatoid factor (RF). Because only 75% of individuals with RA have a "positive" RF and other individuals without RA may also have a positive test, this blood test does not confirm a diagnosis of RA with 100% accuracy.

Living With Your Diagnosis

Rheumatoid arthritis causes joint pain and stiffness that can affect your ability to do daily activities. Rheumatoid arthritis of the hands, wrists, or shoulders can decrease your ability to write, open jars, dress, and carry items. Arthritis affecting hips, knees, or feet can decrease your ability to walk, bend, or stand. If arthritis affects your neck, it may limit your ability to look around. There is no cure for RA. However, with earlier detection, improved medications, and comprehensive treatment, individuals with RA can lead a full life.

Treatment

The best way to manage RA is with a combination of medications, therapies, exercise, education, and "pacing" of activities to prevent fatigue. Medications help decrease the inflammation that causes pain and swelling. Nonsteroidal anti-inflammatory drugs (NSAIDs) are often the first line of therapy. If these medications do not adequately control the pain and swelling, a physician may prescribe "disease modifying" medications that may slow down the RA disease process. These medicines include hydroxychloroquine, methotrexate, and gold shots. Because these medications may take up to a few months to be effective, the doctor may prescribe prednisone. Prednisone is a strong anti-inflammatory medication that works quickly.

All medications can cause side effects. The NSAIDs may cause stomach upset, diarrhea, constipation, ulcers, headache, dizziness, difficulty hearing, or a rash. Hydroxychloroquine may cause nausea, diarrhea, and a rash, and rarely it may affect the eyes. Methotrexate and gold shots may affect your blood, liver, or kidneys and may cause a rash. Prednisone may cause skin bruising, high blood sugar, increased blood pressure, difficulty sleeping, cataracts, weight gain, and thinning of the bones.

Learning about your arthritis is essential because you may have RA for a long time, maybe for the rest of your life. Exercise is important to maintain joint movement and muscle strength. Alternating periods of rest and activity helps to manage fatigue.

The DOs
- Take your medication as prescribed.
- Call your doctor if you are experiencing side effects from medications.
- Ask your doctor which over-the-counter pain medications you may take with your prescription medications.
- Exercise to maintain joint range of motion and muscle strength.

The DON'Ts
- Wait to see whether a possible medication side effect will go away on its own.
- Give up. If one medication doesn't work, discuss with your physician other medicines that might help decrease your pain and stiffness.
- Go on a special diet without the consent of your physician.

- Continue an exercise program that causes pain. If pain after exercise continues, it usually means the exercise program needs to be modified specifically for you.

When to Call Your Doctor
- You experience side effects that you believe are caused by your medications.
- The medication and other treatments are not helping the pain, swelling, or fatigue.
- You believe you may need a referral to a physical or occupational therapist for exercise or joint protection.

For More Information
Contact the Arthritis Foundation in your area. If you do not know the location of the Arthritis Foundation, you may call the national office at 1-800-283-7800 or access information on the Internet at www.arthritis.org.

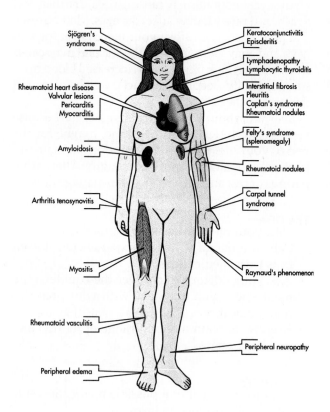

ASBESTOSIS

About Your Diagnosis

Asbestos is a name applied to a group of natural fibrous materials that have been used in a variety of ways because of their durability, flame resistance, and insulation properties. Lung damage can occur as a result of inhalation of asbestos. Significant exposure occurs most commonly in the workplace. Employees at greatest risk include those who mine, mill, or transport unfinished asbestos materials, or those who install, modify, or demolish asbestos products, such as automotive repair and construction workers. Exposures can also occur in individuals whose trades bring them near where asbestos is used (such as painters and carpenters), those who clean the workers' clothes carrying asbestos fibers, or those who live near asbestos factories or mines.

The likelihood of developing lung disease increases with longer and more intense asbestos exposures. There is usually at least a 10-year delay between initial asbestos exposure and the development of disease. Asbestos-related diseases are not contagious. Some types of asbestos fibers are more likely to cause disease than others. Individuals may differ in their sensitivity to asbestos. Fortunately, asbestos-related disease develops in only a minority of workers.

Living With Your Diagnosis

Asbestos exposures can cause a variety of diseases of the lung and pleura (layer of tissue covering the outside surface of the lung):

- Pleural plaques: Areas of thickening of the external lining of the lungs that are often detected when a chest x-ray is done for some other reason. They do not cause symptoms, impair lung function, or increase the risk of cancer, but they may be associated with an increased risk of developing asbestosis.
- Asbestosis: Scarring of the lungs in response to inhalation and accumulation of asbestos fibers over at least a 10-year period. Diagnosis is usually made in the symptomatic patient with prior asbestos exposure who has the characteristic lung examination findings and chest x-rays changes. The scarring may remain stable or progress to involve greater amounts of the lung. Asbestosis results in small, stiff lungs, which explains why shortness of breath is the most frequent symptom. Chronic

cough and phlegm production are also common. Breathing tests are used to assess and follow-up how asbestos is affecting the lungs. Lung cancer may be more common in asbestos workers with asbestosis than those without.

- Lung cancer: By itself, asbestos exposure increases the risk for developing lung cancer. This risk greatly increases if an individual also smokes. Lung cancer usually arises 20 years after initial asbestos exposure.
- Pleural effusion: Fluid that accumulates in the space between the lung and chest wall because of asbestos exposures in the past 15 years. Effusion may be asymptomatic or cause fever, chest pain, and shortness of breath. Effusions do not increase the risk for future cancer but can result in permanent scarring of the pleura.
- Malignant mesothelioma: A rare tumor of the pleura that arises 20–40 years after initial asbestos exposure. Symptoms usually develop slowly and include chest pain, weight loss, and shortness of breath. The tumor may cause other symptoms if it expands to involve structures outside the pleura.

Treatment

Treatment options are limited for asbestos-related lung/pleural diseases. Avoidance of all asbestos is generally recommended when asbestos-related disease is diagnosed, because cumulative exposure appears to increase risk for further disease, and uncertainties remain about what constitutes a safe, low-level exposure.

- Pleural plaques: No treatment is required. However, because plaques are a marker of prior asbestos exposure, regular follow-up is recommended to look for other asbestos-related diseases.
- Asbestosis: There are no treatments that are reliably effective at reversing or preventing the progression of lung scarring. Lung transplantation is considered in certain individuals. Supplemental oxygen may be prescribed to decrease shortness of breath and improve stamina. Inhalers to help open the bronchial tubes may be prescribed if there is also smoking-related lung disease.
- Pleural effusion: Drainage of the fluid as necessary for diagnostic purposes. This is usually done in the doctor's office, but occasionally surgery is required to help exclude cancer. Most effusions resolve on their own over weeks to months, al-

though they may recur over several years.

- Mesothelioma: Prognosis is very poor because there are no consistently effective treatments. Surgery and chemotherapy may be tried. Relief of pain and shortness of breath are the main treatment goals.

The DOs

- Workers in industries with asbestos exposures should follow all recommended procedures, such as wearing protective masks, to decrease asbestos exposures.
- Obtain an influenza vaccination each fall.
- Obtain/update the pneumococcal vaccination.
- Maintain good cardiovascular fitness by participating in an exercise program.
- Maintain close contact with your health care provider.
- No special diet requirements.

The DON'Ts

- If asbestos-related diseases such as pleural plaques or asbestosis are diagnosed, all further asbestos exposures should be avoided.
- Avoid individuals with acute respiratory infections.
- Avoid exposures to other known lung irritants such as smoke, strong fumes, and very cold or very humid air.
- Stop smoking.

When to Call Your Doctor

Call your doctor if any of the following occurs:
- If you suspect you have an acute lung infection as suggested by increased cough, yellow or green sputum production, increased shortness of breath, fever, or chills.
- Blood in the sputum.
- Dusky-colored skin, fingertips, or lips.
- Chest pain.
- New ankle swelling.
- Weight loss.

For More Information
American Lung Association
1118 Hampton Avenue
St. Louis, MO 63139
800-LUNG-USA

ASCARIASIS (ROUNDWORMS)

About Your Diagnosis

Ascariasis is an earthworm-shaped intestinal parasite that can easily be seen without a microscope. The parasite is never transmitted from individual to individual, but the eggs are spread through contaminated water, food, or soil-contaminated hands (such as eating poorly washed raw vegetables grown in contaminated soil). If left untreated, the worms can migrate to other parts of the body such as the lungs. With treatment, ascariasis is usually curable in 1 week. Anybody can be affected, but it is more common in children.

Living With Your Diagnosis

Signs and symptoms include restlessness at night, irritability, fatigue, poor appetite, weight loss, abdominal pain, and sometimes diarrhea and fever. Occasionally worms may be seen in the bowel movement or in the child's bed.

Treatment

Your doctor will prescribe medication to kill the worms. These medications cannot be used if you are pregnant. They may also aggravate a seizure disorder. Side effects of these medications include stomach upset, dizziness, headache, and itching. They may also color the bowel movements red. Wash hands carefully after using the toilet and always before eating. Shower daily with careful attention to cleaning the anal area twice a day. Linens, nightclothes, towels, and washcloths used by someone with roundworms should be boiled or soaked in a solution of 1 cup ammonia to 5 gallons of water. After treatment, bathroom floors and fixtures, including toilet seats, should be scrubbed thoroughly. Toys should be sterilized or scrubbed with the ammonia solution. Other family members should be checked for infection.

The DOs

- Take medication as directed by your doctor. Tell him if you think you might be pregnant or if you have a seizure disorder.
- Wash your hands thoroughly before eating and after using the toilet.
- Keep nails clean and short.
- Shower instead of taking tub baths.
- Boil soiled linens if possible, or soak them in an ammonia solution before washing.
- Sterilize toys or scrub with the ammonia solution, then rinse with clear water.
- Have pets treated for worms, and advise children to avoid strange animals.
- Clean bathroom fixtures thoroughly after treatment.
- Have all family members checked for infection.
- Drink only bottled water when traveling in underdeveloped countries.

The DON'Ts

- Don't eat unwashed vegetables.
- Don't drink water when traveling in economically underdeveloped countries.
- Don't share towels or washcloths.

When to Call Your Doctor

- A high fever develops.
- You have severe abdominal pain.
- Chest pain or shortness of breath occurs.
- After treatment is completed, you continue to have symptoms.

For More Information
Intestinal Disease Foundation
412-261-5888, Monday through Friday from 9:30 AM to 3:30 PM (EST).
National Institute of Allergy and Infectious Disease
301-496-5717

ASTHMA

About Your Diagnosis

More than 15 million Americans have asthma, most with an onset before 20 years of age. The airways inside your lungs are surrounded by a layer of smooth muscle. Inflammation of the airways and smooth muscle constriction make the airways much smaller in individuals with asthma. Individuals with asthma are much more sensitive to certain triggers. Smoke, allergens, exercise, cold air, and infection are some of the common triggers.

Your physician can diagnose asthma by evaluating your symptoms, performing a thorough physical examination, and ordering pulmonary function tests, blood tests, skin tests, and sensitivity tests. Pulmonary function tests look at how well you are breathing and how reactive your airways are. Skin tests may help to identify some of the substances that aggravate your asthma.

Asthma is not curable, but the medications help control the symptoms. Certain cases have a progressive worsening that may lead to serious attacks and even death.

Living With Your Diagnosis

The symptoms of asthma include a sudden shortness of breath that is caused by a specific trigger. Patients with adult-onset asthma may not have a specific trigger that causes an attack. Other symptoms include wheezing and a dry or productive cough. The disease can cause significant changes in lifestyle. Patients should avoid excessive exercise, stress, cold air, smoking, and their identified triggers. Symptoms are often worse at night and may cause disturbances in sleeping. Be sure to carry your inhalers with you at all times because attacks are often unpredictable. Furthermore, you will have to regularly visit your physician to monitor your asthma.

Treatment

Your physician will prescribe certain drugs depending on the severity of your asthma. Many of these drugs will be inhalers. An acute bronchodilating inhaler will provide immediate relief of most asthma attacks. Inhaled steroids offer more long-term effects but do not relieve an attack immediately. All puffers prescribed to you must be inhaled properly to take full effect. Your physician will show you the correct technique. Antihistamines are used to control pollen-induced asthma. If your case is severe, your physician will prescribe oral steroids, oxygen therapy, or other medications.

Continual asthma research has led to the development of several new drugs that may or may not be appropriate for you. Discuss these options with your physician. A peak flow meter should be used daily to track your progress. Make sure you record these values and bring them to your doctor appointments.

Most of the drugs have minimal side effects. Inhaled steroids may cause mouth infections after prolonged use. Oral steroids can cause weight gain, increased infections, and several other side effects. Drugs that can induce an attack include aspirin and Alka Seltzer.

The DOs
- Carry your inhalers at all times.
- Avoid all known triggers.
- Use the peak flow meter regularly.
- Get a yearly flu shot and a pneumococcal vaccine.
- Discuss the need for a written action plan with your doctor.

The DON'Ts
- Do not smoke and avoid second-hand smoke.
- Try to avoid cold air.

When to Call Your Doctor
- If your medications do not control your asthma adequately or you are in the low yellow or red zone.
- If you experience a severe attack that your prescriptions cannot relieve.
- If your peak flow readings are continually decreasing.
- If you begin feeling increasingly tired.

For More Information
One Minute Asthma, Pedipress, 1991.
Take Charge of Asthma, National Institutes of Health, 1994.
National Institutes of Health
Public Information Office
Bethesda, MD 20892
American Lung Association
1118 Hampton Avenue
St. Louis, MO 63139
800-LUNG-USA
www.lungusa.org

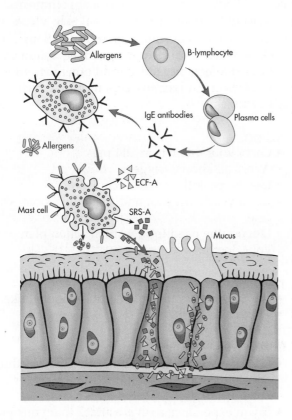

The early phase response in asthma is triggered when an allergen or irritant cross-links IgE receptors on mast cells, which are then activated to release histamine and other inflammatory mediators. (From Lewis SM, Collier IC, Heitkemper MM: *Medical-Surgical Nursing: Assessment and Management of Clinical Problem,* vol. 4. St. Louis, Mosby–Year Book, 1995. Used by permission.)

ATELECTASIS

About Your Diagnosis

Atelectasis refers to the collapse of either part or all of a lung caused by blockage of the air movement through small or large bronchial tubes. Atelectasis can occur abruptly when thick mucous plugs fill the bronchial tubes or when foreign objects, such as peanuts or small toys, are accidentally inhaled. After surgery, atelectasis is especially common because pain and medications prevent patients from taking deep breaths. Atelectasis can develop more gradually when caused by tumors growing inside the bronchial tubes or by processes outside the lung pressing inward, such as tumors, enlarged blood vessels, lymph nodes, or fluid collections. Susceptibility to atelectasis increases with conditions that increase sputum production, such as infection, cystic fibrosis, chronic bronchitis, and bronchiectasis. Impaired ability to cough and take deep breaths caused by chronic illnesses or drugs that decrease alertness also increase vulnerability to atelectasis. Collapse interferes with the lung's ability to supply oxygen to the body.

Living With Your Diagnosis

Some atelectasis may result in chest pain, shortness of breath, and fever. With complete lung collapse, shock may develop as demonstrated by rapid heart rate, low blood pressure, cool and clammy skin, and lethargy. Lung collapse of more gradual onset may not cause symptoms or lead to persistent cough and fever. Diagnosis is made by examination of the chest and by chest x-ray.

Treatment

Ideally, the cause of bronchial tube obstruction should be eliminated. Measures taken to relieve bronchial obstruction depend on the clinical circumstances. Bronchoscopy is a procedure in which your doctor uses a lighted tube to look into your lung air passages. This procedure may be necessary to help diagnose the cause of atelectasis and to relieve any bronchial tube obstructions if, for instance, a strong cough fails to expel a foreign body or clear phlegm. Surgery or radiation therapy may be required to treat large obstructing tumors. Individuals with chronic lung diseases that cause excessive secretions usually perform special maneuvers to help prevent accumulation of phlegm. Some of these maneuvers are also used by respiratory therapists in postop-

erative patients to treat or prevent atelectasis. Antibiotics are prescribed if infection is related to the bronchiectasis. Inhalers are used to open up the bronchial tubes. Atelectasis is usually not life-threatening but, if untreated, may lead to permanent partial lung collapse, pneumonia, or lung abscess.

The DOs

Help prevent atelectasis perioperatively by the following:
- Stop smoking as early as possible before surgery.
- Get out of bed as soon as possible after surgery.
- Use an incentive spirometry hourly while awake (a device that helps expand your lungs by encouraging you to take deep, rapid breaths).
- Work with the nurses and respiratory therapists in their efforts to loosen phlegm from your lungs. They may ask you to turn regularly and cough deeply. They may also administer aerosol treatments and "clap" on your back.

The DON'Ts

- Do not leave small objects, such as peanuts, around small children.
- Avoid dehydration which can thicken lung secretions.
- Avoid overuse of pain medications in the postoperative period that may interfere with the ability to cough and take deep breaths.

When to Call Your Doctor

Call your doctor if any of the following occur:
- Persistent cough.
- Blood in sputum.
- Chest pain.
- Persistent fever.
- Increasing shortness of breath.

For More Information
American Lung Association
1118 Hampton Avenue
St. Louis, MO 63139
800-LUNG-USA
www.lungusa.org

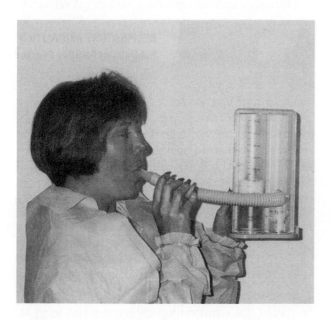

Incentive spirometry device in use. (From Frownfelter D, Dean E:
Principles and Practice of Cardiopulmonary Physical Therapy, vol 3. St.
Louis, Mosby–Year Book, 1996. Used by permission.)

ATHEROSCLEROSIS

About Your Diagnosis

Atherosclerosis causes narrowing in the blood vessels. The inner walls of arteries and veins can become damaged. This causes scarring where the damage has healed. Conditions such as diabetes cause a weakening of the vessel walls, making them prone to damage. Hypertension (high blood pressure) damages the vessels because the blood is pumped through with greater force. Fatty deposits and cholesterol stick to the damaged areas. These areas are called *plaques*. Plaques narrow the opening in the vessel. Blood flow through narrowed vessels is impeded. Small blood clots can form and plug the vessel. This stops blood flow through the vessel. In the heart this means that the heart muscle does not get enough oxygen, causing pain called *angina*. If oxygen is not delivered for excessive amounts of time, that part of the muscle dies. This is called a *myocardial infarction* or a *heart attack*. In the brain, lack of oxygen causes *strokes*.

Atherosclerosis is responsible for most of the coronary artery disease in the United States. The coronary arteries are the vessels that deliver blood to the heart muscle. Heart disease from atherosclerosis is the most common cause of death in the United States. Atherosclerosis of the vessels of the brain may cause strokes. Strokes are the third leading cause of death.

There are no symptoms of atherosclerosis until there is heart disease or damage to other organs. There are several risk factors for heart disease. Persons at risk are:

Men
Women after menopause who are not taking an estrogen replacement
Persons older than 55 years
Persons with a family history of heart disease
Persons who smoke
Persons who are overweight
Persons with diabetes
Persons with hypertension (high blood pressure)
Persons with a high cholesterol level
Sedentary persons (those who do not exercise regularly)
Persons who have diets high in fat and cholesterol

Living With Your Diagnosis

Modification of risk factors is the best approach to managing atherosclerosis and coronary artery disease. You cannot change your age, sex, or family history of heart disease, but you can change many of the other factors.

Treatment

The goal of treatment is to keep atherosclerosis from progressing. Depending on the risk factors, medications may be needed. It is extremely important to take the medicines on time every day. Modifying one's diet to include low-fat and low-cholesterol foods can help considerably. The diet should include high-fiber foods (oat bran, for example) and fruits and vegetables. Taking vitamin C and vitamin E supplements helps ease blood flow in the arteries. An aspirin a day may be prescribed. Aerobic exercise is recommended. The doctor may perform an exercise stress test to determine whether the heart is fit enough for exercise. Exercise should be started easily, and it should be stopped if symptoms develop.

The DOs

- Stop smoking.
- Lose weight if you are overweight.
- Control your blood sugar if you have diabetes. Keep your blood sugar concentration as close to normal as possible through careful monitoring and attention to taking your medications.
- Monitor your blood pressure closely, and take your medication as directed if you have hypertension.
- Choose low-fat, low-cholesterol foods, and take prescribed cholesterol-lowering medications on a regular basis.
- Exercise. Aerobic exercise such as bicycling, swimming, and walking or jogging is needed for 30 minutes a day 3 or 4 days a week to help maintain fitness and lower risk.

When to Call Your Doctor

- If you have new or worsening chest pain, shortness of breath, fainting, or changes in your ability to speak, swallow, see, or move your limbs.

For More Information
The American Heart Association has information on atherosclerosis and other heart conditions. Call 1-800-242-8721 and ask for the literaturedepartment.

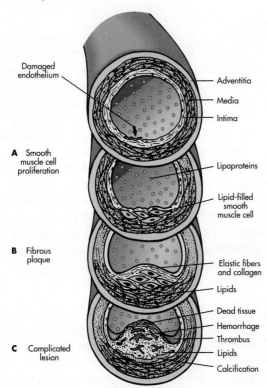

Damaged endothelium

Adventitia

Media

Intima

A Smooth muscle cell proliferation

Lipoproteins

Lipid-filled smooth muscle cell

B Fibrous plaque

Elastic fibers and collagen

Lipids

Dead tissue

Hemorrhage

Thrombus

Lipids

C Complicated lesion

Calcification

Stages of development in progression of atherosclerosis. **A,** smooth muscle cell proliferation. **B,** raised fibrous plaque. **C,** complicated lesion. (From Lewis SM, Collier IC, Heitkemper MM: *Medical-Surgical Nursing: Assessment and Management of Clinical Problem,* vol. 4. St. Louis, Mosby–Year Book, 1995. Used by permission.)

ATRIAL FIBRILLATION

About Your Diagnosis

Fibrillation is a type of abnormal contraction in a muscle. In the heart the atria and ventricles must squeeze in a coordinated way to move the blood effectively. A fibrillating muscle looks as if it is wiggling rather than squeezing and does not move blood the way a normal contraction does. If this occurs in the atrium, the blood inside is not pumped into the ventricle normally and tends to pool. The ventricles can pull most of the blood in and contract to push it out, which allows the heart to perform most of its function. Pooling of blood and inefficient movement of blood through the atrium may cause other problems. If the pooled blood clots, the clots can be sent into the blood stream and can cause heart attacks or strokes.

When the atrium is fibrillating, it is attempting to contract (but the contractions are small) and may signal the ventricle to contract. Because the fibrillation is irregular and fast (wiggling), the contractions are irregular and fast. The ventricles contract when signaled and beat fast. This abnormal rhythm of the heartbeat is *arrhythmia*. Because the ventricles are not filling with blood normally, they must work harder to supply blood to the body and may eventually go into heart failure.

Living With Your Diagnosis

Many things can cause atrial fibrillation. Many persons have atrial fibrillation and never feel it. The most common cause is aging, because the heart becomes more susceptible to changes. Heart and lung disease, other illnesses, and stress also can cause atrial fibrillation. Caffeine, nicotine (cigarettes), and excess alcohol can cause it or make it worse.

Symptoms of atrial fibrillation are commonly the feeling that the heart is beating irregularly or too fast (palpitations). Symptoms of heart failure such as difficulty breathing, chest pain, or fainting may occur. Some persons feel fatigued or have difficulty with exercise. If there has been fibrillation for some time and clots have formed, chest pain or signs of stroke are dangerous and must be evaluated immediately.

Atrial fibrillation is diagnosed on the basis of a particular pattern of pulses and tracings on an electrocardiogram (ECG). The physician may check the motion of the atrium with an echocardiogram (ultrasound examination of the heart). This examination can show whether there are clots in the atrium.

Treatment

Management of atrial fibrillation focuses on the underlying cause. For example, if there is thyroid disease, the patient is treated for this condition. If the fibrillation is caused by too much caffeine, reduction of caffeine intake is recommended. While the cause is being sought or being treated, relief of symptoms depends on what the patient experiences or feels. Heart disease, for example, can be managed, but the fibrillation may not revert to normal.

Fibrillation can be managed with digitalis (digoxin) to help control the rate at which the ventricles contract. It also makes ventricular contractions more efficient. Digoxin therapy often is started in the hospital so that the level of drug in the body and changes in heart rhythm can be monitored. If digoxin therapy continues outside the hospital, the level of the drug in the blood has to be measured periodically.

If clots have formed in the atrium, anticoagulants such as warfarin (eg, Coumadin) may be prescribed. This drug can cause easy bruising or bleeding, and levels are checked periodically.

Arrhythmia may be managed with an antiarrhythmic drug such as verapamil or propranolol. This drug also may lower the blood pressure and cause headaches, dizziness, or nausea.

The abnormal rhythm of the heart from atrial fibrillation sometimes has to be electrically shocked back to normal. This procedure is called *cardioversion*. If you are taking medicine to manage thyroid, heart, or lung disease, for example, the drugs should be taken as directed to avoid more fibrillation.

The DOs

- Stop smoking.
- Reduce your intake of alcohol or caffeine.
- Eat a diet that is healthful for your heart. Decrease fat and cholesterol intake.
- Lose weight.
- Reduce stress in your life as much as possible, because stress can worsen this condition.
- Exercise to your level of tolerance if you are taking the proper medications and have no symptoms.
- Take your medicines as prescribed, and have blood levels of the drugs monitored.

The DON'Ts
- Avoid activities that cause bruising if you are taking anticoagulants.

When to Call Your Doctor
- If you have side effects from your medications or if you have new or worsening symptoms. This includes chest pain, shortness of breath or difficulty breathing, fainting, palpitations, or sudden changes in the ability to speak, eat, walk, or use your limbs.
- If you are taking anticoagulants and sustain a serious cut or head injury.

For More Information
Contact the American Heart Association at 1-800-242-8721 and ask for the literature department.

ATRIAL FLUTTER

About Your Diagnosis

In atrial flutter, the atria of the heart begin to beat in a rapid rhythm because of too many abnormal electrical impulses. The atria may beat up to 300 times per minute. About one half to one fourth of these impulses are passed down to the ventricles. Most of the time this phenomenon is not felt; sometimes there is a feeling of a rapid heartbeat (palpitations). A number of illnesses can cause atrial flutter. Heart or lung disease, thyroid disease, or heart valve disorders are predisposing factors for atrial flutter.

Living With Your Diagnosis

When the atrium is fluttering it is attempting to contract, but the contractions are too fast. The ventricles contract when signaled and beat fast. This abnormal rhythm of the heart is an *arrhythmia*. This rhythm is considered unstable but may revert to normal spontaneously, or it may convert to atrial fibrillation (a more irregular atrial arrhythmia). Because the ventricles are not filling with blood normally, they must work harder to supply blood to the body. This may eventually cause angina (heart pain caused by a reduction in blood supply to the heart muscle) or heart failure (decreased pumping efficiency of the heart). Symptoms of heart failure are difficulty breathing, chest pain, or fainting.

Atrial flutter is diagnosed by a particular pattern on an electrocardiogram (ECG). The motion of the atrium may be evaluated with an echocardiogram, which is an ultrasound examination of the heart. This examination also can show whether there are blood clots in the atrium.

Treatment

Therapy for atrial flutter focuses on the cause of the arrhythmia. While the cause is being sought or treated, acute management of the flutter depends on the symptoms and the suspected cause. Heart disease, for example, should be managed, but the flutter may not revert to normal. The flutter can be treated with digitalis (digoxin) to help control the rate at which the ventricles contract. Digitalis also helps make the contractions more efficient. Digoxin therapy often is begun in the hospital so that the level of drug in the blood stream and changes in heart rhythm can be monitored. If digoxin therapy continues outside the hospital, the level of the medicine in the blood has to be checked from time to time.

If clots have formed in the atrium, administration of anticoagulants such as warfarin (eg, Coumadin) may be started. This medicine can cause easy bruising or bleeding, and levels have to be checked periodically. Sometimes the abnormal rhythm of the heart caused by atrial flutter is electrically shocked to normal. This procedure is called *cardioversion*.

Medicines to manage thyroid, heart, or lung disease are taken as directed to avoid prolonged atrial flutter or fibrillation. Other prescribed medications, should be taken regularly, and levels should be monitored on schedule.

The DOs

- Stop smoking.
- Reduce your intake of alcohol and caffeine.
- Eat a diet for that is healthful for your heart. Decrease fat and cholesterol intake.
- Lose weight if you are overweight.
- Reduce stress in your life as much as possible, because stress may worsen your symptoms.
- Exercise to your level of tolerance if you are taking the proper medications and have no symptoms.

The DON'Ts

- Avoid activities that cause bruising if you are taking anticoagulants.
- Do not forget to take your usual medications.

When to Call Your Doctor

- If you have side effects from your medications or if you have new or worsening symptoms. These include chest pain, shortness of breath or difficulty breathing, fainting, palpitations, or sudden changes in the ability to speak, eat, walk, or use your limbs.
- If you are taking anticoagulants and sustain a serious cut or head injury.

For More Information

Contact the American Heart Association at 1-800-242-8721 and ask for the literature department.

ATRIAL SEPTAL DEFECT

About Your Diagnosis

The atria are the upper chambers of the heart. The septum is the wall of heart muscle that divides the left and right sides. A defect in the septum produces a hole in the heart. These abnormalities develop before birth (congenital) and may persist as holes into adulthood.

The left side of the heart normally pumps under higher pressure than the right side. The defect produces a left-to-right shunt that allows blood from the two sides of the heart to mix. Blood with less oxygen is pumped to the body, and oxygenated blood travels back to the lungs. This may overload the circulation on the right side of the system and cause pulmonary hypertension. Small defects may not cause a problem. Larger defects eventually overload the right heart system, possibly causing heart failure (inefficient pumping of the heart). Heart failure causes fatigue, difficulty breathing, especially with exertion, or chest pain. Cyanosis, a bluish tone to the skin, occurs if poorly oxygenated blood reaches the skin. Abnormal heart rhythms (arrhythmias) may develop.

Atrial septal defects are more common among girls than among boys. Some defects close as the child grows, but others may persist into adulthood. Atrial septal defect is the most common congenital heart defect diagnosed among adults. Persons with small defects or defects that close may never have symptoms and need no treatment. If the defect persists, symptoms may develop that necessitate treatment to correct the defect.

Living With Your Diagnosis

The diagnosis of atrial septal defect is made on the basis of symptoms and findings at physical examination. An electrocardiogram (ECG) may show abnormalities and a chest radiograph (x-ray) is nearly always abnormal, demonstrating enlargement of the lung vessels and an enlarged heart. An echocardiogram (ultrasound examination of the heart) is performed to assess the structure and pumping function of the heart and to measure relative pulmonary versus systemic (to the body) blood flow.

Treatment

Persons with atrial septal defect are referred to a cardiologist. Management of excessive pulmonary flow generally necessitates requires an operation to correct the defect. Heart failure may be managed with diuretics to reduce excess blood volume or digitalis to help the contracting efficiency of the heart. Arrhythmias may be managed with antiarrhythmic drugs. If there is no other heart disease, correcting the defect usually allows a normal life span and lifestyle.

The DOs

- Take all prescribed medications.
- Exercise if allowed by your doctor.

The DON'Ts

- Do not ignore worsening symptoms. Seek medical attention immediately.

When to Call Your Doctor

- If you have symptoms of atrial septal defect.

For More Information

Contact the American Heart Association at 1-800-242-8721 and ask for the literature department.

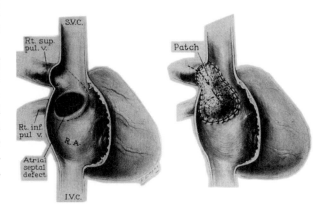

Closure of sinus venosus atrial septal defect. A patch is placed to divide the superior vena cava (SVC) into an anterior systemic venous channel directed into the right atrium and a posterior pulmonary venous channel directed into the left atrium. *inf.,* inferior; *I.V.C.,* inferior vena cava; *pul. v.,* pulmonary vein; *Rt.,* right; *sup.,* superior. (From Giuliani ER, Gersh BJ, McGoon MD, Hayes DL, Schaff HV: *Mayo Clinic Practice of Cardiology, ed 3,* St Louis,Mosby, 1996. Used by permission.)

AUTISM

About Your Diagnosis

Autism is a syndrome of early childhood that results in a lifelong developmental disorder of the brain which interferes with reasoning, social interaction, and communication skills. It is usually discovered during the first 3 years of life, and it occurs in approximately 5–15 of every 10,000 births. Autism is 3–4 times more common in boys.

Although the specific cause of autism is unknown, there appears to be a hereditary pattern in some families, but no gene has yet been identified. Autism is not caused by bad parenting, it is not a mental illness, nor is it a behavior disorder. There is no specific test to detect autism. Instead, a team of health care professionals using different diagnostic tools are required to make the diagnosis.. Although there is no cure for autism, with proper help, your child can learn to cope with the symptoms of this disability.

Living With Your Diagnosis

Your child may not show any signs of autism until about 1–2 years of age. The diagnosis can be suspected early in an infant who does not respond to the parents' caretaking with eye contact, smiling, or cuddling. There is a failure to develop meaningful language and social skills. These infants prefer to remain alone in a crib for many hours, undisturbed and undemanding.

Autistic children tend to be attractive and more graceful in movement, but their attention span is short. They are conspicuously quiet and passive if their environment is undisturbed and their activities uninterrupted. They have a strong need to maintain uniformity, and they may not make eye contact or respond to social cues. Many are overly sensitive to sounds, smells, touch, or taste and may prefer to be alone. They may lack imaginative play. Your child may have frequent temper tantrums with changes in the environment or routine, or for no apparent reason. Self-isolation, screaming fits, and rituals tend to become less frequent after 5 or 6 years of age. Some children are mildly affected whereas others have more severe symptoms. Some children have been capable of normal school education after 10 years of age, and some adults with autism have held jobs and lived independently.

Treatment

To date there is no known cure for autism, but there are many creative ways to help the child cope with the symptoms. These include music therapy, behavior modification, medications, and specific diet therapies.

The DOs
- Provide a highly structured environment with a strict unchanging routine that minimizes opportunities for indulgence in repetitive rituals.
- Enroll your child in a multidisciplinary treatment program.
- Investigate support services and local support groups for parents or caretakers.

The DON'Ts
- Don't deny your child the opportunity to reach his full potential.
- Don't accept traditional therapies as the only way to work with these children—be creative within a structured environment.

When to Call Your Doctor
- If you have questions about your child's health or need information about services available for autistic children.
- If your child has any problem associated with medications.
- If your child's signs or symptoms worsen significantly.

For More Information
Autism Society of America
7910 Woodmont Ave., Suite 650
Bethesda, MD 20814-3015
800-3AUTISM
301-657-0881
Autism Research Institute
4182 Adams Ave.
San Diego, CA 92116
619-563-6840
Therapeutic Nursery for Autistic Children
New Bellevue 21 South
Bellevue Hospital Center
462 First Avenue at 27th Street
New York, NY 10016-9198
212-562-4504
World Wide Web
http://www.autism-society.org/asa_home.html
http://www.autism.org/ari

BALANITIS

About Your Diagnosis

Balanitis is the most common cause of swelling of the penis. It may also involve the foreskin. It can be caused by infection from bacteria or yeast. Sometimes this infection is transmitted by a sexual partner with a yeast infection. It can also be caused by an allergic reaction to clothing, creams, lotions, or medications. Cuts, tears, or wounds of the penis can lead to balanitis. Men with diabetes, poor hygiene, and those with foreskin (uncircumcised) are more likely to get balanitis.

Living With Your Diagnosis

Initially there may be either swelling of the head of the penis or foreskin. Both may occur at the same time. The foreskin can become red, swollen, and tender. If untreated, the shaft of the penis may become involved, and blisters and ulcers can form. Difficulty or burning during urination can occur.

Treatment

Mild cases require bed rest and elevation and an antibiotic cream applied to affected areas. Antibiotics by mouth are frequently given in more severe cases and in diabetics.

Sometimes steroid creams are prescribed to decrease swelling.

The DOs

- Take Tylenol for pain or fever.
- Use an over-the-counter hydrocortisone cream applied twice a day for a few days unless directed otherwise by your doctor.
- If you are a diabetic, maintain excellent diet control and take all diabetic medications as prescribed.
- Avoid vigorous exercise if the balanitis is painful.
- If symptoms are severe, rest and elevation of the penis by lying in bed on your back can be helpful.
- Cleanse the penis with warm water a few times per day.

Once you are able, gently retract the foreskin and cleanse your penis and foreskin with warm water. This should be done every time after you urinate. Once you are better continue to do this a few times per day to prevent recurrences.

The DON'Ts

- Don't take hot baths or showers; this can worsen your symptoms.
- Don't have sex or use condoms while the penis is swollen.
- Don't eat sweets if you are diabetic.

When to Call Your Doctor

- If swelling continues to worsen in spite of treatment.
- If not improved in 3 or 4 days.
- If difficulty producing urine occurs, or if blood or pus is present in the urine.
- If balanitis recurs.

For More Information
American Academy of Dermatology
930 N Meacham Road
Schaumburg, IL 60173
847-330-0230

BASAL CELL CARCINOMA

About Your Diagnosis

Basal Cell Carcinoma (BCC) is the most common type of skin cancer. Although BCC can develop at any age, it occurs more frequently in individuals older than 40 years. Risk increases as age increases. The risk of getting BCC is also higher in fair-skinned individuals, those who have high sun exposure, those who use tanning beds, and those who have had frequent sunburns, especially during childhood. Basal cell carcinoma can occur anywhere, but most occur on the head, neck, or face. The diagnosis may be obvious to a doctor, but a biopsy is usually required to confirm the diagnosis. The biopsy is sent to the laboratory for special analysis under a microscope. Basal cell carcinoma can recur after treatment; if it does retreatment is necessary. Patients who have had one BCC will frequently have additional BCCs develop as they get older. All BCCs should be removed. If you have any risk for skin cancer, you should see your doctor for a skin examination.

Living With Your Diagnosis

There are a few different types of basal cell carcinoma. They are classified by doctors according to their shape, appearance, and color. The most common have a raised, purely white or pink border and a central depression. Others may develop ulcers or erode through the skin. They start off small, less than 1/4 inch, but can become quite large if left untreated. They can spread to other adjacent skin areas and in some cases can grow deeper. This is a particular problem on the face. Very few spread to distant areas on the body.

You should consult your doctor if you have any of the following warning signs of possible skin cancer:

- A suspicious-looking mole or area that concerns you.
- Any area that does not heal or recurrently bleeds.
- A raised skin mole with a central indentation.
- Any mole that changes shape or color.
- Any mole that has irregular or indistinct borders.
- Any mole that is asymmetric; i.e., one side looks different from the other side.

Treatment

Any suspicious-looking mole or abnormal area should be examined by your doctor. If cancer is suspected, your doctor may perform a biopsy or remove the mole or treat the mole by destroying it with freezing or burning. A skin biopsy is performed to remove a sample of the mole. This is usually done by first deadening the area with an anesthetic such as lidocaine. A sample of the mole is obtained using a special biopsy tool or by removal with a sharp, sterile knife. This sample is sent to a laboratory for analysis under a microscope. If the biopsy is positive for cancer, the mole will be completely removed.

At the initial visit, sometimes the mole will be completely removed without first performing a biopsy, especially if the mole is small. Your doctor will remove the entire abnormal area and send it for analysis at the laboratory.

Other methods such as electrosurgery (using an electric needle) and cryosurgery (freezing) are frequently used to treat BCC.

When diagnosed early, BCC is relatively easy to treat and recurrences are less common. When it is extensive, BCC can be more difficult to treat and referral to a specialist may be necessary.

The DOs

- Obtain an annual skin examination from your doctor, more often if recommended by your doctor.
- See your doctor if you have a suspicious-looking mole or abnormal skin area.
- Always wear sunscreen with a sun protection factor (SPF) of 15 or higher when in direct sunlight.

The DON'Ts

- Avoid sunlight during the periods when most intense, especially from 11 AM to 3 PM during summer days. (If you must be in the sun, wear long-sleeve shirts and pants and a hat).
- Avoid sunburns, especially in small children.
- Don't delay seeing your doctor if you have any of the warning signs of skin cancer.

When to Call Your Doctor

- If you have a new mole or a suspicious-looking area on your skin.

For More Information

American Academy of Dermatology
930 N Meacham Road
Schaumburg, IL 60173
847-330-0230

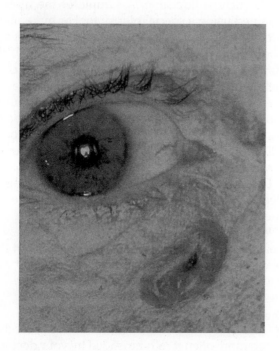

Basal cell carcinoma, nodular type. Note waxy nodule with prominent telangiectasias. (Courtesy of Robert Clark III, M.D., Ph.D. From Goldstein BG, Goldstein AO: *Practical Dermatology,* vol 1. St. Louis, Mosby–Year Book, 1992. Used by permission.)

BELL'S PALSY

About Your Diagnosis

Bell's palsy is a paralysis of the facial nerve, producing distortion on one side of the face; it is the single most common cause of facial paralysis. By definition, peripheral facial nerve palsy is called Bell's palsy when it does not result from a known cause (infection, tumor, or trauma). Because many patients have a viral illness before the symptoms, some believe that Bell's palsy results from facial nerve inflammation caused by the herpes virus.

Living With Your Diagnosis

Bell's palsy can be distressing because the onset is sudden and appears as a weakness or loss of muscle tone to one side of the face, including the eye. Pain behind the ear may precede the development of facial weakness, which sometimes progresses to complete paralysis within hours. In some cases, patients may have an uneven smile, drooling from the weak side of the mouth, pain behind the ear, changes in taste, and an inability to close the affected eye properly. Recovery may take from 2 to 3 weeks to many months; 75% to 80% of patients recover completely. Of those with complete paralysis at the onset, 50% will have incomplete recovery.

Treatment

Some physicians may obtain an electromyogram (EMG) to carefully study the function of the nerve. This may be helpful in forecasting the chances of recovery.

Your physician may prescribe a medication to reduce inflammation and swelling in the nerve. Often steroid medications are used for this purpose because they effectively reduce both pain and inflammation. Your doctor will explain the side effects of the prescribed medication. Protection of the eye is critical. Eye drops may be used for comfort and protection of the affected eye during the day, and eye ointment may be used during the night. In rare cases, surgery may be performed to decrease the pressure on the facial nerve or improve facial movements in patients who do not make a complete recovery.

The DOs

- Take your medications as prescribed.
- PROTECT YOUR EYE. While you sleep, you may need an eye patch to protect your eye.
- During the day, you may need wrap-around lenses to protect against dirt and dust.
- You may wish to avoid bright light or wear dark glasses during the day.
- Apply warmth to the affected side to relieve pain.
- Begin simple muscle exercises and facial massage as strength returns.

The DON'Ts

- Don't reduce your activity level because rest does not improve Bell's palsy.
- Don't stop steroid medications abruptly; these medications must be gradually tapered.

When to Call Your Doctor

- Your eye stays red and irritated or becomes painful.
- You cannot prevent drooling.
- You have any problems associated with the medication.

For More Information
American Academy of Otolaryngology–Head and Neck Surgery (AAO-HNS)
Communications Department
One Prince Street
Alexandria, VA 22314-3357
703-683-5100
Micromedix Medical Information Software
World Wide Web
http://www.rxmed.com/illnesses/bell's Palsy.html
http://www.entnet.org

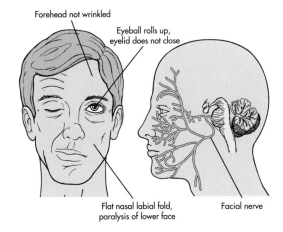

Bell's palsy: facial characteristics. (From Lewis SM, Collier IC, Heitkemper MM: *Medical-Surgical Nursing: Assessment and Management of Clinical Problem*, vol. 4. St. Louis, Mosby–Year Book, 1995. Used by permission.)

BIPOLAR DISORDER

About Your Diagnosis

Bipolar disorder is a psychiatric condition that was formerly known as manic depressive disorder. The main symptom of bipolar disorder involves mood swings between mania or hyperactivity and depression.

Living With Your Diagnosis

During the manic or high stage, you may feel very happy, have a lot of energy, need much less sleep than usual, talk very fast, and have the sensation that your thoughts are running through your head very quickly. You may be unable to turn off your thoughts at night to fall asleep. Often, individuals who are in the high period may get by on only 1 or 2 hours of sleep, and still be able to function the next day. In addition, during the high period, patients often make very bad decisions and use poor judgment; for example, they may gamble, spend money they do not have, make very risky investments, and write bad checks. Many individuals feel that they are more productive during the high or manic episode. However, the manic episode can also involve psychosis; that is, hearing voices, seeing things that aren't there, feeling that one has special powers, and getting overly involved in religion. Frequently when individuals are manic, family members and friends will tell them to slow down and stop talking so fast. Some manic individuals will do things like cleaning the house in the early morning hours to burn off excess energy.

The down period of bipolar disorder is called depression. During this time, the individual will feel very tired all the time, may be sad, may have crying episodes occasionally for no apparent reason, will have difficulty falling asleep, but will feel that they need sleep, may lose their appetite, or less commonly, may eat more. In extreme forms of depression, the individual may be suicidal.

Bipolar disorder often occurs in cycles; you may have an episode once a month, once a week, once a year, once a season, or less commonly once a day. It is difficult to tell how often an individual may go through a mood swing because this depends on the individual. Bipolar disorder is fairly common. It also runs in families, so you are more likely to have it if your parents or grandparents had the condition. In addition, bipolar disorder is more common if your parents or grandparents abused alcohol or had depression. There is no specific laboratory test or x-ray to diagnose bipolar disorder. It is diagnosed by the presence of some of the symptoms mentioned above.

Treatment

The condition is manageable with medications, but bipolar disorder is not curable. The treatment of bipolar disorder involves the use of medications designed to make the mood more stable and to decrease the highs and lows associated with mood swings. The most commonly used drug is lithium, which is very similar to table salt. Some of the side effects from lithium therapy include diarrhea, shaking of your hands, blurred vision, weight gain, and feeling tired. If you have other medical conditions, such as high blood pressure or severe heart disease, you may not be able to take lithium. If your doctor prescribes lithium, it is important to remember that you must not change your intake of salt, nor should you take any salt tablets. However, you should inform your doctor if you are increasing your activity level, especially if done in warm weather where sweating is involved, or if you notice prolonged diarrhea. Anytime you are dehydrated, your lithium level can increase. Patients receiving lithium will have to have blood drawn for a lithium level at different times during their treatment. Your doctor will let you know whether your level is high or low, and will adjust your lithium dose depending on what the blood work shows. If you cannot take lithium, you may have been prescribed Depakote or Tegretol to treat your bipolar disorder. You may also notice that you urinate more frequently while taking the lithium. This is a common effect and generally does not cause problems.

The DOs

- Inform your doctor about all prescription and over-the-counter medications you are taking, while you are receiving medication for bipolar conditions. Drugs such as antihistamines or drugs that contain high amounts of caffeine should be avoided because they may cause a manic episode.
- Avoid drugs of abuse, especially stimulants such as cocaine, amphetamines, or PCP, because they also may produce a manic episode.

The DON'Ts

- Don't change your diet or your intake of salt while you are taking lithium.

When to Call Your Doctor

- If you feel you are getting more energetic or are unable to relax, or your family members or associates have described you as "hyper."
- If you notice any side effects related to the medication you are taking.
- If you intend to change your activity level significantly. • If you notice a decreased need for sleep, or if you have trouble sleeping.

For More Information

Contact your local mental health department, any psychiatric hospital or clinic, or call your crisis center number. You might want to read the book *Moodswing* by Dr. Ronald Fieve, which is available at most bookstores and libraries, or check out the Pendulum Resources Web site @:
http://www.Mindspring.Com/~hugman/pendulum
This Web page also links to the Lithium Information Center.

BITES, ANIMAL

About Your Diagnosis

An animal bite is worrisome because of concerns about infection in the bite wound itself and the possibility of rabies transmission. All animals have germs in their mouths that can cause infection. The animal involved and the location of the bite are important considerations. Bites on the hands, forearms, lower legs, feet, and face are more likely to become infected. The bites of cats are potentially troublesome. Rabies can be transmitted by many mammals. The bites of bats, raccoons, foxes, and skunks are considered high-risk bites for rabies. The bites of well-appearing domestic animals such as dogs, cats, and farm livestock are low-risk bites for rabies transmission, but your physician or health department should be notified at once. Rodents (including rats) and rabbits do not carry rabies.

Living With Your Diagnosis

With proper care, most animal bites do not become infected. Signs of infection include fever, redness and streaking at the bite site, drainage from the wound, pain, and swelling. If bitten on the hand, forearm, leg, or foot, pain with hand or foot movement is also a sign of spreading infection. Rabies is a very serious and often fatal illness. If there is any question or concern about the possibility of rabies in the biting animal, rabies treatment should be started. If safely possible, the biting animal should be captured and quarantined for 10 days.

Treatment

The bite wound should immediately be cleaned with soap and water. Clean water should be allowed to run through the wound (such as under a household faucet). A physician or trained nurse should evaluate the wound promptly. Sutures may be required. The wound should be treated with antibacterial ointment with each bandage change. A dry bandage should be placed and changed when soiled, moistened, or at least once a day. Any sign of infection calls for prompt medical evaluation. You should receive a tetanus shot if more than 5 years has passed since your last shot.

The DOs
- Immediately clean the bite with soap and water.
- Seek medical evaluation promptly.
- Be concerned about rabies if the animal was a fox, bat, skunk, raccoon, opossum, or ill-appearing animal.
- Seek medical care at once if you have had your spleen removed.
- Notify your doctor if more than 5 years has passed since your last tetanus shot.
- Clean the wound every day and apply a clean bandage.
- Seek medical care promptly if signs of infection occur.
- Notify your state or local health department.
- Capture the biting animal if safely possible.

The DON'Ts
- Don't ignore seemingly minor wounds, particularly on the hands and face.
- Don't ignore signs of infection or fever.
- Don't attempt to capture an irritable or agitated animal.

When to Call Your Doctor
- For evaluation of all bites.
- For signs of infection.
- If there is any question of your need for a tetanus shot.

For More Information
Contact your state or local health department.

BITES, HUMAN

About Your Diagnosis

Human bite wounds are usually very "dirty" wounds. The human mouth is heavily laden with germs that are carried into the wound during biting. Infection can easily occur. Human disease can also be transmitted by human bites. Some types of hepatitis and other viruses can be transmitted by biting. The human immunodeficieny virus (HIV) can be transmitted by biting, but this occurs very rarely. Any bite that breaks the skin is at risk for infection or disease transmission. Tetanus prevention is also necessary. Human bite wounds on the hands are a unique problem that requires prompt evaluation and treatment to prevent long-term hand disability.

Living With Your Diagnosis

With proper care, human bite wounds rarely cause serious or lasting problems. Infection is the most serious immediate problem. Bites in areas other than the hand should be watched closely for signs of infection. Human bite wounds to the hand may require surgical exploration and treatment. Redness, streaking, swelling, pain, drainage, and fever may indicate infection. Human bite wounds are also crush wounds, so bruising is also common. Small areas of skin breakdown can occur several days after the bite from the crush injury.

Treatment

Immediate and thorough wound cleansing is extremely important. It is important to seek care for human bites before signs of infection occur. Antibiotics are often prescribed for deep bites or bites in locations such as the hand and face. Antibiotics may be necessary by vein for some injuries. Ice packs and elevation may be used to decrease pain, swelling, and bruising from the crush injury. It is common to avoid or postpone wound repair with sutures in human bite wounds. Surgical consultation is often arranged for human bites to the hand. After evaluation of the risk of disease transmission, special treatments may be indicated.

The DOs

- Promptly clean all human bite wounds with soap and running water.
- Human bite wounds that break the skin should be evaluated promptly by a doctor.
- Take all prescribed medication as directed.
- Make sure you have had a tetanus shot in the last 5 years.
- Change bandages when soiled, moistened, or at least once a day.
- If signs of infection are present, seek care promptly.

The DON'Ts

- Don't ignore human bites to the hand. Seek care urgently.
- Don't stop a prescribed antibiotic until the full course is completed.
- Don't wait for signs of infection to develop before you seek care.

When to Call Your Doctor

- Call your doctor for treatment for any bite that breaks the skin.
- Call your doctor immediately if the area becomes red, swollen, or drains pus.
- Call your doctor if a fever develops.
- Call your doctor if you develop numbness or pain with movements distal to the bite.

For More Information

Call your doctor or local emergency department.

BITES, INSECT (STINGS)

About Your Diagnosis

Biting insects include ants, fleas, ticks, flies, no-see-ums, and mosquitoes. Stinging insects include bees, wasps, and hornets. In general, these are more of a nuisance than anything else. However, some individuals are more sensitive and may have allergic responses to certain bites or stings. In addition, the bites of some insects transmit diseases. Most bites or stings will resolve without further problems, and treatment is available for the diseases transmitted by some insects.

Living With Your Diagnosis

Most of the above bites cause local pain or itching at the time of the bite. Redness, swelling, and itching around the bite itself often follows. Within 1–3 days these have completely resolved. Some potential problems related to specific insects include several different tick fevers such as Rocky Mountain spotted fever and Lyme disease spread by tick bites. Mosquito bites can spread encephalitis. Some individuals are allergic to the bites of specific insects. Any bite can become infected.

Stings likewise cause local pain and swelling, but most resolve within a few days. Multiple stings can be a problem for anyone. They cause systemic effects such as generalized swelling, weakness, confusion, and difficulty in breathing. Systemic effects also include fainting, vomiting, and diarrhea. Kidney failure, cardiac arrest, and death can occur in severe cases.

Treatment

For stings, you should carefully remove the stinger. You should be careful not to squeeze the venom sack if still attached to the stinger, because this will inject more venom. For most bites and stings, application of cold will help decrease itching and swelling, as will steroid creams and antihistamines. Oral steroids are used for severe or multiple bites. Most bites resolve completely within 1–3 days. Except for drowsiness with the antihistamines, there are few side effects of treatment. There are specific antibiotic therapies for the tick fevers. Treatment for the encephalitis carried by mosquitoes is frequently supportive care in the hospital.

Sometimes powdered meat tenderizer from the grocery store mixed with water to make a paste, will help with bee or wasp stings when applied after the stinger is removed. For hives or more severe allergic reactions, you should see your doctor promptly. If you have had significant reactions to stings, you should talk to your doctor about an epinephrine self-injector.

The DOs

The single best treatment for insect bites or stings is avoidance. Insect repellents are effective for most of these insects, and should be used anytime you will be going out where the insects are. Long sleeves and long pants and a hat will help protect you in mosquito- and tick-infested areas. Mosquito screens on houses and tents will help keep mosquitoes, no-see-ums, and flies at bay. Avoidance of ants is the best policy.

Evidence suggests that sweet, floral, or fruity scents may attract some insects (especially bees). If you are in an area with lots of biting or stinging insects, you may want to avoid these scents. If you are sensitive to stings, you must seek medical care rapidly if stung. You may want to carry an epinephrine self-injector.

If you find a tick attached to you, it is important to remove it as soon as possible. Grasp the tick as close to the head as possible without crushing the body. Then remove the tick with a gentle steady pull so as not to jerk the head off, leaving it under the skin where it may cause infection.

The DON'Ts

You should try to avoid unnecessary exposure to biting or stinging insects. With enough bites by any of them, you may have systemic reactions develop. In addition, some may be carriers of infectious diseases.

When to Call Your Doctor

You should call your doctor when there is any sign that any insect bite is becoming infected. You should call when signs of of allergic reactions occur, such as hives, itching at sites other than where bitten, difficulty breathing, and difficulty swallowing or talking. The symptoms of encephalitis include headache, fever, confusion, and drowsiness. The symptoms of the tick fevers depend on the specific fever but include rashes, muscle aches, low-grade fever, headache, and joint pain.

For More Information
Paul Auerbach (ed): *Wilderness Medicine*, ed 3. St. Louis, Mosby–

BITES, MARINE ENVENOMATIONS

About Your Diagnosis

There are literally thousands of venomous animals in the world's oceans, but the majority fall into several classes. These include corals (mostly fire coral in North America), jelly fish and sea nettles, sea urchins and star fish, sting rays, and fish including lion fish, scorpion fish, and stone fish. Most cause envenomation by a sting or by a puncture wound from a spine. Envenomations range from uncomfortable irritations of the skin to potentially life-threatening conditions. You may come in contact with these animals during skin or scuba diving, wading or swimming in shallow waters, or through contact with animals washed up on the beach.

Living With Your Diagnosis

Signs of mild envenomations from fire coral, jellyfish, or sea anemones usually include variable stinging, itching, or pain at the site of contact. This will frequently have a very rapid onset. Especially with jellyfish, there may be tentacles attached to the skin that must be removed carefully to avoid further stings to the victim or the rescuer. Blistering, welts, or swelling (which may last 1–2 weeks) may follow the sting. More severe cases can result in allergic reactions, muscle cramps and spasms, and convulsions. Headache, paralysis, and unconsciousness can occur. Heart irregularities, difficulty breathing, nausea and vomiting, and destruction of tissue with scarring at the site of the sting can also occur.

Puncture wounds from sea urchins, sting rays, and the venomous fishes result in a distinct puncture wound that may contain broken off spines. Most result in rapid pain that is frequently burning. This may spread to include the whole limb. Prolonged bleeding and discoloration around the wound can occur. Severe muscle spasms and cramps, and paralysis of the limb may be seen. Nausea and vomiting, fainting or unconsciousness, difficulty breathing, and delirium are present in severe cases. Infection in the wound is a frequent delayed problem, especially if there are spine fragments in the wound.

Treatment

Treatment falls into two broad categories. For fire coral, anemones, and jellyfish, initial treatment is to flush the area vigorously with vinegar. This will help neutralize the venom and prevent further stings from any stingers left on the skin. You should not use fresh water to rinse. Rubbing alcohol, although suggested in the past, may actually increase stings. Scrape any visible tentacles off with a knife or a razor. Be careful not to touch them with bare skin because you may be stung. After initial treatment, steroids applied either as a cream or given internally may be helpful for severe envenomations. If stung by a sea nettle, a baking powder solution may be better for the initial flushing, but vinegar is best when you are not completely sure what stung you.

For the puncture type of stings, the best initial treatment is to flush the wound with sea water. This is followed by soaking the wound in nonscalding hot water (at around 110°F) for 30–90 minutes or until the pain decreases. You should add hot water as needed to maintain the temperature. If pain recurs, you should soak the wound in hot water again. It is very important to make sure that the water is as warm as can be comfortably tolerated, but not hot enough to scald. Your doctor should examine the wound for any retained spines that need to be removed. Your doctor may need to order x-ray examinations to find spines that are not visible in the wound. Antibiotics may help prevent infection.

The DOs

You should take any medicines as prescribed; these may include antibiotics or steroids. You should decrease activity involving the injured limb until it has recovered. This will decrease swelling and slow spread of any venom present in the wound. The best prevention is to avoid the animals that cause envenomation. If you are going to be diving, swimming, or wading in waters with which you are not familiar, it is wise to consult local experts. These include beach lifeguards or dive shop personnel. Ask them what the local venomous animals are and what to do if you come in contact with them. Especially in Australia and Asia, you may run across animals such as the box jelly fish that can cause rapidly fatal envenomations. Also in Asia, there are such things as sea shells that are venemous.

The DON'Ts

Many sea animals can cause envenomations. Therefore, it is wise not to handle any unknown animals, including sponges, corals, sea worms, jellyfish, sea urchins, and spiny starfish. You should avoid handling sting rays or venomous fishes such as scorpion fish, lion fish, or stone fish. These latter fish are popular in the "underground" tropical aquarium business, and there are many reports of envenomations from aquarium fish. If you are going to keep these fish, you must know the risks involved and take appropriate precautions to avoid injury.

Many fish envenomations affect individuals wading in water in which they can not see the bottom. It is best to avoid this activity but if you must wade, you should shuffle along so as to scare any stingrays or fish out from under your feet before you step on them. You may encounter sea urchins when wading and they can not move, so you have to watch out for them.

When to Call Your Doctor

Because any of these envenomations can have delayed adverse effects, it is prudent to seek medical attention for any envenomation. If you have any signs of infection (such as fever, increasing pain, and increasing swelling, or pus is present in the wound), you should call your doctor.

For More Information

A textbook that your library can get:
Paul Auerbach (ed): *Wilderness Medicine*, ed 3. St. Louis, Mosby–Year Book, 1995.
A spiral-bound softcover book to carry with you:
Paul S. Auerbach: *A Medical Guide to Hazardous Marine Life*, ed 3. Flagstaff, Ariz., Best Publishing Co., 1997.

BITES, SNAKE

About Your Diagnosis

In North America, snakebites can be one of four types. The first type is from nonpoisonous snakes such as rat snakes. These bites require only simple medical attention. The second type of snakebite is from coral snakes. These snakes have a special type of venom that affects the nervous system. Coral snakebite treatment requires hospitalization. The third type of snakebite is from the pit vipers: rattlesnakes, copperheads, and water moccasins. These snakes usually inject venom when they bite, and emergency evaluation is required. The fourth type of snakebite is from imported snakes from other areas. Although rare, they also require emergency evaluation.

Living With Your Diagnosis

Your doctor can usually tell from the appearance of the bite or the snake (if captured) if your bite was from a poisonous or nonpoisonous snake. Fortunately, the pit vipers do not inject venom (envenomate) in about 25% of bites. The signs of envenomation are intense pain, swelling, and discoloration at the bite site. Swelling and pain that extend toward the body from the bite site usually indicate higher degrees of envenomation. Bites from the coral snake and some of the exotic snakes may have no symptoms for the first few hours, and then sudden and rapid paralysis may occur. If you are released without hospitalization, then your doctor is confident that either the snake was nonpoisonous, or no venom was injected during the bite.

Treatment

Wound care is the emphasis of treatment after discharge. The wound should be inspected and cleaned with soap and water at least once a day. Old dressings that adhere to the wound can be removed by soaking with water for several minutes. Hydrogen peroxide can be used to remove clotted blood and debris. After cleansing, allow the wound to dry, then apply an antibiotic ointment as suggested by your doctor. Keep the wound covered with a dry, clean dressing. Change the dressing with each cleansing and more often if it becomes wet or fluid soaks through. If another bite occurs in the future, the following emergency treatments may be beneficial:

- Remain calm and limit movements. Keep activity to a minimum.
- Keep the bitten area still and below the level of the heart.
- Do not attempt to cut the bite or suck poison from the bite with your mouth. Both can cause further injury and increase the risk of infection. Neither has been shown to be effective.
- Seek emergency care as soon as possible.
- Do not risk further bites by capturing the snake.
- If there will be a delay before treatment, a constriction band (such as a shoestring) placed near the bite between the bite and the body may be helpful. It should be loose enough to allow a finger to be introduced snugly under the band.
- Ice is of no proven benefit. Heat should not be used.
- If there is any question of the possibility of envenomation, emergency medical care must be obtained.

The DOs

- Make sure you have an up-to-date tetanus shot.
- Clean and inspect the wound daily. Report concerns promptly.
- Take all your antibiotics as directed (if prescribed).
- Keep your follow-up appointment.

The DON'Ts

- Don't attempt to find the snake. More bites are likely to result.
- Don't ignore your symptoms. If in doubt, call and ask.
- Don't immerse your wound in dirty water.

When to Call Your Doctor

- If you have increasing pain, swelling, discoloration, or bleeding at the wound or in the wounded extremity.
- If you have fever, shortness of breath, become sweaty, or feel bad.
- If you have bleeding from the nose or gums or easy bruising.
- If the wound appears infected (redness, swelling, pain, streaking, pus drains, bad odor).

For More Information
Contact your Poison Control Center.

BITES, SPIDER

About Your Diagnosis

Arachnids are the group of insects that include spiders. The main poisonous biting spiders in the United States are brown recluse spiders, black widow spiders, tarantulas, and hobo spiders. The bite of each produces different symptoms and requires different treatment. Brown recluse spiders are common in the southernmost states but may be found as far north as Wisconsin. The black widow is common in every state except Alaska. Tarantulas live in the South and the Southwest but are also popular pets, so they may show up anywhere. The hobo spider is found in the Pacific Northwest. Although most spider bites are uncomfortable, they are not particularly dangerous and will heal without long-term problems.

Living With Your Diagnosis

Signs and symptoms of brown recluse spider bites often include a stinging sensation at the time of the bite followed by redness and swelling. In severe bites, a blood-filled blister may form in 1–3 days that will then break down into an ulcer which may take 2–5 weeks to heal. Infection can be a problem and if the ulcer is large enough, it may require skin grafts. Symptoms of the hobo spider bite may be similar, but may also include headaches and muscle aches.

Black widow spider bites usually cause an intense burning at the time of the bite. There will not be much to see at the bite. Many times this is all that will happen. In some cases, about 30–60 minutes after the bite, spasms of the abdomen, limbs, and back occur. Elevated blood pressure, sweating, and vomiting may accompany the spasms. All symptoms usually resolve within a few days. Tarantula bites resemble a wasp sting with severe pain, redness, and swelling at the site of the bite that will resolve in a few days without further problems.

Treatment

For brown recluse bites, start treatment with cold packs and elevation if the bite is on a limb. You should get a tetanus shot if you are due for one. If the ulcer has a lot of dead tissue in it, your doctor may cut some of it out (debride it) to allow the ulcer to heal faster. If an ulcer is large, skin grafting may be necessary. There is a medicine called dapsone that may be helpful if an ulcer is forming, to limit its size and to promote healing. Dapsone may have allergic side effects and causes anemia in some individuals. If there are signs of infection in the bite, you may need antibiotics. Treatment for hobo spider bites is similar, but dapsone may not help.

For black widow bites, ice is the first treatment. You should get a tetanus shot if needed. Pain medicines and muscle relaxers will help severe pain or muscle spasms. There is an antivenin available but only for very severe cases, such as when individuals are having trouble breathing or in pregnant women, because antivenin treatment has a high risk of causing allergic reactions. For severe bites, many patients are admitted to the hospital for 1–3 days. They stay until the spasms and elevated blood pressure have resolved.

For tarantula bites, elevation of the limb and oral pain medicines are usually adequate. Some tarantulas have hairs on their bodies that cause severe itching if they get into the skin; steroids and antihistamines may help with the itching. You should get a tetanus shot if needed.

The DOs

If bitten by a spider, you should rest the area bitten, keep it elevated, and consider applying ice. As outlined above, most bites will resolve on their own. You should take pain medicines and antibiotics as prescribed.

The DON'Ts

The best way to treat spider bites is to watch out for the spiders. Most of these spiders are not aggressive, and most try to avoid human contact. The one exception is the hobo spider, which can be aggressive. Be careful when searching in little-used closets, attics, and basements. Especially for the brown recluse, you should shake out and carefully inspect stored bedding or clothes before using them if they have been in storage for any time. If you keep spiders as pets, you should know what the potential for bites is and how to treat them. Remember that many tarantula species can also cause itching if you come in contact with the hairs on their body, so avoid handling those species. The hobo spider lives outside on paths and gardens and can be aggressive if its web is disturbed. If you live in an area where it lives, you should learn to recognize its web so that you can avoid it.

When to Call Your Doctor

If a brown recluse bites you, call your doctor if the ulcer gets larger than about three fourths of an inch in diameter or if it looks as if the ulcer is becoming infected. It may need more treatment, such as with dapsone or an antibiotic. For black widow bites, report any new onset of painful muscle spasms, especially if you are having trouble breathing, are pregnant, or have any chronic health problems.

For More Information

Paul Auerbach (ed): *Wilderness Medicine*, ed 3. St. Louis, Mosby–Year Book, 1995.
Hobo spiders (and a page on brown recluse spiders and one on black widow spiders)
http://www.srv.net/~dkv/hoboindx.html
Tarantulas
http://www.cowboy.net/~spider/ATS.html
All biting insects and spiders
http://entmuseum9.UCR.edu/ent133/ebeling/ebel9-1.html

BLADDER NEOPLASMS

About Your Diagnosis

The bladder is an organ made of muscle; it stores urine before excretion. The inner lining of the bladder is made of cells called *transitional cells*. Nearly 95% of all bladder cancers originate from these transitional cells. Approximately 53,000 new cases of bladder cancer were diagnosed in 1996. No specific cause is known, but certain exposures place people at risk. The two main risk factors for bladder cancer are cigarette smoking and work exposure to certain chemicals. Additional risks are radiation therapy to the pelvic area and infestation by *Schistosoma* parasites.

The only sure way to diagnose bladder cancer is with a tissue biopsy. This procedure usually is performed with a lighted scope placed into the bladder (cystoscopy). The bladder is examined for any abnormal areas. If abnormal areas are found, a biopsy specimen is obtained and examined with a microscope. Sometimes the diagnosis can be made by means of examination of three consecutive morning urine samples for cancerous cells (urine cytology). Bladder cancer detected early has an excellent prognosis.

Living With Your Diagnosis

Blood in the urine is generally the first sign of bladder cancer. Whether the blood is grossly visible or seen with routine microscopic analysis, further evaluation is needed. Other symptoms are frequency, urgency, hesitancy, and pain with urination. Bladder cancer tends to spread locally. The cancer starts off superficially and invades the bladder wall to local structures. This may lead to pain in the pelvic area, obstruction of the ureters (tubes connecting the kidney with bladder), and leg swelling from affected veins and lymph glands.

Treatment

Treatment depends on the extent or stage of the cancer. When cystoscopy is performed to detect and diagnose bladder cancer, tissue that extends beyond the superficial layer to the muscle layer is removed. This tells you the depth of invasion of the cancer. A cystoscope can be used to examine the structures that enter the bladder (ureters) and leave the bladder (urethra) for spread of cancer. Computed tomography (CT) or magnetic resonance imaging (MRI) of the abdomen and pelvis is performed to look for spread beyond the bladder. This staging tells whether the bladder cancer is superficial, invasive, or metastatic (has spread).

Superficial bladder cancer is treated by means of removal of the cancer with a cystoscope and placement of an agent called bacille Calmette-Guérin (BCG) or chemotherapeutic drug directly into the bladder. Side effects are burning with urination, bladder irritation, and urinary frequency.

Invasive bladder cancer (cancer that has invaded beyond the superficial layer to the muscle layer) is managed by means of removal of the entire bladder and surrounding organs (radical cystectomy). Removal of the bladder makes it necessary to form an artificial bladder. In this procedure a piece of small intestine called the *ileum* is attached to the ureters (tubes that connect the kidney to the bladder). The other end of the ileum is attached to an opening in the abdominal wall near the naval where the urine can drain into a pouch. Side effects and complications are infection, kidney stones, blockage or narrowing at the connecting sites, metabolic problems, and impotence.

Metastatic bladder cancer is managed with chemotherapy. Various combinations of drugs are available and are recommended by an oncologist (cancer physician). Side effects of chemotherapy are easy bruising, bleeding, infection, hair loss, nausea, and vomiting.

The DOs

- Remember industries in leather, paint, and rubber may expose you to chemicals that can put you at risk for bladder cancer. Take precautions by wearing protective clothing.
- Ask about environmental safety.
- Remember other occupations such as chimney sweep and dry cleaner also can expose you to chemicals that place you at risk.

The DON'Ts

- Do not smoke.
- Do not be frustrated if superficial cancer returns. This happens often, but the cancer can be controlled with close follow-up care and removal of the lesion with a cystoscope (Fig 1).
- Do not miss follow-up appointments. After superficial cancer is diagnosed, you undergo cystoscopy every 3 months for the first year to see if the cancer returned. Patients who undergo sur-

gical treatment undergo examinations every 3 months to look for recurrence of cancer.

When to Call Your Doctor

- If you have blood in your urine or urinary symptoms of frequency, urgency, hesitancy, or pain.
- If you have pain after your operation.
- If you have excess bleeding, fever, and chills after cystoscopy.
- If you have pain after your operation.
- If you have an abnormal amount of drainage around the urinary diversion site.
- If you have trouble with erections after your operation.
- If you need emotional support.

For More Information

National Cancer Institute (NCI)
9000 Rockville Pike
Bethesda, MD 20892
Cancer Information Service
1-800-422-6237 (1-800-4-CANCER)

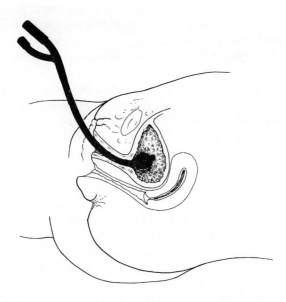

Bladder fulguration. (From Meeker MH, Rothrock JC: *Alexander's Care of the Patient in Surgery*, ed 9, St Louis, Mosby–Year Book, 1991. Used by permission.)

BRADYCARDIA

About Your Diagnosis

Bradycardia is a heart rate that is less than 60 beats per minute. Normal resting heart rates are 60 to 100 beats per minute with an adult average of about 75 beats per minute. Slow heart rates are not necessarily a sign of problems. Among well-conditioned persons such as long-distance runners, it is common to have a slow resting heart rate. For others, such as elderly persons, bradycardia may indicate problems with the sinus node, the site of impulse generation that signals the heart to beat. Medical causes of bradycardia include myxedema (low thyroid hormone), hypothermia (low body temperature), and head injuries. Many drugs can cause bradycardia, including some tranquilizers and blood pressure medications such as beta-blockers.

Living With Your Diagnosis

Bradycardia usually corrects itself when the person begins to exercise. This includes standing up to move around. If the heart rate does not increase with exertion, there may be a feeling of lightheadedness or faintness. Bradycardia may cause low cardiac output of blood, which can cause low blood pressure and low delivery of blood to the brain or heart. This can cause fainting, fatigue, or chest pain. Persons with symptoms usually have normal examinations, and the slow heart rate is found only on an electrocardiogram (ECG). If someone is found to have bradycardia and symptoms of low cardiac output, medications that cause the condition have to be discontinued. All medical conditions that cause bradycardia, such as myxedema, must be managed. Dehydration can worsen the symptoms of low blood pressure.

Treatment

If no cause is found for the bradycardia and the patient continues to have symptoms, a pacemaker may have to be implanted to help the heart beat faster. A pacemaker is an electrical device with a wire to the heart muscle that signals the ventricles to contract regularly (fixed-rate pacers) or to contract faster in response to increased activity (demand pacers). Pacemakers may be external with the wire entering through a vein, or they can be implanted into the patient with a minor operation. Older pacemakers were susceptible to damage from microwaves and strong electronic equipment. New pacemakers are much safer and more reliable. Caution remains against strong magnetic or ultrasonic forces such as those used in some physical therapy settings or in airport security screens. Patients with pacemakers are given instructions by the cardiologist regarding maintenance and care of the pacemaker.

The DOs

- Make sure you have your condition thoroughly evaluated.
- Follow your doctor's advice.

The DON'Ts

- Do not worry. If you have bradycardia and a normal exercise response without symptoms of low cardiac output, no treatment is required.

When to Call Your Doctor

- If you have worsening dizziness, fainting, chest pain, or shortness of breath.

For More Information
Contact the American Heart Association at 1-800-242-8721 and ask for the literature department.

BREAST CANCER

About Your Diagnosis

Breast cancer is the most common cancer among women. More than 180,000 new cases of breast cancer were diagnosed in the United States in 1996. One of every 10 women has breast cancer in her lifetime. The specific cause of breast cancer is not known, but risk factors for breast cancer are as follows:

1. Starting menstrual periods at an early age (11 or 12 years) and going through menopause at a late age (50s).
2. Never having or who having a first child in the mid 30s.
3. Having a relative (mother, sister, or child) with breast cancer.
4. Using birth control pills for a long period of time (8 to 10 years) or before having a first child (possible risk). Using estrogen replacement therapy after menopause (small risk).
5. Eating a high-fat diet and drinking alcohol.

The only sure way to detect breast cancer is by means of biopsy and removal of a suspicious lump that has been detected with mammography (radiograph [x-ray] of the breast) or by means of feeling it. Breast cancer is curable if detected before it has a chance to spread.

Living With Your Diagnosis

A lump in your breast is usually the first sign of a tumor. The tumor sometimes can be detected with a mammogram before you feel a lump. Mammograms have been shown definitely to reduce the chance of dying of breast cancer when the tumor is detected in women older than 50 years. Whether this benefit applies to women in their 40s is controversial.

Breast cancer is a very slow growing cancer and spreads through the lymphatic and circulatory systems to other parts of the body (lymph nodes, bone, lungs, liver, and brain). Other signs and symptoms are nipple discharge, redness of the breast skin, dimpling of the breast skin, and inversion of the nipple. With spread, swollen lymph nodes are felt, and bone pain, shortness of breath, abdominal pain, and neurologic symptoms can occur.

Treatment

Once the diagnosis is confirmed by means of biopsy, a physician stages the cancer and determines whether the cancer has spread. Blood tests, radiography of the chest and breasts, computed tomography (CT) of the head, chest, and abdomen, and bone scans can be ordered to exclude spread of the cancer. If these studies do not reveal spread, a surgical procedure is extremely important in staging. During the operation the surgeon determines the size of the tumor, whether the tumor has spread to the lymph nodes, and whether the cancer has a specific hormone receptor. This information is vital in deciding on the type of treatment.

Management of breast cancer can be surgical therapy, radiation therapy, chemotherapy, hormonal therapy, or a combination of the four. Treatment involves many different specialists working as a team to offer all the treatments. The care is coordinated by the primary care physician.

Side effects of surgical treatment depend on the type of operation. Because many lymph nodes are removed from the armpit area, arm swelling may occur after the operation. Breast deformity depends on the amount of breast tissue and the type of surgical procedure (lumpectomy, mastectomy; Fig 1).

Side effects of radiation therapy include dry, red, and itchy skin over the radiation site. Because radiation is over the chest and armpit area, shortness of breath, coughing, and arm swelling may occur.

Side effects of chemotherapy are nausea, vomiting, hair loss, easy bruising, easy bleeding, infections, and sometimes toxicity of the heart muscle.

Side effects of hormonal treatment are hot flashes, nausea, vomiting, irregular menstrual cycles, vaginal bleeding, and skin rash.

The DOs

- Seek a team of physicians who have experience in all aspects of breast cancer treatment. The management of breast cancer is complex, and you must feel comfortable with the treatment approach you and your team of physicians have decided on. Included in this team of physicians are your primary care physician, oncologist (cancer specialist), surgeon (general surgeon and plastic surgeon if reconstruction of the breast is being considered), and radiation oncologist.
- Remember the importance of nutrition and exercise during and after treatment.
- Educate family members about screening for breast cancer. The American Cancer Society recommends that women between 20 and 39 years of age perform self breast examinations every

month and that a physician perform a breast examination every 3 years. Women 40 to 49 years of age do the same and undergo mammography every 1 or 2 years. Women 50 years and older do the same but undergo mammography once a year.

The DON'Ts

- Do not ignore any lumps in the breast.
- Do not be afraid to ask for emotional support.
- Do not miss follow-up appointments, because this is the time to monitor treatment success and look for tumor recurrence.

When to Call Your Doctor

- If you feel a lump.
- If you have any drainage from the nipple or irregular dimpling of the breast or nipple.
- If you are having back pain, lower leg weakness, or bladder or stool incontinence (leaking).
- If you have fever, nausea, or vomiting after chemotherapy.
- If you feel depressed.

For More Information

American Cancer Society
1599 Clifton Road, N.E.
Atlanta, GA 30329
1-800-ACS-2345

Reference: Murphy G, Lawrence W, Lenhard R: *American Cancer Society Textbook of Clinical Oncology.* 2nd ed. Washington, Pan American Health Organization, 1995, p 198.

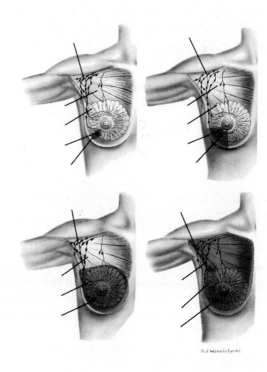

Four ways to deal surgically with cancer of breast. **A,** lumpectomy (tylectomy). **B,** quadrectomy (segmental resection). **C,** total (simple) mastectomy. **D,** radical mastectomy. (From Lowdermilk DL, Perry SE, Bobak IM: *Maternity & Women's Health Care,* vol 6. St. Louis, Mosby–Year Book, 1996. Used by permission.)

BREAST INFECTION

About Your Diagnosis

The majority of breast infections occur after the delivery of a baby when the breasts are actively producing milk. Breast infections can occur in breast-feeding mothers, or in women who have just delivered but have chosen not to breast-feed. Breast infections can occur in women who have not recently delivered, but it is not very common. Sometimes an infection will occur after injury to the breast. Breast infections are usually caused by common skin bacteria.

Breast infections occur in approximately 2% of women in their postdelivery period. It often occurs during the 2–4 weeks after delivery.

Living With Your Diagnosis

Breast infections are easy to recognize. An area of the breast usually becomes red, warm, and very tender, and fever is present. You may feel more tired than usual as if you have the flu.

It is important that the breast be examined and that treatment not be given over the phone, because occasionally an abscess will be present. An abscess has to be drained or it will worsen.

It is important that you keep the follow-up visit to make sure all signs of the infection have resolved because occasionally an infection will hide a breast cancer. Also, a relatively rare type of breast cancer can cause symptoms that are similar to an infection. So if the infection does not clear up as expected, further evaluation should be considered.

Treatment

Breast infections are treated with antibiotics for 10 days, and sometimes heat is recommended. A heating pad can be used or just wrung-out washcloths. If the breast infection has occurred in a breast-feeding woman, usually it is recommended that expression of milk be continued by pumping that breast.

If a breast abscess has been diagnosed, the abscess will have to be opened and drained. Usually, some type of packing is placed into the abscess cavity to allow it to drain for a few days. You may need to return to the doctor's office daily to have the packing changed for a few days.

The DOs

- Take all the antibiotics as prescribed.
- Keep your follow-up appointment. This is important because occasionally breast cancers can have symptoms similar to those of breast infections.

The DON'Ts

- Don't stop the antibiotic early, even if all signs of the infection have gone away. If you stop the antibiotics early, the infection may return.

When to Call Your Doctor

- If the symptoms are not improving; namely, the redness is not decreasing, the fever is not going away, and the tenderness is not decreasing.
- If you are not tolerating the antibiotics or you are having allergic symptoms. Another antibiotic can be prescribed.

For More Information
Understanding Your Body: Every Woman's Guide to Gynecology and Health. Felicia Stewart, M.D., Felicia Guest, M.D., Gary Stewart, M.D., and Robert Hatcher, M.D., Bantam Books, 1987.

BRONCHIECTASIS

About Your Diagnosis

The airways are surrounded by cartilage and muscle that provide support and maintain the shape of the airways. Constant irritation to these two components results in their destruction, causing the airways to enlarge. Bronchiectasis is inflammation and permanent widening of the airways within the lungs.

Severe infection with a virus or bacteria, blockage of an airway, or a defect clearing secretions are common causes of bronchiectasis. The chance of getting this disease depends on the underlying cause.

Your doctor can detect this disease by evaluating the symptoms of your underlying lung disease and ordering specific tests. Cough and sputum production are very common. Common tests include a sputum sample, a chest X-ray, and a computed tomography (CT) scan. The sputum sample allows your doctor to identify organisms causing inflammation and aids in selecting the correct antibiotic. The CT scan allows your doctor to look at the size of your airways and helps establish a correct diagnosis.

The outcome of this disease depends on the cause. Some patients are able to gain back much of their lung function, but others may have a progressive worsening that can lead to death.

Living With Your Diagnosis

Common features of bronchiectasis include fever, constant cough with discolored sputum, wheezing, shortness of breath, and changes in the nails. Many patients often find blood in their sputum. Bronchiectasis is not contagious.

The disease can cause significant lifestyle changes. Because bronchiectasis is a disease of the lungs, you may find yourself quickly becoming short of breath after exertion. Many patients have problems sleeping as a result of secretions accumulating in the lung while lying down. Furthermore, you may notice weight loss and a generalized fatigue. The treatment helps reduce many of the symptoms.

Treatment

Treatment may be medical or surgical. Medical treatment for bronchiectasis involves chest physiotherapy, inhalers, and antibiotics. Chest physiotherapy involves postural changes that allow for better drainage of secretions from the lungs. The inhalers allow for increased airflow through the lungs, and help clear the secretions. Antibiotics reduce some of the inflammation by killing bacteria that have infected the airways. Most patients tolerate the treatment very well. Nevertheless, occasional patients may have resistance develop to an antibiotic.

If your problems are severe and do not respond to conventional treatment, surgery is an option for certain cases. The surgery involves removing affected areas of the lung. Discuss the possibility of surgical removal with your physician before considering this option.

The DOs

- Make sure that you follow all directions for your medications. They are an important part of helping your lungs work well.
- Chest physiotherapy is often time consuming, but it plays an important role in your treatment. Chest physiotherapy allows your lungs to heal faster and breathe easier.
- Get vaccinated for pneumococcal pneumonia and influenza.
- Drink lots of water to loosen secretions in your lungs.
- Exercise regularly.

The DON'Ts

- If you smoke, quitting may slow the progression of the disease and help alleviate the symptoms.
- Do not drink excessive amounts of alcohol.

When to Call Your Doctor

- If you begin to feel another illness (i.e. flu or pneumonia) setting in.
- If treatment is not helping your symptoms.
- If your cough or sputum suddenly increases in quality or quantity.
- If you are coughing up copious amount of blood.

For More Information
Bronchiectasis, *Mayo Clinic Family Health Book*, 1996.
American Lung Association
1118 Hampton Avenue
St. Louis, MO 63139
800-LUNG-USA
www.lungusa.org

BRONCHITIS, ACUTE

About Your Diagnosis

Acute bronchitis generally refers to acute inflammation of the central airways that is usually self-limited and associated with near-complete healing within 4–8 weeks. Viral infections are the most common cause, especially in the winter, but other factors such as air pollution, irritant fumes, and smoke exposure may also produce acute bronchitis. The infectious causes are often spread by aerosol inhalation to other close contacts.

The history is often suggestive of the diagnosis, although a specific cause or precipitant may not always be identified, especially if a viral infection is responsible.

Living With Your Diagnosis

An acute change in cough, especially with colored sputum production, in addition to upper airway symptoms such as sore throat and nasal congestion may be seen. Muscle aches, low-grade fever, and wheezing are also common. Complications of acute bronchitis include bronchopneumonia, cough-related chest wall pain, and sleep deprivation. The severity of the symptoms also depend on the underlying state of the heart and lungs; for example, breathing may be greatly worsened in patients who have severe chronic obstructive pulmonary disease.

Treatment

Rest, oral fluids, and suppression of fever as well as cough are usually adequate to treat most viral infectious flares of acute bronchitis. However, antibiotics may be necessary in patients with concomitant chronic lung disease who have increased volume of colored sputum and fever, or in patients who require hospitalization. Sputum analysis and culture may be helpful in guiding specific therapy. A chest x-ray should be done if bronchopneumonia is suspected or other complications are being considered. Smoking cessation, if relevant, is advised. Use of antibiotics may produce side effects in the form of treatment-related diarrhea or yeast infections.

The DOs

Do rest and take in extra fluid. Contact your doctor if you suspect a noninfectious cause of your acute bronchitis, such as exposure to strong fumes at work or in other places, or if you need help to stop smoking. Complete a full course of antibiotics, if prescribed, even if you feel better after 2 or 3 days.

The DON'Ts

Do not take an antibiotic unless prescribed by your doctor. Cough suppressants should be used cautiously in patients with severe obstructive lung disease. Additional medications and possibly even a course of corticosteroids may be required in patients who have acute bronchitis as well as asthma.

When to Call Your Doctor

You should contact your doctor if your symptoms are not improving; if you have worsening respiratory symptoms with shortness of breath, wheezing, and productive cough; or if you have concerns about any medication side effects. In individuals with asthma or chronic obstructive pulmonary disease, earlier notification of your physician may be required to discuss the need for any additional treatment or hospitalization.

For More Information
American Lung Association
1118 Hampton Avenue
St. Louis, MO 63139
800-LUNG-USA
www.lungusa.org

BULIMIA NERVOSA

About Your Diagnosis

The most important feature in bulimia nervosa is the occurrence of episodes of binge eating. During these episodes, the individual consumes a large amount of food. These episodes of overeating are also associated with a sense of loss of control on the part of the patient. Once the eating has begun, the individual feels unable to stop until a large amount, often an excessive amount, has been eaten. However, patients with bulimia nervosa are able to stop eating if they are interrupted by the unexpected arrival of some individuals. After the overeating, individuals with bulimia nervosa engage in inappropriate behavior to avoid weight gain, such as deliberate vomiting or the abuse of laxatives. In addition, they may misuse water pills, fast for long periods, or engage in strenuous exercise after eating binges.

To establish a diagnosis of bulimia nervosa, the overeating episodes must occur at least twice a week for 3 months and must be accompanied by the behavior designed to avoid gaining weight. In addition, patients with this condition must exhibit an overconcern with their body's shape and weight; that is, they tend to associate much of their self-esteem with how much they weigh. It is important to keep in mind that simple binge eating at times, which is common, does not meet the criteria for bulimia nervosa. There must be the additional sense of lack of control, the overconcern with bodily appearance, and the recurrent behavior designed to lose the weight that may have been gained. There seems to be a high incidence of psychiatric disorder among bulimic patients. Such conditions as anxiety and depression, drug and alcohol abuse, and personality disorders are common.

The cause of bulimia nervosa is uncertain. We do know, however, that it is more common in adolescent girls or young adult women. A personal or family history of obesity and/or depression also appears to be a risk factor, and such factors as society's preoccupation with slimness and physical fitness may also play a role. Bulimia nervosa is 10 times more common among women. It also occurs more frequently in certain occupations, such as modeling, and certain sports, such as wrestling, running, and horse racing. There may be an association between sexual abuse as a child and bulimia

nervosa; however, this has not been scientifically determined.

Bulimia nervosa is associated with a number of physical abnormalities secondary to the condition. These include the development of dehydration, as well as abnormal laboratory test results, caused by deliberate vomiting or the use of laxatives or water pills. Women who have this disorder are more likely to have menstrual problems, and in particular, individuals who engage in self-induced vomiting for many years may develop dental caries, especially of the upper front teeth. The acid from the stomach seems to soften the enamel, which in time disappears, so that the teeth chip more easily and may become smaller. It also may be that this condition is associated with an enlarged stomach and a slowed emptying of the stomach, both of which may increase the likelihood that the individual may be able to tolerate binge eating.

Living With Your Diagnosis

Bulimia nervosa usually occurs after a young woman who sees herself as overweight starts a diet, and after some early success with the diet begins to overeat. She then becomes distressed by her lack of control and her fear of gaining weight, and decides to make up for the overeating by causing vomiting or taking laxatives, usually having heard about these things from her friends or from media reports about eating disorders. After determining that she can successfully induce vomiting, she may feel pleased for awhile that she can eat large amounts and not gain weight. However, the disease is progressive and the binge eating usually increases in size and frequency, and often the sense of lack of control increases as well.

Binge eating tends to occur in late afternoon or evening and almost always occurs in a secretive manner, usually while the patient is alone. Studies suggest that the typical binge meal contains 1,000 or more calories consisting of sweet, high-fat foods that are usually eaten for dessert, such as ice cream, cookies, cake, and candy. The behavior designed to avoid gaining weight usually starts right after the meal is eaten. Some individuals who have bulimia nervosa enjoy being around food whether they are eating or not. They enjoy preparing food for others, enjoy going to restaurants, and often enjoy working in areas where food is prepared. Whenever evaluating someone for bulimia nervosa, it is very important to obtain a specific history to uncover any behavior that might be life-threatening, such as the use of water pills, amphetamines, diet pills, laxatives, and enemas.

Treatment

The goal of treatment in bulimia nervosa is very simple. It is to decrease and then to end the binge eating and the inappropriate behavior afterwards designed to lose weight, as well as to help patients realize that self-esteem should be more appropriately based on factors other than their actual body weight. In general, patients with bulimia nervosa are much easier to treat than those with anorexia nervosa, because the patient with bulimia generally recognizes that there is a problem, so the struggles for control so often seen with anorexic patients are not seen with these individuals. The most common treatment at this time is a combination of cognitive and behavioral therapy. The cognitive component of the therapy concentrates on the abnormal thinking individuals may have about weight, and hopefully allows them to recognize that their self-image is based on other factors. Cognitive/behavioral therapy can be given either in individual sessions or as a group. The behavior aspect of this therapy may also involve positive feedback for desired behavior.

The other commonly used treatment has been drug therapy, particularly with antidepressant medication. Although it was originally thought that antidepressants would be used to treat the depression that was frequently seen among these patients, we have now seen a number of patients without significant depression who have benefitted from antidepressant therapy. The most popular antidepressant drug for treating bulimia nervosa is fluoxetine (Prozac), administered at a dosage of 60 mg a day. It has been studied in many large trials and appears to be effective compared with other alternatives.

There are other special examples of bulimic patients, some of whom may be diabetic and who may purge themselves by omitting insulin dosages. In such particularly hard-to-treat cases, hospitalization may be required. It is important to keep in mind that the consequences of the binge eating and the attempts at purging can in many cases be life-threatening.

The DOs

- You should eat your meals with family members and not eat alone. This will decrease the likelihood of excessive eating.
- Because depression and stress may play a role in the overeating and binge pattern, it is important to reduce stress, perhaps by means of relaxation training or meditation.
- You should contact your physician if any significant mood disorders or suicidal thoughts develop.

The DON'Ts

- You should not go shopping for food when you are already hungry. It is best to have a meal and then go shopping, and it might be a good idea to have someone go shopping with you to decrease the likelihood of buying more of the high-calorie, less nutritious food.
- You should not take any medications without talking to your doctor. You should particularly avoid the use of so-called diet pills, which are usually high in caffeine or contain amphetamines. You should also not use laxatives or enemas unless instructed to do so.
- You should not overexercise. When exercising, it should be of moderate intensity and should be done in the company of someone else to provide some limits to the tendency to overexercise as a way of purging.

When to Call Your Doctor

- If you notice any of the physical complications related to this condition that were previously mentioned.
- If you are feeling the urge to overeat or binge and are unable to control it.

For More Information

Contact the Bulimia Society. There are usually local branches in every state, and your local mental health center or crisis center can also be of benefit. You can also check out the following Web sites:
Eating Disorders @:
http://pathfinder.com/HLC/ lookitup/conditons/eat.htm/
This site contains a list of self-help reading material, and strategies for coping with bulimia.
http://www.well.com/user/selfhelp/bulimia.htm
This site includes contact information for "Overeaters Anonymous."

BUNDLE BRANCH BLOCK

About Your Diagnosis

Bundle branch block is a delay of conduction of electrical signals from the atrium. These signals go through branches of the bundle of His (the electrical wiring of the heart). This bundle carries the electrical signals that tell the ventricles to contract. The block can affect either the left or the right side of the heart. It is generically referred to as *heart block*. There are many different types of blocks of electrical signals in the heart. The atria contract normally, but because the ventricles do not receive the proper signal, they may not contract as often as they are supposed to.

Living With Your Diagnosis

Symptoms of heart block are related to insufficient pumping of blood from the heart. If a block is mild, it may produce no symptoms. Severe blocks can cause dizziness, fainting, angina (chest pain), or stroke (not enough blood flow to the brain).

Heart block is relatively common. About one half of persons with heart block have no known cause. Most of those with heart block have some form of heart disease. They may have had damage to the heart from a heart attack (myocardial infarction), myocarditis (inflammation of the heart muscle), or rheumatic fever (from previous infection with streptococcal bacteria. Heart block also may be caused by overdosing of digitalis (digoxin) or a congenital heart abnormality (one that is present at birth). Heart block is detected with an electrocardiogram (ECG). The patient usually has a slower than normal heart rate.

Treatment

If you have no symptoms and no heart disease, no treatment is required. If you have symptoms because the ventricle not beating fast enough to meet blood demands, a pacemaker may be inserted. A pacemaker is an electrical device with a wire connected to the heart muscle to signal the ventricles to contract more regularly (fixed-rate pacers) or to contract faster in response to increased activity (demand pacers). Pacemakers are battery operated, and the batteries have a long life. Pacemakers can be external with the wire entering through a vein, or they can be implanted inside the patient with a minor operation.

Older pacemakers were susceptible to damage from microwaves and strong electronic equipment. Newer pacemakers are safe and reliable. Caution remains to avoid strong magnetic or ultrasonic forces such as those used in some physical therapy settings or in airport security screens. Patients who need a pacemaker are given instructions by a cardiologist regarding maintenance and care of the pacemaker. Persons with bundle branch block or pacemakers may take medications to manage the heart disease or other medical conditions.

The DOs

- If you are on medications, take them as directed.
- Lower the fat and cholesterol in your diet
- Lose weight
- Stop smoking.
- Exercise as directed by your physician if you have a demand pacer.
- Exercise as tolerated and adopt a healthy-heart lifestyle if you have bundle branch block and no symptoms.

The DON'Ts

- Do not ignore worsening symptoms.

When to Call Your Doctor

- If you have dizziness, fainting, chest pain, or shortness of breath.

For More Information
Contact the American Heart Association at 1-800-242-8721 and ask for the literature department.

BURNS

About Your Diagnosis

Thermal burns are injuries to the skin (and possibly deeper structures) caused by the application of excessive heat or certain types of light. Burns may occur from intense heat for a short time, such as hot grease, or from low levels of heat or light over long times, such as a heating pad or sunburn. The severity of a burn is determined by the depth of tissue injury. The four degrees of thermal burns and the signs and symptoms of each degree are shown in Table 1. Chemicals such as acids and alkali may cause burns from interaction with the body's liquids and molecules. Chemical burns are more complex and difficult to classify.

Table 1. The Classification of Burns

Degree	Depth	Appearance	Painful
1st	Superficial skin	Red. No blisters	Yes
2nd	Deeper skin layers	Blisters, light charring	Extremely
3rd	Full skin depth	Pale, charred, leathery	No
4th	Skin with fat, muscle	Deep charring	No

Living With Your Diagnosis

The diagnosis of a thermal burn is usually obvious to the patient. Pain is the usual initial symptom. First-degree burns may not require attention, nor do some small areas of second-degree burns. Any second-degree burn larger than the size of the patient's palm requires medical attention. Any sized second-degree burn of the hands, feet, face, or genitals, as well as any second-degree burn anywhere on an infant, requires medical attention. All third-degree burns require immediate medical evaluation. Fourth-degree burns are immediately life threatening. Chemical burns should always be evaluated by a physician.

Treatment

Most first- and second-degree burns respond well to local treatment. The injured area requires protection in the form of dressings and antibiotic ointments. Dead layers of skin are gently removed periodically as the burn begins to heal (a process called debridement). The burn is watched closely for signs of infection. Dressings and ointment are changed frequently. All burns deeper than first degree leave scars. Sometimes healing is hastened by the surgical process of skin grafting from uninjured areas to the burn. Some types of burns and large areas of burns require treatment at specialized burn centers.

The DOs

- Change your dressing and apply fresh antibiotic ointment at the prescribed times.
- Elevate the burned area above the heart when possible.
- Use pain medicines as directed. Avoid alcohol.
- Drink a lot of extra fluid. Even small burns cause excessive water loss.
- Eat a healthy balanced diet. Burn healing requires proper nutrition.
- Keep your scheduled follow-up appointments.

The DON'Ts

- Don't ignore second-degree burns. Seek care promptly.
- Don't apply butter or nonprescription creams or ointments to burns.
- Don't allow bandages to become soiled or wet.
- Don't exercise or return to work until instructed by your doctor.
- Don't expose healing burns to sunlight. This will increase scarring.
- Don't try to peal dead skin layers. This leads to infection.

When to Call Your Doctor:

- If you have a fever or chills.
- If you have pus, odor, or red streaking from your wound.
- If you are not urinating regularly, or urine is dark.
- If you are having increasing pain.
- If you have a reaction to your medication.

For More Information

National Burn Victim Foundation
308 Main Street
Orange, NJ 07050
201-731-3112
National Institute for Burn Medicine
909 East Ann St.
Ann Arbor, MI 48104
313-769-9000
First Aid Book
http://www.medaccess.com/first_aid/FA_TOC.htm
First Aid Online
http://www.prairienet.org/%7Eautumn/firstaid/

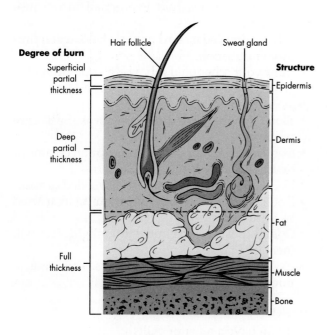

Cross-section of skin indicating the degree of burn and structures involved. (From Lewis SM, Collier IC, Heitkemper MM: *Medical-Surgical Nursing: Assessment and Management of Clinical Problem,* vol. 4. St. Louis, Mosby–Year Book, 1995. Used by permission.)

BURSITIS

About Your Diagnosis

Bursitis is inflammation of a closed sac of fluid known as a bursa. Bursae are located in many areas of the body, usually where tendons and muscles move directly over bony prominences. The bursa helps this motion by providing a gliding surface between the two structures. Several bursae are found in and around the shoulder, elbow, hip, knee, and foot (Fig 1). Overuse injuries and chronic irritation are the usual causes of bursitis; however, direct trauma, systemic disorders such as rheumatoid arthritis and gout, and puncture wounds with subsequent infection may lead to this painful condition.

Localized pain combined with swelling, redness, and tenderness are the usual presenting signs and symptoms. Pain usually worsens when resistance is placed against the muscle that is affected. Radiographs (x-rays) may show calcium deposits in the region around the bursa, but this finding should rarely affect the treatment. Radiographs are helpful for eliminating other possible causes of pain in the area, such as a stress fracture.

Living With Your Diagnosis

Bursitis can become a frustrating diagnosis. It tends to return, even after successful treatment, unless the offending activity is eliminated or altered. A physical therapist, occupational therapist, or athletic trainer may be able to provide retraining for certain activities to minimize the bursitis. Substituting other forms of exercise for those that are producing the symptoms is an important first step.

Treatment

The area is rested by means of discontinuation of the offending activities for at least 2 weeks. Immobilizing the extremity with a splint or cast for 7 to 10 days sometimes is effective. Ice is placed on the acutely inflamed area to reduce swelling and provide pain relief. Anti-inflammatory medications such as aspirin, ibuprofen, or naproxen are available without a prescription and are used to manage mild to moderate cases of bursitis. Prescription-strength anti-inflammatory drugs are used to manage severe bursitis that has not responded to initial treatment and to manage extreme pain.

Aspiration, or removal of fluid from the bursa, can provide temporary relief and gives the physician the opportunity to evaluate the fluid for signs of infection or gout. The fluid may quickly return, however, which may lead to repeated aspiration and possible infection. An injection of steroid medication sometimes can be given to provide temporary relief, but this therapy is used sparingly.

If infection of the bursa is confirmed by means of culture of the fluid, an operation may be required to remove the infected tissue. Intravenous antibiotics may be necessary to cure the infection.

The DOs

- Take as directed over-the-counter anti-inflammatory medications such as aspirin, ibuprofen, or naproxen if the bursitis is mild to moderate. You may need prescription anti-inflammatory drugs to relieve severe symptoms.
- Eliminate the offending activity and allow the affected area to rest for at least 2 weeks. Immobilizing the area may speed recovery.
- Substitute the offending activity with those that do not cause symptoms.
- Return to activity gradually, as long as you are entirely free of pain.

The DON'Ts

- Do not return to activity too soon or too suddenly. Six weeks is the usual time needed for inflammation to subside. Symptoms, not your level of frustration, dictate whether you are ready to resume activity.

When To Call Your Doctor

- If the usual treatments have failed. Your bursitis symptoms may be due to something else, and your doctor should be consulted to rule out other, more dangerous conditions.

For More Information
http://www.merk.com/!!RHnW3FDmtRHuM37hm/pubs/mmanual/html/hhilihej.htm
http://www.mayo.ivi.com/mayo/9506/htm/bursitis.htm

CARDIOMYOPATHY, DILATED

About Your Diagnosis

Cardiomyopathy is a disease of the heart muscle that prevents the muscle from generating the normal force of contraction. The result is that the heart does not effectively pump blood (heart failure). The cardiac chambers may dilate, which means they enlarge inside. The heart muscle may try to thicken to generate more force to keep blood pumping normally from the heart. The heart valves may become affected as the heart chambers enlarge, which may worsen the flow of blood.

The cause of dilated cardiomyopathy is usually unknown. Factors that damage the heart muscle and lead to heart failure can cause it. Toxins such as alcohol, infections, and some connective tissue diseases may cause cardiomyopathy.

Living With Your Diagnosis

Most persons with this condition experience fatigue, decreased ability to exercise, or shortness of breath. You may have swelling of the legs or feet, chest pain, or palpitations (feeling of the heart beating too fast). Symptoms lead to an examination, which may show an abnormal electrocardiogram (ECG) and a heart that looks enlarged on a chest radiograph (x-ray). The examination may show signs of an enlarged heart and heart failure. Echocardiography (an ultrasound examination of the heart) or angiography (radiographic examination performed to assess blood flow through the heart) is used to assess the pumping function of the heart.

Treatment

Therapy for cardiomyopathy is aimed at the symptoms of the heart failure and abnormal heart rhythms (arrhythmias) that occur. A heart valve operation may be needed if the valves are damaged. If damaged valves are present, antibiotics are prescribed for use before and after dental or surgical procedures. If a cause of cardiomyopathy is known, the patient is treated for that condition. Antiarrhythmic medications are prescribed. If pumping function is seriously decreased and the symptoms of heart failure are worsening, heart transplantation is considered for young patients.

The DOs

- Decrease excess sodium (salt) and fluid in your diet.
- Take all medications as prescribed.

The DON'Ts

- Avoid alcohol consumption.
- Avoid strenuous exercise until you have clearance from your physician.

When to Call Your Doctor

- If you have new or worsening chest pain, shortness of breath, swelling in the legs, or fainting.

For More Information

Contact the American Heart Association at 1-800-242-8721 and ask for the literature department.

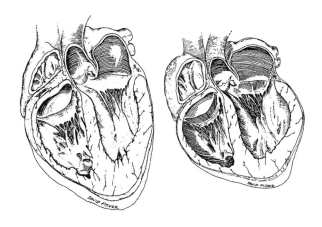

Left: normal heart. Right: dilated cardiomyopathy. (Drawing by David Fisher. From Kinney MR, Packa DR: *Andreoli's Comprehensive Cardiac Care.* vol 8. St. Louis, Mosby–Year Book, 1995. Used by permission.)

CARDIOMYOPATHY, HYPERTROPHIC

About Your Diagnosis

Cardiomyopathy is a disease of the heart muscle that prevents the muscle from generating the normal force of contraction. The result is that the heart does not effectively pump blood. *Hypertrophic* refers to the muscle thickening that occurs in the ventricle. The thickening may occur in the entire left ventricle or only in the portion of the ventricle called the *septum* (the area between the two sides of the heart near where the blood exits the ventricle). A thickened septum eventually grows too large and affects the flow of blood from the ventricle. The thickened muscle usually pumps well but does not fill well. It may become stiff and lead to inefficient pumping of blood to the body. This inefficient pumping of blood is *heart failure*. Because the outflow of blood is compromised, a person with severe hypertrophic cardiomyopathy is at risk for syncope (fainting), angina (chest pain), dyspnea (difficulty breathing), and sudden cardiac death.

Hypertrophic cardiomyopathy usually is caused by genetic inheritance of the condition. It also may occur among elderly persons with long-standing untreated hypertension (high blood pressure).

Living With Your Diagnosis

Most persons with this condition experience fatigue, decreased ability to exercise, or chest pain. With heart failure, there may be swelling in the legs or feet or shortness of breath. There can be palpitations (feeling of the heart beating too fast) from an arrhythmia (abnormal heart rhythm). Symptoms lead to an examination that usually demonstrates an abnormal electrocardiogram (ECG) and a heart that looks enlarged on a chest radiograph (x-ray). The examination may reveal a heart murmur (abnormal sounds in the heart) and usually shows signs of an enlarged heart and heart failure. Echocardiography (an ultrasound examination of the heart) or angiography (radiographic examination performed to assess blood flow through the heart) is used to assess the structure of the heart muscle and the pumping function of the heart.

Treatment

Therapy for cardiomyopathy is aimed at reducing excessive ventricular contraction and address-

ing the symptoms of heart failure and arrhythmia. If the cause of cardiomyopathy is known, the patient is treated for that condition. If there is heart valve damage, antibiotics are prescribed for use before and after dental or surgical procedures to prevent infection of the heart muscle. Antiarrhythmic medications are prescribed. Medications that decrease heart rate and the strength of contractions may be prescribed. These includes beta-blocker (propranolol) or calcium channel blocking (verapamil) medicines. If pumping function is seriously decreased and the symptoms worsen, a pacemaker may be needed.

The DOs
- Take all medications as prescribed.

The DON'Ts
- Do not exercise unless you have clearance from your physician, even if you have no symptoms.

When to Call Your Doctor
- If you have new or worsening chest pain, shortness of breath, swelling in the legs, or fainting.

For More Information
Contact the American Heart Association at 1-800-242-8721 and ask for the literature department.

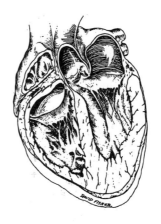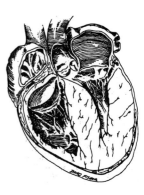

Left: normal heart. Right: hypertrophic cardiomyopathy. (Drawing by David Fisher. From Kinney MR, Packa DR: *Andreoli's Comprehensive Cardiac Care*, ed 8, St Louis, Mosby, 1996. Used by permission.)

CARDIOMYOPATHY, RESTRICTIVE

About Your Diagnosis

Cardiomyopathy is a disease of the heart muscle that prevents the muscle from generating the normal force of contraction. The result is that the heart does not effectively pump blood (heart failure). *Restrictive cardiomyopathy* means the heart is restricted in its ability to contract because the inner lining of the heart becomes stiff. The heart does not expand properly when filling. The heart muscle tries to thicken from the outside to make more muscle for contraction, but improper filling of the heart causes heart failure.

Much of the time the cause of restrictive cardiomyopathy is unknown. It may be caused by diseases such as amyloidosis (abnormal depositing of protein in some body tissues) or sarcoidosis (abnormal inflammation of lymph nodes and other tissues). It may also be caused by an inflammatory or autoimmune condition. Excessive alcohol consumption can worsen cardiomyopathy. Biopsy of the tissues may be performed to confirm the diagnosis. Cardiomyopathy is much less common than heart disease from coronary artery disease or heart valve abnormalities.

Living With Your Diagnosis

Cardiomyopathy can cause heart failure. Most persons with this condition experience fatigue, decreased ability to exercise, and shortness of breath. There may be swelling in the legs or feet, chest pain, or palpitations (feeling of the heart beating too fast). Symptoms lead to an examination that shows an abnormal electrocardiogram (ECG) and a heart that looks enlarged on examination and on a chest radiograph (x-ray). Echocardiography (an ultrasound examination of the heart) or angiography (radiographic test to assess blood flow through the heart) may be performed to assess the pumping function of the heart.

Treatment

Therapy for cardiomyopathy aims at the symptoms of heart failure and abnormal heart rhythms (arrhythmias). If a cause of cardiomyopathy is known, the patient is treated for that condition. Diuretics reduce the fluid in the blood to reduce the workload of the heart.

Antiarrhythmic medications are used for arrhythmias. Medications that suppress immune function or corticosteroid medicines may be used when indicated to fight the condition causing the cardiomyopathy. If pumping function is seriously decreased and the symptoms of heart failure are worsening, heart transplantation may be needed.

The DOs
- Decrease the sodium (salt) and excess fluid in your diet to help this.
- Take all prescribed medications as directed.
- Exercise when you have clearance from your physician.

The DON'Ts
- Avoid alcohol consumption.
- Do not forget to take your medications.

When to Call Your Doctor
- If you have new or worsening chest pain, shortness of breath, swelling in the legs, or fainting.

For More Information
Contact the American Heart Association at 1-800-242-8721 and ask for the literature department.

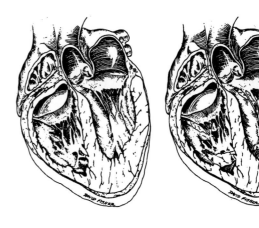

Left: normal heart. Right: restrictive cardiomyopathy. (Drawing by David Fisher. From Kinney MR, Packa DR: *Andreoli's Comprehensive Cardiac Care*, ed 8, St Louis, 1996, Mosby. Used by permission.)

CAROTID SINUS SYNDROME (CAROTID SINUS SYNCOPE)

About Your Diagnosis

Carotid sinus syncope is a brief period of unconsciousness resulting from pressure upon the pressure sensors in the carotid artery (the main arteries supplying blood to the brain).

The carotid sinus (an area within the carotid artery near the branch point) is normally sensitive to blood pressure changes. When the carotid sinus senses pressure, either blood pressure or external pressure, it may send a signal to slow the heart rate or decrease the blood pressure without slowing the heart rate. Syncope may result from stimulation of the carotid sinus pressure sensors by turning the head to one side, by a tight collar, or even by shaving over the region of the sinus in the neck. Spontaneous attacks are also known to occur The majority of reported cases have been in elderly men.

Living With Your Diagnosis

An episode of carotid syncope can be frightening because there is usually no apparent warning sign or symptom. The attack almost always begins when sitting or standing, and unconsciousness rarely last more than a few minutes. Once consciousness is regained, clear thinking generally resumes.

Treatment

If the syncopal episodes recur, your doctor may suggest a medication that will inhibit the signals that otherwise slow the heart rate or reduce the blood pressure. In extremely rare circumstances, surgery to interrupt these inappropriate signals may be beneficial.

The DOs

- Take note of the activity that precedes your attacks; report this to your doctor.
- Take your medications as prescribed.
- Have your carotid arteries scanned for a blockage or constriction of blood flow.

The DON'Ts

- Do not massage your neck or wear shirts with tight collars. Avoid wearing tight neckties.
- Do not wash the front of your neck vigorously.
- DO NOT DRIVE until your doctor approves.
- Do not engage in any activity that may put you or others at risk should you lose consciousness (e.g., climbing a ladder, operating dangerous equipment or tools).
- Do not adjust your medications without your doctor's approval.

When to Call Your Doctor

- If you have recurrent attacks of syncope.
- If you injure yourself during a fall, especially if you strike your head.
- If you have any difficulty related to your medications.

For More Information
World Wide Web
http://www.aan.com
American Academy of Neurology
1080 Montreal Avenue
St. Paul, MN 55116-2325
Phone: 612-695-1940
800-879-1960
Fax: 612-695-2791
E-mail: aan@aan.com

CARPAL TUNNEL SYNDROME

About Your Diagnosis

Carpal tunnel syndrome (CTS) may cause pain or "tingling/numbness" in the hand, the wrist, and sometimes the arm. It is seen four times more often in women than in men, and it occurs most often in middle-aged patients. More than 50% of patients with CTS have it in both hands.

Several nerves travel from the spine, down the arm and into the hand, and help make fine movements of the fingers and hand possible (i.e., handwriting, buttoning, and fine coordination). The nerve affected in CTS is the "median nerve." It travels under the transverse carpal ligament along with the flexor tendons of the wrist and hand through the carpal tunnel, a very small space in the wrist.

Living With Your Diagnosis

Carpal tunnel syndrome may be caused by repetitive motion of the hand or fingers, resulting in inflammation or mild injury of the median nerve. Other medical conditions (obesity, diabetes, hypothyroidism, pregnancy, or tuberculosis) may cause or contribute to CTS. The most common symptoms of CTS are numbness or burning/aching pain (some have no pain) of the hand and/or fingers, which may awaken an individual from sleep or occur while bending the wrist (e.g., when driving or holding a telephone receiver). Also, some patients may have a weak grip and/or wasting of the palm muscles.

Treatment

Several treatment options are available for CTS. Nonsurgical treatments are usually tried first, depending on the stage of the syndrome. Your physician may suggest wearing a wrist splint to keep your wrist in a neutral position to reduce further irritation of the nerve. Fifty percent of patients improve when in early stages of CTS, although relapse is common. A wrist splint may be especially helpful if worn when sleeping. Steroid medication injections into the carpal tunnel may help to reduce the inflammation. Oral anti-inflammatory medications such as aspirin or ibuprofen may be prescribed to help reduce inflammation and relieve symptoms.

Surgery may be considered if conservative treatments have failed to provide adequate long-term symptom relief. A minor surgical procedure may be done through a traditional, small incision in the palm and wrist to release the compression of the median nerve. In some cases, a special endoscope may be used to release the nerve. In either case, it is usually done in outpatient surgery. The patient usually goes home the same day, with the wound bandaged and wearing a sling and/or wrist splint.

The DOs

- If your work requires repetitive wrist or hand action, make sure your wrists and arms have adequate support. Try using a wrist support at the keyboard if you type often. If you begin having symptoms of CTS, rest or divide your work as possible to minimize repetitive wrist or hand action.
- If you are diabetic, try to keep your blood sugar under adequate control.
- Follow your physician's activity and medication instructions.

The DON'Ts

- Avoid striking things with the butt of your palm. This may injure your median nerve and cause CTS.
- Don't allow your weight to exceed or remain above the normal limits for your age and height. This may worsen the symptoms of CTS.
- Don't delay in getting treatment. Once muscle wasting has occurred, the chances of full recovery are significantly reduced.
- Avoid using vibrating hand tools.
- Avoid awkward positions of the hand or wrist.
- Avoid repetitive movements of the hand or wrist, especially forceful grasping or pinching.
- Avoid direct pressure over the palm and wrist.

When to Call Your Doctor

- If the conservative measures prescribed by your doctor have not provided any relief of your symptoms.
- If the pain, numbness, or tingling worsens significantly.
- If your grip becomes weaker.
- If you have any problems associated with your medications.

For More Information
The Neuropathy Association
P.O. Box 2055
Lenox Hill Station
New York, NY 10021
800-247-6968
e-mail: info@neuropathy.org
World Wide Web
http://www.neuropathy.org

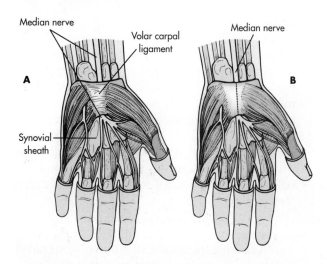

A, wrist structures involved in carpal tunnel syndrome. **B,** decompression of median nerve. (From Lewis SM, Collier IC, Heitkemper MM: *Medical-Surgical Nursing: Assessment and Management of Clinical Problem*, vol. 4. St. Louis, Mosby–Year Book, 1995. Used by permission.)

CATARACTS

About Your Diagnosis

A cataract is a clouding of the natural lens within the eye. Cataracts often occur with increasing age but can be seen at any age, including infants. The cause of most cataracts is unknown; however, cataracts can be caused by long-term steroid use, intraocular inflammation and infections, and systemic illness such as diabetes.

Living With Your Diagnosis

The symptom of cataracts is blurred vision or occasionally double vision. At times, distance vision will be blurred more than reading vision, while at other times the reverse will be true.

Treatment

Cataracts do not damage the eye. They only cause a blurring of vision. If patients are still happy with their overall visual function, then cataract surgery is not necessary. Once patients reach a point where they are no longer satisfied with their overall ability to see, then cataract surgery needs to be considered to improve vision. At times it is possible, with early cataracts, to improve vision with glasses; however, as the cataract progresses, changing the glasses will not improve vision.

In most instances, cataract surgery can be performed as an outpatient procedure. There are usually minimal restrictions on activities after surgery. Cataract surgery is never performed on both eyes at the same time. It is usually recommended that patients have cataract surgery performed on their weaker eye first, so that they can have the stronger eye to depend on while the operated eye is healing.

The DOs

There are no specific medications, diet, or exercise that would be helpful for patients with cataracts.

The DON'Ts

There are also no specific restrictions when patients have cataracts. In general, cataract surgery is considered an elective operation. This means that the surgery should only be performed if patients desire to improve their overall visual function. In rare instances, when the cataract is so advanced that it is no longer possible for the doctor to examine the inside of the eye, it may be recommended that surgery be performed.

When to Call Your Doctor

Patients should always call their doctor when they notice that their vision is decreasing. There are no "normal" causes of decreased vision. If a patient has a cataract and notices that the vision has gotten worse, they should still be reexamined because there could be other problems occurring in their eyes besides the cataract.

For More Information

To request the pamphlet "Cataracts" or to obtain additional information, contact the American Academy of Ophthalmology by calling 415-561-8500, or access the information on the Internet at www.eyenet.org.

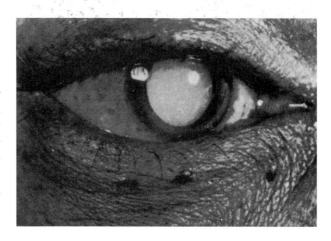

Cataract, visible as the large white area behind the pupil.

(From LaFleur-Brooks ML: *Exploring Medical Language—A Student Directed Approach.* vol 3. St. Louis, Mosby–Year Book, 1993. Courtesy of Havener WH: *Synopsis of Ophthalmology,* ed. 6. St. Louis, Mosby, 1984. Used by permission.)

CAT-SCRATCH DISEASE

About Your Diagnosis
Cat-scratch disease is an infection believed to be caused by a bacteria that is carried on the claws of a cat. The infection spreads to the lymph glands nearest the scratch. It is common in children and young adults who have contact with cats.

Living With Your Diagnosis
Signs and symptoms appear a few days after the injury. First a lump with or without pus or fluid forms at the site. From 1 to 3 weeks later, the lymph glands nearby begin to swell. There may be a low-grade fever, fatigue, and headache.

Treatment
Symptoms usually resolve in 1–2 weeks without specific treatment. Your doctor may prescribe antibiotics. Rest until the fever subsides and your energy returns. No special diet is needed, although fluid intake should be increased during the fever.

The DOs
- Rest until the fever subsides and energy returns.
- If antibiotics are prescribed, take them until finished.
- Observe scratches from a cat for signs of infection.
- Use caution when handling cats. Teach young children to avoid strange animals.
- If possible have cats declawed.

The DON'Ts
- Don't skip doses or stop antibiotics if they have been prescribed.
- Don't isolate the individual infected because the disease is not spread from individual to individual.
- Don't handle strange animals.

When to Call Your Doctor
- A high fever occurs (temperature of 102°F or above).
- The lymph gland becomes red and painful.
- Red streaks appear near the site of the scratch.

For More Information
National Institute of Allergy and Infectious Diseases
9000 Rockville Pike
Bethesda, MD 20892
301-496-5717
Internet Sites
www.healthfinder.gov (Choose SEARCH to search by topic.)
www.healthanswers.com

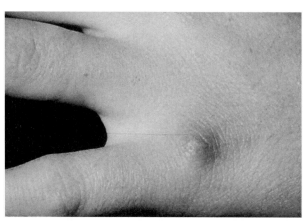

Primary lesion of cat-scratch disease is a tender papule occurring 3–10 days after a scratch. (From Noble J: *Textbook Primary Care Medicine,* vol 2. St. Louis, Mosby–Year Book, Inc., 1995. Used by permission.)

CELIAC DISEASE

About Your Diagnosis

Celiac disease is also known as nontropical sprue and gluten enteropathy. It is an allergic condition of the small intestine that causes malabsorption. An allergic reaction to gluten causes this condition. Gluten is a protein found in wheat, rye, oats, and barley. This allergic condition causes the small intestine lining to lose its ability to absorb nutrients. It also causes the digestive enzymes normally made by the small intestine to be no longer produced.

Celiac disease affects about 50–75 in 100,000 individuals. It is a congenital disorder. It occurs most commonly in two age groups: children younger than 1 year and adults older than 60 years. It usually appears in children once they start eating cereals.

Examining the stool for excessive amounts of fat helps in diagnosing this condition. A biopsy of the small intestine done through an endoscope (a lighted flexible tube used to view the stomach and small intestine) will confirm the diagnosis. The condition is not curable but can be controlled with a gluten-free diet.

Living With Your Diagnosis

Celiac disease usually presents with foul-smelling diarrheal stools. Abdominal pain and bloating are common. Weight loss or slowed weight gain, especially in children, is observed. Children can have a mild bowing of the legs associated with a complication of this disease known as rickets. Adults will have bone pain and tenderness. This is associated with diseases known as osteomalacia. Anemia can be present with the symptoms of paleness and fatigue.

Treatment

The treatment for celiac disease is elimination of gluten from the diet. Because of the malabsorption, vitamin and mineral supplements are needed to correct any deficiencies.

The DOs

- Strictly adhere to the gluten-free diet.
- See a dietician to help with diet instruction.
- Substitute with rice, corn, or soybean flour.
- Take vitamin and mineral supplements as prescribed.

The DON'Ts

- Avoid foods containing gluten.

When to Call Your Doctor

- If you or your child have symptoms of celiac disease.
- If symptoms do not improve after 3 weeks of diet modification.
- If fever develops.
- If your child fails to gain weight after starting the diet.

For More Information

American Celiac Society/Dietary Support Coalition
58 Musano Court
W. Orange, NJ 07052
201-325-8837
Celiac Disease Foundation
13251 Ventura Blvd. #3
Studio City, CA 91604
818-990-2354
Gluten Intolerance Group
P.O. Box 23053
Seattle, WA 98102-0353
206-325-6980

CELLULITIS

About Your Diagnosis
Cellulitis is an infection of tissue beneath the skin. It is not contagious. It is usually caused by staph or strep bacteria, which invade the skin through a break in the skin that may not be visible. Cellulitis can occur anywhere on the body, but usually occurs on the face or lower legs. It is curable in 7–10 days with treatment.

Living With Your Diagnosis
Signs and symptoms include sudden redness, swelling, and tenderness in the skin. The area grows rapidly, sometimes with a red line developing that extends toward the heart. Fever is sometimes present along with chills and sweats.

Treatment
Your doctor will prescribe antibiotics to fight the infection.

You should rest in bed until the fever and symptoms subside. If cellulitis is present in the lower leg, elevation and warm soaks can relieve pain and swelling. No special diet is needed. Extra vitamin C can help healing.

The DOs
- Take antibiotics until finished.
- Apply warm soaks to the area to reduce pain and inflammation.
- Elevate the affected area to reduce swelling.
- Rest and take Tylenol for fever.
- Increase fluid intake if fever occurs.
- Take vitamin C supplements to aid healing.

The DON'Ts
- Don't skip doses or stop the antibiotics until finished.
- Don't resume your normal activities until swelling and pain subside.
- Don't swim if you have a skin wound.

When to Call Your Doctor
During the treatment you experience:
- High fever.
- Vomiting.
- Headache.
- Blisters over the affected area.
- Red streaks that don't go away.

For More Information:
National Institute of Arthritis, Musculoskeletal and Skin Disorders of the NIH
301-495-4484
National Health Info Center
800-336-4797, Monday through Friday from 9 AM to 5 PM (EST).
Internet Site
www.healthanswers.com

CEREBROVASCULAR ACCIDENT

About Your Diagnosis

Cerebrovascular disease is the most common cause of neurologic disability in the United States. Most cerebrovascular illnesses are caused by artery disease and high blood pressure, or a combination of both. A "stroke" or CVA may be caused by a partial or complete blockage of a blood vessel supplying part of the brain, and in this case there is generally no bleeding. Or, a stroke may result from a ruptured blood vessel with bleeding in or around the brain.

Living With Your Diagnosis

The symptoms and signs of a stroke reflect the area of brain that is damaged and not necessarily the specific artery that is diseased. The symptoms of a stroke tend to occur abruptly. If it is a bleeding stroke, it may have a catastrophic onset. Symptoms are almost always limited to one side of the body. Strokes may cause facial weaknesses, difficulty with speech, difficulty swallowing, or weakness of the arm and/or leg. The symptoms of a stroke are usually worst in the first 24–72 hours.

The neurologic deficit after a stroke may range from mild to debilitating, depending on the area of the brain that is affected; however, the degree that one may recover or adapt often will not be know for months to years. Many individuals who have strokes will require some form of rehabilitation. This may include speech therapy, physical therapy, and occupational therapy.

Treatment

In addition to treating the underlying conditions (high blood pressure, diabetes, tobacco abuse, sedentary lifestyle, and high cholesterol levels), the treatment is aimed at preventing further strokes. For many individuals this will include medications to prevent blood clots from forming in the heart or blood vessels supplying the brain. For others it will mean controlling high blood pressure and reducing their other risk factors for stroke.

Depending on the nature and extent of a stroke, you may be treated as an outpatient or inpatient. Often this is as simple as taking a small amount of aspirin each day. However, if you continue to have transient ischemic attacks (TIAs) and/or strokes while on medication, a more potent "blood thinner" may be necessary, which usually requires admission to the hospital.

Some TIAs and strokes are caused by plaques or clots in the large arteries of the neck. An ultrasound study of the arteries in your neck may be necessary to determine the probable cause of your symptoms and whether surgery is necessary to remove the blockage. The following are some of the more common symptoms of a TIA or stroke:

- Weakness or numbness on one side of the face or body (face, arm, leg).
- Changes in vision.
- Confusion.
- Dizziness.
- Binocular blindness.
- Double vision.
- Slurred speech, inability to talk, or difficulty swallowing.
- Loss of coordination or balance.

In 70% of cases, the symptoms of a TIA will resolve in less than 10 minutes, and in 90% they will resolve in less than 4 hours. Those deficits that persist beyond 24 hours are regarded as a stroke or CVA. Remember, a TIA is a warning sign that you are at risk for a stroke.

The DOs

- Take note of the conditions and symptoms when you have a TIA:
  What kind of activity were you doing when it occurred?
  Exactly what symptoms did you have?
  How long did your symptoms last?
  When did they occur?
- Take only the medications prescribed by your doctor. Some of these medications may require you to get blood tests on a regular basis.
- If you have other medical problems, such as diabetes, a high cholesterol level, or high blood pressure, be sure that your physician is aware of those problems and that they are being managed as well.
- Keep your follow-up appointments with your doctor.

The DON'Ts

- Don't use tobacco products; these promote and accelerate vascular disease, and they will increase your risk of stroke.
- Don't eat a high-fat diet.
- Don't use alcohol.
- Avoid driving or doing any activity in which a

sudden onset of symptoms described above could put you or others in danger.

- Don't delay in reporting recurrent symptoms to your doctor.
- Avoid strenuous activities and exertion.

When to Call Your Doctor

- If you have another TIA or stroke after beginning medication.
- If you have an unusually severe headache.
- If you have any problems associated with your medication.

For More Information

National Stroke Association
96 Inverness Drive East, Suite I
Englewood, CO 80112-5112
303-649-9299
World Wide Web
http://neuro-www.mgh.harvard.edu/
Robert's Neurology Listings on the Web
http://mediswww.meds.cwru.edu/dept/neurology/robslist.html
Stroke Connection
800-553-6321

CERVICAL CANCER

About Your Diagnosis

The cervix is located at the end of the vaginal canal. If is a button-like structure with a narrow opening that leads into the uterus (womb). Cancer of the cervix or cervical cancer was at one time the most common cause of cancer death among women, but this risk has declined considerably over the years because of early detection with Pap smears (Papanicolaou smear). Approximately 60,000 new cases are diagnosed each year, and most are in the earliest stage, meaning the likelihood of cure is high.

Risks for cervical cancer include the following: sexual intercourse before 18 years of age, many sexual partners, smoking, use of oral contraceptives (birth control pills), having a mother who took diethylstilbestrol (DES) during pregnancy to prevent miscarriage, infection with human papillomavirus (HPV), which is sexually transmitted.

Pap smears are 95% accurate in the detection of early cervical cancer. They are recommended for all women older than 20 years or sooner if sexually active and should be performed annually (some organizations recommend every 3 years).

If a Pap smear is abnormal, a primary care physician makes a referral to a gynecologist for colposcopy (microscopic examination of the cervix with a lighted tube). With this method, tissue can be removed and examined by a pathologist. If this does not give definitive evidence of cancer, a cone biopsy may be performed. In this procedure a cone-shaped sample of tissue is removed to detect cancer.

Living With Your Diagnosis

Patients with cervical cancer usually have no symptoms until the cancer has invaded nearby tissue. The most common symptom is vaginal bleeding or bleeding after sexual intercourse. Vaginal bleeding after menopause is cause for concern. Increased vaginal discharge may be another symptom. The cancer usually spreads locally to invade other nearby structures and can cause symptoms such as back pain, urinary frequency, and bowel changes.

Treatment

Treatment usually depends on the stage of the cancer. Staging a cancer means to find out whether the cancer has spread, and if so, where has it spread?

A physician performs a pelvic examination and orders blood and urine tests, radiographs (x-rays), including an intravenous pyelogram (IVP), to examine the kidneys, bladder, and ureter (the tube that connects the kidney with the bladder) to exclude any spread. Computed tomography (CT) is performed to exclude spread to lymph nodes. Cystoscopy and proctosigmoidoscopy (examinations with lighted scopes passed into the bladder and rectum, respectively) also may be performed.

Staging is as follows: Stage 0, cancer only at the site; stage I, cancer confined to the cervix; stage II, cancer invasion but not to the lower third of the vagina; stage III, cancer invasion beyond the cervix to the lower third of the vagina; stage IV, cancer invasion of the bladder or rectum.

Treatment includes surgical, radiation, and chemotherapy. Most patients can be treated with surgical therapy or surgical and radiation therapy. Stages 0 and I cancer can be managed by means of surgical removal of the uterus (hysterectomy). Radiation therapy can be used in place of surgical therapy for stage I disease. Radiation is the preferred therapy for stages II through IV cancer. Chemotherapy has not been effective but is are tried for cancer in advanced stages.

Side effects of surgical treatment include pain, infection, vaginal drainage, urinary discomfort, and bowel changes. Side effects of radiation therapy, because it is in the lower abdomen and pelvic area, include diarrhea; loose, bloody stools; dry, itchy, red, burning skin; nausea and vomiting; and urinary burning, pain, and frequency. Side effects of chemotherapy include easy bruising and bleeding, fever, nausea, vomiting, and hair loss.

The DOs

- Undergo yearly Pap smears.
- Educate your children (girls and boys) about early sex, multiple partners, and sexually transmitted diseases.
- Understand that early detection usually results in cure.
- Understand the importance of nutrition after surgical, radiation, or chemotherapy.
- Understand that depending on the stage of disease, you are treated by a team of physicians, including a primary care physician, gynecologist, oncologist, and radiation oncologists.

The DON'Ts

- Do not miss follow-up appointments because repeat Pap smears, pelvic examinations, and other laboratory studies are performed to make sure the cancer has not returned.
- Do not forget to stay active. Exercising daily helps you deal with the disease.
- Do not be afraid to ask about emotional support groups.
- Do not forget about social workers who can help with services such as rehabilitation, home care, finances, and transportation.

When to Call Your Doctor

- If you have any abnormal vaginal bleeding.
- If you have any pain after surgical treatment.
- If you have any bowel or urinary problems after surgical treatment or radiation therapy, such as bloody diarrhea, urinary frequency, or pain.
- If you have any excess vaginal drainage or fever after surgical treatment.
- If you are experiencing hot flashes, vaginal dryness, or vaginal pain with intercourse.

For More Information

National Cancer Institute (NCI)
9000 Rockville Pike
Bethesda, MD 20892
Cancer Information Service 1-800-422-6237 (1-800-4-CANCER)
American Cancer Society
1599 Clifton Road, N.E.
Atlanta, GA 30329
1-800-ACS-2345

CERVICAL DISC DISEASE

About Your Diagnosis

The neck (cervical) portion of your spinal column is made of seven vertebrae separated by cartilaginous discs. These discs are the "shock absorbers" of the head and neck. They act as a cushion between the bones and allow some of the bending movements of the head and neck. Degenerative changes or trauma may rupture the annulus fibrosus, the tough band of cartilage surrounding each disc, and disc material may bulge or herniate into the spinal canal or nerve root canal. The herniated or bulging piece of the disc or degenerative bone spur may compress the spinal cord or nerve root, causing pain in the neck or "tingling and numbness" that may radiate to the shoulder, upper back, arm, or hand. Some patients also have weakness, clumsiness, and difficulty walking.

Living With Your Diagnosis

The pain from a bulging or herniated disc is worse on movement and may be worsened by coughing, laughing, or straining when having a bowel movement.

Degenerative changes in the discs are a normal process as we age. Tobacco abuse, poor posture, and strenuous work with poor lifting technique may accelerate the degenerative changes. The discs gradually become worn, less plump, and eventually flattened. When the disc space becomes narrow enough that the vertebrae rub one another, then wear and tear changes develop at the edges of the vertebrae. This wear and tear causes bone spurs to develop that may begin to press on the spinal cord or nerve root. As the nerve becomes irritated, it may cause pain, tingling, numbness, or weakness.

Treatment

If your physician suspects that you have a cervical disc that is causing a problem, one or more of the following tests may be ordered: computed tomography (CT) scan (special x-ray pictures of the neck); magnetic resonance imaging (MRI: special non–x-ray pictures of the neck); myelogram/CT (x-ray of the spinal canal and nerve roots); or an electromyogram/nerve conduction velocity test (EMG/NCV: an electrical test of the nerves and muscles). Conservative treatments such as physical therapy, localized heat, cervical traction, and special exercises are usually performed by a trained physical therapist. Injection of steroids and an anesthetic medication into the cervical spinal canal is usually performed by anesthesiologists with special training in pain control. Generally, surgery is the final option if conservative treatments have failed to relieve the symptoms. Your surgeon will discuss the risks and benefits of surgery.

The DOs
- Perform gentle stretching and bending of your neck.
- Maintain good posture while sitting and walking.
- Always wear a seat belt when traveling in a motor vehicle.
- Place a pillow under your head and neck when lying in bed.
- Participate in a daily exercise program approved by your physician.

The DON'Ts
- Don't use tobacco. This causes cumulative injury to your spine by damaging the normal repair process in the discs and vertebrae.
- Don't make a habit of "popping" your neck.
- Don't slouch in a chair or bed.
- Don't return to work without clearance from your physician.
- Don't engage in any strenuous activities until cleared with your physician.
- Don't resume driving until pain free without pain medication.

When to Call Your Doctor
- If you have any problems associated with your medications.
- If your symptoms become much worse or if you have new weakness.
- If you have difficulty walking, have weakness or inability to move your limbs, or have loss of control of your bowels or bladder.

For More Information
North American Spine Society
6300 North River Road, Suite 500
Rosemount, IL 60018-4231
847-698-1630
e-mail: nassman@aol.com
World Wide Web
http://www.webd.alink.net/nass/

CERVICAL DYSPLASIA

About Your Diagnosis

Cervical dysplasia means that the cervical tissue is growing abnormally. This condition is sometimes called "precancerous changes." The degree of abnormal tissue growth can be "mild," "moderate," or "severe." If severe dysplasia is not treated, it can progress to cancer of the cervix.

The Pap smear is a screening test for cervical dysplasia. This means that when a Pap smear is abnormal, actual abnormal tissue may or may not be actually present. To diagnose abnormally growing tissue, an office procedure called "colposcopy" has to be performed, in which the cervix is examined very closely using a colposcope. The colposcope is a very large microscope that magnifies the view of the cervix. The physician looks for abnormal tissue growth patterns. If an area looks abnormal by colposcopy, a biopsy of the cervix is performed by pinching off a small piece of the cervix. Local anesthesia is not required. The biopsy will feel like a sharp pinch or cramp, but it only lasts for a moment. The biopsy specimen of the cervix is sent to the pathology laboratory where it will be examined very carefully. The laboratory will determine whether "dysplasia" (abnormally growing tissue) is present. The report will also state whether the dysplasia is mild, moderate, or severe.

Cervical dysplasia cannot be transmitted sexually or in any other manner. However, the human papillomavirus, which is sexually transmitted, can increase the risk of developing dysplasia and cervical cancer. Cigarette smoking may increase the risk of developing cervical dysplasia. Other risk factors include sexual activity (intercourse) at an early age and multiple sexual partners.

Living With Your Diagnosis

Cervical dysplasia does not cause any symptoms. It is usually discovered by a Pap smear. Very rarely, if the dysplasia is very advanced, abnormal bleeding will occur.

If you have been diagnosed with dysplasia, it is important that you keep your follow-up appointments so that the dysplasia can be followed carefully. If you smoke cigarettes, you should try to quit.

Treatment

Cervical dysplasia can be treated by several methods. The most commonly used method is the loop cone biopsy (this procedure goes by many different names). This procedure is performed in the office under local anesthesia. There is minimal discomfort from the procedure. Some patients may experience mild cramping after the procedure for 1–2 days. Vaginal discharge is increased for 1–2 weeks after the loop cone biopsy. The success rate is 85% to 90%, which means that the cervical dysplasia only recurs in 10% to 15% of patients.

Cervical dysplasia can also be treated by "cryosurgery," which is simply freezing the cervix. When the cervix is frozen, the abnormal tissue dies and falls off. This is an office procedure as well. Patients usually experience mild-to-moderate cramping with this procedure. Vaginal discharge is usually increased for 2–4 weeks after the procedure.

Occasionally, your gynecologist will recommend that the cone biopsy be performed in the operating room as an outpatient procedure. This means that you come in on the day of your procedure and go home on the same day.

The DOs

- Keep your follow-up appointments as scheduled. It is better to treat cervical dysplasia in the early stages.
- Practice "safe sex." Protecting yourself from sexually transmitted diseases, especially the human papillomavirus, can decrease your risk of developing cervical dysplasia.

The DON'Ts

- Don't miss your follow-up appointments if you have been told you have dysplasia.
- Don't miss your follow-up appointments if you have a cone biopsy. Cervical dysplasia can recur, so it is very important that you have follow-up Pap smears and colposcopy after the cone biopsy.

When to Call Your Doctor

- If you experience persistent bleeding, longer than a week, after a cervical biopsy.
- If you experience more bleeding or vaginal discharge than expected after the loop cone biopsy.
- If you have fever after the loop cone biopsy.

For More Information

Understanding Your Body: Every Woman's Guide to Gynecology and Health. Felicia Stewart, M.D., Felicia Guest, M.D., Gary Stewart, M.D., and Robert Hatcher, M.D., Bantam Books, 1987.

CERVICAL POLYPS

About Your Diagnosis
Cervical polyps are growths of tissue that usually start growing from inside the cervical canal (the entrance into the uterus). It is felt that cervical polyps grow because of inflammation. Cervical polyps are very common. Almost all cervical polyps are benign (not cancerous). Often polyps are found at the time of a routine gynecologic examination (when the Pap smear is being performed). Sometimes polyps can cause spotting. Polyps do not cause any pain. Polyps are easily removed in the office.

Living With Your Diagnosis
Many polyps do not cause symptoms. Therefore, they are often discovered at the time of a routine gynecologic examination when a Pap smear is taken. Sometimes a polyp will be diagnosed because it has caused abnormal spotting or bleeding after intercourse. Polyps do not cause any pain or discomfort.

Treatment
Cervical polyps are easily removed in the office. No anesthesia or pain medication is necessary. The polyp is simply grasped and twisted gently off or taken off with a biopsy instrument. The procedure only takes a few minutes and usually is painless; occasionally, it may cause mild cramping. The polyp is sent to the pathology laboratory for examination to make sure there is no sign of cancer or any type of precancerous abnormality.

The DOs
- Do keep your appointment with your health care provider to have the polyp removed. Even though the vast majority of polyps are benign (noncancerous), cancerous polyps do occur rarely.
- You can continue your usual activities. Most of the time strenuous activities can be continued as usual, unless you notice that it causes bleeding or spotting.

The DON'Ts
- If you have experienced bleeding after intercourse and a polyp has been diagnosed, you may want to avoid intercourse to avoid further bleeding.

When to Call Your Doctor
- If you have vaginal bleeding after menopause or between periods.
- If you have pain in the pelvic area.
- If you have bleeding after intercourse.
- If you have prolonged or unusually heavy menstrual periods.

For More Information
Understanding Your Body: Every Woman's Guide to Gynecology and Health. Felicia Stewart, M.D., Felicia Guest, M.D., Gary Stewart, M.D., and Robert Hatcher, M.D., Bantam Books, 1987.

CERVICAL SPONDYLOSIS

About Your Diagnosis

Cervical spondylosis is a term used to describe one of the causes of neck pain. It usually involves arthritis at the level of the vertebral bodies in the neck and may cause pressure on the nerves or spinal cord. This can make the condition difficult to differentiate from disk herniation or rupture. Pain may be present in the neck and may radiate to the shoulder blades, arm, and hand and fingers. Weakness in the arms may develop gradually and only be discovered during a physical examination.

Living With Your Diagnosis

Cervical spondylosis can begin as an intermittent problem or become apparent with severe pain on awakening. Numbness and tingling may develop in the arm and fingers. There is usually no history of injury. The acute neck pain usually responds to rest and use of medication. Partial paralysis sometimes develops and necessitates surgical decompression.

Treatment

Limitation of neck motion with a collar or neck brace generally helps to decrease the pain. Most patients dislike the collar at fist; some, however, actually become dependent on the collar and do not want to go without it. Acute painful episodes are treated with rest and medications such as analgesics and anti-inflammatory drugs. Muscle relaxants are used sparingly and only for short periods of time. When the acute pain subsides, neck exercises are started and are used with the collar (Fig 1). Traction may be an option for some patients, although some may not be able to tolerate it, and a few become worse with it. Exercises in which patients actively move their necks are recommended for increasing motion and strength. Spinal manipulation is not recommended for this diagnosis. In rare instances an operation is necessary to relieve pressure on the nerves or spinal cord. This is usually recommended after nonsurgical treatment has not provided relief.

The DOs

- For acute, painful episodes, rest, immobilize the neck, and take as directed medications such as analgesics and anti-inflammatory drugs.
- Perform as directed exercises that focus on active neck motion and strengthening.

The DON'Ts

- Do not undergo spinal manipulations if you are experiencing acute pain.

When To Call Your Doctor

- If pain has not responded to rest and medication. Sudden muscle weakness or paralysis should be dealt with immediately.

For More Information

Mayo Clinic Health Letter, August 1993
http://www.mayo.ivi.com/mayo/9308/htm/neck_qa.htm

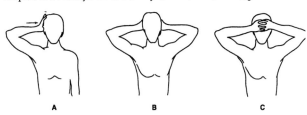

Isometric neck exercises. A, The hand is placed against the side of the head slightly above the ear, and pressure is gradually increased while resisting with the neck muscles and keeping the head in the same position. The position is held 5 seconds, relaxed, and repeated five times. B, The exercise is performed on the other side and then C, from the back and front. The exercise should be performed three to four times daily.(From Mercier LR: *Practical Orthopedics*, vol 4. St. Louis, Mosby–Year Book, 1995. Used by permission.)

CERVICITIS

About Your Diagnosis

Cervicitis is inflammation of the cervix. (The cervix is the structure that makes up the opening into the uterus.) Cervicitis can be caused by infections such as gonorrhea, chlamydia, or *Trichomonas*. Viral infections such as herpes or the virus that causes genital warts (human papillomavirus [HPV]) can also cause cervicitis. Sometimes cervicitis can be caused by a foreign body such as an intrauterine device (IUD), or by a forgotten tampon, diaphragm, or pessary. Cervicitis is very common. It is usually easily curable once the cause is diagnosed and the appropriate treatment instituted.

Living With Your Diagnosis

Cervicitis may not cause any symptoms and may only be discovered at a routine gynecologic examination. Sometimes cervicitis can cause increased vaginal discharge, which may appear yellow or creamy colored. Also, very slight vaginal bleeding may occur that may appear as a pinkish or brownish discharge.

If cervicitis is caused by chlamydia or gonorrhea and the infection spreads into the fallopian tubes, it can cause pelvic pain and infertility. If cervicitis is caused by *Trichomonas*, you may experience itching, irritation, and increased vaginal discharge. Generally, *Trichomonas* does not cause pelvic pain or infertility. If cervicitis is caused by herpes, you probably will not have any symptoms. Herpes generally only causes symptoms if the herpes infection is external, on the vulva.

Treatment

The treatment of cervicitis depends on the cause. If cervicitis is caused by chlamydia, gonorrhea, or *Trichomonas*, antibiotics are prescribed. Viruses cannot be cured, although a medication such as acyclovir can lessen the severity and shorten the duration of the symptoms.

If an antibiotic is prescribed, sometimes a vaginal yeast infection will follow. Taking antibiotics can make it more likely to develop a yeast infection because the antibiotic "kills" the "healthy, protective" bacteria. Lack of the healthy bacteria allows the yeast to grow. Medications that are used to treat herpes are generally well tolerated.

The DOs

- Take all your medication as prescribed, even if your symptoms resolve.
- If symptoms of a vaginal yeast infection develop, use an over-the-counter medication.
- Protect yourself from sexually transmitted diseases such as gonorrhea, chlamydia, *Trichomonas*, herpes, and the wart virus (human papillomavirus [HPV]); know your partner and have your partner use a condom.

The DON'Ts

- If metronidazole (Flagyl) is prescribed for a *Trichomonas* infection, do not drink any alcoholic beverage. Combining metronidazole and an alcoholic beverage can cause severe nausea.

When to Call Your Doctor

- If you continue to have symptoms such as increased vaginal discharge or slight vaginal bleeding after the medication has been completed.
- If a fever or pelvic pain develops while you are taking medication.
- If you do not tolerate the medication for any reason (e.g., the medication causes nausea), or you have allergic symptoms or signs develop (e.g., a rash).

For More Information
Understanding Your Body: Every Woman's Guide to Gynecology and Health. Felicia Stewart, M.D., Felicia Guest, M.D., Gary Stewart, M.D., and Robert Hatcher, M.D., Bantam Books, 1987.

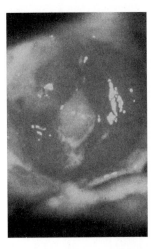

Cervicitis. Like gonococcal urethritis in men, gonococcal cervicitis usually produces a mucopurulent discharge from the cervical os (**A**). Chlamydial infection, on the other hand, may be asymptomatic or result in significant cervical edema and discharge (**B** and **C**). (From Noble J: *Textbook Primary Care Medicine,* vol 2. St. Louis, Mosby–Year Book, Inc., 1995. Used by permission.)

CHALAZION/HORDEOLUM

About Your Diagnosis

Chalazia and hordeolums are lesions that occur in the eyelid and are commonly referred to as "sties." These occur when oil glands in the eyelid become clogged, creating a lump or pustule similar to a boil in the skin. These are quite common, and patients will often have multiple chalazia/hordeolums during a several-month period. There are a number of treatments for chalazia and hordeolums, and they can virtually always be eliminated.

Living With Your Diagnosis

The signs and symptoms of a chalazion/ hordeolum are a painful, swollen lump in the eyelid. After this has been present for some time, the pain may decrease and patients will still be left with a rubbery-to-firm lump in the lid. The chalazion/ hordeolum can cause local pain in the eyelid, pus on the eyeball, and distorted vision. In addition, these lumps are often cosmetically unappealing.

Treatment

Approximately 80% of chalazia/hordeolums will resolve during a 4- to 6-week period when treated just with warm compresses.

If there is just a small, isolated lump and the rest of the eyelid is normal, antibiotic drops and ointments are not necessary to treat these lid lesions. If, however, the entire lid becomes inflamed, it may be necessary to use antibiotics.

If the chalazion/hordeolum does not resolve with warm compresses, it can be treated with a steroid injection. This will often allow the swelling to resolve during the next several weeks. In African Americans and individuals with darkly pigmented skin, the steroid injection can cause abnormal lightening of the skin and therefore is often contraindicated.

If the chalazion/hordeolum does not go away with conservative treatment, then surgical excision can be performed. This is a brief in-office procedure that can be done under local anesthesia.

The DOs

Warm compresses are the mainstay of treatment for this condition. The more patients use these, the greater the chance that the lid bumps will go away on their own. To apply the warm compress, patients should take a washcloth and run it under warm water. The cloth is then applied for 5–10 minutes. It is best to avoid using very hot water because this can irritate the sensitive skin around the eye. The water should just be warm enough so it is comfortable. Patients can apply these compresses four or five times a day or even more frequently.

The DON'Ts

Patients should avoid directly squeezing or manipulating the lid lesions because this can cause greater irritation.

When to Call Your Doctor

You should call your doctor if the lesions appear to be increasing in size, if pain from the lesions is worsening, or if the entire eyelid and surrounding skin are becoming red. In addition, if the lid lesions do not resolve with conservative treatment during a 4- to 6-week period, then they are unlikely to go away on their own. At this point, either a steroid injection and/or excision could be considered.

For More Information

To request the pamphlet "The Red Eye" or to obtain additional information, contact the American Academy of Ophthalmology by calling 415-561-8500, or access the information on the Internet at www.eyenet.org.

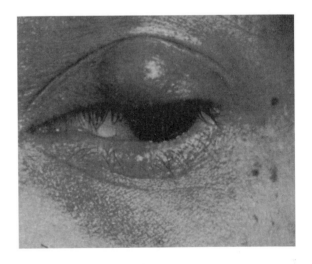

Chalazion, appearing on the upper lid; a hordeolum, or sty, appears on the lower lid. (From LaFleur-Brooks ML: *Exploring Medical Language—A Student Directed Approach.* vol 3. St. Louis, Mosby–Year Book, 1993. Courtesy of Havener WH: *Synopsis of Ophthalmology,* ed. 6. St. Louis, Mosby, 1984. Used by permission.)

CHANCROID

About You Diagnosis

Chancroid is an acute sexually transmitted disease that produces painful ulcers involving the skin of the genital area. In women there may be no external signs of infection. It is caused by a bacteria and is transmitted by direct contact with the open lesions. Diagnosis is made by culturing the lesions.

Living With Your Diagnosis

Signs and symptoms of the disease appear in 4–7 days after exposure. Multiple raised lesions that are surrounded by redness appear. These lesions rapidly break down and become painful ulcers.

Lymph nodes in the groin area may enlarge on one side. There may be fever, headache, chills, and fatigue.

Treatment

Antibiotics such as erythromycin must be taken for at least 7 days. Pain medications may be prescribed. The lesions should be washed three times a day with soap and water and kept dry. No creams, lotions, or oils should be used on or near the lesions because this increases the chance of spreading the lesions. Testing for other sexually transmitted diseases should be done. Sexual contacts should be tested also. Sexual relations should not be resumed until after a follow-up examination shows complete healing, which usually occurs in 2–3 weeks.

The DOs

- Take antibiotics until finished.
- Take pain medications if needed.
- Wash the areas with soap and water three times a day and dry thoroughly.
- Notify sexual contacts so they can receive treatment.
- Avoid sexual relations until an examination by your doctor shows that it is safe to do so.
- Get tested for other sexually transmitted diseases.

The DON'Ts

- Don't skip doses or stop taking the antibiotics before finished.
- Don't apply creams, lotions, or oils on or near the lesions.
- Don't have sexual relations until cleared by your doctor.

When to Call Your Doctor

- If fever continues after antibiotics are finished.
- If pain is not relieved with over-the-counter pain medication.
- If any lesion appears infected.

For More Information

The CDC National STD Hotline
800-227-8922, Monday through Friday from 8 AM to 11 PM (EST).
American Social Health Association
800-972-8500, to request pamphlets about sexual health or information about support groups.
Internet Site
http://sunsite.unc.edu/ASHA/

CHARCOT'S JOINT

About Your Diagnosis

Charcot's joint is a destructive process that primarily affects joints in the weight-bearing extremities, such as the feet, ankles, knees, and possibly hips. Many times Charcot's joint can be confused with an infection involving these areas, and it may be difficult for your physician to differentiate these two conditions. By definition, a patient with Charcot's joint has decreased sensation in the affected area and peripheral neuropathy, which is most commonly due to diabetes. There are other causes of peripheral neuropathy. However, they are much less common than diabetes. As a result, it is common for persons with diabetes to experience peripheral neuropathy first, which is followed by Charcot's joint. A high index of suspicion is generally required to make the diagnosis early in the disease process.

A person with Charcot's joint experiences swelling, pain, and increased skin temperature over the affected joint or joints. These are the same signs and symptoms that occur with infections, so this cause has to be considered as well. The use of weight-bearing or standing radiographs (x-rays) is essential not only to establish the diagnosis but also to determine the degree of destruction of the joints. Most patients with Charcot's joint have acute inflammation without a history of trauma or cut or break in the skin, which would suggest an infection. Charcot's joint is generally considered treatable but not curable.

Living With Your Diagnosis

Prevention is the key to minimizing the deformities that can occur. At the earliest onset of swelling, redness, and increased skin temperature directly over an affected joint or joints, contact your doctor. Ignoring the warning signs may lead to destruction of the joints with disintegration of the bones and collapse (Fig 1). Many times Charcot's joint is an extremely painful condition, even though it occurs in areas affected by peripheral neuropathy. Persons with this severe pain usually seek treatment sooner than persons with little pain, who often do not seek treatment until the deformity becomes severe.

Treatment

There are no medications available specifically to treat Charcot's joint. The acute inflammatory phase is managed with immobilization of the extremity and use of crutches or a walker to decrease weight bearing or eliminate weight bearing through the extremity. It can take as long as 6 weeks for the acute inflammation to subside. After the inflammation subsides, the joint or joints are braced and likely require bracing or other support to prevent further flare-ups and destruction of the joints.

The DOs

- Control your diabetes with proper medication, diet, and exercise.
- Should Charcot's joint develop, modify the exercise program to eliminate weight bearing. Substitute non–weight-bearing forms of exercise, such as cycling or water exercises.

The DON'Ts

- Do not begin an aggressive walking or running program immediately after being fitted with braces or splints.

When to Call Your Doctor

- If you notice the recurrence of swelling, heat, or redness around any weight-bearing joint, particularly if it recurs in a joint that was treated.

For More Information
http://www.merk.com/!!tKbSq1RNKtKbSq1RNK/pubs/mmanual/html/qmifigdb.htm
http://bio-3.bsd.uchicago.edu/~cppweb/cases/Neuropathicarthritis.html

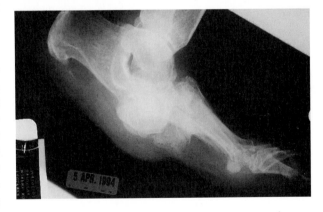

Charcot foot deformity. A, Lateral radiograph demonstrating severe midfoot osteoarthropathy with collapse of the cuboid and medial cuneiform. B, Clinical photo of same foot with plantar ulceration underlying the abnormal prominences of the midfoot. (From Noble J: *Textbook Primary Care Medicine,* vol 2. St. Louis, Mosby–Year Book, Inc., 1995. Used by permission.)

CHICKENPOX

About Your Diagnosis

Chickenpox is a highly contagious disease caused by the varicella-zoster herpes virus. It is common in children aged 2–8 years. It affects the skin and mucous membranes. It is spread from individual to individual by contact with respiratory secretions and airborne droplets, or contact with the skin lesions of an infected individual. Symptoms usually appear 7–21 days after exposure. The disease is usually contagious 1–2 days before the appearance of the rash and up to 6 days after the blisters form. Recovery takes 7–10 days. It may be more severe in adults and last longer.

Living With Your Diagnosis

Fever, fatigue, abdominal pain, and loss of appetite may appear 1–2 days before the rash.

The rash is raised and itchy, appearing on the face, scalp, and trunk. It then progresses to a blister-like stage. Within 24 hours the blisters collapse and start to form scabs. A new crop of blisters will erupt every 3–4 days. Complications are possible and include infection of the blisters, scarring, pneumonia, Reye's syndrome (associated with aspirin use during a viral infection), arthritis, and eye infection.

Treatment

There is no specific medications for chickenpox, but relief of the symptoms can be obtained. Nonaspirin products such as Tylenol or Advil can be used to reduce the fever. DO NOT give aspirin to a child with chickenpox. Antihistamines such as Benadryl can be used to reduce the itching, although it will also cause drowsiness. Lotions such as calamine can be used on the lesions. Colloidal oatmeal baths (such as Aveeno) may also help reduce the itching and dry the lesions. Encourage liquids and rest during the fever period. Keep away from others until the blisters are crusted to prevent spreading the disease.

The DOs
- Rest, but allow quiet activity.
- Use a nonaspirin product for the fever.
- Encourage fluids during the period when fever is present.
- Keep the environment cool (heat and sweating increase itching).

- Notify the school nurse and parents of playmates that may have been exposed during the contagious period.
- Keep away from others until the crusts disappear (about 1 week). It is especially important to avoid exposing individuals who are immunosuppressed (e.g., patients with AIDS, patients who have received an organ transplant, and those receiving chemo-therapy).
- Use cool sponge baths with baking soda, along with antihistamines, to reduce itching.

The DON'Ts
- Don't give aspirin to a child younger than 16 years because of the risk of Reye's syndrome.
- Don't scratch the blisters to prevent infection and scarring. Use soft mittens or white gloves on a very young child.
- Don't expose others unnecessarily. Keep the child out of school until all blisters are crusted.

When to Call Your Doctor

- If the temperature increases to more than 103°F.
- If signs of infection occur, such as severe skin pain with burning and purulent drainage.
- If weakness, headache, or sensitivity to light develops.
- If vomiting with restlessness and irritability occurs, together with a progressively decreased level of consciousness. These could be signs of Reye's syndrome.

For More Information
National Institute of Allergy and Infectious Diseases of the NIH
9000 Rockville Pike
Bethesda, MD 28892
301-496-5717
The American Academy of Pediatrics
141 NW Point Blvd.
Elk Grove Village, IL 60007-1098
Send a business-sized, self-addressed stamped envelope with your request for information about chickenpox.
Internet Sites
www.healthfinder.gov (Choose SEARCH to search by topic.)
www.healthanswers.com

CHLAMYDIA INFECTION

About Your Diagnosis

Chlamydia infection is a sexually transmitted disease caused by a bacteria that inflames the urethra, vagina, and reproductive organs. It is spread by vaginal or anal intercourse. It is detected by examining a vaginal, rectal, or urethral smear in the laboratory. Possible complications include a secondary infection or sterility in the female.

Living With Your Diagnosis

During the early stages of the disease there may be no symptoms. Later, females may have a vaginal discharge and redness of the vagina, whereas males may have a urethral discharge and redness of the top of the penis. Both males and females may have fever; abdominal pain; and pain on urination.

Treatment

Antibiotics such as tetracycline must be used for 2 weeks. Sexual partners must also be treated. Tetracycline must not be taken with milk or antacids. Keep the genital area clean. Use unscented soaps and avoid tub baths. Sexual relations should be delayed until treatment is completed and all symptoms are gone. No special diet is needed except for the avoidance of milk if taking tetracycline.

The DOs
- Take antibiotics as directed and until finished.
- Notify sexual partners so they can be treated also.
- Take showers instead of tub baths, and use unscented soaps.
- Keep the genital area clean and dry. Always wipe from front to back after urinating or having a bowel movement.
- Wear cotton underpants and avoid tight-fitting clothes.
- Keep follow-up appointments with your doctor to make sure the infection is cleared and no other treatment is needed.
- Be tested for other sexually transmitted diseases.

The DON'Ts
- Don't skip or stop taking your antibiotics before finished.
- Don't take tetracycline with milk or antacids.
- Don't take tub baths.
- Don't wear underwear that is nonventilating (e.g., nylon underwear).

- Don't have sexual relations until your treatment is completed and there are no symptoms.

When to Call Your Doctor
- If you have any unusual bleeding or swelling during your treatment.
- If your symptoms worsen after starting treatment or your symptoms last longer than 1 week.

For More Information
National STD Hotline of the CDC
800-227-8922, Monday through Friday from 8 AM to 11 PM (EST).
National Womens Health Network
202-628-7814, Monday through Friday from 9 AM to 5 PM (EST).
American Social Health Association
800-972-8500, to request pamphlets about sexual health or information about support groups.
Internet Sites
http://sunsite.unc.edu/ASHA/
www.healthfinder.gov (Choose SEARCH to search by topic.)

CHOLELITHIASIS

About Your Diagnosis

You have cholelithiasis, also known as gallstones. This means that you have stones that have developed in your gallbladder. Your gallbladder is the small sack attached to the underside of your liver. These organs sit in the right upper portion of your abdomen, or belly. Your gallbladder stores the bile that your liver makes. Your gallbladder then squirts the bile into your bowels whenever you eat a meal, especially if the meal contains much fat. Bile helps in the digestion of fats in the food you eat. Under the right conditions and over time, gallstones can form in your gallbladder.

Gallstones are common: 10% to 20% of men and 20% to 40% of women get gallstones during their lifetime. Women are more likely to get gallstones because of the effects of estrogen (a female hormone) on bile. Being overweight increases your risk of getting gallstones, as does getting older. Prolonged fasting causes bile to stagnate in the gallbladder, making stones more likely to form. The actual cause of stone formation is a loss of balance between the various chemicals in bile, which include cholesterol, bile salts, and others.

Ultrasound detects 95% of gallstones and is usually the first test performed. A special x-ray test also will detect stones. Gallstones can be cured by surgically removing the gallbladder. Treatment is recommended only if you have symptoms.

Living With Your Diagnosis

Most gallstones cause no symptoms and may never cause any problems for you. However, gallstones can cause severe pain, as well as other problems. If a gallstone gets stuck in the bile duct that empties bile from the gallbladder into the bowel, the gallbladder will squeeze harder and harder, and the duct may contract around the stone. This will cause severe, crampy pain in the right upper part of your abdomen, or perhaps between your shoulder blades. The pain gets worse for a few hours before it gets better. You will likely feel sick to your stomach and may vomit. The symptoms go away if the stone either falls back into the gallbladder, or moves all the way through the bile duct and into the bowel. If the stone stays in the bile duct long enough, you may have other problems such as inflammation or infection in the gallbladder or pancreas.

Treatment

Gallstones that do not cause symptoms rarely need treatment. If you have had symptoms from your gallstones, treatment will probably be necessary, especially if the stones have caused other problems. The usual treatment is surgery to remove the gallbladder and stones. In some cases your doctor may ask you to take medicine to try to dissolve the stones, but this does not always work. Surgery usually cures gallstone disease, and once you recover from surgery you will not miss your gallbladder. Your body will function well without it.

The DOs

Maintain a normal weight. If you are overweight, ask your doctor to help you with a weight loss program. You should try to lose weight at a slow, steady rate. If you have pain that you think gallstones may be causing, take some pain medicine, rest, and do not eat anything. Call your doctor if the pain lasts for more than 3 hours, or if you get a fever.

The DON'Ts

Don't eat meals high in fat. Fat foods cause the gallbladder to contract strongly, which may cause a stone to get squeezed into the bile duct. It is even more important to avoid meals high in fat once you have been on a low-fat diet for awhile. Avoid extra large meals and foods that cause indigestion. Do not fast for prolonged periods or go on a crash diet.

When to Call Your Doctor

Call your doctor if you think you are having symptoms from gallstones. If you have had gallstones diagnosed and have had symptoms before, you should call your doctor if the symptoms last more than 3 hours, or if you get a fever.

For More Information

If you want to understand gallstones in more detail, go to the public library and ask for a textbook on internal medicine or surgery. Look in the book under "cholelithiasis," "gallstones," and "cholecystitis."

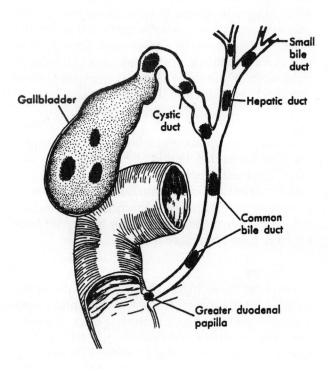

Common sites of cholelithiasis and choledocholithiasis (stones in the bile duct). (From LaFleur-Brooks ML: *Exploring Medical Language—A Student Directed Approach*, vol. 3. St. Louis, Mosby–Year Book, 1993. Used by permission.)

CHRONIC OBSTRUCTIVE PULMONARY DISEASE

About Your Diagnosis

Chronic obstructive pulmonary disease is characterized by the inability of your lungs to ventilate properly. The two types of COPD are chronic bronchitis and emphysema. Most cases of COPD are a mixture of both diseases. Chronic bronchitis is defined as excessive mucous production on at least 3 months of 2 consecutive years. Emphysema is caused by destruction of the air sacs in the lungs. These diseases cause inhaled air to remain trapped in the lungs. Therefore, effective air exchange does not take place.

Chronic obstructive pulmonary disease is not a contagious disease. It is most often the result of longtime smoking, but some cases of emphysema may be hereditary. Other less common causes include air pollution, childhood infections, and inhalation injury.

Your physician can diagnose COPD by evaluating your symptoms, performing a complete physical examination, and ordering pulmonary function tests, a chest x-ray, and arterial blood gases. In emphysema, pulmonary function tests show large lung volumes and difficulties expiring air. Patients with chronic bronchitis may have the same features but also have a chronic, productive cough. The chest x-ray allows the physician to look at changes in the lung as a result of this disease. Arterial blood gases measure how much oxygen and carbon dioxide is carried in your blood. Abnormal arterial blood gas values are often found in these diseases.

Chronic obstructive pulmonary disease is usually a progressive disease and not curable. However, smoking cessation and medications can help prolong life.

Living With Your Diagnosis

Chronic bronchitis is characterized by a chronic productive cough and episodic shortness of breath. The disease may cause sleep disturbances that are caused by mucous collecting in the airways. Other symptoms include lung infections, wheezing, weight gain, and a bluish tinge to the lips or skin.

Emphysema is associated with shortness of breath and little cough or sputum production. Other manifestations are a "barrel-shaped" chest and weight loss. These diseases are progressive and can lead to increased strain on your heart.

Treatment

Treatment includes smoking cessation, exercise, airway dilators, hydration, vaccinations, oxygen, antibiotics, decongestants, breathing exercises, and lung transplant. Decongestants help loosen mucus in the airways. The breathing exercises allow for controlled expiration and easier breathing. Postural changes will allow for enhanced drainage of mucus. Antibiotics and vaccinations decrease the number of infections that you can acquire. Medical treatment generally has few complications. Lung transplant is usually an option for patients with the inherited form of the disease. Discuss the options with your physician to find out what is best for you.

The DOs

- Perform breathing and regular exercises.
- Have an influenza vaccination annually.

The DON'Ts

- Stop smoking. This is a priority.

When to Call Your Doctor

- Your shortness of breath or cough is not relieved with medications.
- You are feeling continuously fatigued or losing a lot of weight unintentionally.
- You notice a bluish tinge in your lips or nails.

For More Information

Chronic Bronchitis and Emphysema Handbook, John Wiley & Sons, 1990.
COPD (Chronic Obstructive Pulmonary Disease), Mayo, 1992.
Facts About Chronic Bronchitis, American Lung Association, 1992.
Facts About Emphysema, American Lung Association, 1990.
Understanding Oxygen Therapy: A Patient Guide to Long Term Supplemental Oxygen, National Association for Medical Direction of Respiratory Care, 1996.
Requirements for Traveling with Oxygen, American Association for Respiratory Care, 1992.
Facts About A1AD Related Emphysema, American Lung Association, 1994.
American Lung Association
1118 Hampton Avenue
St. Louis, MO 63139
800-LUNG-USA
www.lungusa.org

CIRRHOSIS

About Your Diagnosis

Cirrhosis is chronic scarring of the liver. The scarring prevents the liver from functioning normally. There are many causes of cirrhosis. Alcoholism is the most common cause in the United States. Inherited diseases such as Wilson's disease, hemochromatosis, and cystic fibrosis are also known causes. Chronic viral hepatitis and exposure to toxic substances can also cause cirrhosis. Primary biliary cirrhosis, which causes blockage of the bile duct, can likewise cause this condition.

Cirrhosis is one of the top 10 causes of death in the United States. It is more common in men. History and physical examination are key in detecting this condition. Blood work and a liver biopsy may also help in the diagnosis. The prognosis is dependent on the amount of liver damage done and its cause; the more damage, the worse the prognosis. If the cause is treatable and the liver damage stops, the prognosis is good. However the liver damage is not reversible.

Living With Your Diagnosis

The early stages of cirrhosis are associated with fatigue, nausea, decreased appetite, and weight loss. Physical signs in the early stages are enlargement of the liver and redness of the palms of the hands. In the later stages of the disease, jaundice, diarrhea, and dark urine are present. Spider blood vessels (fine vessels spreading out from a central point) of the skin, easy bruising and bleeding, enlargement of the breasts in men, and hair loss are present also. Physical signs in the late stages are enlargement of the spleen, fluid accumulation in the abdomen (ascites) and legs (edema), mental confusion, and coma. Complications such as gastrointestinal (GI) bleeding from portal hypertension (high blood pressure within the liver), kidney failure, and infections can occur.

Treatment

The key to treatment is removing the cause. After removal of the offending cause, the primary treatment is supportive. A high-calorie diet may help. Salt (sodium) and/or fluid restriction may be necessary to control fluid accumulation. If the ascites or edema is severe, diuretic medications can be given to remove the fluid. Medications can also be given to help with the mental confusion and coma.

The treatment of portal hypertension is dependent on its severity. Medications are the first option. Endoscopy (a lighted flexible tube used to view the esophagus, stomach, and small intestines) with sclerosing of the bleeding areas is an option if bleeding is occurring. If severe, surgery is an option. A portacaval shunt is done to relieve the pressure on the blood vessels. Liver transplantation is a final option.

The DOs

- Eat a well-balanced diet. Protein may need to be avoided in the diet because the liver may not be able to break down the protein.
- Modify activity according to the symptoms. A good fitness program may help with the fatigue.
- If alcohol abuse is the cause, seek treatment through an alcohol rehabilitation program.
- Obtain prompt treatment for hepatitis.
- If there is a family history of cirrhosis or inherited diseases that cause cirrhosis, family members should be observed for sign of cirrhosis.
- If exposed to blood and body fluid on the job, use proper protective equipment such as gloves and eye protection to lessen the chance of accidental exposure.
- If you are in a high-risk group, you should receive the hepatitis B vaccine. High-risk groups are health workers, homosexual men, and household contacts of carriers.

The DON'Ts

- Avoid alcohol.
- Avoid medications that can be harmful to the liver such as acetaminophen, sedatives, and tranquilizers.
- Avoid chemicals and other substances that could be harmful to your liver.

When to Call Your Doctor

- If you have symptoms of cirrhosis.
- If during treatment for cirrhosis you have vomited blood, have passed a black stool or bright red blood, have mental confusion, or have fever or other signs of infection.

For More Information

Alcoholism

Alcoholics Anonymous World Services
P.O. Box 459
Grand Central Station
New York, NY 10163
212-686-1100

Liver Disease

American Liver Foundation
1425 Pompton Avenue
Cedar Grove, NJ 07009
1-800-223-0179
National Digestive Diseases Information Clearinghouse
2 Information Way
Bethesda, MD 20892-3570
www.niddk.nih.gov
nddic@aerie.com

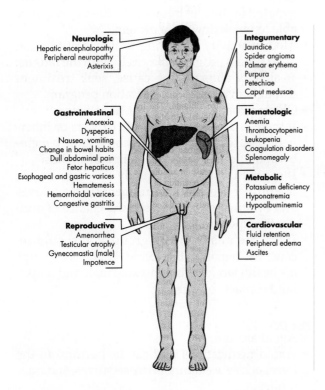

Systemic clinical manifestations of liver cirrhosis. (From Lewis SM, Collier IC, Heitkemper MM: *Medical-Surgical Nursing: Assessment and Management of Clinical Problem,* vol. 4. St. Louis, Mosby–Year Book, 1995. Used by permission.)

CIRRHOSIS, PRIMARY BILIARY

About Your Diagnosis

Primary biliary cirrhosis is a chronic liver disease. With this disease, the bile ducts in the liver become inflamed, blocked, and scarred, preventing the excretion of bile. This leads to liver inflammation and scarring, and eventually to cirrhosis of the liver.

The cause of this condition is not known. It does not appear to be inherited, but it does tend to be more common in families where one member has previously been affected. The role of the immune system is not clear but may be a factor in the cause. The incidence is 8 cases per 100,000 individuals. It is most commonly found in 35- to 60-year-old women. Detection usually comes during a routine blood test that shows abnormal liver function. A liver biopsy will confirm the diagnosis. The prognosis is dependent on the age of the patient and the degree of liver damage. Individuals who show no symptoms at the time of diagnosis often remain symptom free for more than 10 years.

Living With Your Diagnosis

Initially most individuals do not have symptoms. As the disease slowly progresses, pruritis (itching) develops involving the hands and feet and, in time, the entire body. Symptoms of liver damage, jaundice, abdominal pain, and dark urine then develop. Sun sensitivity is present. Steatorrhea (large, foul-smelling, bulky stools) will occur because of fat malabsorption in the gastrointestinal tract. This can lead to malnutrition. Physical signs of primary biliary cirrhosis include enlargement of the liver and spleen. In addition, small, yellow fatty deposits (xanthelasma and xanthoma) form around the eyes. This is a reflection of the elevated cholesterol level that is common in this condition. There is an increased risk of spontaneous fractures because of osteoporosis and osteomalacia; both are conditions that complicate this disease.

Treatment

There is no specific treatment for this condition. Research is ongoing. The nutritional deficiencies must be treated. A low-fat diet with vitamin supplementation is necessary. You should take calcium supplements to lessen the chance of spontaneous fractures. You can help control the itching associated with liver disease with cholestyramine, a prescription medication. For individuals with severe liver failure, liver transplantation is an option.

The DOs

- Eat a low-fat, well-balanced diet.
- Vitamin A, D, and K supplements may be needed.
- Calcium and zinc supplements may be need.

The DON'Ts

- Avoid drugs, foods, and toxins that are potentially harmful to the liver.
- Avoid alcohol.

When to Call Your Doctor

- If prolonged itching of the skin develops that is not related to other causes.
- If jaundice or other symptoms of cirrhosis develop.
- If during treatment for cirrhosis you have vomiting of blood, pass a black stool or pass bright red blood through the rectum, have mental confusion, or have fever or other signs of infection.

For More Information
American Liver Foundation
1425 Pompton Avenue
Cedar Grove, NJ 07009
800-223-0179

COLON CANCER

About Your Diagnosis

Colon cancer, colorectal cancer, and adenocarcinoma of the large intestine (bowel) are the same thing. Colon cancer is the most common cancer of the gastrointestinal tract. The cancer commonly involves the lower rectum and sigmoid portion of the colon but also can be found at the beginning of the colon (the cecum).

Approximately 160,000 people will be found to have colon cancer this year. Although not completely understood, environmental and hereditary factors are believed to lead to colon cancer. A high consumption of saturated fat (animal fat) and a low-fiber diet are leading theories of a dietary cause of colon cancer. The main risk factors for colorectal cancer are age older than 50 years, long-standing inflammatory bowel disease (ulcerative colitis, Crohn's disease), genital or breast cancer, and a family history of colon cancer or familial polyposis.

Colon cancer is usually detectable by means of colonoscopy (a scope is passed through the rectum to visualize the entire colon). Biopsies are easily performed on any suspicious areas, and any polyps (growths from the surface of the colon that can transform into malignant cancer) can be removed.

Colon cancer can be cured if detected early, before it has had the chance to spread (metastasize). The best way to detect colon cancer early is by means of screening (see below).

Living With Your Diagnosis

Signs and symptoms to be aware of are change in bowel habits, such as constipation; change in the caliber of stools (e.g., pencil-thin stools); black tarry stools; frank rectal bleeding; and abdominal pain.

Sometimes you may not have any symptoms but may be found to have iron deficiency anemia. This usually necessitates evaluation to exclude colon cancer. Colon cancer if undetected or untreated usually spreads through the wall of the intestine into the surrounding areas and also into the liver. Sometimes it can spread to the lungs and bone.

Treatment

The best treatment is prevention by means of screening. Screening guidelines include the following: a digital rectal examination annually after 40 years of age; testing of stools for occult blood annually after 50 years of age; and flexible sigmoidoscopy every 3 to 5 years after the age of 50 years.

Once the diagnosis of colon cancer is made, treatment depends on the extent of spread of the cancer. Abdominal and pelvic computed tomography (CT) is performed to determine whether the tumor has spread to the liver or outside the colon to regional lymph nodes. This information is important because it is used to decide whether chemotherapy is needed.

Surgical intervention is the best therapy for complete removal of the tumor and the best chance for cure if there is no evidence of spread. Also with surgical treatment, additional information is found about local extension of the tumor within the layers of the wall of the colon and within regional lymph nodes. This information is important because chemotherapy and radiation therapy may be recommended after surgical treatment.

Side effects and complications of surgical treatment include pain and infection. Radiation therapy may cause colitis with diarrhea and bloody stools. Chemotherapy can lead to bone marrow suppression making one prone to infection, bleeding, and anemia. Other side effects of chemotherapy include nausea, vomiting, diarrhea, hair loss, and mucositis (pain and redness) of the eyes and mouth.

The DOs

- Understand the importance of colon screening for all persons older than 50 years and for all family members of patients with colon cancer.
- Make sure your diet is high in fiber and low in animal fat.
- Make sure that once your cancer is diagnosed and you are treated and cured, you undergo colonoscopy 1 year postoperatively and every 3 years thereafter.
- Understand that there is a blood test called carcinoembryonic antigen (CEA) measurement that is usually performed once the diagnosis of colon cancer is made and after surgical treatment to detect recurrence.

The DON'Ts

- Do not forget the importance of screening.
- Do not miss follow-up appointments with your primary care physician, oncologist (cancer specialist), radiation oncologist if radiation therapy was provided, and general surgeon for wound care and colostomy care if you have a colostomy.

- Do not be afraid to ask your primary care physician about emotional support groups.
- Do not forget the importance of nutrition after surgical treatment.

When to Call Your Doctor

- If you have change in bowel habits, bloody or black stools, diarrhea, or constipation.
- If you have new abdominal pain or back pain with lower leg weakness.
- If you note skin color change such as jaundice.
- If you have a fever during chemotherapy.
- If you note abnormal drainage from within or around the colostomy site.
- If you continue to have no appetite and weight loss.
- If nausea and vomiting persist.

For More Information
National Cancer Institute
9000 Rockville Pike
Bethesda, MD 20892.
Cancer Information Service
1-800-422-6237 (1-800-4-CANCER)
American Cancer Society
1599 Clifton Road, N.E.
Atlanta, GA 30329
1-800-ACS-2345

CONCUSSION

About Your Diagnosis

A concussion is an injury to the brain caused by a blow to the head, or by striking the head on another object. It may result in loss of consciousness or confusion. It may also cause amnesia or loss of memory about the event that related to the concussion as well as a variable amount of time before or after. A history of loss of consciousness, amnesia, or confusion after a blow to the head is diagnostic of this injury. In addition, a neurologic examination, which may include a computed tomography (CT) scan or a magnetic resonance imaging (MRI) scan, reveals normal findings. The effects of a concussion usually resolve completely in a few hours or days.

Living With Your Diagnosis

The signs and symptoms of concussion include temporary unconsciousness, short-term amnesia (including events shortly before the blow to the head), dizziness, headache, confusion, mild lack of coordination, nausea and vomiting, and inability to concentrate.

All of these symptoms are short-term (hours to at most a few days) and should show steady improvement after the initial symptoms.

Treatment

Treatment consists of rest and careful observation. The initial symptoms of a concussion are similar to that of a head injury with bleeding into the brain. The difference is that the symptoms related to a concussion show improvement over a short period. If symptoms are worsening or not showing improvement, there is cause to worry about swelling or bleeding inside the skull. You can safely observe most individuals with a concussion at home. Indeed, a family member or close friend may notice changes in normal behavior that a medical person who did not know the patient might miss.

The DOs

Medications such as acetaminophen may be helpful for any headache. A light diet is appropriate. Many individuals with a concussion have nausea. If you are nauseous, you should stick mostly to small amounts of food or fluids; let your appetite be your guide.

Many individuals will have a headache. Vigorous activity may make it worse. You probably do not need to be at bed rest, but you should keep your activity light and get plenty of rest until you are feeling normal. Ask your doctor about when you may return to work or athletic competition. An ice pack to the area struck by the original blow may help with pain.

It is important to be watched for signs of increasing injury. Symptoms include increasing confusion, drowsiness, loss of coordination, loss of memory, or nausea and vomiting. You should not be alone. Someone should check on you every couple of hours for the first 24 hours or until you are feeling back to normal.

The DON'Ts

You should avoid any medicines or substances that cause drowsiness or changes in level of consciousness, including narcotic pain medicines, alcohol, sleeping pills, muscle relaxants, tranquilizers, or recreational drugs. The symptoms produced by all of these drugs are similar to those of increasing pressure within the brain, and may mask important symptoms of a worsening condition. You should avoid a heavy diet because this may lead to vomiting. You should avoid strenuous activity because this will usually result in a more severe headache. In addition, you should avoid operating dangerous machinery. Many individuals with a concussion will be dizzy, have a decrease in muscle coordination, have a decrease in ability to concentrate, or have a decrease in memory. These symptoms would make operation of machinery hazardous.

You should be very careful to avoid another concussion in the near future. Although a concussion usually resolves completely with no long-term effects, there is evidence that repeated concussions over time (especially within 3 months) may result in permanent brain damage and even death. Therefore, it is prudent to refrain from football, boxing, or full contact martial arts for a period of 3 months after a concussion to avoid another concussion.

When to Call Your Doctor

You should call your doctor if you have any increase in symptoms or if you are not improved within about 24 hours. Symptoms to be especially aware of include an increasingly severe headache; repetitive vomiting; increasing confusion; increasing drowsiness, including an inability to be wakened from sleep; muscle weakness on one or both sides; difficulty walking; unequal pupils or abnormal eye movements (which may cause double vision); and convulsions.

All the above symptoms will be an obvious change from normal for anyone that was familiar with the injured individual. All of these symptoms may be symptoms of a closed head injury with increasing pressure from swelling and bleeding. If you experience any of them, you must contact your doctor or the Emergency Medical System promptly.

For More Information

Brain Injury Association (formerly the National Head Injury Foundation)
1-800-444-6443
http://www.biausa.org

CONDYLOMA ACUMINATUM

About Your Diagnosis

Condyloma acuminatum are warts that appear in the genital area, including in the urethra and rectum. They are caused by the same human papillomavirus as other warts but are much more contagious. They can be easily passed from the skin of the infected individual, and are usually sexually transmitted. After exposure, the warts will appear in 1–6 months. They are curable with treatment.

Living With Your Diagnosis

There usually are no symptoms. These warts appear on moist surfaces such as the penis, and the entrance to the vagina and the rectum. They grow in clusters. Although the warts are small, the clusters can become very large. Complications of untreated genital warts can include cervical cancer in females and urinary obstruction in males.

Treatment

These warts need to be treated by a doctor. Small warts can be treated with a topical solution; larger warts may be treated with liquid nitrogen. Some may need laser treatment or surgical excision. Recurrence is common so treatment may need to be repeated. Your doctor may prescribe the ointment for you to apply at home.

The DOs

- Apply medication as instructed.
- Keep follow-up appointments until all warts are gone.
- Notify sexual partners so they can be examined and treated.
- Avoid sexual relations until the warts are completely gone; then use latex condoms during intercourse.
- Maintain proper hygiene.
- Be tested for other sexually transmitted diseases.

The DON'Ts

- Don't apply the medication to moles or birthmarks, or to warts that are bleeding.
- Don't have sexual relations until warts are gone and healing is complete.
- Don't skip follow-up appointments. The warts can recur and a different treatment may be needed.

When to Call Your Doctor

- You have signs of recurring warts.
- Treated areas show signs of infection—redness, swelling, tenderness, or a foul smell.

For More Information

The CDC National STD Hotline
800-227-8922
The American Social Health Association
800-972-8500
National Institute of Allergy and Infectious Diseases Office of Communications
Bldg 31 Rm7A-50
9000 Rockville Pike
Bethesda, MD 20892
Write for a free STD pamphlet.
Internet Sites
www.healthfinder.gov
www.healthanswers.com
http://sunsite.unc.edu/ASHA/

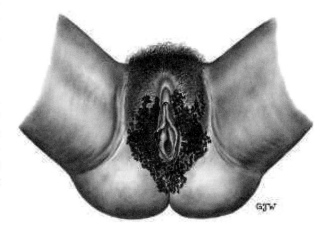

Human papillomavirus (HPV) infection. Condyloma acuminatum. (From Lowdermilk DL, Perry SE, Bobak IM: *Maternity & Women's Health Care*, vol 6. St. Louis, Mosby–Year Book, 1996. Used by permission.)

CONGESTIVE HEART FAILURE

About Your Diagnosis

Heart failure means the heart is failing to pump enough blood to the organs and tissues. One side of the heart (or both) cannot force enough blood out, so blood backs up into the system on the other side. This causes congestion in the tissues or organs. *Congestion* means that fluid leaks from the blood vessels into the tissues or organs, and blood does not move through the system well. If the left side of the heart fails, the system on the right side becomes congested, and vice versa. The congested side of the heart must work harder to move blood, and it also may eventually fail.

Living With Your Diagnosis

If the left side of the heart is in failure, the system on the right side becomes congested, causing fluid to leak back into the lungs. This causes fatigue, difficulty breathing (especially at night), coughing, or shortness of breath. If the right side of the heart fails, the left system becomes congested. This causes the liver to swell, which may cause pain in the abdomen. There may be swelling in the legs and feet.

Heart failure is relatively common; any disease that stresses the heart muscle can cause heart failure. Examples of conditions that cause heart failure are high blood pressure, heart attack, heart muscle disease, heart valve problems, infections, arrhythmias, anemia, thyroid disease, pulmonary disease, or fluid excess in the body. Congestive heart failure is detected with an examination for physical changes such as swelling in the legs or crackling breath sounds. It can be detected with a chest radiograph (x-ray) because the heart looks enlarged and there may be signs that fluid has leaked into the lungs.

Curing heart failure means curing the condition that caused the failure. You can manage congestive heart failure if you aggressively control your symptoms and monitor your breathing, swelling, and weight.

Losing weight means lowering the fat and calories in your diet. Needing to rest makes exercise difficult, but going for an easy walk can burn a few extra calories and help reduce stress and keep you moving. Ask your doctor if it is safe to exercise. Some patients with heart failure benefit from a nap during the day just to give their heart a break and can do well with normal activities through the rest of the day. Reducing salt and fluid intake means stop adding salt to your meals and choose low-sodium foods. Dieticians and nutritionists can help you plan a diet.

Treatment

The goal of treatment is to manage the initial symptoms so the failing ventricle does not have to work as hard. It is also important to manage the condition that caused the heart failure. To reduce its workload, the ventricle has to rest, pump less blood, and contract more efficiently. Resting helps reduce the workload. Decreasing fluid and salt in the diet reduces excess fluid in the blood and decreases blood volume. Additional oxygen eases the workload on the lungs. More oxygen is available for the blood, and less blood is needed.

Weight loss is important. It means less tissue to pump blood through, less blood volume, and less weight for the muscles to move. This reduces the work of the heart. Smoking also makes the heart work harder. If a heart valve problem is the cause, an operation may be needed to repair or replace the valve.

Medications may be prescribed to reduce fluid in the body or help the ventricle contract better. Diuretics help remove fluid. Nitrates help open blood vessels so blood flows more easily. Digitalis helps the ventricle contract efficiently. Blood pressure medications may be used to help reduce the pressure at which the heart has to pump. All these medications have side effects. Diuretics can cause dehydration or decrease electrolyte levels. Levels of digitalis have to be monitored. Digitalis causes low blood pressure, which may cause fatigue, dizziness, fainting, nausea, and vomiting.

The DOs

- Take your medications properly.
- Lose weight.
- Stop smoking.
- Decrease salt and extra fluid in your diet.
- Rest
- Decrease the stress in your life.
- Get your family involved in your care. It is important that they understand the lifestyle changes that you must make so they can help.

The DON'Ts

- Do not forget to take all your medications as directed.

When to Call Your Doctor

•If you have side effects from your medications.

•If you have new or worsening symptoms, such as increasing shortness of breath, chest pain, or fainting. You will see your doctor often during the early part of treatment. Ask other questions about diet and exercise as your condition improves.

For More Information

Contact the American Heart Association at 1-800-242-8721 and ask for the literature department.

CONJUNCTIVITIS

About Your Diagnosis

Conjunctivitis is an inflammatory condition of the outer lining of the eye where the outer part of the eye becomes red and irritated. Often there is an associated discharge.

Common causes of conjunctivitis are viral, bacterial and allergic. Most cases of viral conjunctivitis are caused by the same "cold virus" that causes a common cold, but instead of the virus infecting the mucous membrane lining of the nose and throat, it infects the mucous membrane lining of the eye. Viral conjunctivitis is highly contagious through direct contact with the tears. It is diagnosed by examination and its treatment is outlined below.

Bacterial conjunctivitis can be caused by a number of infectious organisms. It is diagnosed both by examination and by taking a culture. It is also transmitted by direct contact can be treated with antibiotics.

Allergic conjunctivitis produces a red irritated eye which also itches. The itching is the clinical sign that allows for the diagnosis of allergic conjunctivitis.

Living with Your Diagnosis

Conjunctivitis produces a red irritated eye with either a watery discharge (allergic and viral) or mucopurulent (bacterial). Conjunctivitis causes local discomfort and irritation. Serious sight threatening consequences are extremely rare.

Treatment

Viral conjunctivitis is treated with symptomatic treatment. Just as there is no "cure" for a common cold, there is no "cure" for viral conjunctivitis. Cool compresses often relieve the associated itching and burning. Topical decongestant drops can also provide relief.

Allergic conjunctivitis can be treated either with systemic (oral) allergy medications or topical eye drops specifically designed for allergic conjunctivitis.

Bacterial conjunctivitis is treated with topical antibiotic eye drops.

Although eye drops can cause local stinging and irritation, there are no significant side effects or complications associated with treatment of conjunctivitis.

The DOs

- Medications should be used as directed. If using more than one eye drop, wait five minutes between instilling each drop so that the second drop does not "wash" the first drop out.
- Patients with conjunctivitis should wash their hands frequently to avoid transmitting their infection to either their other eye, friends or family members.

The DON'Ts

- Patients with conjunctivitis should avoid touching their eyes and should not share towels, pillow cases, etc. with others since the infection can be transmitted this way.

When To Call Your Doctor

You should call your doctor if your conjunctivitis is associated with any of the following:

- Severe pain
- Fever
- Blurred vision

For More Information
American Academy of Ophthalmology, telephone #415-561-8500
Pamphlet , "The Red Eye" or
American Academy of Ophthalmology Website, "www.eyenet.org"

CONTRACEPTION

There are several different methods of preventing pregnancy available to couples. Many couples may have to try several methods of contraception to find out which method suits them. Lifestyle, frequency of sexual activity, and personal preference will affect one's choice of contraception. Many couples will use different types of birth control throughout their life. Choice of birth control method may also depend on the reason a birth control method is desired. For example, a couple may desire to space out their children, or a couple may need a birth control method while either the woman or the man is taking a medicine.

How Pregnancy Occurs

It is helpful to understand how a pregnancy occurs, to understand how a pregnancy can be prevented. Every month, approximately 12–16 days after a woman's period, the ovary produces an egg (this is called "ovulation"). The egg is released from the ovary and travels into the fallopian tube, which is connected to the uterus. Pregnancy occurs when the egg is fertilized by the sperm in the fallopian tube.

Therefore, pregnancy can occur if intercourse occurs around the time of ovulation. When the man ejaculates (or climaxes), sperm are released into the vaginal canal. The sperm travel through the cervix (the opening of the uterus) into the uterus, then into the fallopian tubes. If the sperm fertilizes the egg, pregnancy occurs.

Pregnancy can be prevented in three ways:
1. Prevent ovulation (the production of an egg from the ovary).
2. Prevent the sperm from traveling to the egg in fallopian tube.
3. Alter the lining of the uterus (the "endometrium") so it is not suitable for pregnancy.

Methods of Birth Control

Birth Control Pills

Birth control pills contain hormones that are very similar to the hormones produced by the ovaries. The hormones prevent ovulation, the release of an egg from the ovary each month. Because there is no egg than can be fertilized, pregnancy cannot occur.

Birth control pills are the most commonly used birth control method. They are easy to use—one pill is taken daily—and the method is very effective. Also, for most women, birth control pills are safe and cause few side effects.

Women that smoke, have high blood pressure, are obese, or have a family history of blood clotting disorders may have an increased risk of stroke, heart attack, or blood clot by taking birth control pills. These women should discuss their possible increased risks with their physician when deciding on an appropriate method of birth control.

Possible side effects of birth control pills include mild nausea and mild headache in the first 3 months. However, in most women, after the first 3 months, these side effects resolve. Other side effects include weight gain or weight loss, breakthrough bleeding (bleeding in between periods), persistent headaches (after the first 3-month adjustment period), and depression.

Birth control pills can be safely taken for years and stopped only 1 or 2 cycles before pregnancy is desired. Most women conceive easily after the pill is stopped.

Levonorgestrel Implants

Implants are one of the newer birth control methods in the United States. They are a safe, effective form of birth control that will last up to 5 years. Six slim capsules are inserted just under the skin on the inside of the upper arm. This procedure is performed under local anesthesia in the office. The capsules contain levonorgestrel, a synthetic progestin, which is released very slowly during the 5 years. This hormone prevents ovulation, in a manner similar to that of birth control pills.

The advantages of the implants are that they are convenient to use, and that their effects are completely reversible by removing the implants at anytime. Most women will become pregnant as easily as women who never used this method.

Possible side effects include irregular bleeding, headache, nervousness, nausea, dizziness, and removal difficulties.

Injectable Progesterone

Injectable progesterone is a progesterone-only form of contraceptive that is injected every 3 months. This hormone prevents ovulation in a manner similar to that of birth control pills and the implant contraception. It is very effective and safe for most women.

Women who may choose this form of contraception are those who should not take estrogen, who would like a form of birth control that they do not have to take daily, or who would prefer not to insert any device before intercourse.

Side effects include irregular bleeding. Most women who use this form of contraception will experience a change in their periods, such as irregular bleeding, spotting, and occasionally heavy periods. This irregularity will usually resolve for about 50% of users in 1 year, at which time the periods stop completely.

Injectable progesterone may have a prolonged contraceptive effect even after the medication is discontinued. Therefore, it may take 10 months, on average, to get pregnant once the medication is discontinued.

Intrauterine Device (IUD)

The IUD is a small device that is inserted into the uterus by a health care provider. The IUD alters the endometrium, making it unfavorable for implantation of the fertilized egg, or creates a reaction that prevents fertilization of the egg in the fallopian tube. There are two types of IUDs currently available. The "Copper T" is a small T-shaped plastic device with copper wrapped around it. This IUD only has to replaced every 8 years. Another type of IUD secretes the hormone, progesterone. This IUD has to be replaced every year, but it may decrease menstrual flow and cramps, so it may be useful for some women.

The IUD is often very useful for women who have had their family but do not want a permanent form of sterilization. The IUD is not recommended for women who have not had children, because they have an increased risk of pelvic infection from the IUD. The IUD may also increase menstrual flow and cramping, so women who already experience heavy periods and severe cramping may want to choose another form of birth control.

Barrier Methods

Barrier methods include (1) condoms, (2) diaphragms, and (3) cervical caps. All barrier methods should be used with a spermicide, otherwise the effectiveness of the method is decreased.

The condom is a thin covering made of rubber or animal membrane that is placed on the penis before intercourse. The condom prevents the sperm from entering the vaginal canal. Condoms should always be used in conjunction with a spermicide such as vaginal suppositories or vaginal foam to increase the effectiveness of the condom. Condoms can help decrease the risk of contracting a sexually transmitted disease.

The diaphragm is a rubber dome-shaped device that is placed into the vaginal canal over the cervix (the opening into the uterus). Spermicide jelly is place in the diaphragm before placing it in the vagina. The diaphragm helps to prevent the sperm from getting into the uterus, and it holds the spermicide jelly against the cervix so that any sperm that get past the diaphragm are inactivated by the spermicide. If the diaphragm method is used properly, it is a very effective method of birth control and it is very safe. Side effects from the diaphragm are rare.

The cervical cap is a small rubber device that fits right on the cervix to prevent sperm from entering the uterus and to hold spermicide against the cervix. It prevents pregnancy in a manner very similar to that of the diaphragm. The advantages of the cervical cap are that it is smaller than the diaphragm, so some couples feel they have more sensation with the cervical cap, and the cap can be left in place for 48 hours. (The diaphragm is usually taken out 6–8 hours after intercourse.) The disadvantages of the cap are that it is more difficult to learn how to correctly place the cap into the vagina on the cervix, and not all women can be fitted with a cap because it only comes in four sizes.

Permanent, Surgical Birth Control Methods

There are two "permanent" methods of birth control available currently. A tubal ligation ("tying the tubes") can be performed in the woman, or a vasectomy can be performed in the man. Although theoretically both methods can be reversed surgically, these methods should be thought of as permanent procedures because reversal of the procedures does not work in many cases.

A tubal ligation is performed by doing laparoscopic surgery. A very small (less than 1 inch) incision is made in or underneath the umbilicus (the belly button), and another incision is made just above the pubic bone. Instruments are placed that can either cauterize the fallopian tube or place a clip across it, thus closing it. This will prevent the egg from being fertilized by the sperm. The surgery is usually performed under general anesthesia, although sometimes it can be performed under local anesthesia. It is "day surgery," so you come in and go home the same day.

A vasectomy is a minor surgical procedure in which tubes in the testes are tied off so the sperm can not enter the ejaculate fluid. This procedure is often performed under local anesthesia in the office or in same-day surgery.

Couples may choose tubal ligation or vasectomy when they are sure they do not desire any more children or do not desire any children in the first place. Sometimes the woman may have a medical condition that makes it dangerous to get pregnant, so she may desire a very effective, permanent form of birth control.

Periodic Abstinence/"Rhythm" Method

Pregnancy is avoided by not having intercourse around the time of ovulation (release of the egg). This method only works if the woman has fairly regular cycles (the time from one period to the next). Ovulation can be estimated by counting the days from the previous period, watching for changes in the cervical mucus, and watching for changes in body temperature (the "basal body temperature" must be taken).

Statistically, this method is not very reliable. However, some couples are very successful in using it as their primary form of birth control.

Decision Making

Some couples may choose to use more than one form of birth control; for example, using the diaphragm to prevent pregnancy, but also using the condom to decrease the risk of transmitting sexually transmitted diseases. You may also use one form of birth control and then change to another type of birth control if desired. Many couples use different forms of birth control throughout their life depending on many factors.

You may want to consider the following when choosing a birth control method:
- How each method is used.
- Your age and health.
- How frequently you are sexually active.
- Your partner's feelings about birth control methods.
- How important it is that you avoid pregnancy.

Finally, sometimes it can be difficult to find a birth control method that will suit you. However, if you work with your health care provider and persist, most couples can find a birth control method that they can feel comfortable and safe with.

CORNEAL ABRASION

About Your Diagnosis

The cornea functions as a "clear window" on the front of the eye. A corneal abrasion is a scratch on the surface of the cornea. This is no different than a scratch on the skin in any other location on the body; however, because of the extreme sensitivity of the cornea, abrasions are extremely painful.

Living With Your Diagnosis

The signs and symptoms of a corneal abrasion are a red, painful eye often associated with blurred vision. Although the pain can be severe, there are very few long-term effects from the abrasion and the vision in almost all instances returns to normal.

Treatment

An antibiotic ointment is usually used to treat a corneal abrasion. The antibiotic helps prevent infection, and the ointment lubricates the corneal surface so that each time the eyelid blinks it does not rub against the irritated area.

Abrasions will heal with or without patching the injured eye shut. At times, patching may be used to help large abrasions heal more quickly. Contact lens wearers with a corneal abrasion should never be patched because of an increased incidence of infection with corneal abrasions in contact lens wearers.

There are no potential side effects or complications from the treatment of corneal abrasions. However, until the abrasions heal completely there is always a risk that the abrasion can get infected. Abrasions caused by organic material such as plant matter, or gardening equipment at a high risk for developing an infection.

The DOs

If the injury was caused by a severe blow to the eye, then a complete eye examination should be done to look for any other injuries. Patients with a corneal abrasion may use ice compresses and oral analgesics to help with pain relief. The antibiotic ointment should be applied at least two to three times during the day and definitely at bedtime to keep the ocular surface moist and well lubricated. If the eye is not patched, patients will often be more comfortable keeping the eye closed.

The DON'Ts

Topical anesthetics should never be used in treating corneal abrasions because they will prevent the abrasion from healing and can cause an infection.

When to Call Your Doctor

Corneal abrasions should always be evaluated by a physician and re-evaluated if they are slow to heal or the pain from them worsens.

For More Information
American Academy of Ophthalmology, telephone #415-561-8500
Pamphlet, "Eye Injuries" or
American Academy of Ophthalmology Website, "www.eyenet.org"

CORNEAL FOREIGN BODY

For More Information
American Academy of Ophthalmology, telephone #415-561-8500
Pamphlet, "Eye Injuries" or
American Academy of Ophthalmology Website, "www.eyenet.org"

About Your Diagnosis

The cornea functions as a "clear window" on the front of the eye. A corneal foreign body occurs when a foreign object hits and remains on the cornea. It commonly occurs when people are using power tools or hand tools. (In all these types of activities, people should always wear protective goggles.) If the foreign body is just on the surface of the eye, it can be removed easily in the office. If, however, the foreign body is deeply embedded, it may require surgical removal.

Living with Your Diagnosis

A corneal foreign body causes the eye to be red, painful and light sensitive. The vision may be blurred.

Treatment

A corneal foreign body should be evaluated as soon as possible by a physician. This will help determine the best method of removal. When the foreign body is removed, there will be a defect or scratch on the corneal surface. The eye will still hurt until the scratch is healed. The scratch will be treated with either an antibiotic ointment or antibiotic eye drop.

It is not always possible to remove the entire foreign body at one time. This is especially common with metallic foreign bodies which can leave a "rust stain." If the entire foreign body cannot be removed at once, the residual pieces can be removed in a day or two.

The DOs
- Seek medical treatment as soon as possible
- Follow directions for using antibiotic medication
- Wear safety glasses when working with hand tools, power tools, and machinery

The DON'Ts
- Do not use topical anesthetic for pain relief — it will prevent the eye from healing.

When to Call Your Doctor
- Increasing pain or redness
- Worsening vision

COSTOCHONDRITIS

About Your Diagnosis

The ribs are connected to the sternum (breast bone) by cartilage. This connection is called the "costochondral junction," which means the joining of bone and cartilage. Costochondritis is chest pain and tenderness in this region of the chest. One type of costochondritis caused by swelling of the cartilage is called "Tietze's syndrome." It can occur anywhere in the chest but usually on the left side.

Costochondritis is a common cause of pain in the front of the chest. No one knows what causes costochondritis, but certain forms of arthritis may cause chest pain in this area. Costochondritis is diagnosed by a medical history and physical examination. Tenderness over the cartilage is a common finding. Although there are no specific blood tests or x-rays for costochondritis, your doctor may order other tests to be sure you do not have another condition.

Living With Your Diagnosis

Individuals with costochondritis have pain and tenderness in the chest. The pain may be mild or severe and may last for several days or longer. Coughing, sneezing, deep breaths, and certain movements can make the pain worse. Some individuals feel anxious because of the pain and may feel short of breath.

Treatment

Costochondritis usually goes away on its own. Nonsteroidal anti-inflammatory drugs (NSAIDs) such as ibuprofen may be particularly helpful. Other treatments include heat and stretching exercises. If these treatments do not relieve the pain, a cortisone injection might be tried. Potential side effects of NSAIDs include stomach upset, ulcers, constipation, diarrhea, headaches, dizziness, difficulty hearing, and skin rash. Cortisone injections usually work quickly but require injecting a needle through the skin.

The DOs

- Take your medicines as prescribed.
- Follow your doctor's treatment instructions.
- Ask your doctor which over-the-counter medications you may take with your prescription medications.

The DON'Ts

- Wait to see if side effects from medications will go away.
- Leave a heating pad on for more than 20 minutes at a time.
- Continue an exercise program that causes pain most of the time.

When to Call Your Doctor

- You experience any medication side effects.
- You develop a new, unexplained symptom with your chest pain.
- You experience worsening warmth or redness of the skin after a cortisone injection.

For More Information

Contact the Arthritis Foundation in your area. If you do not know the location of the Arthritis Foundation, you may call the national office at 1-800-283-7800 or access the information on the Internet at www.arthritis.org.

CROHN'S DISEASE

About Your Diagnosis

Crohn's disease is a chronic inflammatory disease of the gastrointestinal tract. The most common areas it affects are the ileum, the lower portion of the small intestine, and the colon. Granulomatous ileitis and regional ileitis are other names for this disease. It is one of two disorders grouped in the condition called inflammatory bowel disease. The other disorder is ulcerative colitis. Crohn's disease causes inflammation of the entire thickness of the bowel wall. The cause of Crohn's is not known, but it is aggravated by bacterial infections and inflammation. Crohn's affects women slightly more often than men and appears to run in some families. About 1–5 per 10,000 individuals have Crohn's disease. The most commonly affected individuals are between the ages of 15 and 25 years.

Detection of Crohn's is by a flexible sigmoidoscopy, a procedure where a lighted flexible instrument is inserted into the rectum to view the lower portion of colon and rectum. Tissue samples are taken from the colon and sent for microscopic examination. Alternative detection methods are colonoscopy, a procedure similar to a flexible sigmoidoscopy but with a longer instrument, or barium enema x-ray. This is a lifelong condition in most individuals, but the disease course varies. Many individuals will not have symptoms after the first couple of attacks. Others will have recurrent symptoms. The majority of individuals with Crohn's can carry on a normal life but can expect a shorter total life expectancy. Medications can control the symptoms. This condition often requires surgery.

Living With Your Diagnosis

Abdominal pain and chronic diarrhea are the most common symptoms of Crohn's disease. The abdominal pain is usually right sided or around the navel. Eating may make the pain worse. The diarrhea can sometimes be bloody. It also can be severe enough to cause malnutrition. Other symptoms include fatigue, weight loss, loss of appetite, and fever. Symptoms are not limited to the gastrointestinal tract. About 20% of individuals will have joint pains. Others will have skin lesions.

Complications of Crohn's are many and varied. Bowel obstructions (blockages) are common. Fistulas and fissures in and around the anus and rectum can form. A fistula is an abnormal passage between two parts of the intestine or the intestine and the skin, bladder, or vagina. A fistula between two portions of bowel allows food to bypass certain areas of the bowel and causes malabsorption. A fistula between the intestine and the skin, bladder, or vagina causes continuous drainage of bowel contents onto the skin or into the bladder or vagina. This can cause infections. Fissures are cracks in the skin. Infections can be a complication of both of these conditions.

Treatment

The goal of treatment is to relieve symptoms, control the inflammation, and prevent complications. No treatment is necessary if there are no symptoms present. Mild symptoms of diarrhea are controlled with antidiarrheal agents and dietary fiber. If symptoms are more severe, anti-inflammatory drugs such as sulfasalazine and corticosteroids are given. If infections are present from fistulas and fissures, antibiotics such as metronidazole may be effective. Pain relievers and a hot water bottle can provide relief from the abdominal pain and cramping. If malnutrition is present, vitamin and mineral supplements are needed.

About 70% of individuals with Crohn's disease will require surgery for the disease at some point in their life. During surgery, a portion of the bowel is removed. An ileostomy, with a plastic pouch to collect stool, is generally done. The surgery is often done to control the complications.

The DOs

- Maintain normal physical activity except when symptoms require bed rest.
- Take medications as prescribed.
- A heating pad or hot water bottle placed on the abdomen may help with the pain and cramping.
- To relieve the pain of a rectal fissure, sit in a warm tub of water.
- See your physician regularly.

The DON'Ts

- Avoid fat in the diet.
- Avoid spicy foods, coffee, and alcohol. They can cause the diarrhea symptoms to worsen.

When to Call Your Doctor

- If you have symptoms of Crohn's disease.
- If you begin leaking stool through the skin or vagina.
- If fever or chills develop.
- If the number of bowel movements increase or if bleeding starts.
- If your bowel movement has a tarry appearance.
- If the abdomen becomes distended.

For More Information
National Foundation for Ileitis and Colitis
444 Park Avenue S, 11th Floor
New York, NY 10016-7374
800-343-3637
National Digestive Diseases Information Clearinghouse

CRYPTOCOCCOSIS

About Your Diagnosis

Crytococcosis is a disease caused by a fungus that usually starts in the lungs without causing symptoms, then spreads to the nervous system, kidneys, bone, or skin. It is more serious for individuals with underlying conditions. It can be life threatening for those with leukemia, Hodgkin's disease, transplant patients taking antirejection drugs, and AIDS patients. The fungus may be spread through the air by dust particles contaminated by pigeon droppings. It can be detected by laboratory studies and x-rays. It is curable with treatment.

Living With Your Diagnosis

Signs and symptoms include dull chest pain and a cough that may produce blood-streaked sputum; severe headache; fever; blurred vision; confusion; red facial rash; and skin ulcers.

Treatment

Mild cases in a healthy individual may require no treatment. Those with a suppressed immune system may need hospitalization.

Antifungal medications such as Diflucan will be prescribed. Side effects of the medication are nausea, vomiting, and headache. Tylenol can be used for minor pain and fever. No special diet is needed. Bed rest may be needed until fever and cough disappears.

The DOs

- Rest until the fever and cough subside.
- Take Tylenol for minor pain and fever.
- Take the antifungal medication until finished.
- Maintain adequate fluid intake and nutrition. Try small frequent meals if nausea is a problem.
- Keep follow-up appointments. Frequent visits to your doctor are needed to detect recurrence of the disease.

The DON'Ts

- Don't skip doses or stop taking the antifungal medication.
- Don't miss follow-up appointments with your doctor.

When to Call Your Doctor

- If you cannot tolerate the medication because of nausea and vomiting.
- If unexplained weight loss occurs.
- If a high fever develops during treatment.
- If a severe headache, neck stiffness, or blurred vision occurs.

For More Information

National Heart, Lung and Blood Institute Information Line
800-575-WELL
National Institute of Allergy and Infectious Disease
9000 Rockville Pike
Bethesda, MD 20892
301-496-5717
Internet Site
www.healthfinder.gov (Choose SEARCH to search by topic)

CUSHING'S DISEASE AND SYNDROME

About Your Diagnosis

Cushing's syndrome results from exposure of tissues to excess cortisol circulating in the bloodstream over time. Cortisol is a hormone produced by the adrenal glands. It is important for the maintenance of blood pressure, especially in times of stress. The amount of cortisol produced is tightly regulated by adrenocorticotropic hormone (ACTH) released from the pituitary gland.

The extra cortisol may come from medications prescribed by doctors for the treatment of other conditions such as asthma, bronchitis, or arthritis. Alternatively, certain tumors in the body may manufacture excess cortisol. These tumors may arise in the pituitary gland (Cushing's disease), the adrenal gland, or elsewhere in the body.

Cushing's syndrome is an uncommon disorder with approximately 2,500 new cases per year in the United States.

Cushing's syndrome is detected by performing a complete medical history and physical examination, and then measuring excess cortisol in a 24-hour urine collection or in the blood. For the blood test, a 1-milligram dose of dexamethasone is taken at midnight, and then a fasting blood cortisol level is measured the next morning at 8 AM. Once detected, the next step is to find out the cause. An ACTH blood level may provide a clue. If the ACTH level is low, the Cushing's syndrome is caused by a problem of the adrenal gland, and a computed tomography (CT) scan of the abdomen is performed. More commonly, however, the ACTH level is elevated, suggesting either a pituitary source or another source of the problem. A high-dose dexamethasone suppression test may then be ordered. Dexamethasone is given every 6 hours for 48 hours with a 24-hour urine collection before the test, after day 1 of the test, and after day 2 of the test. Patients with a pituitary source typically have a marked decline in cortisol levels in their urine over time. Others will have less of a decrease. Based on these test results, your doctor will suggest further imaging studies. These tests will generally localize the suspicious lesion in the pituitary or the chest. Occasionally, further testing is required. Once the tumor is localized, the treatment is to surgically remove the tumor.

Most cases of Cushing's syndrome are curable by eliminating the medication causing the disease or by surgical removal of the tumor. If it cannot be found, rarely patients may require removal of their adrenal glands to prevent extra cortisol from being produced. These patients must then take hydrocortisone to replace the missing cortisol.

Living With Your Diagnosis

Symptoms of Cushing's syndrome include increased weight and increased fat (especially upper body fat), facial flushing and rounding, increased blood pressure, frequent urination, poorly healing wounds, purple streaks on the abdomen, brittle bones, easy tiredness and weakness, personality changes, increased hair growth in women, and irregular menstrual periods.

Cushing's syndrome may predispose patients to diabetes, hypertension, osteoporosis, and obesity.

Treatment

The dosages of medications that cause Cushing's syndrome should be minimized. Tumors must be surgically removed. Surgery carries the risk of anesthesia, bleeding, or infection. Postoperatively, patients require hormone replacement therapy until the remaining gland recovers. For patients who are not surgical candidates or in whom tumor tissue remains postoperatively, radiation therapy is an option. For others, medications such as mitotane or ketoconazole may help control symptoms but may cause nausea or increased liver function tests.

The DOs

- Inform your doctor if you have a history of depression or drink alcohol every day. These may give a falsely elevated dexamethasone suppression test in an individual who actually does not have Cushing's.
- Find an experienced surgeon if you require surgery for your disease.
- Watch your intake of fat and calories to minimize weight gain.
- Have regular checkups for blood sugar, blood pressure, and bone density to ensure early treatment of diabetes, hypertension, and osteoporosis.

The DONT'S

- Don't begin an unsupervised exercise program until your blood pressure, blood sugar, and bones have been evaluated.
- Don't overeat.

- Don't take phenytoin (Dilantin) or phenobarbital for 1 week before dexamethasone suppression testing because this may cause a falsely normal test.
- Don't obtain radiologic studies until you have confirmed Cushing's syndrome with a blood or urine cortisol test and a blood ACTH level. This will prevent unnecessary studies or procedures.

When to Call Your Doctor

- You have a fever or infection.
- You have excessive weight gain or increased bruising.
- You are feeling weak or dizzy postoperatively. You may need to increase your replacement dose of hydrocortisone.

For More Information

Cushing's Support and Research Foundation, Inc. 65 East India Road, 22B Boston, MA 02110
617-723-3824 or 617-723-3674
Pituitary Tumor Network Association 16350 Ventura Boulevard #231 Encino, CA 91436
805-499-9973
National Institute of Diabetes and Digestive and Kidney Diseases
http://www.niddk.nih.gov/CS

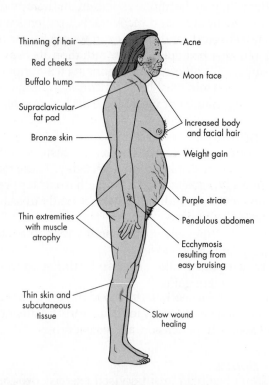

Common characteristics of Cushing's syndrome. (From Lewis SM, Collier IC, Heitkemper MM: *Medical-Surgical Nursing: Assessment and Management of Clinical Problems*, vol. 4. St. Louis, Mosby–Year Book, 1995. Used by permission.)

CYSTIC FIBROSIS

About Your Diagnosis

Cystic fibrosis is an inherited disease resulting from the abnormal transport of sodium and chloride (salt) within certain cells (epithelial cells) that form the mucus and sweat glands of the body. Because of this abnormality, thick and sticky mucus is produced that clogs the airways of the lungs, producing frequent infections. This disorder can also cause blockage of certain areas of the pancreas, preventing enzymes made by the pancreas and necessary for absorption of nutrients from reaching the small intestine. The lack of these enzymes can cause poor absorption of necessary nutrients.

Cystic fibrosis is the most common fatal genetic disease in the United States. It is more common in Caucasians, occurring in 1 of every 2,000 births. Approximately 1,300 new cases are diagnosed each year. Currently there are more than 30,000 individuals affected with CF in the United States.

Cystic fibrosis is an autosomal recessive disorder. This means that for a child to have CF, he must inherit a CF gene from each parent. There are more than 12 million Americans (1 in 20) who are asymptomatic carriers of the CF gene. Each time a child is conceived by two carriers, there is a 50% chance that the child will be a carrier and a 25% chance that the child will have CF.

If your physician suspects CF, a "sweat test" will be performed. It is a painless test that measures the amount of salt in the child's sweat. An abnormally high level of salt confirms the diagnosis. Siblings of any children with CF should also be tested.

Living With Your Diagnosis

Children with CF have chronic cough and recurrent bronchitis and pneumonia caused by obstruction of the lung airways. Chronic diarrhea, bulky foul-smelling stools, and excessive appetite (but poor weight gain) are also common because of deficiency of pancreatic enzymes. Intestinal blockage in the newborn caused by increased thickness of the first stool (meconium) may be the first sign of CF. Abnormalities of the sweat glands also cause "salty-tasting skin," usually noted by parents when kissing the affected baby.

Treatment

The type of treatment will depend on the stage of the disease and which organs are involved.

Postural drainage and chest percussion are often used to dislodge thick mucus from the lungs.

Medications are also available to thin thick mucus and prevent clogging of the airways.

Antibiotics are also often prescribed for suspected infections.

Pancreatic enzyme preparations to supply missing digestive enzymes, and special diets (high protein, low fat) may be used to improve nutrition.

The DOs

Some broad considerations for drug therapy include the use of (1) antibiotics, either nebulized, intravenous, or oral, adjusted for the susceptibility of the organisms found for each patient; (2) inhaled bronchodilators; (3) pancreatic enzyme supplements; (4) high-calorie nutritional supplements; (5) mucus-thinning agents such as acetylcysteine (Mucomyst) or DNAse; and (6) insulin, in a few cases. Family and patient education is very important because of the many questions and problems encountered.

The DON'Ts

- Don't forget to take proper precautions to avoid infections and excessive dehydration.
- Don't miss appointments scheduled by your doctor.
- Don't stop your antibiotics early or forget to perform chest physical therapy if advised by your doctor.

When to Call Your Doctor

The time to see or call your doctor differs for each patient with CF. A close partnership is required between family and caregivers to live as normal a life as possible.

For More Information
The National Institutes of Health
Public Information Office
Bethesda, MD 20892
Facts About Cystic Fibrosis, 1995.
Cystic Fibrosis Foundation
6931 Arlington Road
Bethesda, MD 20814
800-344-4828 or look in the phone book for your local CF chapter.

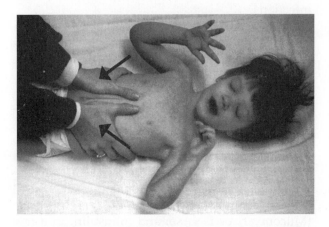

Manual lowering of the rib cage. Note: *arrows* indicate direction of therapist's hand movement (caudal and medial). (From Frownfelter D, Dean E: *Principles and Practice of Cardiopulmonary Physical Therapy*, vol 3. St. Louis, Mosby–Year Book, 1996. Used by permission.)

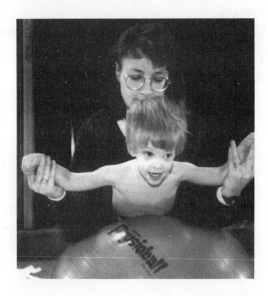

Handling to facilitate active upper thoracic extension, as a means of actively opening the anterior chest and lengthening rectus abdominis while supporting the lower rib cage on the ball. (From Frownfelter D, Dean E: *Principles and Practice of Cardiopulmonary Physical Therapy,* vol 3. St. Louis, Mosby–Year Book, 1996. Used by permission.)

DEPRESSION, MAJOR

About Your Diagnosis

Depression is a very common psychiatric complaint affecting at one time or another about 80% of individuals. In the medical sense, depression is not the same thing as being temporarily sad when bad things happen. This is normal. However, if sadness lasts for a matter of days or weeks, or prevents you from doing things such as working or being involved with your family, or involves any thoughts of hurting or killing yourself, then psychiatric evaluation for depression is indicated.

Depression is more common in women than in men. It can occur at any age, either after something happens in an individual's life or for no apparent reason.

Living With Your Diagnosis

One of the features of depression is trouble sleeping. This can be difficulty falling asleep, but more likely it is awakening early in the morning for no reason. Patients who are depressed often are wide awake at three or four in the morning, and are unable to fall asleep again. Less commonly, depression can involve too much sleep, where the individual might sleep most of the day. In addition to sleep problems, depression also involves changes in appetite. Some individuals do not eat when they are depressed and may lose a lot of weight. Others eat more when they are depressed. Other features of depression include losing interest in things that you once liked to do; being unable to concentrate on reading or watching television because your mind is wandering to other topics; feeling sad; having crying spells, often times for no reason; feeling badly about yourself, or feeling like your future is not going to be any better; being very agitated or restless, or moving and speaking very slowly; and losing interest in sexual activity. In severe forms, depression involves suicidal thoughts—that is, wanting to kill yourself—or homicidal thoughts—wanting to kill someone else. Or it may involve thinking about death all the time, dreaming about death, or wishing you were dead without actually planning to take your own life. Occasionally depression also involves psychotic features such as hearing voices, seeing things that aren't there including individuals who may have previously died, and

feeling that individuals are following you or talking about you behind your back (paranoia).

Depression can also be caused by certain drugs such as alcohol or "downers," such as Librium, Valium, Ativan, barbiturates, and similar drugs. There are also other medications that can cause depression. The list of these medications is very long, so you should always check with your doctor to see whether any medication you may be taking has been associated with depression.

There are also some medical conditions, such as thyroid disease and stroke, that are frequently associated with depression.

There are no specific laboratory or x-ray tests to diagnose depression. It is diagnosed on the basis of some of the symptoms mentioned earlier.

Treatment

Depression is treatable; therefore it is important to alert your family or your doctor if you experience any of the symptoms of depression. The treatment of depression usually involves using medications and talking to a therapist or a psychiatrist, usually at least once a week. The medications that are used to treat depression are called antidepressants, and there are many of them. Some of the more commonly used drugs are Zoloft, Prozac, Paxil, Elavil, Effexor, Sinequan, and Wellbutrin. Your doctor will have chosen an antidepressant that is designed to treat whatever particular symptoms of depression you may have. Some of these drugs will increase your sleep and appetite, but you should keep in mind that it takes about 2–3 weeks before you will begin feeling the effects of these drugs on depression. So, do not expect relief from the depression right away when starting antidepressant medication.

There are some side effects to the treatment of depression, and they depend on the drug that is used. However, some of the more common side effects include weight gain, sexual problems, oversedation, and nausea and diarrhea. If you have any side effects, let your doctor know because you may be able to take a different drug.

The DOs
- Decrease your exposure to stress.
- Make sure your diet is healthy.
- Exercise regularly.

The DON'Ts
- Don't use alcohol or drugs, because these will increase your depression or interfere with some of the medications that are being used to treat depression.
- Don't take any prescription or over-the-counter medication without first discussing it with the doctor who prescribed your medication for depression.

When to Call Your Doctor
- If your depression symptoms get worse.
- If you have any side effects from the medication you are taking.
- Call immediately if you have any suicidal thoughts or thoughts about killing or hurting someone else.
- Call immediately if you have any psychotic features, such as hearing voices or seeing things that are not there, or feeling paranoid.
- If depression related to grief involves suicidal thoughts. Depression can normally occur as part of grief—that is, after the death of a loved one. This depression related to grief usually gets somewhat better as time passes.

For More Information
Contact your family doctor, your local mental health center, your local crisis center hot line, or check out the following Web sites:
Clinical Depression Screening Test
http://sandbox.xerox.com/pair/ cw/testing.htm/
Depression and Mental Health Links
www http://drycas.club.cc.CMU.edu/~maire/depress.htm/ for a live chat with a counselor on depression on AOL Keyword depression.

DERMATITIS, ATOPIC

About Your Diagnosis

Atopic dermatitis is a skin inflammation caused by increased skin sensitivity to the environment. It often runs in families and may occur with hay fever, asthma, or nasal allergies as well. Atopic dermatitis is very common, affecting 1% of adult Americans, and 5% to 10% of American children. It is not contagious and is not transmitted by any known organism.

The increased skin sensitivity causes an "itch" sensation, which in turn causes the patient to scratch. Scratching, however, often provokes worsened itching. Scratching can also break the skin barrier, increasing the risk of infection.

Atopic dermatitis is treatable, and with appropriate medications and skin care, symptoms can be minimized or even eliminated. Without treatment, however, the skin inflammation may worsen and become complicated by scarring or infection.

Living With Your Diagnosis

Signs and symptoms of atopic dermatitis include reddened, inflamed, sensitive skin that feels dry and itchy. A slight burning sensation may also be noted. With oral and topical therapy, the dryness and itching can be reduced.

Treatment

The treatment of atopic dermatitis consists of moisturizing skin care and anti-inflammatory medications. Although a simple, nonmedicated moisturizing cream may be used on a daily basis, steroid creams are prescribed for severe episodes of itching. Use these carefully and only as directed by your physician. Do not use steroid creams on the face unless specifically directed to do so by your physician.

Oral medicines minimize the itch as well. One type, antihistamines, provide relief from the itch by calming the nerve endings in the skin. Unfortunately, most of these antihistamines also calm other nerves as well and can be very sedating (sleep inducing). Check with your doctor about which type of antihistamines you should use, and whether you should limit your activity (avoid cooking, driving, etc.) while taking them.

The second type of medicine taken orally is a form of steroid. Often prescribed in "dose-pack" or tapering regimens, steroids stop the inflammation, reduce redness, and minimize the itch. Although they work well, side effects limit their use to severe episodes. Long-term side effects from steroids (taken orally) include ulcers, bone loss, weight gain, and hormone imbalances, so the medicines must be used and tapered exactly as prescribed.

The DOs

- Do moisturize your skin on a daily basis, even when symptoms are not present. You may use an oil-based cream or ointment, and it is best applied immediately after bathing, while the skin is still slightly damp. Lotions are generally drying and do not moisturize as well as creams or ointments. Avoid products with fragrances (they may cause increased sensitivity) and multiple components (if your skin worsens after using them, you won't know which component caused the worsening). Use hypoallergenic products when possible. When itching becomes severe despite moisturizing, a very mild over-the-counter steroid cream (1% hydrocortisone) may be used in addition to your usual regimen. If no improvement occurs, it's time to call your doctor.

- Do use oral medicines as recommended by your doctor for the full course of treatment. Do not stop medicines sooner than recommended unless your doctor approves.

- Do avoid any type of food in which you may be allergic. Keeping a "food diary" may help you identify foods that cause your skin to worsen. If food allergies are present, avoidance of those foods may improve your skin disease somewhat. Ask your doctor for help in obtaining testing for allergies if you have a history of asthma or nasal allergies as well.

- Do exercise on a daily basis. Be careful to avoid excessive dryness and irritation that may result from the use of deodorant soaps afterward, and be sure to protect your skin from sun drying and damage with an appropriate sunblock (SPF 15 or greater). After showering with warm, not hot, water and mild soap, be sure to apply your usual lubricants.

- Do monitor the dryness in your home. Heated homes in the winter can become dryer than the desert! A home humidifier may help prevent excessive environmental skin drying.

- Do keep fingernails very short, to minimize the damage that may be done by absent-minded scratching. Wearing long pants and sleeves will also minimize random irritation.

- Do wash clothing and linens in fragrance-free soap, and double rinse when possible, to minimize irritating soap or detergent residues.

The DON'Ts

- Don't allow the skin to become excessively dry.
- Don't forget your daily skin regimen even if you are feeling well. Often flares occur during vacations, moves, etc., when the usual routine is broken. Plan ahead for trips by saving a supply of your usual skin care products and keeping them readily available.
- Don't drive, cook, or operate machinery while using antihistamines that cause drowsiness.

When to Call Your Doctor

- If you have fever, chills, nausea, or generalized aches.
- If you have signs of infection (worsening redness, pus).
- If you are wheezing or having difficulty breathing.
- If you have a severe stomachache or bone pain when using oral steroids.

For More Information
Asthma and Allergy Foundation of American
1-800-727-8462
National Eczema Association
1221 S.W. Yamhill, #303
Portland, OR 975205
503-228-4430

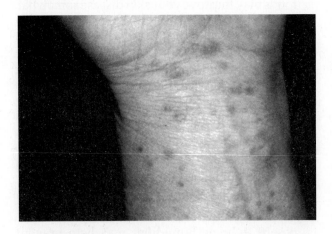

Atopic dermatitis. Classic distribution of lesions in children and adults. (From Goldstein BG, Goldstein AO: *Practical Dermatology*, vol 1. St. Louis, Mosby–Year Book, 1992. Used by permission.)

DERMATITIS, CONTACT

About Your Diagnosis

Contact dermatitis is a skin irritation that may be dry, red, and can blister. It is caused by skin contact with material that either irritates the skin or causes skin allergies. Contact dermatitis is very common. More than 50% of adult Americans have had at least one case. Many have contact dermatitis every time they are exposed to an allergen (like poison ivy). Contact dermatitis is not contagious. It can be treated with topical creams and lotions, by oral medicines, and by avoiding contact with the irritating materials.

Living With Your Diagnosis

Signs of contact dermatitis include dry, red, or blistery areas of skin. Symptoms may include itching, dryness, or mild pain. Contact dermatitis does not cause a fever. Wheezing or nausea may occur if the irritating substance was inhaled or swallowed, or if severe allergy occurs. Usually proper treatment causes rapid improvement in the redness and blistering, as well as the itch. Because the skin is fragile, repeated scratching may lead to infection, which may require use of an antibiotic.

Treatment

The best treatment is avoidance. If the offending substance can be identified, exposure to it should be eliminated as much as possible. For example, if you are allergic to wool, avoid buying wool clothes and blankets, and protect your feet if your carpeting is wool. If you are allergic to poison ivy, learn how to recognize it, then avoid contact as much as possible. Wearing gloves, long sleeves, and long pants when gardening will prevent accidental exposure.

Other treatment options include anti-inflammatory medications (steroids) to be used orally or topically, antihistamines to reduce itching, and immunotherapy (desensitization) to minimize the reaction.

Steroid medicines are powerful anti-inflammatory drugs and will quickly reduce swelling and irritation, but they also carry the risk of serious side effects. These may include stomach irritation, bone loss, and confusion, if the drug is taken orally. Topical use (creams or lotions) can produce thinning of the skin or worsening of bacterial infection if inappropriately used. For these reasons, steroids are usually prescribed for short periods (7–10 days). If longer use is required, your doctor will ask you to taper the dose slowly, because your body will need time to begin making its own steroids.

Other medications that may be used include antihistamines to reduce itching, and antibiotics to fight possible infection. Antihistamines can be very sedating (sleep inducing), so be sure not to drive, cook, or use machinery when taking them. Anti-itch lotions such as calamine are very soothing for oozing, blistery rashes, and may be used as needed. Oatmeal baths are soothing as well, but use with care because they make the bathtub slippery.

The DOs

- Do be sure to use your oral steroid and antibiotics each day as directed. Oral antihistamines can be used as needed and may be skipped if the itching improves.
- Do use steroid ointments and creams on clean, dry skin, and repeat 2 or 3 times per day as directed.
- Do use anti-itch lotions as needed, but avoid using them during the first hour after applying the steroid medications. (Give the steroid time to soak in first!)
- Do keep good nutritional habits while contact dermatitis is being treated. If you suspect an allergy to food, keep a diary of your meals and your skin symptoms to discuss with your doctor.
- Although exercise is important, hot, sweaty skin will itch more. Do wash and cool the skin soon after exercise.
- Do use a mild soap or cleanser (baby bath works well) to keep skin clean. Avoid any extra irritation that might be caused by deodorants or fragrances in the soap.

The DON'Ts

- Don't skip doses of steroid or antibiotic medicines. You will not lower your risk of side effects, and your dermatitis may worsen.
- Don't use antihistamine lotions or creams. These can cause rashes themselves!

When to Call Your Doctor

- If fever is present.
- If vomiting or diarrhea occur.
- If the rash worsens despite treatment, or a new or different rash occurs.
- If cough or wheezing is present.

For More Information

Asthma and Allergy Foundation of American
1-800-727-8462
American Academy of Dermatology
930 N. Meachum Road
Schaumburg, IL 60173
847-330-0230

DERMATITIS, DIAPER

About Your Diagnosis

Diaper dermatitis, commonly referred to as diaper rash, affects most infants at least once. It can be caused by irritants, yeast, or bacteria trapped against the infants' skin by diaper materials. In some cases, the diaper materials (synthetic absorbents, germ-killing rinses, etc.) cause irritation as well. It can be treated, and recurrences can be prevented by simple changes in diapering methods and proper medication.

Living With Your Diagnosis

Signs of diaper dermatitis include redness and irritation in the diaper area. Often this begins with faint, raised, pink spots, which seem to enlarge and to soon cover the diaper area if untreated. In extreme cases, the skin may look red and begin to peel. Skin folds may become raw as well. Baby is usually fretful and fussy, and may cry, especially after voiding or moving the bowels. Diaper dermatitis does not normally cause a fever.

Treatment

The best treatment for diaper dermatitis is prevention. By keeping baby's diaper area as dry as possible, outbreaks can be minimized. Once the dermatitis occurs, it requires treatment with topical creams as well as frequent diaper changes.

Many topical creams and ointments can be used for diaper dermatitis. If irritation from urine is the primary problem, a simple ointment containing zinc oxide will often be enough to provide relief. It should be applied at each diaper change after the diaper area is gently cleansed with lukewarm water and patted dry.

If the diaper dermatitis persists despite careful use of zinc oxide and frequent diaper changes, changing the type of diaper used may provide relief. Some babies are sensitive to chemicals in cloth diaper rinses, and others are irritated by synthetic materials in disposables. Switching brands or double-rinsing cloth diapers may eliminate the problem. Commercial diaper wipes are another source of irritation.

If yeast (*Candida*) has caused the dermatitis, your doctor may prescribe nystatin or clotrimazole ointments. Often yeast dermatitis occurs after antibiotic treatment for ear infections, and it may be accompanied by thrush (oral yeast infection). If so, your doctor may also prescribe oral nystatin drops to treat the thrush as well.

The DOs

- Do leave the skin open to fresh air as much as possible.
- Diaper loosely and change baby frequently.
- Do use lukewarm water with a soft washcloth for cleaning the diaper area after urination. A small amount of baby bath can be used on the washcloth for cleansing after bowel movements.
- Do reapply zinc oxide or antiyeast ointment at each diaper change.

The DON'Ts

- Do not wait for a physician visit to begin treating diaper dermatitis. If the diaper area appears reddened, immediately begin frequent (hourly) diaper checks, and change if any dampness is noted.
- Do not use commercial diaper wipes on a baby with diaper dermatitis because they will worsen the irritation.
- Do not use over-the-counter antibacterial ointments unless specifically recommended by your doctor. These can cause irritation and rash themselves and are rarely needed.

When to Call Your Doctor

- If body temperature is greater than 101°F (rectal) or 100°F (axillary).
- If rash worsens despite home treatment, or rash is expanding beyond the diaper area
- If baby refuses breast or bottle.
- If vomiting or diarrhea occur.

For More Information
American Academy of Dermatology
930 N. Meachum Road
Schaumburg, IL 60173
847-330-0230

DERMATITIS, HERPETIFORMIS

About Your Diagnosis

Dermatitis herpetiformis is a chronic, recurrent skin disorder characterized by clusters of itchy, small vesicles (blisters) and papules (red bumps).

The specific cause is unknown. It is likely autoimmune (i.e., a condition in which your immune system mistakenly attacks normal parts of the body, resulting in tissue injury or disease).

Dermatitis herpetiformis is uncommon. It typically affects adults between 20 and 60 years of age, although it may erupt in children. It occurs in males twice as often as in females.

This condition is hereditary but not infectious or cancerous. Other members of your family may have a history of dermatitis herpetiformis. Hot, humid weather may trigger an eruption of the skin lesions. Some individuals with this condition have gluten sensitivity and celiac disease, genetic disorders of the small intestine in which an individual cannot normally digest gluten, a major protein in wheat.

Diagnosis is usually based upon the appearance of the skin lesions. Your doctor may perform a skin biopsy (i.e., removal of a small piece of skin or other tissue) for laboratory evaluation to assist in diagnosis. Your doctor may also order blood tests to check for certain immune markers that may aid in the diagnosis.

Dermatitis herpetiformis is a chronic condition in which episodes may persist for days, weeks, months, or even years. Periods of remission occur between episodes. Treatment can control symptoms and may lessen the severity and duration of the skin lesions, but does not cure the disease.

Living With Your Diagnosis

Skin lesions are very itchy and may occasionally cause a burning or stinging sensation. Lesions appear as clusters of blisters that are typically symmetric (i.e., develop simultaneously in similar patterns on both sides of your body). Scratching the lesions can cause abrasions, crusting, and secondary bacterial infections. Lesions typically involve the scalp, face, elbows, forearms, knees, shoulder blades, lower back, and buttocks.

Scratching may cause secondary bacterial infections requiring antibiotic therapy. After healing, the skin may show spots of darker pigmentation. If you also have celiac disease (see above), you may or may not have symptoms. Symptoms include diarrhea, weight loss, fatigue, and abdominal gas, which can cause cramping and bloating. Diagnosis of celiac disease usually requires a biopsy of the small intestine and blood tests for immune markers. You may also experience social embarrassment because of your skin's appearance.

Treatment

Specific treatment of dermatitis herpetiformis depends upon its location and severity, the impact it has on the quality of your life, and your response to therapy. Treatment lessens the severity of your condition and prevents complications, but it does not cure dermatitis herpetiformis. Treatment includes the avoidance of precipitating factors, general measures, and medications.

General measures include:
- Cool-water soaks to soothe irritation and decrease itching.
- Restricting gluten in your diet, which can suppress dermatitis herpetiformis or may allow you to decrease the dosage of your medication.

Your doctor may prescribe a variety of medications to reduce inflammation, improve symptoms such as itching, and lessen the severity and duration of your dermatitis herpetiformis. These medications include:
- Topical steroid creams, lotions, and ointments to reduce inflammation. These medications are effective. Exercise caution when using topical steroids because they may be absorbed through your skin into your bloodstream and cause toxic effects.
- Calamine lotion and similar agents can reduce itching and irritation.
- Antihistamines reduce itching and may allow you to rest more easily. They may cause drowsiness, so use these agents cautiously when driving or performing other activities in which you must be awake and alert.
- Dapsone or sulfapyridine may be prescribed to reduce skin eruptions and blistering. You will probably need to take one or both of these agents for an extended time. Your doctor will likely monitor for side effects by checking periodic blood tests. Side effects include hemolytic anemia, peripheral neuropathy (tingling, numbness, or loss of feeling), muscle weakness, and liver toxicity.

The DOs

- Take medications as prescribed by your doctor. Inform your doctor of all other medications, including over-the-counter medicines, that you are now taking. Continue these medications unless your doctor instructs you to stop them.
- Read the labels of medicines and follow all instructions. Consult your doctor if you have any concerns or if you have side effects caused by the medication.
- Eliminating or restricting gluten in your diet may improve your condition or may allow you to reduce the dosage of medications used to treat dermatitis herpetiformis.
- Avoid activities that cause overheating and excessive sweating or moisture. If you perform activities that result in excessive moisture, immediately shower and cleanse the skin lesions.
- Maintain good skin hygiene to reduce the risk of secondary bacterial infection.
- Keep scheduled follow-up appointments with your doctor. They are essential to monitor your condition, your response to therapy, and to screen for possible side effects of treatment.
- Monitor your skin for healing and for evidence of secondary bacterial infection. Signs and symptoms of infection include redness around the skin lesions, purulent discharge (pus), increased pain or swelling of the skin lesions or lymph nodes, and fever.
- Frequently wash clothing, towels, and linens as skin lesions are oozing, crusting, or may be infected. This action reduces the risk of transmission of infection.

The DON'Ts

- Do not stop your medicine or change the prescribed dose without consulting your doctor. Do not exceed recommended doses of medicines, because higher doses may increase your risk of toxic effects.
- Do not use potent topical steroids on the face or genitals because these areas are most prone to skin injury and atrophy (thinning and wasting of the skin associated with wrinkling and abnormal, small blood vessels).
- Do not drive or perform other potentially hazardous activities when taking medication that can cause drowsiness or sedation (e.g., antihistamines).

- Avoid activities that can cause overheating, sweating, or excessive moisture, because these conditions can trigger or aggravate your dermatitis herpetiformis.
- Avoid activities that can cause infection of the skin lesions.

<#4>When to Call Your Doctor

- If any signs or symptoms of infection develop (see above).
- If you notice that lesions are becoming worse or if new lesions appear despite appropriate therapy.
- If new or unexplained symptoms develop that may indicate a complication of your condition or a side effect of treatment.

For More Information

Consult your primary care physician or your dematologist to learn more about dermatitis herpetiformis. You may also contact: American Academy of Dermatology
Attention: Communications Department
930 N. Meacham Road
Schaumburg, IL 60173
847-330-0230

DERMATITIS, STASIS

About Your Diagnosis

Stasis dermatitis is a chronic inflammation and irritation of the skin, usually in the lower legs, resulting from poor circulation of blood and lymphatic fluids. It is caused by conditions that slow normal fluid return from the feet to the heart. Common causes include lack of movement, obesity, and congestive heart failure. It is very common, affecting 50% of Americans with these risk factors.

Living With Your Diagnosis

Signs and symptoms of stasis dermatitis include reddened, swollen feet and lower legs. Often the skin appears shiny. The feet may become painful as swelling worsens. Small sores or ulcers may appear on the feet or lower legs, and may not heal well. The effects of the swelling and skin breakdown include predisposition to infection, which may be limited to an ulcer or become so extensive that deeper tissues (muscle or bone) may be involved. Severe pain and swelling also limit a patient's activity, as walking becomes more painful. This decrease in exercise worsens the condition further and results in progressive disease if not corrected.

Treatment

Treatment consists of reducing the fluid trapped in the feet and lower legs. Mechanical devices such as hospital-grade support hose or leg compression pumps are very effective in improving fluid return from the legs if used consistently. Some patients may also benefit from diuretics (water pills). Because diuretics may cause potassium or calcium losses, or result in fluid imbalance, it is essential that they only be used if prescribed by your physician. Not all patients can use diuretic therapy.

The DOs

- Do take diuretics exactly as prescribed. Your doctor will need to check your potassium, calcium, and kidney function periodically while on these medicines. Check with your doctor for the schedule of testing right for you.
- Do use your mechanical devices such as support hose or compression pumps every day. Compression hose should be ordered specifically for you. Your nurse will check your thigh and leg-length measurements to ensure the proper size is ordered. Hose should be bought in sets of two pairs, so one can be worn while the other is laundered. Put the hose on first thing in the morning after bandaging any ulcers or sores carefully. They should be removed at night for sleeping.
- Do learn to use your compression pump properly. Your home health nurse will instruct you in the care of the inflatable cuffs as well as safe use of the pump. Pumps should be used as directed by your doctor for several sessions each day. Be sure to follow instructions carefully to ensure proper fit of the cuffs and adequate time for them to work.
- Do eat a low-fat, low-cholesterol diet and avoid excess salt. Ask your doctor how much salt you may have each day. In general, more than 4 grams (4,000 mg) of sodium will increase foot swelling, and some patients must limit their intake to even lower levels. Local bookstores have many books about diet to help you calculate your daily fat, cholesterol, and salt intake. These are helpful to plan meals, and the best ones will list the values for typical fast-food choices as well. Also ask your doctor whether you need to limit water intake. Although most individuals need 8 glasses of water per day, patients with stasis dermatitis may need slightly less. Check with your doctor to be sure.
- Do exercise daily. Twenty minutes of mild-to-moderate exercise (walking), if approved by your doctor, will improve circulation and fluid return from the legs. If walking is too difficult because of swelling, physical therapy may be used to improve strength and range of motion. When seated or reclining, elevation of the legs may be helpful as well.

The DON'Ts

- Don't take diuretics prescribed for other individuals.
- Don't use more that 4 grams of salt per day.
- Don't miss blood tests for potassium and kidney function.
- Don't exercise without your doctor's permission.
- Don't sit for prolonged periods with your legs crossed or your feet hanging down.

When to Call Your Doctor

- If you notice new sores, ulcers, or redness in the feet or legs.

- If you have increased swelling in the legs despite use of hose or pumps.
- If you have fever, chills, or shortness of breath.

For More Information

American Heart Association
1-800-242-8721
American Cancer Society
1-800-227-2345
American Academy of Dermatology
930 N. Meachum Road
Schaumburg, IL 60173
847-330-0230

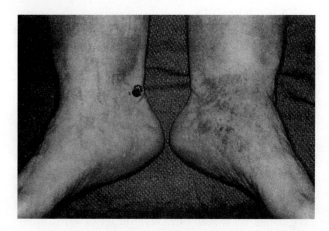

Moderate stasis dermatitis with hyperpigmentation and bilateral venous insufficiency. (Courtesy of Department of Dermatology, University of North Carolina at Chapel Hill. From Goldstein BG, Goldstein AO: *Practical Dermatology,* vol 1. St. Louis, Mosby–Year Book, 1992. Used by permission.)

DIABETES INSIPIDUS

About Your Diagnosis

Diabetes insipidus is a disorder resulting from a decreased amount or action of the antidiuretic hormone (ADH), also known as vasopressin. Antidiuretic hormone is normally secreted by the posterior pituitary into the bloodstream where it acts upon the kidneys to maintain normal water balance.

There are two main types of diabetes insipidus, central and nephrogenic. Central diabetes insipidus is caused by decreased production of ADH by the posterior pituitary. In nephrogenic diabetes insipidus, the production of ADH is normal or increased, but the kidneys are resistant to the effects of the hormone.

Diabetes insipidus is a rare disorder except in certain circumstances. Patients with hypothalamic or pituitary tumors or infections may have central diabetes insipidus as a result of compression or as a side effect of surgical exploration. Patients with head injuries or meningitis may have central diabetes insipidus as well. Nephrogenic diabetes insipidus may be a hereditary disorder or a result of medicines such as lithium.

Diabetes insipidus is usually suspected in patients who have a large volume of dilute urine output and excessive thirst. A 24- hour urine collection is obtained to document the volume of urine produced. Special tests are performed on the urine and blood to determine whether the kidneys are excreting a normal amount of water. One test is the specific gravity. The specific gravity of urine is inappropriately low in diabetes insipidus.

Once diabetes insipidus is diagnosed, the next step is to figure out the cause. If the medical history and physical examination do not reveal the answer, a vasopressin (ADH) level may be measured. In central diabetes insipidus, the vasopressin level is low. In nephrogenic diabetes insipidus, the vasopressin level is normal or high. Some patients may require a water deprivation test to see whether ADH is released normally in response to dehydration. If central diabetes insipidus is suspected, a magnetic resonance imaging (MRI) scan of the posterior pituitary will be performed, revealing an absence of the normal posterior pituitary bright spot.

Diabetes insipidus is generally curable if it is caused by pressure on the posterior pituitary by a tumor. The cure is to remove the tumor. It may also be merely a transient condition after pituitary surgery that resolves spontaneously. If it is caused by a medicine and the medicine is stopped, the diabetes insipidus usually resolves. In other cases, however, the condition may be permanent. The symptoms may be ameliorated with certain treatments.

Living With Your Diagnosis

Symptoms include frequent urination of high volumes of very dilute, watery urine, urinating at night, extreme thirst (especially a desire for cold water), or dehydration with dizziness upon standing. Family members may notice behavioral changes if the patient has been unable to obtain enough water.

Untreated diabetes insipidus may lead to markedly elevated blood sodium, mental confusion, seizures, and death.

Treatment

Patients with nephrogenic diabetes insipidus must stop any drugs that are exacerbating the condition and maintain a liberal intake of water whenever thirsty. Patients are able to autoregulate their serum sodium to normal levels based only on their thirst. Any attempts to restrict patients from access to water may result in severe elevation of sodium levels.

Central diabetes insipidus is responsive to DDAVP (desmopressin) subcutaneously or as a nasal spray. This medicine is usually started once a day, although some patients require twice-a-day administration. Complications from this medicine include a decreased sodium from overtreatment. Serum electrolytes must be closely monitored.

The DOs

• Drink water whenever thirsty. You are the best person able to regulate your serum sodium based on your natural thirst mechanism.
• Take your medicine as prescribed.
• Allow several hours of increased urination and thirst at least every few days to avoid complications of hyponatremia (low serum sodium) from overtreatment with DDAVP.
• Find an experienced surgeon if you require surgery, to help minimize the risk of permanent diabetes insipidus.

The DON'Ts

• Don't drink lots of high sodium-containing fluids such as soft drinks to relieve your thirst. This

may lead to worsening symptoms. Instead, choose water.
- Don't confuse diabetes insipidus with diabetes mellitus. Both may cause frequent urination, but diabetes mellitus is associated with a high blood sugar, whereas diabetes insipidus is not.

When to Call Your Doctor

- You notice unquenchable thirst.
- You or a family member notices a change in your ability to think.
- You have worsening frequency of urination despite treatment.
- You have high fever, diarrhea, or sweats.
- You are about to undergo elective surgery.

For More Information

Pituitary Tumor Network Association   16350 Ventura Boulevard   Encino, CA 91436
1-800-642-9211 or 805-499-9973
The Endocrine Society
4350 East West Highway, Suite 500
Bethesda, MD 20814-4410
1-888-ENDOCRINE

DIABETES MELLITUS, TYPE I

About Your Diagnosis

Type I diabetes is a disease of the insulin-producing cells of the pancreas that results in the inability of the body to metabolize nutrients normally.

Type I diabetes is caused by a lack of insulin. Insulin is a hormone produced by special cells in the pancreas called beta cells. In most individuals with type I diabetes, beta cells are destroyed by the body's own natural defense system, the immune system. Researchers do not know what causes the body to attack its own beta cells. Without insulin, the body is unable to normally use carbohydrates from the diet for energy. The result is a buildup of sugars in the bloodstream called glucose. Type I diabetes may develop in other patients as a result of certain diseases, such as cystic fibrosis or hemochromatosis. Type I diabetes may also result from surgical removal of the pancreas or severe inflammation of the pancreas.

Type I diabetes is slightly more common in men than women and has a peak age of onset at 12–15 years. Most cases are diagnosed before 30 years of age. It is more common in Caucasians of European descent than in other ethnic groups. There are currently more than 300,000 individuals in the United States with type I diabetes.

There currently is no cure for diabetes, except under special circumstances, in which patients receive a pancreas transplant operation. It is generally reserved for only those few patients with advanced kidney disease, who are receiving a simultaneous kidney transplant.

Living With Your Diagnosis

Symptoms of type I diabetes include frequent urination (especially at night), excessive thirst, increased hunger, rapid weight loss, and extreme fatigue. Blurry vision, slow-healing sores in the skin, or numbness in the hands or feet may develop.

Type I diabetes may lead to decreased vision and blindness. Kidney failure requiring dialysis may occur. Nerve damage may also occur. These complications generally happen after many years of type I diabetes, especially if poorly controlled. Patients with type I diabetes are also at increased risk of coronary heart disease and peripheral vascular disease.

Treatment

The best treatment for type I diabetes involves a team approach of medical professionals who specialize in the care of diabetes, including a registered dietician, a certified diabetes educator, and a physician. The dietician will establish a meal plan with predictable quantities of carbohydrates and calories eaten at specific times of the day. The diabetes educator will teach insulin administration techniques, home blood glucose monitoring, and the treatment of high and low blood sugars. The physician will take a complete medical history, perform a physical examination, and prescribe insulin. Long-term studies have proven that individuals who undergo intensive insulin therapy using multiple injections of insulin a day, or an insulin pump, are able to achieve better control of their blood sugar levels and have fewer complications from their diabetes. Additional members of the health care team that may be consulted include an exercise physiologist, a psychologist, a podiatrist, a nephrologist, and an ophthalmologist.

Hypoglycemia, or low blood sugar, is the most common side effect of diabetes treatment. Occasionally a severe hypoglycemic reaction may occur in which the patient becomes unconscious or has a seizure. Other possible side effects from treatment include fat atrophy at the insulin injection site, leading to poor insulin absorption over time. Very rarely an allergic reaction to insulin may occur.

The DOs

- Follow your diet, eating regular meals at regular times.
- Learn how exercise and food affects your blood sugar levels.
- Take your insulin as prescribed.
- Monitor your blood sugar levels at home.
- Obtain an annual eye examination by an ophthalmologist if you have had type I diabetes for more than 5 years.
- Obtain annual urine testing for protein.
- Obtain a hemoglobin A1c blood test every 3–6 months as an indicator of your long-term blood sugar control.
- Instruct family members in the use of glucagon administration in the case of low blood sugar emergencies.

The DON'Ts
- Don't skip doses of your insulin, especially when you are sick.
- Don't run out of your insulin.
- Don't drink excessive amounts of alcohol because this may lead to unpredictable low blood sugar reactions.
- Don't forget that exercise will lower your blood sugar level.

When to Call Your Doctor

- If you have a fever or nausea and vomiting and are unable to keep down any solids or liquids.
- You are having high or low blood sugars that you cannot explain.
- You are overdue for your eye examination or urine protein test.

For More Information
Joslin Diabetes Center
One Joslin Place
Boston, MA 02215
617-732-2400.
American Diabetes Association
1-800-232-3472
http:\\www.diabetes.org.
National Institute of Diabetes and Digestive and Kidney Diseases
http:\\www.niddk.nih.gov.

DIABETES MELLITUS, TYPE II

About Your Diagnosis

Type II diabetes is a disease in which the amount of insulin produced by the pancreas is inadequate to meet the body's needs. Insulin is a hormone that is vital to proper metabolism of glucose. In type II diabetes, glucose is not taken up normally from the blood into body tissues. The tissues are insulin resistant. Initially the pancreas is able to compensate for this extra blood glucose by increasing insulin production. Eventually, the pancreas cannot supply enough insulin to meet the body's demand, and blood sugars begin to rise. This early rise in blood sugars is known as impaired glucose tolerance (IGT). Diabetes will develop in 1% to 5% of individuals per year with IGT.

Insulin resistance may also develop in pregnant women, especially late in pregnancy. When this leads to elevated blood sugars, it is called gestational diabetes mellitus (GDM). Gestational diabetes mellitus usually resolves at the end of the pregnancy. These women are at higher risk of developing diabetes later in life.

Eight million adults in the United States have received a diagnosis of type II diabetes; another 8 million remain undiagnosed. Type II diabetes occurs more commonly in individuals with IGT, obesity, and in certain ethnic populations (African Americans, Native Americans, and those of Hispanic origin).

According to 1997 American Diabetes Association guidelines, type II diabetes is detected by a fasting blood sugar greater than 126 mg/dL measured on two or more occasions, or two random blood sugar levels greater than 200 mg/dL, or one blood sugar level greater than 200 mg/dL in an individual with symptoms of diabetes.

An oral glucose tolerance test (OGTT) may also be used to diagnose diabetes. A glucose level of 200 mg/dL or more 2 hours after drinking 75 grams of glucose defines diabetes in the OGTT. For pregnant women, a 50-gram glucose drink is followed by a blood test 1 hour later. If the blood glucose level is 140 mg/dL or greater, a follow-up test with 100 grams of glucose that lasts 3 hours is performed. If any two or more of the following values are elevated, the patient is considered to have GDM: fasting, greater than 105 mg/dL; 1 hour, greater than 190 mg/dL; 2 hour, greater than 165 mg/dL; or 3 hour, greater than 145 mg/dL.

There is no cure for type II diabetes, but every year new treatments are becoming available.

Living With Your Diagnosis

Signs and symptoms of type II diabetes include excessive thirst, frequent urination (especially at night), and increased appetite. Blurry vision and numbness in the toes or fingers may also occur. Most patients feel tired and may have slow-healing sores. Many individuals have no symptoms early in their disease.

Type II diabetes is the leading cause of blindness in working adults in the United States. It is also a leading diagnosis of patients with end-stage renal disease who are receiving dialysis. It is a major cause of amputations and places patients at increased risk for coronary heart disease.

Treatment

Patients should follow a low-fat, low-calorie diet. Aerobic exercise under physician guidance is beneficial. Many oral medications are now available for the treatment of diabetes, each with its own benefits and risks. Finally, insulin may be used for patients whose diabetes is not well controlled despite all the above measures. Insulin may also be temporarily used for patients who are sick or undergoing surgery.

Risk factors for heart disease must be controlled. Blood cholesterol, blood pressure, and body weight should be normalized. Cigarette smoking must be discontinued.

Complications of diabetes must also be prevented. An annual eye examination by an ophthalmologist is recommended for all patients with type II diabetes. A urine test for protein is performed once a year. A foot examination is conducted regularly to detect early nerve damage.

The DOs
- Monitor your blood sugars at home and record these in a log.
- Follow your diet.
- Begin a medically supervised exercise program.
- Obtain annual eye examinations and urine tests for protein.
- Examine your feet at home.
- Learn your cholesterol level.

The DON'Ts

- Don't exercise if your blood sugar levels are very elevated. This may lead to a temporary worsening of your blood sugar levels.
- Don't enroll in a fad diet.
- Don't skip your insulin if you feel ill.

When to Call Your Doctor

- You have a high or low blood sugar level you cannot explain.
- You have a fever or are otherwise sick.
- You are scheduled for surgery or a radiology procedure that requires intravenous dye.
- You notice an abrupt change in your vision.
- You have a nonhealing ulcer on your foot.

For More Information

Joslin Diabetes Center
One Joslin Place
Boston, MA 02215
617-732-2400
American Diabetes Association
1-800-232-3472
http:\\www.diabetes.org
National Institute of Diabetes and Digestive and Kidney Diseases
http://www.niddk.nih.gov

DIFFUSE INTERSTITIAL PULMONARY DISEASE

About Your Diagnosis

The term "diffuse interstitial pulmonary disease" is a collective name for a group of many different lung diseases that have varying causes and manifestations. These diseases are linked together because they all cause inflammation of the area surrounding the air sacs of the lungs. This inflammation can result from inhalation of environmental or job-related irritants, medications, radiation, inflammatory diseases outside the lung, or for unknown reasons. The inflammation often leads to lung scarring (fibrosis) that significantly impairs lung function. These conditions are not contagious. There are no preventive vaccines, and they are generally difficult to treat because cures are not available in most circumstances.

A typical interstitial lung disease is idiopathic pulmonary fibrosis. The term "idiopathic" means that the cause of the lung scarring is unknown. This is a chronic disease of middle-aged men and women that is characterized by a steady decline in exercise tolerance as the lung scarring progresses. Fifty percent of patients will die within 3–5 years of the onset of chest symptoms. Some patients will decline rapidly, whereas others will stabilize over time. Spontaneous remissions are very rare.

Diagnosis begins with a history and physical examination conducted by your health care provider. Questions will be asked regarding your job history, smoking history, whether you have had diseases outside the chest, the nature of any prior medical treatments, and whether there is a family history of interstitial lung disease. With lung scarring, the physical examination may reveal crackling breath sounds, which resemble the sound made by a piece of Velcro being released. The fingertips may take on a clubbed-like appearance. The chest x-ray is usually abnormal and can reveal a variety of changes, including a honeycomb-like appearance. A chest computed tomography (CT) scan is often obtained to further define the patterns of lung inflammation. If the diagnosis remains unclear, biopsy specimens can be obtained by bronchoscopy, a procedure by which your doctor uses a lighted tube to look down into your lungs. It may be necessary for a chest surgeon to perform the lung biopsy while the patient is receiving general anesthesia.

Breathing tests are performed to assess how the interstitial lung disease is affecting function.

Living With Your Diagnosis

Because interstitial lung disease includes a group of many different diseases, the symptoms may vary. However, nearly all produce shortness of breath and dry cough that usually start gradually and slowly worsen over time. In those cases where the lung inflammation is part of a disease affecting other organs, symptoms outside the lung may predominate. Abrupt chest pain may signal lung collapse. Fever and changes in cough raise the possibility of bacterial or viral pneumonia. Coughing up blood may occur with some interstitial lung diseases or may be caused by a cancer. Heart failure may occur as the illness worsens.

Treatment

Treatment options vary depending on the specific interstitial lung disease. Smoking cessation is recommended in all cases and may be all that is necessary with some diseases. Inhalers may be prescribed to open the bronchial tubes if there is also smoking-related lung disease. If the interstitial lung disease is felt to be caused by environment exposures, avoidance measures are indicated (such as working with protective breathing masks). Frequently, a decision must be made about the use of potent anti-inflammatory drugs. The most commonly prescribed drug in this regard is the steroid, prednisone. Side effects include:

- Rapid mood swings.
- Weight gain resulting from water retention and a strong appetite.
- Facial puffiness.
- Easy bruising, especially over hands and forearms.
- High blood pressure.
- Poor blood sugar control.
- Cataracts.
- Bone loss.
- Increased susceptibility to infections.

Because the interstitial lung diseases are potentially life threatening, your doctor may feel that the benefits of using drugs like prednisone outweigh the risks. Months to years of therapy may be necessary, but generally the prednisone dose is tapered to the lowest possible dose. The prednisone may be combined with other anti-inflammatory agents. Response to therapy is judged by changes in symptoms, chest x-ray findings, and breathing tests.

Unfortunately, treatment of lung fibrosis is often unrewarding. Treatment options are limited, and there are no drugs that reliably reverse lung scarring. Supplemental oxygen may be used to decrease shortness of breath and improve stamina. Lung transplantation is considered in certain patients.

The DOs
- Obtain an influenza vaccination each fall.
- Obtain/update the pneumococcal vaccination.
- Maintain good cardiovascular fitness by participating in an exercise program.
- Maintain close contact with your health care provider.

The DON'Ts
- Avoid all further exposures to any inhaled material felt to be responsible for your interstitial lung disease.
- Avoid individuals with acute respiratory infections.
- Stop smoking.

When to Call Your Doctor
Call your doctor if any of the following occur:
- If you suspect that you have a lung infection as suggested by an abrupt worsening of cough, yellow or green phlegm production, increased shortness of breath, fevers, or chills.
- Blood in your sputum.
- Dusky-colored skin, fingertips, or lips.
- Chest pain.
- New ankle swelling.
- Any problems with medications.

For More Information
American Lung Association
1118 Hampton Avenue
St. Louis, MO 63139
800-LUNG-USA
www.lungusa.org

DISK HERNIATION

About Your Diagnosis

Disk herniation usually refers to protrusion of the soft, rubbery material that sits between the vertebral bodies in the spinal column that act as shock absorbers. When they begin to bulge or protrude, the disks can apply pressure to the nerves as they exit the spinal cord. This can produce pain, numbness, and possibly weakness, extending down the arms and into the hands and fingers or down the leg and into the feet and toes. The causes of disk herniation are varied but most commonly are related to a degenerative, arthritis-like process. Improper bending and improper lifting technique can lead to disk herniation, particularly lifting of heavy objects. This is a relatively common condition and usually can be managed.

Living With Your Diagnosis

The signs and symptoms of disk herniation include pain somewhere along the spinal column, whether it be in the neck or back, with radiation of the pain into either the arms or legs. The pressure of the disk on the nerve can actually cause weakness in some muscles or paralysis.

Treatment

Most disk protrusions can be treated with rest, medication, and time. Sometimes, however, disk herniation does not respond to conservative measures, and surgical intervention may be needed. Medications typically used for the new onset of back pain and pain down into the arms or legs include nonsteroidal anti-inflammatory drugs (NSAIDs), muscle relaxants, and pain relievers.

A concern with back pain that does not respond quickly to medical therapy is the potential for addiction to narcotics and other medications. These medications are to be used for short periods of time, and are generally not recommended for long-term use. The side effects of conservative treatment are generally related to the use of medications. Possible complications of surgical treatment include permanent damage to the nerve and wound infection.

Relative rest is recommended until the pain begins to subside, which may take 2 weeks or more. Should the pain symptoms subside, treatment is directed at rehabilitation and re-education on proper lifting techniques (Fig 1). Many cities now have back centers that focus on rehabilitation and retraining in proper lifting techniques. For low back difficulties, including herniation, elastic low back supports may be of benefit.

The DOs
• Rest and take your medications as prescribed.
• Use proper lifting techniques.

The DON'Ts
• Avoid lifting heavy objects, particularly using inappropriate lifting techniques.

When to Call Your Doctor
• If you notice partial paralysis of muscles or loss of bowel or bladder control, this may represent a surgical emergency.

For More Information
http://www.medfacts.com/d_disk.htm

DISSEMINATED INTRAVASCULAR COAGULATION

About Your Diagnosis

Hemostasis is the natural phenomenon of keeping the blood in a fluid state by means of keeping a fine balance between coagulation and anticoagulation. Pathologic processes that alter the normal balance among normal hemostatic determinants can lead to either inadequate hemostasis, which results in hemorrhage, or excessive hemostasis, which produces thrombosis.

The process of coagulation involves a group of plasma proteins, platelets (blood cells that help blood to clot), and cells that line the walls of the blood vessels (endothelial cells). The coagulation proteins are normally in an inactive state. Activation of these proteins results in a cascade of events that lead to conversion of prothrombin to thrombin. Once it is generated, thrombin can initiate intravascular clotting, which causes consumption of thrombin-susceptible plasma proteins and formation of fibrin and platelet aggregates.

Disseminated intravascular coagulation (DIC) is a phenomenon characterized by activation of procoagulants. This results in generation of thrombin and failure of the natural coagulation inhibitory mechanisms that neutralize thrombin. Fibrin strands in the vessels may develop and cause mechanical damage to red blood cells, producing microangiopathic hemolytic anemia and thrombocytopenia (low platelet count). DIC is not a disease; it is a phenomenon that results from many different diseases, such as infections, malignant diseases, trauma, and some obstetric problems. The incidence of DIC ranges from 12 to 49 patients per year at most medical centers.

The possibility of DIC is usually considered when patients with infections, certain malignant diseases, open head injuries, and obstetric complications start bleeding from multiple sites. Spontaneous bruises, oozing from venipuncture sites, and spontaneous bleeding into the gastrointestinal tract, central nervous system, or lungs may occur.

Abnormal results of laboratory tests usually consist of broken red blood cells, very small red blood cells, disfigured red blood cells, and decreased numbers of platelets on a peripheral blood smear. Results of tests of coagulation such as prothrombin time (PT), partial thromboplastin time (PTT), and thrombin time are prolonged. Levels of coagulation proteins such as fibrinogen and factors V and VIII are decreased. Platelet count is decreased. In most instances, changes in three or more laboratory values and a low platelet count are consistent with DIC. DIC is always secondary to another problem. The prognosis depends on the underlying condition.

Living With Your Diagnosis

DIC presents itself as generalized bleeding from different body sites, such as the gastrointestinal tract, lungs, and urinary tract. Shock (blood pressure that cannot be measured) out of proportion of bleeding occurs with severe forms of DIC.

DIC causes disturbances in the fine balance between hemostasis and fibrinolysis. This results in formation of generalized microclots in the circulation. Red blood cells are injured mechanically during their passage through the microcirculation, resulting in microangiopathic hemolytic anemia. Coagulation factors and platelets are consumed in this generalized clotting process, resulting in deficiency of coagulation proteins and thrombocytopenia, which increases the tendency to bleeding.

Treatment

Management of the underlying condition remains the cornerstone of therapy for DIC. Patients with DIC are usually admitted to the hospital, and they are quite ill. Intensive replacement therapy is provided with blood products (packed red blood cells, platelets, and coagulation factors). Once the diagnosis of DIC is made and if there is any evidence of bleeding, blood products should be transfused to replace the deficient products accordingly. Heparin (an anticoagulant drug that inhibits the activated coagulation factors) is useful in certain cases of DIC.

Transfusions of blood products are safe. The likelihood of transmission of infection is low. Fluid overload can develop if transfusions are too rapid. Patients can stop responding to platelet transfusions by making antibodies against the transfused platelets.

The DOs

- Adhere to any dietary restrictions depending on the underlying condition.
- Exercise as tolerated once your general condition improves.

The DON'Ts

- Do not take medications, such as aspirin or non-steroidal anti-inflammatory drugs (NSAIDs), which can increase the tendency to bleed, without consulting your physician.
- Do not exercise until your condition stabilizes.

When to Call Your Doctor

- If you start bleeding from the nose or gums, notice bloody urine, or find spontaneous black and blue spots on your skin.

For More Information
National Heart, Lung, and Blood Institute Information Center
P.O. Box 30105
Bethesda, MD 20824-0105
301-251-1222
MedWeb Hematology: http;//www.gen.emory.edu/medweb.hematology.html
MedMark Hematology: http//medmark.bit.co.kr/hematol.html

DIVERTICULITIS

About Your Diagnosis

Diverticuli are herniations of the colon mucosa through the muscular layer of the colon. This produces a small saclike swelling in the colon wall. Diverticulitis occurs when diverticuli become inflamed and infected. Small abscesses form and then rupture causing symptoms.

Diverticulitis occurs during lifetime in about half of the individuals who have diverticuli. Roughly 3,000 cases per 100,000 individuals occur annually. It is not a contagious or cancerous condition. A barium enema x-ray examination is used to detect this condition. Diverticuli may also be found on colonoscopy or flexible sigmoidoscopy (lighted flexible tubes used to examine the colon). With treatment the prognosis is good. Relapses do occur, however.

Living With Your Diagnosis

The initial symptoms of diverticulitis are intermittent cramping and abdominal pain that becomes constant. The location of the pain is usually in the left lower abdominal area. Fever and chills can occur, as well as constipation or diarrhea. There is generally a loss of appetite and nausea. Examination may reveal tenderness and a mass over the painful area. An elevated white blood cell count is usually present. Complications of diverticulitis include hemorrhage (bleeding), perforation (rupture), bowel obstruction, and abscess formation.

Treatment

Treatment is generally outpatient unless the symptoms are severe and there are signs of widespread infection or complications. Bed rest, stool softeners, a liquid diet, and oral antibiotics are the basis of outpatient treatment. If hospitalized, the treatment is similar. You are put at bed rest and intravenous fluids are given. Intravenous antibiotics are started, and analgesics are given for pain control. Initially you may not be allowed to eat. As the symptoms resolve, your diet is slowly returned to a high-fiber, low-fat diet.

If the case is severe or complicated, surgical resection of the affected area of colon is an option. Surgical resection is a treatment option for frequent reoccurrences.

The DOs

- Take medications as prescribed.
- Eat a high-fiber, low-salt, low-fat diet between attacks.
- Drink plenty of fluids between attacks.
- Maintain proper physical activity between attacks.
- Maintain proper weight. Try to lose weight if overweight.
- Maintain proper bowel habits by trying to have a bowel movement daily.
- Watch for signs of blood in the stool or dark tarry bowel movements.
- Watch for signs of reoccurrences and other complications, such as abdominal pain and fever.

The DON'Ts

- Do not strain with bowel movements.
- Avoid laxatives.

When to Call Your Doctor

- If you have blood in the stool.
- If abdominal pain develops or becomes worse.
- If a fever develops and you have abdominal pain.

For More Information
National Digestive Diseases Information Clearinghouse
Box NIDDC
Bethesda, MD 20892
www.niddk.nih.gov
nddic@aerie.com

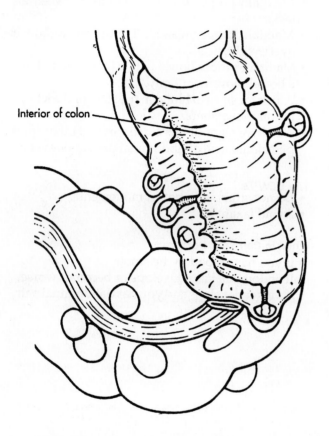

Interior of colon

Diverticula are outpouchings of the colon. When they become inflamed, the condition is diverticulitis. The inflammatory process
can spread to the surrounding area in the intestine. (From Lewis
SM, Collier IC, Heitkemper MM: *Medical-Surgical Nursing: Assessment and Management of Clinical Problem*, vol. 4. St. Louis, Mosby–
Year Book, 1995. Used by permission.)

DIVERTICULOSIS

About Your Diagnosis

Diverticulosis is caused by the herniation of the colon mucosa through the muscular layer of the colon. This produces a small saclike swelling in the colon wall (diverticula). The most common locations for diverticuli are in the sigmoid and distal colon. The exact reason for the herniation is not known. Up to 20% of the general population is affected with diverticulosis. Older individuals tend to have diverticuli more often than younger individuals. Up to 50% of individuals at age 50 will have them. Individuals who eat a low-fiber diet are much more apt to form diverticula. A barium enema x-ray examination is used to detect this condition. Diverticuli may also be found on colonoscopy or flexible sigmoidoscopy (lighted flexible tubes used to examine the colon). The condition is a lifelong problem. Complications such as infection (diverticulitis) and bleeding can occur.

Living With Your Diagnosis

Diverticulosis usually does not have any symptoms. About 10% to 20% of individuals with the condition will have mild,

left-sided abdominal cramping. A bowel movement or passing gas often relieves the cramping. Constipation may be an occasional problem.

Treatment

No treatment is necessary unless there are symptoms. For symptoms a change in diet and stool softeners will help.

The DOs

- Eat a high-fiber, low-salt, low-fat diet.
- Drink plenty of fluids.
- Maintain proper physical activity.
- Maintain proper weight. Try to lose weight if overweight.
- Maintain proper bowel habits by trying to have a bowel movement daily.
- Watch for signs of blood in the stool or dark tarry bowel movements.
- Watch for signs of diverticulitis and other complications such as abdominal pain and fever.

The DON'Ts

- Do not strain with bowel movements.
- Avoid laxatives.

When to Call Your Doctor

- If you have blood in the stool.
- If abdominal pain develops or becomes worse.
- If a fever develops and you have abdominal pain.

For More Information

National Digestive Diseases Information Clearinghouse
Box NIDDC
Bethesda, MD 20892
www.niddk.nih.gov
nddic@aerie.com

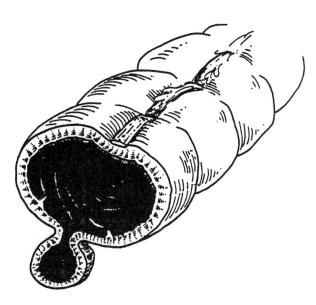

Divertibulum of the large intestine. (From LaFleur-Brooks ML: *Exploring Medical Language—A Student Directed Approach.* vol 3. St. Louis, Mosby–Year Book, 1993. Used by permission.)

DOWN SYNDROME (TRISOMY 21, MONGOLISM)

About Your Diagnosis

Down syndrome is a hereditary condition that is characterized by moderate-to-severe mental deficiency. Children with Down syndrome are born with extra genetic material on chromosome 21. Other names for this condition are trisomy 21 and mongolism. Dr. John Down, a British physician, first identified this condition in 1866.

Down syndrome occurs in approximately 1 of every 800–1,000 live births. Although any woman may give birth to a child with Down syndrome, the age of the mother is a strong influencing factor. The older the mother when she becomes pregnant, the greater the risk of having a child with Down syndrome. The risk of a woman younger than 25 years of having a baby with Down syndrome is 1 in 1,400. At age 35, the risk increases to 1 in 350, and at age 40, the risk is 1 in 100. There are tests that a pregnant woman may have to determine whether her unborn baby has Down syndrome.

Living With Your Diagnosis

Children with Down syndrome are different from other children their age both mentally and physically. They typically tend to be placid and rarely cry. Other characteristics include a small head, various degrees of mental retardation, delays in development, slanting eyes, and small, low-set ears. The tongue appears too big for the mouth, and their muscles seem floppy. They have short and broad hands with a single palmar crease. Although there is no cure for Down syndrome, individuals with this condition can live well into their 60s. Their life expectancy may be somewhat decreased by heart disease (found in 35% of patients with Down syndrome) and susceptibility to acute leukemia. Regular health check-ups are important so that problems may be discovered and treated early.

The DOs
- Enroll your child in an early intervention program.
- Seek information and assistance from local and national support groups.
- Keep scheduled health care appointments.
- Explore educational, developmental, and vocational options as your child becomes older.
- All parents should seek genetic counseling.

The DON'Ts
- Don't underestimate your child's ability. Enroll your child in a multidisciplinary teaching program.
- Don't allow your child to be unsupervised.

When to Call Your Doctor
- If you have questions about your child's health or need information about services for children with Down syndrome.
- If your child becomes increasingly ill or confused.
- If your child has any problems associated with medications.

For More Information
A Parent's Guide to Down Syndrome: Toward a Brighter Future. Baltimore, Paul H. Brookes Publishing Co.
National Down Syndrome Congress
1605 Chantilly Drive, Suite 250
Atlanta, GA 30324-3269
800-232-6372
National Down Syndrome Society
666 Broadway, 8th Floor
New York, NY 10012-2317
800-221-4602
212-460-9330
World Wide Web
http://www.ndss.org

DUMPING SYNDROME

About Your Diagnosis

Dumping syndrome is a complication of stomach surgery. The stomach contents are rapidly moved into the small intestines after meals. This causes patients to have abdominal pain, vomiting, and the other symptoms of dumping syndrome. The symptoms are caused by at least two factors. The first factor is blood flow changes; there is an increased blood flow to the gastrointestinal tract to aid in digestion. The second is increased insulin release in response to the meal. Most patients who undergo stomach surgery will have some minor symptoms for 1–6 months after the procedure. Only a small percentage, 1% to 2%, will have serious problems. Detection of the condition is made with an upper gastrointestinal series. The barium given with this study will move rapidly from the stomach into the small intestine. Most individuals with this condition recover with time, and the prognosis is favorable.

Living With Your Diagnosis

The symptoms of dumping syndrome can be categorized by when they occur, either early or late. In early dumping syndrome, the symptoms begin a few minutes to 45 minutes after eating and are caused by increased blood flow to the intestines. Symptoms include weakness, sweating, flushing, dizziness, and fainting. The heart rate increases and the blood pressure drops. Some individuals become short of breath. Symptoms of nausea, vomiting, abdominal cramps, and explosive diarrhea also occur.

In late dumping syndrome, the symptoms begin 2–3 hours after meals. It is caused by excess insulin release, which causes the blood sugar to drop. Symptoms of sweating, anxiety, shakiness, and fainting occur. The blood pressure tends to drop and a headache may develop.

Treatment

This condition can generally be treated on an outpatient basis. Diet modification is the key. Vitamin and mineral supplementation may be necessary to correct deficiencies. In early dumping syndrome, lying down until the symptoms have passed may help. In late dumping syndrome, eating candy or drinking sweetened drinks may help raise the blood sugar and relieve symptoms. It may also help to add soluble fiber such as pectin or gaur gum to the diet.

The DOs

- When having symptoms, lie down and rest.
- Eat six small meals a day that are low in carbohydrate and high in protein.
- Restrict fluids to between meals.
- Take vitamin and mineral supplements as prescribed.
- If symptoms are not controlled with simple measures, consider adding fiber in the form of pectin (found in fruits and vegetables) or gaur gum (a filler in ice cream and other food) to your diet.

The DON'Ts

- Avoid fluids with meals. Fluids can speed up the passage of food from the stomach to the small intestines.
- Avoid simple and refined sugars. Simple sugars are found in fruits.

When to Call Your Doctor

- If symptoms are not relieved by simple treatments.
- If you have signs of gastrointestinal bleeding, such as vomiting blood, dark tarry stools, or bright red blood with bowel movements.

For More Information
National Digestive Diseases Information Clearinghouse
2 Information Way
Bethesda, MD 20892-3570
www.niddk.nih.gov
nddic@aerie.com

DYSFUNCTIONAL UTERINE BLEEDING

About Your Diagnosis

Dysfunctional uterine bleeding (DUB) is irregular bleeding during a menstrual cycle that is caused by hormonal irregularities. The most common hormonal irregularity occurs because the ovary did not ovulate (the ovary did not produce an egg during that particular cycle). This is called an "anovulatory cycle." Anovulation is very common. Many women have one or two anovulatory cycles each year. Sometimes the anovulation will cause irregular bleeding. You may have bleeding between normal periods; bleeding can last from one period to the next, or for a prolonged period.

If you have abnormal bleeding, it is important to determine that other causes of abnormal bleeding are not responsible for the irregularity. Other causes include uterine fibroids (myomas, benign tumors of the uterus), endometrial polyps, cervical abnormalities, miscarriage of an early pregnancy, or uterine cancer (this mostly applies only to perimenopausal and postmenopausal women). If other causes are not found and the periods return to normal after the abnormal bleeding occurs, then DUB is diagnosed.

In the majority of cases, DUB is self-limiting so no treatment is necessary. If bleeding has been continuous since the previous period or there is bleeding between periods, the abnormal bleeding will usually stop after the next period. If it is a prolonged period, usually the period will stop without treatment. However, sometimes the bleeding is very heavy and does not slow down; this type of DUB requires treatment.

Living With Your Diagnosis

Dysfunctional uterine bleeding can occur in many different ways. Sometimes the bleeding is continuous from one period to the next; other times it may be a flow or it may be just spotting. The DUB may occur as intermittent bleeding between periods—that is, bleed for a few days, stop for a few days, then bleed again—until the next period. Other times, DUB will be a prolonged period; instead of bleeding for 4 or 5 days, the period lasts for 10–14 days. Sometimes the period will be heavier with clots.

You may have increased premenstrual symptoms during a cycle in which you are having DUB. These symptoms include increased breast tenderness, feeling bloated, and increased irritability.

Treatment

Most DUB is self-limiting, so no treatment is necessary. The abnormal bleeding will stop after the next period. However, sometimes the bleeding can be very heavy and can cause significant blood loss. In these cases, treatment is necessary to prevent serious blood loss. In most cases, the flow can be reduced by taking a hormone. One of the more commonly used hormones is Provera. Also, birth control pills (two or three pills taken daily) can be used temporarily to control heavy DUB. In occasional cases, a minor procedure called "dilatation and curettage" (D&C) is necessary to control the bleeding. During a D&C the lining of the uterus, the endometrium, is scraped out. This helps the uterus to shed the endometrium all at once so the bleeding stops.

Side effects from progestins include feeling bloated, breast tenderness, lower backache, irritability, and mild depression. However, usually the progestin has to be taken for only 7–10 days, so although the side effects may be difficult to tolerate, it is only for a short while. Taking two or three birth control pills a day can cause mild nausea. If vomiting occurs, then another way of controlling the DUB will have to be prescribed.

The DOs

- If a medication is prescribed, do take it as directed.

The DON'Ts

- Don't stop the medication early (even if the bleeding stops) unless directed by your health care provider.

When to Call Your Doctor

- If your period lasts longer than 7 or 8 days.
- If your period is much heavier than usual, i.e., soaking through maxi pads or super tampons every 2 hours, or passing large (walnut size or larger) clots.
- If you have bleeding between periods.
- If the bleeding doesn't slow down or stop as expected.
- If you are bleeding heavily and are feeling dizzy or weak. These may be symptoms of severe ane-

mia, so you should have your blood cell count
checked.
- If there is any chance you could be pregnant.

For More Information
*Understanding Your Body: Every Woman's Guide to Gynecology and
Health.* Felicia Stewart, M.D., Felicia Guest, M.D., Gary Stewart, M.D.,
and Robert Hatcher, M.D., Bantam Books, 1987.

DYSMENORRHEA

About Your Diagnosis

Dysmenorrhea is uterine cramping that occurs in association with a period. It is felt to be caused by a high level of prostaglandin production (a substance produced by the uterus) in some women.

In other women, the presence of fibroids, adenomyosis, or endometriosis may be the cause. Dysmenorrhea is very common. Many women have mild-to-moderate cramps associated with their periods; severe dysmenorrhea occurs in approximately 15% of women.

Dysmenorrhea can be treated with medication (see below). Sometimes it spontaneously disappears or becomes much less bothersome after the delivery of a baby. In some cases, it lessens with age.

Living With Your Diagnosis

Although most women with dysmenorrhea have cramps, some women have sharp, stabbing pains and others have a sensation of dull pressure. Women may have the discomfort or pain in the lower abdomen, the lower back, or in both the front and the back.

Dysmenorrhea can be accompanied by nausea, vomiting, diarrhea, and on some occasions, sweating, shaking, and headache. The severity of the symptoms can vary from month to month; sometimes the cramping may be mild, other times severe.

Treatment

Over-the-counter ibuprofen can be very effective in relieving the cramps. Over-the-counter ibuprofen comes in 200-milligram tablets. You can start with 2 tablets every 4 hours. However, if this does not relieve the cramps enough, you can take 3 tablets (600 milligrams) every 6 hours or 4 tablets (800 milligrams) every 8 hours. You should always take ibuprofen with some food on your stomach to avoid stomach irritation. (Obviously, you should not take ibuprofen if you have an allergy to it, have been told you should not take it or aspirin-like products, or have a history of ulcer or gastritis.)

Prescription medication may be prescribed for you if over-the-counter ibuprofen does not seem to be effective.

If ibuprofen and ibuprofen-like medications do not treat your dysmenorrhea effectively, birth control pills may be prescribed if appropriate. Birth control pills can be very effective in decreasing dysmenorrhea with the additional benefit of making the periods lighter.

If you take ibuprofen or ibuprofen-like medications for your dysmenorrhea, watch for stomach irritation. Taking too much ibuprofen, taking it on an empty stomach, or having a sensitivity to it may cause a stomach ulcer.

The DOs

- If medication has been recommended, it is very important to take the medication before the dysmenorrhea becomes severe. • Your doctor may recommend that you start the medication even before the cramps began.
- Take ibuprofen and ibuprofen-like medications with some food in your stomach to avoid stomach irritation and decrease the risk of ulcer.
- Exercise may help decrease dysmenorrhea.
- Heat, such as a heating pad, hot water bottle, or soaking in a hot tub may relieve some symptoms.

The DON'Ts

- Don't take ibuprofen or ibuprofen-like medications on an empty stomach.
- Don't take more medication than recommended or prescribed.

When to Call Your Doctor

- If the medication is not relieving the dysmenorrhea satisfactorily.
- You are not tolerating the medication.
- Your dysmenorrhea is becoming progressively worse despite current treatment.

For More Information
Understanding Your Body: Every Woman's Guide to Gynecology and Health. Felicia Stewart, M.D., Felicia Guest, M.D., Gary Stewart, M.D., and Robert Hatcher, M.D., Bantam Books, 1987.

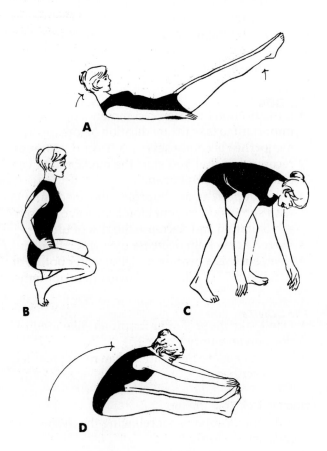

Sitting-up exercises for dysmenorrhea. **A,** Supine position with head and legs raised simultaneously; arms should be kept at side and legs straight. **B,** Deep knee bends; back should be kept straight. **C,** Monkey walk; keep hands flat on floor and walk about on hands and feet. **D,** Toe touching; keeping back straight and the legs straight, bend and touch toes with hands. (From Hood GH, Dincher JR: *Total Patient Care: Foundations and Practice of Adult Health Nursing,* vol 8. St. Louis, Mosby–Year Book, 1992. Used by permission.)

ECZEMA

About Your Diagnosis

Eczema is a chronic skin condition characterized by reddened, dry, itchy, scaly skin. Several types of eczema are known, the most common being atopic dermatitis, hand eczema, and nummular eczema. These may result from hypersensitive skin or chronic irritation; however, often no clear cause can be determined. Eczema is not contagious, but some cases do "run in families." It is not curable, but careful treatment can minimize the itching and dryness of the skin, and prevent complications such as infection. Various forms of eczema affect between 5% and 10% of all Americans each year.

Living With Your Diagnosis

Eczema may first appear in infancy or childhood. Reddened, scaly patches appear on the face, forearms, and lower legs. After school age, patches are more common behind the knees and in the folds of the elbows. Eczema almost never affects the back.

Hand eczema usually involves the fingers and palms. Nummular eczema can occur on any body surface but is most common on the chest, arms, and abdomen.

Symptoms of eczema include intense itching and irritability. Often no visible rash is noted until after the patient has begun scratching. If untreated, the skin will be damaged by the scratching and can become thickened with scars. Infection can also occur because the scratching can decrease the skin's ability to fight bacteria.

Treatment

All treatment is aimed at breaking the itch-scratch cycle. Avoid irritants such as hot water, detergents, and other chemicals as much as possible. Keep children's fingernails short, and put mittens on young infants to prevent scratching. Antihistamine medicines, taken by mouth, can decrease the itching. However, these medicines are very sedating (sleep inducing), and you must be careful to avoid driving, cooking, or working with machinery while using them. Use antihistamines cautiously in children as well, because school performance may suffer if the child is too sleepy in class.

Other treatments include lubricating and moisturizing the skin, which also helps minimize the itching. Use mild, hypoallergenic, over-the-counter skin creams or ointments to prevent excessive skin dryness. Use prescription steroid creams for more resistant cases of irritation and scaling as directed by your doctor. (Do not use these creams on your face unless specifically prescribed for facial rash. The facial skin is fragile and can be thinned by overuse of steroid creams.)

Occasionally your doctor may prescribe oral steroids (tablets or syrup) for a severe episode of inflammation. These are powerful anti-inflammatory drugs and can have serious side effects if used frequently. These side effects include stomach irritation, ulcers, and osteoporosis. Be sure to use these medicines carefully and exactly as directed by your doctor.

If infection is present, your doctor will prescribe oral antibiotics to fight the bacteria. Over-the-counter antibiotic creams will not fight the infection adequately, so be sure to complete your oral antibiotics as prescribed.

The DOs

- Do follow a daily skin wellness regimen, even when your skin is free of itching.
- Do lubricate your skin after each exposure to water.
- Do use the mildest soap and shampoo available.
- Do keep fingernails short, and bandage areas of severe itching if possible to keep the risk of scratching minimal.
- Do use long sleeves and long pants to help prevent the itch-scratch cycle, especially in children.
- Do double-rinse clothing to minimize irritation.

The DON'Ts

- Don't bathe with hot water because it will dry the skin and increase irritation.
- Don't use steroid products on the face or near the eyes unless specifically directed to do so by your doctor.

When to Call Your Doctor

- If you have fever or chills.
- If you have nausea or vomiting.
- If you have increased redness, bleeding, or discharge around the rash.

For More Information

American Academy of Dermatology
930 N. Meachum Road
Schaumburg, IL 60173
847-330-0230
National Eczema Association
1221 S.W. Yamhill, #303
Portland, OR 97205
503-228-4430

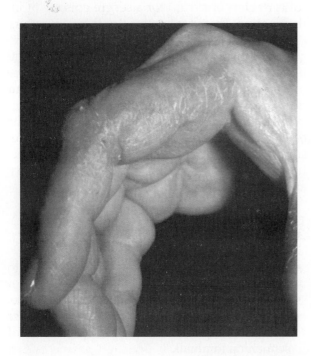

Inflamed hand eczema with early fissure. (From Goldstein BG,
Goldstein AO: *Practical Dermatology*, vol 1. St. Louis, Mosby–Year
Book, 1992. Used by permission.)

EJACULATION, PREMATURE

About Your Diagnosis

Premature ejaculation (PE) is a relatively common disorder seen primarily in heterosexuals. It occurs in about 25% to 40% of men at different points in their sexual life. It is characterized by an inability to maintain an erection during sexual intercourse for a long enough time to satisfy the individual. Because the problem does involve such an intimate part of a relationship, premature ejaculation can lead to social isolation and psychological distress. If, however, the man's partner does not complain about the premature ejaculation, it is unlikely that the man will seek professional help about this problem.

Living With Your Diagnosis

In most instances, the ejaculation comes less than a minute after entering the vagina. Rarely, ejaculation can occur either immediately before or immediately after vaginal entry. However, in either case, the ejaculation occurs before the individual or his partner would desire it. One should not, however, be preoccupied with the length of time. The real deciding factor in diagnosing premature ejaculation is that both the patient and his partner are dissatisfied with this aspect of their sexual functioning. It is also important to keep in mind that most men ejaculate prematurely, but generally not all the time as do individuals with this disorder.

In assessing the individual with premature ejaculation, the following questions should be asked:

- Why is the patient seeking therapy now?
- What is the couple's length of sexual experience?
- Are there any other emotional aspects that might be affecting their sexual behavior?
- Are their expectations for sexual intercourse reasonable? • Is the man desperate about losing his partner because of rapid ejaculation?
- Does sexual activity occur under secretive conditions where the couple might be interrupted?
- Does the sexual partner have some form of sexual disorder, such as an unusual amount of pain during sexual activity or a decreased interest in sex?

The answers to these questions will allow the individual evaluating the man with premature ejaculation to determine whether this condition is acquired or lifelong, and also to determine what other psychosocial factors need to be addressed to help treat the condition.

Usually, men who have premature ejaculation are able to delay an orgasm during masturbation but not during sexual intercourse. To be considered abnormal, premature ejaculation must cause distress for the patient or difficulties with a relationship, and must not be related to any drugs the patient may be taking. In particular, withdrawal from some narcotics causes premature ejaculation.

There are different types of premature ejaculation. PE is classified according to the onset, whether it is lifelong or acquired later, and by context, whether it is generalized or just situational. PE can be caused by a psychological condition or by a combination of factors. As young males become more sexually experienced with age, the majority learn how to delay orgasm. However, some men continue to have premature ejaculation, and they are the ones who may seek help for this disorder. In lifelong premature ejaculation, the problem begins with the first sexual intercourse and continues throughout all the patient's relationships until treatment is sought. When premature ejaculation occurs after there has been a period of normal sexual functioning, it is usually because of a decreased frequency of sexual activity or intense performance anxiety with a new partner. Some men who have stopped regular use of alcohol may have premature ejaculation because they relied on their drinking to delay organism, instead of learning from experience how to do so.

Treatment

The treatment of premature ejaculation can involve a range of therapy, from simply reassuring the patient and providing him with realistic expectations about sexual activity, to the use of medications. In particular, the use of clomipramine in a dose of 25–50 mg has been shown, in some cases, to increase the time before ejaculation by an average of 250%. In addition, other serotonin drugs, such as Zoloft, Paxil, and Prozac, may also be of some benefit. In general, those individuals who respond to clomipramine or other medications will have a reoccurrence of the disorder if the medication is stopped.

Much attention has been focused on the so-called squeeze technique for the treatment of premature ejaculation. In this technique, the male will focus his attention on the sensations he is obtaining through his penis during intercourse, and then he will signal his partner to stop moving or to apply a firm squeeze to the penis in an attempt to interrupt ejaculation. This obviously requires excellent communication between an individual and his partner, which probably improves functioning as well. It is important to remember that in premature ejaculation, as with any sexual dysfunction, the primary concern is not what is "normal sexual behavior" but what sexual difficulties are adversely affecting the pleasure and enjoyment of both partners involved. It is those conditions that merit treatment.

The DOs

If you have premature ejaculation, it is important to create an appropriate atmosphere for sexual activity. Fear of interruption and clandestine (secret) sexual activity increase chances of premature ejaculation. You should also communicate with your partner to allow for both of you to express your feelings and expectations regarding sex. Together you might develop techniques (e.g., squeeze technique) that may prolong an erection. Most important, try to relax. Anxiety (especially performance anxiety) only makes this condition worse.

The DON'Ts

Because your ejaculation may be rapid and unpredictable, avoid such risky "birth control" methods as withdrawal before ejaculation. Do not feel embarrassed to discuss this condition with your physician.

When to Call Your Doctor

You should call your physician if you are unable to achieve an erection, if you have a bloody or foul-smelling discharge, pain on intercourse, or significant depression secondary to premature ejaculation.

For More Information

Consult your local library, or ask your physician for a referral to a sexual disorder treatment center. Helpful information can also be found online @:
http://www,doctors-10tv.com/alt/men/men.htm
http:www.catalog.com/ie/ hr.htm
http://www.cei.net/~impotenc

ENCOPRESIS

About Your Diagnosis

Encopresis is the repeated passage of stool or feces into inappropriate places such as the clothing or floor, whether intentional or involuntary. To be diagnosed with encopresis, an individual must be at least 4 years of age, and the encopresis must occur at the rate of at least one episode a month for 3 months or more. Finally, the encopresis cannot be due solely to the direct effect of a substance (for example, a laxative), or a medical condition. Encopresis can occur with or without constipation.

Less than one third of children in the United States have finished toilet training by their second birthday. Generally, control of bowels is achieved before bladder control. Because about 95% of children have acquired stool continence (the ability to control their bowels) by the age of 4 years, that age is usually established as the normal age by which continence is acquired. As with continence of urine, girls achieve bowel control earlier than do boys.

In terms of looking at who has this condition, one study shows that the prevalence of encopresis in children aged 7–8 years is about 1.5% of all children in that age group, with boys being more commonly affected than girls. In this and other studies, by the age of 16 years, the rate of bowel incontinence is almost zero. Of patients who have encopresis, 80% to 90% have associated constipation. The children who have encopresis and constipation often have distention of their colons and can have significant impaction with hard feces.

Living With Your Diagnosis

We don't really know what causes encopresis, but it may occur after an episode of constipation, after an illness, or it may occur after a change in diet. Stressful events such as the birth of a sibling, starting a new school, or moving have been associated with up to one quarter of cases of secondary encopresis. Excessive stress during the toilet-training period, leading to increased anxiety and so-called "pot phobia" have all been associated with higher rates of encopresis.

Hersov has listed three types of identifiable encopresis in children. In the first, it is known that the child can control defecation, but he chooses to defecate in inappropriate places. In the second, there is true failure to gain bowel control, and the child is either unable to prevent the soiling or is unaware of it. In the third case, the child's soiling is caused by excessively liquid feces, whether from constipation and overflow, or from anxiety. Of course, these three mechanism of encopresis can also overlap. Unlike urinary incontinence, fecal incontinence rarely occurs during the night, and if it does, represents a poor sign for recovery.

In the first type of encopresis where the child has some control over the behavior, the encopresis tends to be temporary and often resolves after the stress—such as a new sibling, move, or change in school—is no longer acute. In some families where there is an especially large amount of chaos or overstrict punishment, the feces may even be deposited in places designed to cause anger or irritation, and may even be smeared on furniture or walls.

In the second group, where there is failure to learn bowel control, the stool is deposited fairly randomly in clothes, at home, or other places. In these children, there may be some other medical illness, either some kind of brain damage or intellectual deficiency, that has retarded their ability to learn how to control their bowel.

In the third group, where there is excessively fluid feces, the child may have a condition that usually produces diarrhea, such as ulcerative colitis, or may just have constipation with overflow diarrhea. The child is extremely self-conscious of their liquid feces and will go to elaborate lengths to avoid having a bowel movement in public.

Assessing a child with encopresis obviously involves a complete medical examination with appropriate laboratory and x-ray studies. Most of these medical evaluations will be negative in that there is very rarely a physical cause of the encopresis; however, there may be consequences of the behavior, such as colon dilatation. Ulcerative colitis, Crohn's disease, and Hirschsprung's disease should all be ruled out. It is also important to do a psychiatric and psychosocial and family interview to obtain more information about the developmental history, as well as what behaviors or events may have preceded the encopresis.

Treatment

The management and treatment of encopresis involve four stages.

The first stage consists of an assessment to determine whether encopresis is primary or secondary. Also, physical causes are looked for, as well as any other factors that might be contributing to the encopresis.

In the second stage, advice is given. This is mainly an educational phase regarding diet and toileting. Also an attempt is made to reduce the parent's practice of punitive behavior toward the child, as well as to transmit some optimism to the child and the family.

The third stage is focused on toileting. It includes focusing on positive achievements related to toilet training, eating a high-fiber diet, and toileting after meals for a maximum of 15 minutes. Also, those patients with "pot phobia" are gradually exposed to toileting. This stage may also involve the use of laxatives, and Senokot and Lactulose syrup are often used. If there is no benefit from laxatives, enemas may be used if the bowel is excessively full of very hard feces. Bisacodyl can often be used for this purpose.

The fourth stage consists of biofeedback, and this is done only in those cases where there is a relapse after training.

There are a number of other therapeutic tools that are used. Behavior treatments are very popular, including the use of positive reinforcement. It is very important to work with the families because often they are obsessively concerned with the encopretic behavior and make it the center of the family's attention. Therefore it is very important to shift the family's focus away from the encopresis. Instead the family should be encouraged to notice and mention positive behavior. This may defuse tension and decrease hostility. Frequently the increased attention that a child gets, and the escape from the usual responsibilities (e.g., not attending school) may provide secondary gain for the encopresis behavior. While mild consequences may be used such as telling the child to clean himself after soiling, it should be pointed out that one must be careful not to carry punitive behavior to the extreme. Generally, behavioral therapy combined with laxatives is effective in about 75% of the cases, in decreasing the encopretic episodes. Finally, biofeedback for external sphincter control has also been effective.

Medications for this condition are primarily the ones that we have mentioned: the laxatives and sometimes enemas. Excessive use of laxatives should be avoided because of the potential for drug dependency. It is important for the child to maintain a healthy diet. A high-fiber diet is often recommended. This can be done by adding bran to cereals, fruit, or milkshakes. There are few complications related to the medications used to treat encopresis if they are used appropriately.

When to Call Your Doctor

- If your child has a fever, begins to have nausea or vomiting, or has particularly hard stools.
- If your child has diarrhea and becomes excessively dehydrated.
- If you see any blood in your child's stool or blood around the rectum, call immediately.

For More Information
Contact your family physician or your local pediatric association.

ENDOCARDITIS, INFECTIVE

About Your Diagnosis

Endocarditis is an infectious and inflammatory process that affects the lining of the heart and valves. It can affect individuals of all ages and is curable with treatment. The disease can be detected by performing blood cultures and an echocardiogram (a type of ultrasound). The usual cause is a bacteria such as staph or strep, but it can also be caused by a fungal infection. The bacteria or fungus can enter the bloodstream from infections elsewhere in the body (e.g., the urinary tract, gastrointestinal tract, or the skin), or as a result of any surgical or dental procedure.

Living With Your Diagnosis

Signs and symptoms of the disease include fever, fatigue, weakness, chills and night sweats, muscle and joint pain, and a heart murmur. Later there may be swelling of the feet and legs, and shortness of breath with an irregular heartbeat.

Treatment

Antibiotics will be needed for 4–6 weeks. If intravenous antibiotics are prescribed, a home health nurse will be arranged to continue intravenous antibiotics at home. Bed rest is needed until recovery is complete. Non-aspirin medications such as Tylenol can be used for fever and minor pain. A regular diet can be followed as tolerated. Fluid intake should be increased while fever is present. Good dental hygiene is needed to prevent infection.

The DOs

- Take the antibiotics until finished.
- Use nonaspirin products for fever and minor pain.
- Increase fluid intake especially during the fever.
- Maintain bed rest as ordered.
- Move your legs and change position frequently while in bed.
- Resume normal activity gradually as your strength allows.
- See your dentist regularly. Use a soft-bristled toothbrush.

The DON'Ts

- Don't skip doses or stop the antibiotics until you have finished a complete treatment course of antibiotics, or your doctor tells you to stop the antibiotics.
- Don't try to keep your normal schedule; bed rest is needed to have a full recovery.
- Don't have dental work or surgical procedures in the future without notifying the doctor of your history of endocarditis.
- Don't floss your teeth because it may introduce bacteria from the gums. See your dentist frequently for proper gum care.

When to Call Your Doctor

After your treatment you have:
- Fever.
- Loss of appetite or weight gain without diet changes.
- Blood in your urine.
- Chest pain or shortness of breath.
- Sudden weakness in the muscles of the face or limbs.

For More Information

National Heart, Lung and Blood Institute Information Line
800-575-WELL
Internet Site
www.healthanswers.com

ENDOMETRIAL CANCER

About Your Diagnosis

The uterus, or womb, is located between the bladder and the rectum. The inner layer of the uterus is called the *endometrium*. Endometrial cancer is cancer of the cells of this layer. More than 30,000 new cases of endometrial cancer are diagnosed each year in the United States. The cause is not known. The cancer usually occurs among women between 55 and 70 years of age but can occur among younger women before they go through menopause. Women at risk for endometrial cancer are obese, have diabetes, and have never been pregnant or given birth. Another risk is taking estrogen as replacement therapy for the effects of menopause.

The only sure way to diagnose endometrial cancer is to obtain tissue by means of biopsy and examine it with a microscope. This is usually done because a woman reports abnormal vaginal bleeding. Endometrial cancer detected early can be cured.

Living With Your Diagnosis

Vaginal bleeding after menopause is the primary symptom for nearly 90% of patients. If you go through menopause and start bleeding again, this is abnormal and should be evaluated. For women who have not yet gone through menopause, any abnormal vaginal bleeding (heavy bleeding, minimal bleeding, bleeding between menstrual cycles) should be evaluated.

Endometrial cancer if left untreated spreads locally to nearby structures, causing a foul vaginal discharge, pain in the pelvic area, bloating, bowel symptoms such as constipation and blood in stools, and urinary symptoms such as frequency, urgency, or pain with urination. If the cancer continues to spread, it can cause local swollen lymph glands and an abdominal mass and eventually involve the liver, lung, and bone.

Treatment

To confirm the diagnosis of endometrial cancer for a woman with abnormal vaginal bleeding, a biopsy specimen is obtained from the uterus by means of a procedure called dilation and curettage (D & C). The cervix is dilated (widened) and a curette (a small spoon-shaped instrument) is inserted to remove tissue. Once the diagnosis is confirmed, a physician determines the extent of cancer (staging).

Staging tells whether the cancer has spread. Blood tests, chest radiographs (x-rays), and computed tomographic (CT) scans of the abdomen and pelvis are obtained to look for any spread.

Treatment can be surgical, radiation, hormonal, or chemotherapy. The treatment used depends on the stage of the cancer (stage I, tumor confined to the uterus; stage II, tumor invading the cervix; stage III, tumor involving the vagina, ovary or abdominal cavity; stage IV, tumor invading the bladder and intestine). Most endometrial cancers are in the early stages (I or II), and surgical removal of the uterus, fallopian tubes, and ovaries (hysterectomy and bilateral salpingo-oophorectomy) generally is recommended. Radiation may be given after the operation if the cancer extends beyond the uterus. The patient and physicians must discussed this.

Side effects of surgical treatment include pain and soreness in the pelvic area and difficulty in emptying the bladder or moving the bowels. Side effects of radiation therapy are red, dry, itchy skin, fatigue, diarrhea, discomfort with urination, dryness of the vagina, and pain with intercourse.

The hormone called progesterone may be recommended if the cancer has spread extensively or has returned after treatment. Chemotherapy also may be recommended in this situation. Side effects of hormonal therapy include breast tenderness, leg swelling, acne, nausea, and headaches. Side effects of chemotherapy include nausea, vomiting, hair loss, easy bruising and bleeding, and infections.

The DOs

- Remember that sexual intercourse and desire are not affected by hysterectomy. Sexual intercourse and normal activity can be resumed 4 to 8 weeks after the operation.
- Remember you will no longer have periods (menstrual cycles). If your ovaries are removed or damaged by irradiation, menopause occurs, and you can experience hot flashes, sweating, and other symptoms of menopause.
- Keep all your follow-up visits during and after treatment. It is important to undergo examinations to look for response to treatment or recurrence of cancer.

The DON'Ts

- Do not ignore any vaginal bleeding after menopause.
- Do not ignore any abnormal vaginal bleeding

(excess, between periods) before menopause.

- Do not forget the risk of using estrogen replacement, and discuss this with your physician.
- Do not forget the importance of exercise and diet both before the diagnosis and after therapy for endometrial cancer.
- Do not forget there is evidence that shows the use of birth control pills may decrease risk for endometrial cancer, presumably because of the progesterone in the pill.

When to Call Your Doctor

- If there is any vaginal bleeding or abnormal vaginal bleeding.
- If you have any abnormal vaginal discharge (smell, quantity, color).
- If you need emotional support after treatment.
- If you have any side effects of treatment (surgical, radiation, hormonal, or chemotherapy).

For More Information

Cancer Information Service 1-800-4-CANCER
American Cancer Society
1599 Clifton Road, N.E.
Atlanta, GA 30329
1-800-ACS-2345

ENDOMETRIOSIS

About Your Diagnosis

Endometriosis is a condition in which tissue similar to the lining of the uterus, the endometrium, grows in abnormal places in the abdominal cavity, usually the pelvic area. The most common sites for endometriosis to grow are the ovaries, the fallopian tubes, and the lining (the peritoneum) of the pelvis, especially behind the uterus. The cause of endometriosis is unknown although there are several theories. Endometriosis may be familial. Endometriosis can be found in 5% to 15% of women of reproductive age.

Sometimes a presumptive diagnosis is made by the presence of certain symptoms. However, the only way endometriosis can be diagnosed definitively is by laparoscopy. This is a minor surgical procedure in which a telescope-like instrument is placed through a small incision into the abdominal cavity to visualize the endometriosis. Sometimes biopsy specimens may be taken to confirm the presence of endometriosis, especially if the appearance of the endometriosis is not typical.

Endometriosis can be very effectively treated with birth control pills or other medications. If you have been diagnosed with endometriosis, you will always have the possibility of developing problems from it until you go through menopause. Endometriosis is stimulated by estrogen, so when your estrogen levels decrease in menopause, the endometriosis is no longer a problem.

Living With Your Diagnosis

Endometriosis may not cause any symptoms. Many women have endometriosis and have no symptoms, and it is only discovered because they have surgery for some other reason (e.g., a tubal ligation).

The most common symptoms are:
- Dysmenorrhea (pain in association with periods).
- Pelvic pain that is associated with periods.
- Painful intercourse, usually deep pelvic pain.
- Infertility.

Endometriosis can cause scar tissue to form around the pelvic organs, the uterus, fallopian tubes, and ovaries. The scar tissue can cause pelvic pain and infertility by blocking the fallopian tubes. Occasionally, the scar tissue can block bowel (intestines) or the ureters (the tubes that connect the kidneys to the bladder).

Treatment

Birth control pills are a very effective way to treat endometriosis. Birth control pills are not risky for most women and are usually well tolerated. Also, women can stay on birth control pills for many years, as long as necessary, to keep the endometriosis suppressed. If pregnancy is desired, then the birth control pills are discontinued and attempts to conceive are started right away (discuss with your doctor).

Danazol is also a very effective treatment. Some of the common side effects include weight gain, oily skin or acne, hot flashes, deepening of the voice, emotional lability, facial hair, and water retention.

Gonadotropin-releasing hormone agonists, such as Lupron or Synarel, are also very effective in treating endometriosis. These types of medications turn off the ovaries so menopause is induced. Without estrogen, the endometriosis is no longer active. The most common side effects are hot flashes and vaginal dryness. A potential complication is osteoporosis, a loss of bone density, so it is usually only prescribed for 6 months at a time.

Often laparoscopy is used to diagnose and treat endometriosis. At the time of surgery, the endomet some type of medical treatment after surgery.

The DOs
- If you are started on birth control pills or on medication, do take it as directed.
- If your endometriosis causes cramping with your periods, exercise may help relieve some of the cramps.
- Ibuprofen and ibuprofen-like medications can also help relieve painful periods.

When to Call Your Doctor
- If your treatment is not helping your symptoms.
- If you are not tolerating your medication or birth control pills. Sometimes another medication will be better tolerated.
- Don't take any herbal therapies without checking with your doctor. Some of the herbal remedies may have estrogen-like molecules and may stimulate your endometriosis.

For More Information:
The Endometriosis Association
8585 North 76th Place
Milwaukee, WI 53223
414-355-2200
800-992-ENDO
Breitkopf LF, Bakoulis MG: *Coping With Endometriosis.*
New York, Prentice Hall Press, 1988.
Understanding Your Body: Every Woman's Guide to Gynecology and Health. Felicia Stewart, M.D., Felicia Guest, M.D., Gary Stewart, M.D., and Robert Hatcher, M.D., Bantam Books, 1987.

ENURESIS

About Your Diagnosis

Enuresis, commonly called "bed-wetting," is defined as the intentional or involuntary passage of urine into bed or clothes by children aged 4 years or older who do not have any physical abnormality. Acquiring the ability to hold one's urine is the final stage of a very consistent developmental process. Usually the beginning of this process is bowel control during sleep, followed by bowel control during waking hours. Control of the bladder during the day occurs next, followed by nighttime control of the bladder. Most children are able to control their bladder at night by the age of 3 years. However, as children get older, the likelihood that they will stop bed-wetting becomes much less.

Living With Your Diagnosis

Bed-wetting is as common in boys as it is in girls until the age of 5 years, but by age 11 years of age, boys outnumber girls by two to one. In fact, not until 8 years of age are boys able to hold their urine at night as well as girls do by 5 years of age. This appears to be because boys mature at a slower rate than girls do. Interestingly, however, daytime wetting occurs more commonly in girls than in boys and has a much higher incidence of associated emotional problems.

In evaluating enuresis, it is important first to consider medical factors that might be causing the condition. This would include an investigation of any abnormalities in the urinary tract (e.g., a bladder that is unable to carry a full amount of urine), any abnormalities in hormone secretion, some abnormal sleep patterns, the fact that it may run in the individual's family, and also, any overall delays in the development of the child. There also seems to be a relationship between children who get frequent urinary tract infections (UTIs) and enuresis. However, it is now believed that the (UTIs) found in these individuals are probably more a result of the bed-wetting than the cause of it. Although the size of the bladder and the level of sleep of the patient may or may not be related to enuresis, it does seem that enuresis may be inherited. About 70% of children who have nighttime bed-wetting have a relative who has or has had this condition. Also, stress may play a role in those patients who have enuresis after a period of being dry at night. In particular, the birth of a younger sibling, frequent early hospitalizations, and head injury can lead to secondary enuresis.

In many instances, families have attempted to treat the nighttime bed-wetting at home. These treatment attempts have included fluid restriction, especially after dinner, night lifting, and a system of rewards and punishments. Although rewarding children may be somewhat beneficial in treating enuresis, usually punishing them for enuresis merely makes the condition worse. It may also lead to even more self-esteem problems for the children.

The evaluation of the patient should include both a physical examination and a mental status examination, as well as any x-ray studies, urinalysis, and blood tests that are needed to be sure that a physical cause is not responsible for the enuresis.

Treatment

Most studies suggest that the majority of children with enuresis never come to the attention of health care professionals. It seems that most families consider bed-wetting part of normal childhood development. Initially, after obtaining a good history, treatment is aimed at reassuring the child that enuresis can be treated, and that a number of children have enuresis. About 10% of patients who undergo this first evaluation visit will improve without further treatment. Other therapies involve waking the child and fluid restriction.

A number of medications have been used to treat enuresis. These have included hormonal drugs and antidepressants, especially the antidepressant imipramine (Tofranil). Imipramine has been shown to be very effective in treating bedtime enuresis, and it definitely reduces the frequency of bed-wetting in about 85% of bed-wetters and eliminates it entirely in about 30%. However, there are many side effects from imipramine treatment of enuresis, including dry mouth, constipation, headache, and dizziness. There is also some concern about whether drugs like imipramine cause arrhythmias that may contribute to sudden infant death syndrome. Stimulant drugs such as dextroamphetamine have also been used, as well as other drugs that reduce the frequency of urinating.

There are also psychosocial treatments for enuresis, one of which is the night alarm. This system initially used two electrodes that were separated by some bedding connected to the alarm. When the child wet the bed, the urine completed the electrical circuit, sounding the alarm and awakening the child. Since the initial alarm system, other devices have been used. A vibrating pad beneath the pillow can be used instead of a bell or a buzzer, or the electrodes can be made into a single unit. They can be miniaturized so it can be attached to nighttime or daytime clothing. With such treatment, full elimination of enuresis can be expected in about 80% of the cases. If the alarm system is used, it is important to be patient because it usually is not until the second month after the alarm has been used that enuresis begins to decrease. Relapse after successful treatment of any kind usually takes place within 6 months after the treatment is stopped, and it seems that about one third of all children relapse.

Unlike nighttime bed-wetting, daytime enuresis is much more likely to be associated with urinary tract problems including urinary tract infection, and also with other psychiatric disorders. It seems that nighttime bed-wetting can often be kept a secret, whereas daytime enuresis is almost impossible to hide from other individuals. The most appropriate intervention for daytime enuresis may be regular trips to the bathroom before the enuresis occurs. This may require some help from the teacher, who might remind the student about going to the bathroom. Often, students with enuresis are ashamed to ask to go to the bathroom for fear of calling attention to themselves. As mentioned earlier, there are also portable systems that can be worn on the body during the day, or a sensor in the underwear that can serve as an alarm to the patient. A simpler intervention is to buy the child a digital watch with a countdown alarm timer. Unlike nighttime bed-wetting, the use of anti-depressants such as Tofranil or imipramine are not effective for daytime enuresis. Daytime wetters may respond to the use of drugs that actually slow down the function of the bladder. It is, of course, important to appreciate the tremendous psychosocial distress that daytime enuresis can cause. The child will need reassurance, and the parents and family will have to exercise patience to avoid long-term effects on the child's self-confidence.

The DOs
- If your child has enuresis, you should avoid excessive criticism of him/her.
- Your child should avoid liquids in the evening, and urinate at specified times (e.g., after dinner, before leaving house, before bedtime).
- Give your child positive reinforcement for "dry" nights.

The DON'Ts
- Don't "baby" or smother your child (infantilization) because this will only increase dependency.

When to Call Your Doctor
- If daytime wetting occurs in a child who initially only wet the bed at night.
- If urine produced is foul smelling, blood tinged, or associated with pain.
- You should also call your doctor if the bedwetting stops. He likes to hear good news too!

For More Information
Contact your pediatrician or visit your local library.

EPIDIDYMITIS

About Your Diagnosis

Epididymitis is an infection and inflammation of the epididymis, which is an oblong structure at the upper area of each testicle. It is usually a complication of a bacterial infection elsewhere in the body, such as a urinary tract infection. It may also be caused by a scrotal injury. It is curable with treatment. Possible complications of the disease include sterility; blockage or narrowing of the urethra causing urinary difficulty if the infection involves both testicles; and constipation, because bowel movements may aggravate the pain.

Living With Your Diagnosis

For mild pain, over-the-counter medications may be used. If pain is moderate to severe, your doctor may need to prescribe a stronger pain medication. Stool softeners are useful to prevent constipation and to decrease pain associated with bowel movements. Bed rest may be necessary until the fever, swelling, and pain improve. While in bed, elevating the scrotum on a rolled towel may help. Activity should be increased gradually, and an athletic supporter should be worn. Sexual relations should be put on hold until 1 month after symptoms disappear.

Treatment

Antibiotics are needed to fight the infection.

The DOs

- Rest in bed until the fever, swelling, and pain improve.
- Place a soft, rolled towel under the scrotum while in bed.
- Apply an ice pack to the scrotal area to help reduce swelling and pain.
- Wear an athletic supporter when your activity increases.
- Take antibiotics until finished.
- Take nonprescription pain medication.
- Eat foods that are natural laxatives, such as fresh fruits, nuts, prunes, and whole grain cereals to prevent constipation.
- Increase your fluid intake but avoid carbonated, caffeinated beverages and alcohol.

The DON'Ts

- Don't skip doses or stop your antibiotics.
- Don't drink alcohol, carbonated beverages, tea, or coffee because they can irritate the urinary tract.
- Don't resume sexual relations until several days after symptoms are completely gone.

When to Call Your Doctor

- A high fever develops during treatment.
- Your pain is not controlled with nonprescription medications.
- You become severely constipated.
- Your symptoms don't improve in 3 or 4 days after your treatment starts.

For More Information:
National Kidney and Urologic Disease Information Clearinghouse
301-654-4415
Internet Sites
www.healthfinder.gov (Choose SEARCH to search by topic)
www.healthanswers.com

EPIGLOTTITIS

About Your Diagnosis

Epiglottitis is an inflammation of the epiglottis (a small flap of tissue that covers the entrance to the lungs when swallowing), which causes the epiglottis to swell. It can be mistaken for the croup, but is much more dangerous and life threatening. Children aged 2–12 years are usually affected, although adults without immunity to the *Haemophilus influenzae* bacteria have been known to develop it. It is usually caused by a bacteria such as *H. influenzae*, or occasionally by streptococcus. Prevention is now available with the *Haemophilus influenzae* type B (Hib) vaccine.

Living With Your Diagnosis

Epiglottitis has a sudden onset. Symptoms and signs include severe sore throat, muffled voice with hoarseness, fever, drooling caused by difficulty swallowing saliva, and increased difficulty breathing. Children with epiglottitis will tilt their neck back and lean forward, trying to inhale more air.

Treatment

Hospitalization is usually needed for oxygen and intravenous antibiotics. Close observation is needed in case the airway becomes totally obstructed and an emergency airway is needed. Death can occur if untreated. With treatment, improvement of symptoms is seen in 24 hours, with complete relief of swelling in 72 hours.

Children with suspected epiglottitis should be kept in an upright position to aid breathing. Keep them calm until reaching the hospital because breathing becomes more difficult if they panic. After hospitalization it will be necessary to continue antibiotics for at least 10 days. A cool-mist humidifier will be helpful at night for several weeks; remember to change the water and clean the unit daily.

The DOs

- Have your child immunized with the Hib vaccine early.
- Seek emergency treatment if epiglottitis is suspected.
- Continue antibiotics as directed, usually at least 10 days.
- Resume activity gradually after all symptoms disappear.
- Encourage fluids and follow a normal diet as tolerated.
- Continue using a cool-mist vaporizer at the bedside for several weeks. Remember to change water and clean unit daily.

The DON'Ts

- Don't delay treatment because death can occur if the infection is not treated.
- Don't skip doses or stop antibiotics before they are finished.

When to Call Your Doctor

- There are signs of a respiratory infection and your child has had epiglottitis in the past.
- During a respiratory infection there is any difficulty breathing.
- After treatment, fever or sore throat recurs.

For More Information:
American Academy of Otolaryngology
One Prince Street
Alexandria, VA 22314
703-836-4444, Monday through Friday from 8:30 AM to 5 PM (EST).
National Institute of Allergy and Infectious Diseases of the NIH
Office of Communications
9000 Rockville Pike
Bethesda, MD 20892
301-496-5717
Internet Sites
www.healthfinder.gov (Choose SEARCH to search by topic.)
www.healthanswers.com

EPISTAXIS

About Your Diagnosis

Epistaxis is a nosebleed. Rupture of blood vessels somewhere in your nose causes a nosebleed. This may result from an injury such as a blow to the nose. Other causes include chemical irritants, infections, or abnormalities of the blood vessels of the nose. Diseases such as elevated blood pressure or bleeding abnormalities may cause a nosebleed. The most common cause is excessive drying of the nasal passages from dry air, especially in the winter. Most individuals will have at least one nosebleed during their lives. They are twice as common in children. Most resolve with direct pressure on the nose, although some may need further medical intervention such as packing or cautery.

Living With Your Diagnosis

The signs and symptoms of epistaxis include bleeding from one or both nostrils. There also may be bleeding down the back of the throat with spitting of blood, coughing of blood, or vomiting of blood. Swallowed blood irritates the stomach, frequently causing vomiting. Most nosebleeds do not result in sufficient blood loss to cause significant problems. However, a very prolonged, vigorous nosebleed may result in anemia. If you have had a significant nosebleed recently, you may notice dark or tarry bowel movements; these indicate that you have swallowed a significant amount of blood.

Treatment

The first-line treatment for epistaxis is direct pressure. Grasp the nose firmly between the thumb and forefinger and squeeze it for 10–30 minutes without releasing the nose or peeking. Some feel that placing an ice pack on the neck or on the bridge of the nose may be helpful in slowing the blood flow to the nose. Lean forward so that any blood running down the throat may be spit out rather than swallowed. This may help prevent vomiting.

If this is not successful, it may be necessary to pack the nose. Your doctor will pack absorbent gauze into the nose so as to place pressure on the bleeding site. It may be necessary to cauterize the bleeding site. The main side effects of packing are discomfort and the inability to breathe through your nose. Complications include an increased risk of sinus infection with packing. In some elderly individuals, slowed pulse rate or decreased blood pressure can be a result of packing, and your doctor may recommend hospitalization for close monitoring of the elderly individual. With cautery, there is a risk of perforation of the septum, the tissue that separates one nostril from the other.

The DOs

If your nosebleed is caused by elevated blood pressure, you should work with your doctor to get your blood pressure under good control. If you are prone to nosebleeds, you should probably avoid aspirin products because they may slow clotting. Humidification of the air in your home and, if possible, at work may prevent nosebleeds caused by dry air. Other useful treatments may include placing a small amount of petroleum jelly inside the opening of the nostril to protect it from drying. A scarf or cloth mask may be helpful if you must be out in cold, dry air. Salt water nasal sprays may be helpful. If irritating chemicals or dusts are a problem, avoidance or a filter-type mask may help. Your doctor may prescribe a steroid nasal spray if infections or allergies are a problem.

The DON'Ts

If bleeding is stopped by direct pressure, it is important not to blow the nose vigorously or to pick at any clots, because this may restart the bleeding. If you find that you are prone to nosebleeds, you should try to avoid factors that cause them. Decongestant nasal sprays can be a problem, and you should discuss their use with your doctor. Dry air and picking of the nose cause the majority of nosebleeds. Avoiding both of these situations will help prevent nosebleeds.

When to Call Your Doctor

You should call your doctor if your nose is gushing or if you are having repeated episodes of vomiting from swallowed blood. You need medical attention if applying direct pressure to your nose for 30 minutes does not control the bleeding. Also, call your doctor if you are having more than three or four nosebleeds a day. You should call your doctor if you know that your nosebleeds are caused by elevated blood pressure or a bleeding problem such as hemophilia or leukemia. You should call if you are on blood thinners such as heparin or coumadin. You should call your doctor if you have a temperature of greater than 102°F, especially if your nose was packed or cauterized.

For More Information

Robert Kelly (ed): *Family Health and Medical Guide*. Dallas, Word
Publishing, 1996.

ERECTILE DYSFUNCTION

About Your Diagnosis

Erectile dysfunction, commonly referred to as male impotence, can have both physiologic and psychological causes; however, much more attention has been devoted to the physiologic causes of this disorder. Erectile dysfunction increases dramatically in later life, from about 10% of men in their 60s to 30% by their 70s. It increases even further in men between 70 and 80 years of age. Most of the patients with erectile dysfunction in this age group have heart and blood vessel disease; however, many cases are medication induced. It can also be caused by a neurologic disturbance, radiation, diabetes, hypertension, smoking, being overweight, and being sedentary (not exercising).

By definition, erectile dysfunction is persistent or recurrent inability to get or to keep an adequate erection until completion of sexual activity. As do most sexual disorders, male erectile dysfunction causes marked distress and difficulties with interpersonal relationships.

Psychogenic erectile dysfunction, which is caused by emotional and not physical reasons, is more difficult to diagnose. An important finding in making the diagnosis of emotional or psychosocial impotence would be that the individual may have reliable, firm erections under some circumstances and be impotent in other situations. In evaluating the individual with erectile dysfunction, the doctor will inquire about the relative firmness and length of time of erections under the following circumstances: masturbation, sex other than intercourse, sex with female or other male partners, stimulation with explicit materials such as sexually arousing movies or pornography, erections in the middle of the night, or in particular, erections upon arising from a night's sleep. Most males, particularly those who are younger, awaken with an erection. Obviously, in the absence of diseases that are known to cause impotence, and if an individual can have an erection with masturbation or early morning awakening, then the likelihood of psychogenic impotence is very high.

Living With Your Diagnosis

Erectile dysfunction can be lifelong or acquired later in life. It can be generalized or associated with specific situations, and it can be caused by psycho-logical factors or a combination of psychological and physical factors. In psychiatric terms, lifelong male impotence typically involves some kind of anxiety or confusion about sexual identity, including such issues as transvestism, homosexuality, or a psychiatric diagnosis that increases the patient's fear of being sexually close to a partner (e.g., schizophrenia or schizoid and avoidant personality disorders). Occasionally, a physician may not ask you about your sexual functioning. Although you may be hesitant or somewhat embarrassed to discuss it, it is very important that you mention sexual dysfunction to your psychiatrist or family doctor because many of these conditions can be successfully treated. Obviously, for the man with lifelong impotence, the earlier he is into treatment the better. Individuals who are anxious about their first sexual encounter and have impotence secondary to that have particularly good outcome with treatment. The outlook for success among older men who have had lifelong erectile dysfunction is poor. In contrast, men who have had long-established good potency, who have recently lost their erectile abilities, so-called acquired psychogenic impotence, have a much better prognosis than those with a lifelong pattern. These men can be treated individually or in couples therapy, and the psychiatrist will try to identify the cause of the impotence and suggest treatment for it. Often, an affair outside of marriage, or some discord in the relationship is responsible for secondary or acquired impotence. Potency is frequently lost after a separation or divorce, as well as after the death of a spouse (so-called widower's impotence). Other risk factors for impotence include the crumbling of a man's financial or occupational life, the occurrence of a serious new physical illness, such as a heart attack or stroke, or when the man's wife becomes seriously ill. Regardless of what stressor may have caused secondary impotence, the basic problem is still one of performance anxiety. The anxiety that a man who is impotent feels involves initially a fear that he will not be able to obtain an erection, and if he does, worrying whether it will be maintained long enough or is hard enough for the completion of sexual activity. Needless to say, such preoccupation diminishes the satisfaction of any sexual intercourse.

Treatment

The most basic treatment for this form of anxiety is to ask the man to make love with his partner without trying intercourse on several occasions, just to show him how different lovemaking can feel when he is not overly concerned with failure of potency. Often this enables the man to relax and concentrate on lovemaking, and refocuses attention on pleasing his partner and obtaining pleasure for himself. This technique is known as sensate focus.

One of the major problems in our culture that leads to impotence has to do with the belief that men should be able to perform intercourse with anyone, anywhere, and in any circumstance. It is impossible for most men to live up to this expectation. Physicians who are not psychiatrists have three basic treatments to offer men with impotence. They often prescribe (1) the use of a vacuum pump; (2) the injection of a substance into the penis that causes blood vessels to open up, thereby increasing blood flow to the penis; or (3) surgical implantation of a penile prosthesis. This last procedure is often done in patients who have sexual dysfunction from diabetes. Although some may be hesitant to admit it, most men at some point during their sexual lives are unable to get and/or keep an erection. It is only when this function is persistent and causes significant distress that the patient generally is referred to a physician.

The DOs

It is important to discuss this condition with your physician. As mentioned previously, the physician may not ask about your sexual functioning; however, you should not be too embarrassed to discuss any problems you are having. Secondly, make sure you tell your physician all the medications you are taking because many medications, including many of the antidepressants, can cause sexual dysfunction. Thirdly, talk to your partner. It is very easy for some partners to assume that a male's difficulty with erection is somehow related to the fact that they are less pleasing and less desirable, and so some feelings of guilt may arise. Keep the lines of communication open. Common-sense measures including regular exercise and a healthy diet are very helpful in normal sexual functioning. However, the most important thing to remember in acquired impotence is to relax. Like many conditions in the field of psychiatry, worrying about it only makes it worse. There are many activities that can be engaged in that are part of making love that do not have as high a degree of performance anxiety.

The DON'Ts

You should be realistic about your sexual ability. Do not expect to have completely normal sexual functioning during periods of high stress or during periods of grieving or significant depression. Impotence during these times is temporary, and becoming anxious about it only makes it worse. Do not engage in drastic actions like having an affair or getting a divorce.

When to Call Your Doctor

Contact your doctor if you notice blood or discharge from your penis, if sexual intercourse becomes painful, if you have a long-lasting erection that persists after intercourse, or if your concern about this condition leads to severe depression or suicidal thoughts.

For More Information

For more information about erectile dysfunction, contact your physician for referral to a sexual disorders clinic or a urologist. If you believe medication may play a role, consult the Physician's Desk Reference (PDR) under the "Adverse Effects" section for the drugs you are taking.
You can also check out the following Web sites:
Impotence Information Page
http://www.demon.co.uk/hernia/nfo/mcd.html
Impotence: Its Reversible
http://www.cei.net/~impotenc
Successfully Treating Impotence
http://www.impotent.com

ERYSIPELAS (ST. ANTHONY'S FIRE)

About Your Diagnosis

Erysipelas is an infection of the skin and its deep layer, caused by bacteria called beta-hemolytic stretococcus. Sometimes the staphylococcal bacteria are involved. It was a very common infection in the preantibiotic era and became somewhat more prevalent again in the late 1980s.

Because erysipelas is a bacterial infection, it would be thought to occur more frequently in settings such as hospitals, nursing homes, and day-care centers. However, most of the cases are isolated. The infection most frequently occurs in the very young, the elderly, and patients who are infected with the human immunodeficiency virus (HIV-positive patients) as well as those who have acquired immunodeficiency syndrome (AIDS). Diabetics and alcoholics are also more likely to get the infection. It can occur in wounds after surgery. It may also occur in patients without any other medical problems.

Living With Your Diagnosis

The skin abruptly becomes painful and then develops redness and swelling with a very distinct edge. The affected area is tender and hot. Small or large blisters may develop in the area of the redness. The classic area for this infection to develop is on the face; however, it now occurs more frequently on the leg. It is commonly seen in the area of the vein that has been taken for use in coronary artery bypass surgery.

Other sypmptoms are fever, chills, and headache. Tiredness, loss of appetite, and abdominal pain also occur. There are frequently swollen lymph nodes in the area of the infection.

Your doctor may do some laboratory tests such as cultures of your nose and throat for streptococcal bacteria. Blood tests for evidence of a streptoccocal infection and a white blood cell count may also be done.

Without treatment, abscesses, infection in the veins, and gangrene can develop. These complications are also more likely to occur in patients with diabetes, alcoholism, previous blood clots in the leg, and AIDS.

Treatment

Penicillin and some of its related drugs are the treatment of choice for this infection. If you are allergic to penicillin, then erythromycin and its related drugs also work well. Individuals with complicating conditions may have to be treated in the hospital with intravenous antibiotics.

The most common side effect of antibiotics is an allergic rash. If hives, shortness of breath, and swelling of the tongue and eyes occur, contact your doctor or the emergency department of the hospital immediately. Some individuals do not tolerate erythromycin very well. It can cause diarrhea and abdominal cramps. Women may get a vaginal yeast infection after taking antibiotics.

Unfortunately, some individuals get recurrences of this infection. If this becomes frequent or very severe, long-term treatment with low-dose antibiotics may be recommended.

The DOs

- You may use warm soaks to improve the blood flow to the infected area. If you are diabetic, be very careful about the heat of the soak.
- If the infection is in your leg, elevate the leg to help with the swelling.
- If there are others in the household, separate your towels, wash cloths, and bedding from other household laundry. Wash these in very hot water.
- Take all of your antibiotics, even after the skin has apparently cleared.

The DON'Ts

- Do not stop your antibiotic, even if the area of infection has greatly improved. Erysipelas is a serious infection. You must complete the antibiotic that your doctor has given you.
- Do not put any salves, creams, or lotions on the area of the infection. If the area weeps a little, dress it with plain gauze.
- Do not allow other family members to use your towels or wash cloths while you have this infection. Any serum that the skin weeps may contain bacteria, and you can give the infection to other family members.

When to Call Your Doctor

- If you seem to be having a reaction to the antibiotic that your doctor has prescribed.
- If your rash and redness continue to spread.
- If you have fever, chills, or other alarming signs

such as dizziness when you stand up and a rapid
heart rate.

For More Information
World Wide Web
http://www.housecall.com/aafp
American Medical Association Family Medical Guide, 3rd edition.
*American Academy of Family Physician's Family Health and Medical
Guide*. Word Publishing, 1997.

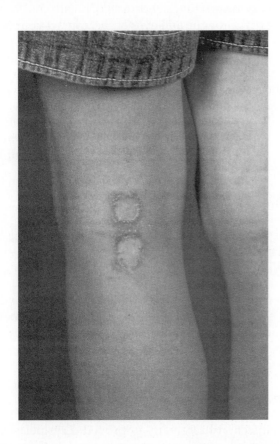

Erysipelas. Note well-demarcated erythematous plaque on arm.
(Courtesy of Department of Dermatology, University of North Carolina at Chapel Hill. From Goldstein BG, Goldstein AO: *Practical
Dermatology*, vol 1. St. Louis, Mosby–Year Book, 1992. Used by permission.)

ERYTHEMA MULTIFORME

About Your Diagnosis

Erythema Multiforme is a relatively common disorder that affects the skin and sometimes the internal organs. The extent of involvement of the internal organs varies greatly, but widespread or severe involvement is rare. There are many causes of erythema multiforme. These include viral and bacterial infections, certain chronic diseases, pregnancy, cancer, and others. In more than half of all cases a cause cannot be found. The diagnosis can usually be made on examination by a doctor, but a biopsy is frequently done to confirm the diagnosis. Most cases of erythema multiforme resolve with treatment, but severe cases may require hospitalization.

Living With Your Diagnosis

In the minor form of erythema multiforme, there are round, red bumps and blisters on both sides of the body that occur on the arms, legs, face, and lips. These bumps can take on the appearance of red or pink targets, or they can become large blisters. The rash itches a lot and may develop into hives. It usually affects children and young adults and lasts from 2 to 4 weeks. Fever and muscle and joint aches may be present. It can recur during the first few years.

Erythema multiforme major, also called Stevens-Johnson syndrome, is a more serious illness with high fever, large blisters, and ulcers on membranes of the mouth, nose, eyes, genital area, arms, and skin. There may be severe itching and occasionally lung involvement. If there are no complications, symptoms resolve in 4 weeks, but mouth sores can persist for months. Untreated eye involvement can lead to blindness. Severe cases require hospitalization.

Treatment

Mild cases of erythema multiforme may not require any treatment. Prednisone may be used if necessary. If your doctor suspects a medication you are taking may have caused your problem, the medication will be stopped. Antibiotics are used when a secondary infection occurs. Any medical illness causing erythema multiforme should be treated as appropriate. Steroid creams applied to skin may be prescribed. Erythema multiforme associated with herpes simplex virus can recur, and preventive medications are frequently used. Itching can be controlled with antihistamines such as Benadryl. Mouth pain is frequently treated with lidocaine rinses. Eye involvement may require a consult with an eye specialist.

The DOs

- Apply cool wet Burow's compresses to blisters, or just a cool wet cloth can be used.
- Call your doctor immediately if any vision changes occur.
- Take acetaminophen for pain unless otherwise directed by your doctor.

The DON'Ts

- Don't apply skin creams or ointments to broken or bleeding skin.
- Don't take hot baths or hot showers. These can make the skin itch more. Cool or lukewarm baths may help.
- Avoid strenuous or vigorous activities if ill with fever, headaches, or malaise.

When to Call Your Doctor

- Call immediately if any decreased vision or eye pain develops during treatment.
- If persistent vomiting or diarrhea occur.
- If new symptoms occur during treatment, or if symptoms worsen significantly.

For More Information

American Academy of Dermatology
930 N. Meacham Road
Schaumburg, IL 60173
847-330-0230

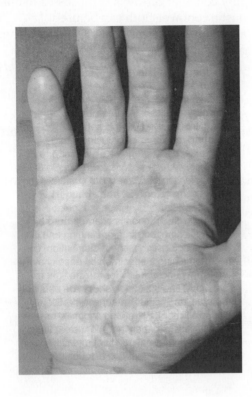

Mild erythema multiforme. Note target lesions and no bullae. (Courtesy of Department of Dermatology, University of North Carolina at Chapel Hill. From Goldstein BG, Goldstein AO: *Practical Dermatology*, vol 1. St. Louis, Mosby–Year Book, 1992. Used by permission.)

ERYTHEMA NODOSUM

About Your Diagnosis

Erythema nodosum (EN) is a rash that occurs in a number of different conditions. It almost always occurs on the front of the lower legs (over the shin bones) but can also occur in other places. Erythema nodosum is more common in women than men. Although anyone can get EN, it usually occurs in individuals in their 20s and 30s.

Erythema nodosum is caused by inflammation of the fat under the skin. The most common causes of EN are certain medications (in particular, birth control pills and "sulfa" medicines) and infections. Sarcoidosis, ulcerative colitis, Crohn's disease, thyroid conditions, lupus, and pregnancy can also cause EN. In many individuals the cause of EN is not known.

Erythema nodosum is usually diagnosed by the typical way it looks. However, a skin biopsy specimen is sometimes needed to make the diagnosis. A medical history, physical examination, chest X-ray, and certain blood tests may help determine whether there is a specific cause.

Living With Your Diagnosis

Erythema nodosum causes painful, bright-red nodules (or bumps) under the skin. It usually occurs on both legs. Sometimes individuals have fevers, chills, fatigue, and joint pain before the rash begins.

Treatment

Treatment of the condition causing erythema nodosum usually will help improve the rash. Otherwise, it usually improves on its own in about 6 weeks. If your doctor believes the EN is from a medication, it will be necessary to stop that drug. Nonsteroidal anti-inflammatory drugs (NSAIDs) may help reduce the pain and inflammation of EN. Occasionally, a more potent anti-inflammatory medicine such as prednisone, a cortisone-like medicine, is necessary. Potential side effects of NSAIDs include stomach upset, ulcers, constipation, diarrhea, headaches, dizziness, difficulty hearing, and skin rash. Potential side effects of cortisone-like medicines are increased appetite, weight gain, difficulty sleeping, easy bruising, and stomach upset.

The DOs
- Take your medicines as prescribed.
- Follow your doctor's treatment instructions.
- Ask your doctor which over-the-counter medications you may take with your prescription medications.

The DON'Ts
- Wait to see if side effects from medications will go away.

When to Call Your Doctor
- You experience any medication side effects.
- The treatment is not decreasing your symptoms in a reasonable amount of time.
- You develop new, unexplained symptoms.

For More Information
Contact the Arthritis Foundation in your area. If you do not know the location of the Arthritis Foundation, you may call the national office at 1-800-283-7800 or access the information on the Internet at www.arthritis.org.

ESOPHAGEAL TUMORS

About Your Diagnosis

The esophagus is the part of the digestive tract that connects the throat with the stomach. Cancer of the esophagus is more common in Asia and China than in the United States. Approximately 12,000 new cases of esophageal cancer were diagnosed last year in the United States. The cause of esophageal cancer is unknown, but there are risk factors, such as heavy alcohol and tobacco use, that increase your chances of getting this cancer. Acid reflux (back up) from the stomach to the esophagus that occurs over a long time can lead to Barrett's esophagus, which can convert to esophageal cancer.

Esophageal cancer is not contagious. The cancer is detected by means of one of two radiographic (x-ray) studies, a barium swallow examination or esophagography. The easiest way for a physician to diagnose esophageal cancer is to obtain tissue with an endoscope (a lighted tube passed through the mouth into the esophagus). The tissue is examined with a microscope.

Living With Your Diagnosis

Most cancers of the esophagus occur in the lower part of the esophagus. Difficulty in swallowing solid foods is the typical symptom. As the tumor grows, liquids become difficult to swallow, and you can have pain with swallowing. The cancer usually spreads to nearby structures (lung, windpipe, lymph glands, and liver). This can cause hoarseness, coughing, coughing of blood, vomiting of blood, and chest pain.

Treatment

Once the diagnosis is made, you undergo a staging process. Staging of esophageal cancer tells you the extent of the disease and whether it has spread. Staging usually includes a physical examination, blood tests, radiographs (x-rays) of the chest, and computed tomography (CT) of the chest and abdomen. Laryngoscopy (examination with a lighted tube passed into the voice box) can be performed if it looks like the cancer has spread into the larynx (voice box). Bronchoscopy can be performed if it is believed the cancer has spread into the lungs or the tubes that lead into the lungs (trachea and bronchi).

Esophageal cancer is a difficult cancer to cure unless it is detected in its earliest stage. Therapy for esophageal cancer depends on the extent of disease; it can include surgical, radiation, and chemotherapy.

An operation on the esophagus is called *esophagectomy.* In the operation the surgeon removes the part of the esophagus with the tumor and nearby lymph glands. If the cancer completely blocks the esophagus, tubes are placed to reopen the esophagus and allow nutrition. Complications of surgical treatment are infection, pneumonia, and breathing and swallowing problems.

Radiation therapy is used instead of surgical treatment when the tumor is too large to remove or when the patient cannot withstand an operation. The side effect of radiation therapy is dry, red, itchy burning skin over the treated area. If the irradiation was over the neck and chest, dry mouth, sore throat, cough can occur.

Chemotherapy can be used with radiation if surgical treatment is not possible. Sometimes radiation and chemotherapy are tried before surgical intervention. The patient and oncologist decide this together. Side effects of chemotherapy can be easy bruising, bleeding, fever, nausea, vomiting, and hair loss.

The DOs

- Report any symptoms of pain or difficulty swallowing.
- Ask for second opinions.
- Ask about your prognosis. This is a difficult cancer to cure.
- Understand that nutrition is important both before and after the operation. Because there are difficulty and pain with swallowing, marked weight loss occurs before and especially the days to weeks after the operation. It is important to eat high-calorie foods and nutritional supplements. A nutritionist can be a good resource.
- Ask for emotional support groups, psychiatrists, and social workers to help with coping, rehabilitation, travel, financial issues, and home care.

The DON'Ts

- Do not smoke.
- Do not drink alcohol in excess.
- Do not miss follow-up appointments with your physicians. You have a team of physicians and health care providers, including a primary care physician, surgeon, oncologist, radiation oncologist, nutritionist, physical therapist, and social worker.

When to Call Your Doctor

- If you are having pain with swallowing, difficulty swallowing, or food becoming stuck after eating.
- If you cough up blood or vomit blood.
- If you are short of breath, coughing, and have a fever.
- If you have a fever after chemotherapy.
- If you cannot eat and continue to lose weight.
- If you have pain.

For More Information

National Cancer Institute (NCI)
9000 Rockville Pike
Bethesda, MD 20892
Cancer Information Service
1-800-422-6237 (1-800-4-CANCER)
American Cancer Society
1599 Clifton Road, N.E.
Atlanta, GA 30329
1-800-ACS-2345

FEMORAL NECK FRACTURE

About Your Diagnosis

A femoral neck fracture is a break of the thigh bone at the hip. This may be caused by a severe fall or an auto accident in younger individuals, but it is much more commonly seen in older individuals, particularly women. A femoral neck fracture usually results from osteoporosis or thinning of the bone associated with increasing age. If the bone of the hip is thin enough, even twisting can result in a break. Indeed, in many elderly individuals, they may twist while standing, which causes the break, and then they fall. As many as one fourth of all women older than 75 years may have severe enough osteoporosis to experience a hip fracture. Hip fractures are diagnosed by physical examination and an x-ray. Many individuals have a complete recovery after surgery.

Living With Your Diagnosis

The symptoms of a hip fracture are pain in the hip, buttock, or pubic area, especially with movement of the hip or leg. A frequently seen sign is shortening of the affected leg when compared with the other leg. In addition, the foot of the affected leg will frequently turn in. A later sign may be bruising on the hip, especially in thin individuals.

Treatment

Treatment is nearly always surgical. There are a variety of surgical options depending on where the hip fracture is located and on the condition of the bone. These range from placing pins across the fracture to using metal plates and screws to hold the bone fragments together. Other choices include replacing the ball of the hip joint with a metal one, or replacing the socket as well as the ball. At times, if the patient is in very poor health and cannot tolerate surgery, the treatment may be bed rest to try to allow the fracture to heal. This has a very poor success rate with many complications and is reserved for individuals who simply cannot tolerate surgery. The main side effects of surgery are those seen with any surgery: namely, infection and bleeding. Sometimes, the surgery fails to stabilize the joint, usually because the remaining bone is too thin for the artificial joint or the screws or pins to hold.

The DOs

Your doctor will prescribe medications for pain. After most of the surgeries done now, a physical therapy program is started, which will have the patient out of bed within a few days after surgery. This is important to prevent weakening of the muscles. Pain medicines will make this more comfortable and should be used appropriately to speed recovery. An adequate diet to provide protein and calcium will speed healing of the bone. Exercise in the form of physical therapy is a crucial part of recovery from surgery. Most individuals will achieve a total recovery if they are diligent in the physical therapy regimen.

The prevention of hip fractures is crucial. It is possible to slow or even reverse osteoporosis with appropriate diet, exercise, and medical therapy, including hormone replacement therapy (estrogen) for women who have gone through menopause. The stronger the bone, the less likely you are to sustain a hip fracture. If osteoporosis is present, there are medicines that may help reverse the process. You should discuss this with your doctor. In addition, there are things to do in the home that will decrease the chance of falls. These include adequate lighting and avoiding tripping hazards such as loose rugs and poor-fitting shoes. Many home health agencies can offer help in making the home safer.

The DON'Ts

Medications that have side effects of dizziness or drowsiness may increase the risk of falls. Medicines such as steroids, thyroid medicines, and diuretics may increase osteoporosis and should only be used if the benefits outweigh the risks of osteoporosis. Alcohol and tobacco use increase the risk of osteoporosis, as does lack of weight-bearing exercise. A diet low in calcium and excessive in protein increases risk. A living environment with poor light and lots of tripping hazards increase the risk of a fall.

The most significant long-term adverse effects of hip fractures have been pneumonia or blood clots to the lungs because of prolonged bed rest. Indeed, this is largely why the outcome of nonsurgical treatment is poor. With advances in surgical techniques that allow ambulation to start within a few days after surgery, these adverse effects have decreased. However, failure to comply with a physical therapy program, as well as prolonged bed rest, will increase these risks.

When to Call Your Doctor

You should call your doctor if you have any increasing pain in your hip after surgery. This could be a sign of infection, bleeding, or loosening of the hip replacement or screws. You should also call if you are having increasing difficulty walking, because this also can be a sign of loosening of the hip replacement. You should also call when signs of infection are present, such as fever, or swelling or redness of the incision line. Any shortness of breath and coughing should be reported to your doctor because they could be signs of pneumonia or a blood clot to the lungs, which can be complications of a hip fracture.

For More Information

Description of fractures and of surgical repairs
http://www.medmedia.com/oo4/156.htm
Description of surgery and recovery
http://www.depuy.com/PatientEd/Hip/Hip.htm
Information on osteoporosis
http://www.oznet.ksu.edu/dp_fnut/NUTLINK/pages/bones.htm
Osteoporosis and Related Bone Diseases National Resource Center1-800-624-BONE

FIBROCYSTIC BREAST DISEASE

About Your Diagnosis

Breasts that are "fibrocystic" have an exaggerated response to the hormonal fluctuations of the menstrual cycle. After ovulation, 1–2 weeks before the period, the breasts develop cysts, retain fluid, and enlarge. They may also become tender and sometimes very painful. The pain can radiate into the axilla (the armpit) or even into the shoulder area. After the period, the breasts will shrink in size, and become less lumpy and less tender.

Fibrocystic breasts are diagnosed by the symptoms that occur before the period and by examination. Many women with fibrocystic breasts have cysts that can be felt by examination. If you are undergoing mammograms, the mammogram findings may also indicate fibrocystic changes.

It is estimated that 50% of all women have some degree of fibrocystic changes of the breast.

Fibrocystic breasts are usually symptomatic between the ages of 20 and 50 years. Once a woman has gone through menopause, the fibrocystic changes are less symptomatic or not symptomatic at all. However, if the woman starts on hormone replacement therapy, sometimes the fibrocystic breasts will continue to be symptomatic because of the hormonal stimulation.

Living With Your Diagnosis

The most common symptoms are that both breasts become tender or painful and engorged 1–2 weeks before the period. The tenderness or pain is often in the outer, upper sides of the breasts (toward the armpit). However, sometimes the tenderness or pain can occur in other areas of the breast as well. If the breasts are examined, they may feel thicker and lumpy as if examining a mound of peas clumped together. Occasionally, a breast cyst will grow larger than usual, up to 2.5 inches, and will cause pain in one particular spot and can be felt as a distinct lump.

The tenderness and/or pain can range from very mild to very severe. However, most of the time pain medication is not necessary. If you have fibrocystic changes, try not to examine your breasts before your period. Do your self-breast examination as recommended, only after your periods. Otherwise, you may feel "lumps" and become unnecessarily alarmed. However, despite your best efforts, you may find that you visit your doctor more often than someone who doesn't have fibrocystic breasts to get a lump checked out.

Treatment

Most women will not need medication to treat their fibrocystic breast symptoms. If some medication is needed, often over-the-counter ibuprofen can be effective in relieving some of the symptoms. If more relief is needed, your doctor may prescribe a mild diuretic to start with. If your symptoms do not respond to ibuprofen or a diuretic, your doctor may refer you to a breast surgeon or gynecologist for further medical treatment. Sometimes birth control pills are prescribed. Other medications that may be prescribed are danazol, bromocriptine or tamoxifen.

Decreasing the amount of caffeine and nicotine (if you are a smoker) may decrease the severity of the symptoms. One study of women with fibrocystic changes demonstrated that 92% had less severe symptoms when they decreased their caffeine and/or nicotine intake. Although, other studies have not confirmed this finding, it may be worthwhile to decrease caffeine and nicotine intake to see whether your symptoms lessen.

Evening Primrose Oil capsules may also lessen symptoms from fibrocystic breasts. In a study looking at premenstrual symptoms, it was observed that women receiving Evening Primrose Oil capsules had milder breast symptoms than women not taking Evening Primrose Oil. The amount recommended is 1.5–2.0 grams of Evening Primrose Oil twice each day 10–14 days before each period. Usually, it can be purchased at a health food store. No side effects have been reported.

The DOs
- Take as directed any recommended or prescribed medication.
- Wear a good supportive bra.
- Have a yearly breast examination, and have mammograms performed when recommended.

The DON'Ts
- Don't take in excessive caffeine or nicotine.

When to Call Your Doctor
- If your symptoms are not relieved by the recommended treatment, another medication may be prescribed.

• If you feel a lump in your breast.

For More Information
Understanding Your Body: Every Woman's Guide to Gynecology and Health. Felicia Stewart, M.D., Felicia Guest, M.D., Gary Stewart, M.D., and Robert Hatcher, M.D., Bantam Books, 1987.

FIBROMYALGIA

About Your Diagnosis

Fibromyalgia (FM) means pain in the muscles, tendons, and ligaments. In FM, there are specific areas of pain in the body called tender points (Fig 1). We do not know the cause of FM. However, research has looked at sleep, levels of chemicals called serotonin and substance P, as well as muscle and growth hormone as possible important factors in the cause of FM.

It is estimated that FM may occur in up to 2% of the population. It is about eight times more common in women than men. Fibromyalgia usually occurs in individuals between the ages of 20 and 50 years, although it is also common in women older than 60 years. Although we do not know the cause of FM, it is not an infectious illness. A physician is able to diagnose FM by obtaining a medical history and performing an examination of the joints and muscles. Most blood tests and x-rays show no abnormalities. However, your doctor may perform blood tests to determine whether your pain and fatigue result from other diseases that may cause similar symptoms, and x-rays may be done to look for any bone or joint abnormalities.

Living With Your Diagnosis

Individuals with FM experience pain and fatigue. Pain is usually worse in the areas of the upper back and neck, and the lower back and hips, although pain can occur around any of the tender points. The fatigue can be severe. Individuals with FM may also have headaches, numbness or tingling in the hands or feet, abdominal bloating, diarrhea or constipation, and forgetfulness. Fibromyalgia may affect your activities at work and at home because of the pain and fatigue. Although there is no cure for FM, individuals with this diagnosis can feel better with appropriate therapies. Treatment focuses on managing the symptoms with medications, exercise, stress management, and fatigue management.

Treatment

The best way to manage FM is through a combination of sleep improvement, exercise, stress management, and medications. Medications can improve the amount and quality of sleep. Individuals with FM often awaken frequently throughout the night and wake up feeling tired. This interrupted sleep pattern prevents them from reaching the deepest form of sleep. A physician may prescribe a medicine to reach this deeper stage of sleep. By improving sleep, the pain will also decrease. The most common medications include amitriptyline, nortriptyline, and cyclobenzaprine. These medications are used in large doses to treat depression, but to manage pain and sleep the medications are used in small doses. The most common side effects from these medications are grogginess upon awakening, dry mouth, constipation, weight gain, and rash.

Appropriate exercises are very helpful in decreasing pain. Stretching and posture exercises should be done every day to maintain good body alignment and prevent pain. Endurance exercises should be done three or four times a week and can include walking, biking, or water therapy. This type of exercise will improve your ability to do activities for a longer length of time. It is important to *begin exercise slowly and to increase gradually.*

Although stress does not cause FM, it is more difficult to manage daily life when you hurt and are tired. Often individuals with FM have forgotten how to "relax." You should look at your life realistically and explore whether family or financial problems or depression is interfering with your ability to feel better. A counselor can offer services that range from relaxation therapy to family counseling.

The DOs
- Call your doctor if you are experiencing side effects from medications.
- Ask your doctor what over-the-counter pain medications you may take with your prescribed medicines.
- Work with your health professionals. Management of FM may be difficult but not impossible. Communication and follow-up are key factors in feeling better.

The DON'Ts
- Expect medications alone to decrease your pain and fatigue from FM. Feeling better involves improved sleep, exercise, and stress management.
- Take any diet supplement without discussing it first with your physician
- Stop exercising.

When to Call Your Doctor

- Experience side effects from your medications.
- Continue to wake frequently throughout the night.
- Need a counselor to help with family or financial problems.
- Need additional exercise instruction.
- Need an occupational therapist to help you manage your fatigue.

For More Information

Contact the National Arthritis Foundation in your area. If you do not know the location of the Arthritis Foundation, you may call the national office at 1-800-283-7800 or access information via the Internet at www.arthritis.org. You may also contact the Fibromyalgia Network at 1-800-853-2929.

FIFTH DISEASE

About Your Diagnosis

Fifth disease is a mild, infectious viral illness that occurs in outbreaks often during the winter and spring. It is named for its position on a list of childhood diseases developed in the early 1980s. It is caused by a virus called the human parvovirus B19. It spreads by airborne particles. Symptoms generally appear 4–14 days after exposure. It affects mostly children aged 5-14 years. There is no prevention, and the child is no longer contagious after the rash appears.

Living With Your Diagnosis

A fiery red rash appears on the cheeks—the so called "slapped cheek" appearance. The rash spreads to the rest of the body and usually has a "lacy" pattern. It may fade and reappear for several days. Slight fatigue, headache, and itching may occur. Fever is uncommon. Adults may experience mild joint pain and swelling. Many cases show no symptoms at all.

Complications are rare in healthy individuals. Children with

sickle cell anemia have an increased risk of complications. There is a small risk of miscarriage in a pregnant woman if she is infected during the first trimester.

Treatment

There is no specific treatment for fifth disease. Symptoms can be controlled. Nonaspirin products such as Tylenol can be given if a fever is present or for aches. DO NOT give aspirin to a child with fifth disease because of the risk of Reye's syndrome. The symptoms usually last 5–10 days.

The DOs

• Rest during the initial phase of the illness.
• Encourage fluid intake; no special diet is needed.
• Use cool compresses or calamine lotion if the rash itches.

The DON'Ts

• Don't give aspirin to a child with a viral infection. There have been studies that show an increased risk of Reye's syndrome when aspirin is given during a viral infection.

• Don't be concerned if the rash recurs after the illness is over, especially during exposure to the sun and temperature changes.

When to Call Your Doctor

• If symptoms worsen with normal treatment.
• If symptoms of Reye's syndrome occur, such as vomiting, restlessness, irritability, and a progressive decrease in the level of consciousness.

For More Information
National Institute of Allergy and Infectious Diseases of the NIH
Office of Communication
9000 Rockville Pike
Bethesda, MD 20892
301-496-5717
The American Academy of Pediatrics
141 NW Point Blvd.
Elk Grove Village, IL 60007-1098
Send a business-sized, self-addressed stamped envelope when requesting information.
National Institute of Child Health and Human Development
31 Center Drive
MSC 2725 Building 31/2A32
Bethesda, MD 20892
301-496-5133
www.nih.gov/nichd

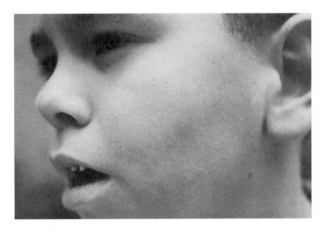

The slapped cheeks appearance of fifth disease. (From Noble J: *Textbook Primary Care Medicine*, vol 2. St. Louis, Mosby–Year Book, Inc., 1995. Used by permission.)

FOLLICULITIS

About Your Diagnosis

Folliculitis is a common skin infection of the hair follicles (base of the hair). It is usually a mild infection caused by staphylococcal bacteria after a break in the skin. Certain bacteria in hot tubs or pools can lead to folliculitis. Pseudofolliculitis resembles folliculitis but is actually a reaction to shaving with razors, and is treated differently than folliculitis. A doctor can usually make the diagnosis with visual inspection of the skin, but sometimes a sample of a pustule is taken for culture. Mild folliculitis may resolve without treatment, but antibiotics may be required to quicken the cure. The risk of folliculitis is higher in patients with diabetes, poor hygiene, and certain chronic illnesses.

Living With Your Diagnosis

In patients with folliculitis, there are many small, white, pus-filled bumps (pustules) surrounded by red or pink skin. Hairs may be seen near or in a pustule. Folliculitis can occur anywhere on the body. Sometimes the pustules can be painful. Although there are no long-term effects of folliculitis, recurrences are common.

Treatment

Mild cases are treated with antibiotic creams such as over-the-counter bacitracin or Burow's solution. In moderate-to-severe cases, antibiotics by mouth clear the infection in 1–2 weeks with minimal side effects.

The DOs

- Bathe at least once per day during and after treatment.
- Use an antibacterial soap.
- Gently remove crusts or pustules with a washcloth while bathing.
- After drying off apply medication.
- Clean and wash clothing and bedding regularly.
- Replace old razors. They can worsen the problem.
- If you are diabetic, follow your diet carefully and take your medication.

The DON'Ts

- Don't scratch affected areas. This can cause the infection to spread. Use cool compresses to help with itching.
- Don't shave red, tender, or swollen areas until they are healed.
- Don't share towels or clothing while infected because this can spread infection to others.

When to Call Your Doctor

- If fever develops during treatment.
- If the infection spreads or a pus pocket develops during treatment.
- If folliculitis recurs after treatment.

For More Information
American Academy of Dermatology
930 N. Meacham Road
Schaumburg, IL 60173
847-330-0230

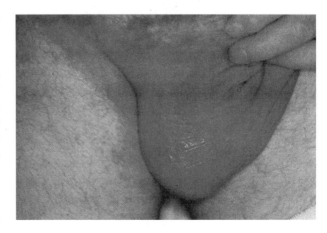

Primary papules and pustules with secondary erythema in a patient with folliculitis. Note a hair piercing several pustules. (Courtesy of Beverly Sanders, M.D. From Goldstein BG, Goldstein AO: *Practical Dermatology*, vol 1. St. Louis, Mosby–Year Book, 1992. Used by permission.)

FOOD POISONING, BACTERIAL

About Your Diagnosis

Bacterial food poisoning is an illness resulting from eating contaminated food. It is a common condition caused by a variety of bacteria (Table 1). The diagnosis is usually made by the symptoms and the fact that a group of individuals who ate the same foods have similar symptoms. It is generally a self-limited disease that will resolve in a few days. One form of food poisoning, botulism, is life-threatening, however.

Living With Your Diagnosis

Symptoms of bacterial food poisoning generally develop within 48 hours of eating the contaminated food. Nausea and vomiting with abdominal cramps develop. Diarrhea is common and, depending on the causative organism, may have blood in it. Fever may also be present. In severe cases, shock and electrolyte abnormalities can develop because of the diarrhea and vomiting.

Treatment

The key to treatment is the replacement of fluids and electrolytes. Oral fluids such as clear broth or special oral glucose-electrolyte preparations can be given. Take small, frequent sips even if vomiting continues. If symptoms are severe, hospitalization and intravenous fluids may be necessary. If the causative agent is known, antibiotics may be of benefit in treating certain organisms.

The DOs

- Bed rest with ready access to bathroom or bedpan is necessary.
- Continue to try to take oral fluids even if vomiting continues.
- Advance to a soft, bland diet as tolerated. Then gradually return to a normal diet over 1 or 2 days.
- Avoid dairy products and antacids containing magnesium if diarrhea is present.
- Save any samples of recently eaten food that may help identify the cause.
- Contact the local health department if multiple individuals are affected. They can help identify the source of the infection.
- Maintain proper hygiene while preparing foods. Wash hands between the handling of different foods. Keep the cooking area and all utensils clean.
- Properly cook and store foods. Throw out foods that do not "smell right" or are in bulging cans.
- Wash the hands after using the bathroom.

The DON'Ts

- Avoid raw seafood or meat.
- Avoid fresh vegetables that have not been properly washed.
- Avoid unpasteurized food products.
- Avoid drinking water and eating raw foods when traveling in foreign countries. Fruits that are peeled before eating are generally safe.

When to Call Your Doctor

- If young children or older adults have symptoms of food poisoning.
- If symptoms worsen after treatment begins.
- If vomiting is so severe that you are unable to keep liquids down.

For More Information
Food Safety and Inspection Service
Office of Public Awareness
Dept. of Agriculture
Washington, DC 20205
202-447-9351

Table 1.

Organism	Source	How is it transmitted?
Campylobacter jejuni	Milk and poultry	Eating undercooked poultry, meat, or raw dairy products.
Salmonella	Eggs and meat, especially poultry	Eating undercooked poultry, eggs, meat, or raw dairy products.
Clostridium perfringens	Spores in food	Eating contaminated meat, gravies, dried foods, and vegetables.
Staphylococcus aureus	Food contaminated by humans	Eating contaminated foods. Especially high-protein foods, egg salad, cream-filled pastries, poultry, and ham.
Bacillus cereus	Spores in food	Eating contaminated cereals, fried rice, dried foods, and herbs.
E. coli	Varies	Eating raw vegetables and other foods. Drinking contaminated water.

FROSTBITE

About Your Diagnosis

Frostbite is the result of freezing of living human tissues. It can be a very serious injury. It is commonly caused by exposure of bare or poorly protected skin, hands, and feet to subfreezing temperatures. Increasing wind speed, known as "wind chill," is often a factor. Alcohol consumption, fatigue, and dehydration increase the risk of frostbite. Once frostbite occurs, it is irreversible. Recovery can take weeks, and loss of skin, fingers, and toes, as well as deformity and discoloration, are possible. The best treatment, therefore, is prevention.

Living With Your Diagnosis

The signs of impending frostbite are pain, decreasing ability to sense touch, and redness upon exposure to cold. If recognized and treated at this stage, mild swelling and peeling of the skin may be the only effect. As the process progresses, the affected area becomes pale and firm. As the area is rewarmed, large blisters, blood blisters, and an obvious appearance of dead tissue (black, blue, or dark gray) can occur.

Treatment

The best treatment is prevention! Dress adequately for conditions. Protect and monitor small children closely! Drink plenty of nonalcoholic and noncaffeinated fluids. Plan ahead. Limit exposure when possible. If injury is suspected, immediately seek shelter and warmth. The best treatment is immersing the injured area in warm water (optimally 104°F). Do not use hot water because this may cause more injury. If possible, rewarm the entire body, encourage fluid intake, and elevate the affected area after rewarming. If blistering occurs, do not rupture the blisters. Wrap the area in dry, clean bandages and seek emergency care.

The DOs

- Do anticipate weather conditions and dress accordingly.
- Do drink plenty of nonalcoholic fluids.
- Do seek shelter at the first sign of symptoms.
- Do protect and monitor small children closely in adverse weather.
- Do elevate the injured area after rewarming.
- Do warm the entire body when able.
- Do remove all wet clothing as soon as possible.
- Do seek emergency care immediately if blisters or dead tissue appear.

The DON'Ts

- Don't rub the injured area with snow! This worsens the injury.
- Don't consume alcohol before exposure to subfreezing cold.
- Don't become fatigued or dehydrated in subfreezing cold.
- Don't ignore frostbite's early symptoms: pain, numbness, and redness.
- Don't rupture any blisters that form if at all possible.
- Don't allow frostbitten areas to refreeze.

When to Call Your Doctor

- Call if you suspect frostbite injury.

For More Information
First Aid Book
http://www.medaccess.com/first_aid/FA_TOC.htm
Cold Injuries
http://www.nols.edu/School/Pubs/FirstAid/EX9Cold#HYPO
Your local American Red Cross chapter

FROZEN SHOULDER

About Your Diagnosis

Frozen shoulder, also known as adhesive capsulitis, usually develops without any identifiable cause. It is a painful condition that almost universally results in decreased range of motion of the shoulder joint. It may develop gradually, preventing one from realizing the magnitude of the problem. On the other hand, the symptoms can be quite sudden and severe with nearly complete loss of shoulder motion. Adults in their forties and fifties are most at risk; however, anyone with a previous shoulder injury may be affected. Persons with a history of diabetes are at greater risk for adhesive capsulitis than are persons who do not have diabetes. The condition can often be present in both shoulders and may resist all forms of treatment.

Radiographs (x-rays) usually are needed to rule out other possible causes of shoulder stiffness, such as degenerative arthritis, tumors, and shoulder dislocation.

Living With Your Diagnosis

Frozen shoulder has been termed a "benign" process because it tends to improve over the course of 1 to 3 years. Unfortunately, many patients cannot endure the pain or the limitation of motion while they wait for the symptoms to resolve. As a result, physical therapy plays an important role in the conservative management of this condition.

Treatment

When frozen shoulder develops spontaneously, without a prior shoulder injury or operation, conservative management with physical therapy is preferred. However, when this condition develops after an operation on the shoulder, a more aggressive treatment plan, including possible further surgical intervention, may be necessary. Analgesics and anti-inflammatory drugs may help to reduce pain, but use of these drugs has to be combined with a supervised therapy program for maximum relief. Injection of steroid-type medications into the joint itself often is helpful.

The DOs
- Take your medications as prescribed.
- Undertake a supervised therapy program that combines range of motion exercises with strengthening exercises.

The DON'Ts
- Do not discontinue your physical therapy without consulting your doctor.

When to Call Your Doctor
- If you notice shoulder pain that is not responding to rest and is associated with a decrease in the overall range of motion of the shoulder joint.

For More Information
http://www.vir.com/frankenstein/faq/shoulder/frozen.faq.html

FURUNCULOSIS

About Your Diagnosis

Furunculosis is a condition causing deep sores of the skin, also known as boils. Furuncles are painful, deep bacterial infections of hair follicles.

The usual cause is infection, usually from *Staphylococcus* bacteria, that begins in the hair follicle and penetrates into deeper skin layers.

Furunculosis is very uncommon in young children, but it occurs more frequency after puberty. Transmission from individual to individual can occur if contact is made with drainage of pus from a furuncle.

The furuncle begins as a deep, tender, firm, red papule which enlarges rapidly into a tender, deep-seated nodule that remains painful.

With appropriate treatment, the infection can be eradicated.

Living With Your Diagnosis

Pain becomes more intense as the furuncle enlarges. Furuncles can appear suddenly and are usually 1/2 to 1 inch in diameter; some are larger.

The furuncle either remains deep and reabsorbs or it will rupture through to the surface of the skin. The point of rupture heals with scarring. Without treatment, the infection may enter the bloodstream and spread to other body parts.

Treatment

Warm moist compresses provide comfort and encourage localization and pointing of the abscess; apply three or four times daily for 20 minutes each time.

Your physician may incise and drain the furuncle when the skin over the furuncle becomes thin and the mass underneath is soft. Without treatment, the furuncle will heal in 10–20 days. With treatment, furuncles will heal in less time and symptoms will be less severe.

A potential complication of treatment is that the pus that drains when the furuncle opens spontaneously may contaminate nearby skin, causing new furuncles.

The DOs

- Do take prescribed antibiotics.
- Do decrease activity until the infection heals. Avoid sweating and contact sports while furuncles are present.
- Do keep the skin clean.

The DON'Ts

- Don't use nonprescription antibiotic creams or ointments on the furuncle's surface because they are ineffective.
- Don't share towels, washcloths, or clothing with other household members.

When to Call Your Doctor

- If fever occurs or symptoms do not improve in 3 or 4 days, despite treatment.
- If new furuncles appear or furuncles develop in other family members.

For More Information
American Academy of Dermatology
930 N. Meachum Road
Schaumburg, IL 60173
847-330-0230

GASTRITIS

About Your Diagnosis

Gastritis is an inflammation of the lining of the stomach. Numerous factors cause this illness. Many are caused by lifestyle excesses: excess smoking, excess alcohol, excess caffeine, and excess eating. Gastritis is also a side effect of many medications. Aspirin and nonsteroidal anti-inflammatory drugs are well-known causes. Bacterial and viral infections are also a cause, as is stress from surgery, severe burns, and trauma. These factors tend to produce gastritis by causing an increased acid production in the stomach. One known cause of gastritis that is not caused by increased acid production is atrophic gastritis, in which the stomach lining becomes wasted and acid is not produced.

Gastritis is a common condition. It affects virtually everyone at some point in their life. The diagnosis of gastritis is made by the history. Occasionally an upper gastrointestinal x-ray study or upper endoscopy (viewing the stomach through a lighted flexible tube) is done. Most cases of gastritis are short-term and have no lasting effects.

Living With Your Diagnosis

The main symptoms of gastritis are upper abdominal pain and cramps. The pain is many times made worse by eating. Many individuals will have a decrease in appetite. The pain may radiate to the chest causing the patient to think it is related to the heart. Many will have a burning acid taste in the mouth. Nausea and vomiting occasionally occur. Occasionally bleeding will complicate gastritis.

Treatment

Treatment of gastritis focuses on the symptoms and elimination of the cause. Mild symptoms are controlled with antacids. The liquid form of antacids is better than the tablet form in providing relief. Over-the-counter histamine-2 (H_2) blockers are available. These medications relieve the symptoms by causing a decrease in acid production. These medications are also available in prescription strength. Other medications that protect the stomach lining are available from your health care provider. If the cause of the gastritis is associated with the bacterial infection from *Helicobacter pylori*, antibiotics may be prescribed. If the gastritis is severe and bleeding is present, hospitalization may be needed. Intravenous fluids and medications are given to control the symptoms, decrease stomach acid production, and protect the stomach lining.

The DOs

- Eat regularly and in moderation.
- Use antacids and over-the-counter H_2 blockers for mild symptoms.

The DON'Ts

- Stop smoking.
- Avoid alcohol.
- Avoid foods that are hard to digest.
- Avoid medications that can irritate your stomach, such as aspirin and nonsteroidal anti-inflammatory drugs.

When to Call Your Doctor

- If the abdominal pain becomes severe.
- If symptoms do not improve after 3–5 days of treatment.
- If chest pain is severe, radiates to the neck, jaw, or arm, and is associated with sweating or shortness of breath.
- If there is blood with bowel movements or dark tarry stools.
- If you vomit blood.

For More Information
National Digestive Diseases Information Clearinghouse
2 Information Way
Bethesda, MD 20892-3570
www.niddk.nih.gov
nddic@aerie.com

GASTROESOPHAGEAL REFLUX DISEASE

About Your Diagnosis

Gastroesophageal reflux disease or GERD is more commonly known as acid indigestion or heartburn. It is a burning feeling behind the breastbone. This feeling can move up into the throat and also give a sour or bitter taste in the mouth.

Gastroesophageal reflux disease is caused by stomach acid moving from your stomach up into your esophagus (the tube that connects the mouth and stomach). This may happen if the muscle between the stomach and esophagus is weak. There are conditions that may aggravate this. They include diabetes mellitus, pregnancy, and medications used to treat high blood pressure and heart conditions.

Gastroesophageal reflux disease is very common. About 5% of individuals have symptoms every day. About 15% have symptoms every week. Almost half of all individuals have symptoms at least once a month.

Gastroesophageal reflux disease is diagnosed most commonly by history. If the symptoms do not improve with treatment or the pain is severe or chronic, further studies are needed. An upper gastrointestinal (GI) series is a special x-ray used to show the esophagus, stomach, and upper part of the intestine. The upper GI does not provide a lot of information about GERD, but it helps identify other disorders that can cause a similar pain. Endoscopy, using a small light tube with a tiny video camera on the end, can be done to identify irritation in the esophagus.

Living With Your Diagnosis

The most common symptom of GERD is heartburn. The burning, pressure or pain of GERD can last as long as 1 or 2 hours and is often worse after eating. Lying down or bending over can also make the pain worse. The pain associated with heartburn can be mistaken for the pain of a heart attack or angina. However, the pain associated with the heart is usually aggravated by exercise and relieved by rest. Heartburn pain is usually not associated with physical activity.

Treatment

In most cases, GERD can be relieved through diet and lifestyle modifications. For immediate relief, antacids can neutralize the acid and stop the heartburn. However, there are side effects with the long-term use of antacids. These include diarrhea, altered calcium metabolism, and excess magnesium buildup in the body.

Over-the-counter and prescription strength histamine-2 (H_2) blockers are also available. These medications inhibit the secretion of acid by the stomach. Another type of prescription drug is a proton pump inhibitor. These drugs inhibit an enzyme needed for acid secretion. Other drugs are available to strengthen the muscle and quicken stomach emptying.

A small number of individuals may need surgery because of severe GERD or poor response to medications. The surgical procedure increases the pressure in the lower esophagus, preventing acid from backing up from the stomach.

The DOs

- Lose weight if overweight.
- Avoiding lying down after meals.
- Sleep with the head of the bed elevated 6 inches by putting blocks of wood under the two legs at the head of the bed.
- Take medications with plenty of water.
- Eat four or five small meals a day.

The DON'Ts

- Avoid alcoholic beverages and caffeine products (coffee, tea, cocoa, cola drinks).
- Avoid fried, spicy, and fatty foods, citrus juices and fruits, tomato products, peppermint, and spices that aggravate the symptoms of GERD.
- Do not bend over or lie down immediately after eating.
- Do not smoke.
- Avoid tight-fitting pants, belts, and undergarments.

When to Call Your Doctor

- If the symptoms worsen or do not improve after using general measures.
- If you have pain that happens with shortness of breath, sweating, or nausea.
- If you vomit blood or have recurrent vomiting.
- Symptoms do not improve after 1 month of treatment.

For More Information
National Digestive Diseases Information Clearinghouse
2 Information Way
Bethesda, MD 20892-3570
www.niddk.nih.gov
nddic@aerie.com

GIARDIASIS

About Your Diagnosis

Giardiasis is an intestinal infection caused by a parasite (a protozoa). It is spread through contaminated food or water. The parasite causes destruction of the intestinal lining, resulting in poor absorption of food. It is commonly found in children and can spread through a day-care center or a preschool. Giardiasis can be detected by examining the stools for the parasite. Recovery occurs faster with treatment.

Living With Your Diagnosis

Symptoms occur 1–3 weeks after ingestion. This is the time it takes for the inflammation to start causing symptoms. Symptoms include sudden abdominal cramps with explosive, loose, frequent stools (2–10 times a day); nausea; slight fever; fatigue; and weight loss. Dehydration is the most common complication.

Treatment

A child should be kept home from school or day care until the infection has cleared. Hand washing is essential in preventing the spread of the infection. Medications such as metronidazole or quinacrine may be prescribed. Side effects of these medications include headache, dizziness, a metallic taste, and nightmares. Alcohol should not be taken with these medications. Fluid intake needs to be increased to prevent dehydration. A liquid diet may be needed if nausea is a problem. Other family members should be tested for the infection.

The DOs

- Keep the child home from day care or school until symptoms are gone.
- Maintain adequate fluid intake.
- Wash hands thoroughly and frequently to prevent spreading the disease.
- Use a heating pad to help relieve abdominal pain.
- Follow-up with your doctor to make sure the infection has cleared.

The DON'Ts

- Take the medication prescribed until finished.
- Don't drink alcohol while taking the medication; severe side effects can occur.
- Don't give medications for the diarrhea. These may mask symptoms and delay recovery.
- Don't forget to wash your hands before you eat.
- Don't drink water from streams or lakes when camping or traveling unless it has been purified.
- Don't eat uncooked foods that may have been washed in contaminated water.

When to Call Your Doctor

- A high fever occurs after treatment has started.
- The medication can't be tolerated because of the side effects.
- There are signs of dehydration such as dry wrinkled skin, coated tongue, and decreased urination.

For More Information
National Institute of Allergy and Infectious Disease
9000 Rockville Pike
Bethesda, MD 20892
301-496-5717
Internet Site
www.healthfinder.gov (Choose SEARCH to search by topic.)

GILBERT'S DISEASE

About Your Diagnosis

Gilbert's disease is a relatively common and benign liver disorder. You are born with this condition. It appears that Gilbert's disease is hereditary. The condition occurs when the liver is not able to change bilirubin into bile efficiently. Bilirubin is a yellow pigment excreted by the liver and is the byproduct of red blood cell breakdown. When the liver is not able to change bilirubin into bile, the bilirubin levels increase in the blood.

Males have this condition more frequently than females. The diagnosis is made most commonly when you are in your teens or early adulthood. The diagnosis is with a blood test. An elevated serum bilirubin level is obtained. Many times individuals with Gilbert's disease are unaware that they have the disease. They may only find out when they go to donate blood, have incidental laboratory studies done, or go through a mass screening at a health fair. The bilirubin levels in Gilbert's disease increase if you do not eat and when you have a fever or other illness such as influenza. Typically the other liver function tests are normal. About 3% to 7% of the adult population has Gilbert's disease.

Living With Your Diagnosis

Gilbert's disease is characterized by a mild, fluctuating increase in the serum bilirubin levels. There are usually no signs or symptoms of the disease. On occasion a slight yellow color (jaundice) to the skin or whites of the eyes may be noted. Rarely you may experience tiredness, loss of appetite, or upper abdominal pain.

Treatment

Gilbert's disease does not require treatment. It will not interfere with a normal lifestyle.

The DOs

- Maintain a healthy lifestyle with exercise and proper diet.
- Make yourself aware of your condition. Inform your health care provider. This may prevent unnecessary medical evaluations in the future.

The DON'Ts

- Avoid alcohol in excess.
- Avoid tobacco products.

When to Call Your Doctor

- If you believe your skin looks yellow.

For More Information
American Liver Foundation
1425 Pompton Avenue
Cedar Grove, New Jersey 07009
800-223-0179

GINGIVITIS

About Your Diagnosis
Gingivitis is an inflammation of the gum tissue surrounding the teeth. It is caused by poor oral hygiene and poor nutrition.

Living With Your Diagnosis
Signs and symptoms include swelling and redness of the soft areas around the teeth, which become tender; bleeding of the gums; and constant bad breath.

Treatment
Frequent checkups by your dentist are needed. If an infection is present you may need antibiotics. Vitamins may be prescribed if you have a deficiency. A fluoride mouthwash may also be prescribed. Careful brushing of the teeth with a soft-bristled toothbrush and flossing daily are important. Avoid foods high in sugar because they stimulate the production of acid that attacks the teeth. Eat a well-balanced diet. In severe cases, the dentist may have to perform surgery to remove infected tissue.

The DOs
- Visit your dentist regularly.
- Follow proper brushing techniques to maximize the cleaning of the area between the gums and teeth.
- Floss daily.
- Eat a well-balanced diet.
- Take a vitamin supplement.
- Avoid foods high in sugar.
- Change your toothbrush frequently.

The DON'Ts
- Don't brush with a hard-bristled brush that may irritate the gums.
- Don't stop taking antibiotics before they are finished if your doctor or dentist has prescribed them.

When to Call Your Doctor
- If a high fever develops.
- If excessive bleeding from the gums occurs.
- If pain in the gums or teeth is present.

For More Information
American Dental Association
Department of Public Education and Information
211 E. Chicago Avenue
Chicago, IL 60611
Write to request information or visit their Internet site:
www.ada.org/
National Oral Health Information Clearinghouse
301-402-7364, Monday through Friday from 9 AM to 5:30 PM (EST), for brochures, pamphlets, and fact sheets on oral health.

GLAUCOMA, PRIMARY OPEN ANGLE

About Your Diagnosis

Primary open angle glaucoma is a condition where the pressure inside the eye (intraocular pressure) is greater than normal. If the intraocular pressure were to be measured in everyone across the country, the average pressure would be 16 mm Hg. A pressure above 21 mm Hg is considered elevated. There are some patients with intraocular pressures of between 21 and 25 who do not go on to develop glaucoma. However, these patients need to be watched closely.

The exact causes of primary open angle glaucoma are not well understood. Aqueous fluid is constantly produced within the eye and travels throughout the eye, ultimately draining through a trabecular meshwork to be reabsorbed back into the rest of the body. It is believed that in individuals with glaucoma, the trabecular meshwork does not allow the fluid to leave the eye as quickly as in "normal" patients and as a result, the pressure in the eye becomes elevated. Primary open angle glaucoma can be detected on examination. Except in advanced cases, there are no symptoms associated with it.

One of the tests which is helpful for diagnosing glaucoma is called a visual field test. In this test, the patient stares at a screen and lights flash in different positions to check the patient's peripheral vision. In glaucoma, the first sign of damage to the eye is a decrease in peripheral vision. Therefore the visual field test can be examined by the patient's eye doctor to assess whether there is early damage to peripheral vision. In addition, the patient's eye doctor will carefully examine the inside of the eye to look at the appearance of the optic nerve. As glaucoma worsens, there is a central depression or a "cup" in the optic nerve that will enlarge.

Glaucoma can be treated with medications, laser surgery, or formal glaucoma surgery.

Living With Your Diagnosis

In the early stages, there are no signs or symptoms of glaucoma. The usual damage that occurs from glaucoma can occur slowly over time, so it is often not until years later that patients will finally notice that their vision is reduced. Unfortunately, once vision has been damaged from glaucoma, it is not possible to restore.

Treatment

Glaucoma can be treated with eye drops, laser surgery, or formal glaucoma surgery. The type of treatment used depends on the degree of glaucoma present when the diagnosis is first made, and how difficult it is to normalize the intraocular pressure. The mainstay of all glaucoma treatment is to lower the elevated intraocular pressure to a more normal range. In some patients, this can be accomplished through the use of one or two different eye drops, whereas in other patients, eye drops alone are ineffective. In these instances, either laser surgery or sometimes formal surgery is recommended.

The eye drops used to treat glaucoma can have systemic side effects. Eye drops that fall into the class of beta blockers should be used only with great care in patients with asthma, breathing problems, or cardiac problems.

Laser surgery for glaucoma can be quite effective. Unfortunately, not all patients who have laser surgery for glaucoma have their pressure normalized. In many instances, patients need to continue using eye drops after the laser surgery.

Surgery for glaucoma involves creating a new "drain" for the eye to allow the aqueous to filter out faster, thereby lowering the eye pressure. As with any operation on the eye, there are potential complications that can occur which could ultimately lead to worsening of vision or complete loss of vision.

The DOs

If patients are going to be treated medically for glaucoma, it is important that they use their drops exactly as directed and do not miss using the medication. The drops only work when used. If patients have an elevated intraocular pressure, the drops will not cure the problem but will help control it. Therefore once patients begin medication, they typically will use it indefinitely.

Patients who have glaucoma can exercise in most normal fashions but should avoid yoga and other exercise that involve "standing on the head."

The DON'Ts

It is important for patients to use their medications as directed. They should let their internist and other physicians know what eye drop medications they are taking inasmuch as these medicines can have systemic side effects. In addition, some cold remedies can aggravate glaucoma, and before using these or any medication, patients should check with their eye doctor.

When to Call Your Doctor

When there is worsening of vision, pain, or redness in the eye, the doctor should be called.

For More Information

To request the pamphlet "Glaucoma" or to obtain additional information, contact the American Academy of Ophthalmology by calling 415-561-8500, or access the information on the Internet at www.eyenet.org.

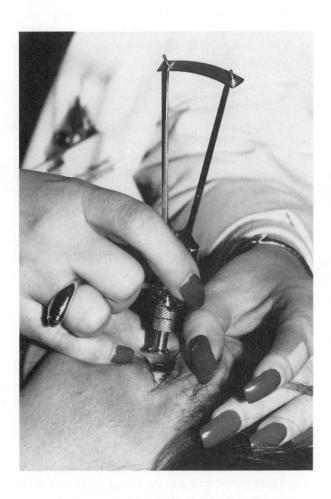

GLOMERULONEPHRITIS, ACUTE

About Your Diagnosis

Glomerulonephritis is the term used to describe a group of diseases that cause inflammation of the part of the kidney that filters blood. The inflammation in turn causes damage to the kidney, and it cannot get rid of the waste products and extra fluid in the body. Sometimes the kidneys may stop working completely. There are two forms of this condition, acute and chronic. The acute form develops suddenly, whereas the chronic form may develop silently over many years. You may get acute glomerulonephritis after an infection in your throat or skin, although this is not always the case. It may also be caused by some other illnesses, including lupus, Goodpasture's syndrome, Wegener's granulomatosis, Henoch-Schönlein purpura, and polyarteritis nodosa. On the other hand, in many cases of chronic glomerulonephritis the cause is not known. In some cases the disease runs in the family. This kind shows up in young men who also have associated hearing loss. Some forms are caused by immune system changes. An episode of acute glomerulonephritis may be followed by chronic disease years later. The diagnosis is made by clues from your history. Urine showing protein and blood cells is a further clue. Blood tests help your doctor determine the cause of your glomerulonephritis in some cases, as well as how much your kidneys have been damaged. Sometimes your doctor will need to do a kidney biopsy (take a tiny piece of your kidney with a special needle) to help determine the best form of treatment.

Living With Your Diagnosis

With acute glomerulonephritis, you will feel ill and go to the bathroom less often. Your urine is red, smoky, or rusty because blood is in it. Your face, eyelids, and hands may be swollen in the morning, and your ankles may be puffy in the evening. You may be short of breath and cough because of extra fluid in your lungs. Your blood pressure may be high. One or all of these symptoms may be present. With chronic glomerulonephritis, you may have long periods with no symptoms, but your kidneys are still being damaged. You may have protein and blood in your urine as the only sign. As the disease worsens, you have symptoms such as swelling of your face and ankles, loss of appetite, vomiting, and feeling very tired. Your skin may become dry and itchy, and you may have muscle cramps at night.

Treatment

Occasionally the glomerulonephritis may not need any treatment and go away by itself. Sometimes you may need high doses of medicines that affect your immune system, or you may need to have a special blood filtering process called plasmapheresis. Antibiotics may be used for treatment of infection that may in turn have caused the glomerulonephritis. Temporary treatment with an artificial kidney machine may be required for removal of extra fluid and poisons that build up in the body with glomerulonephritis. There is no specific treatment for the chronic form of the disease. Your doctor may ask you to eat less protein, salt, and potassium, and to take blood pressure pills and calcium supplements.

The DOs

- Good hygiene, "safe sex," and avoiding intravenous drugs are helpful in preventing infections that could lead to this type of illness.
- Do follow dietary advice because it is very important in preventing complications from your disease.
- Do keep to the fluid restriction you have been advised because otherwise you could have fluid build up in your lungs. This could be dangerous to your immediate health.
- If you have the chronic type of glomerulonephritis, it is very important to control your blood pressure; it is *the single most important thing that may slow down kidney damage.* Therefore do take your blood pressure medicine regularly.
- Do exercise within your capacity to do so.

The DON'Ts

- Don't stop taking your medication before checking with your doctor.
- Don't take over-the-counter medication unless you have checked it with your doctor. Some of these medicines may not be safe with your kidney condition.
- Don't take any herbal preparations that you may find at health food stores. Some of these preparations have been known to cause kidney disease.
- Don't hesitate to ask your doctor any questions

about your disease or any concerns about the treatment that you may have.

When to Call Your Doctor

- Always call your doctor if you feel unwell. He may be able to assess whether you need to be seen right away or whether a change in medication is necessary.

For More Information

Many patients with kidney failure are able to live normally again after getting used to their treatment. Your national Kidney Foundation affiliate can give you further information about types of treatment available. Their address can be obtained from your doctor or The National Kidney Foundation, Inc., 30 East 33rd Street, New York, NY 10016.

GLOSSITIS

About Your Diagnosis

Glossitis is an inflammation of the tongue. It may be acute or chronic. It may be a condition in and of itself or may be a symptom of another disease. It is a common condition that affects individuals of all ages. It does seem to occur more commonly in men. There are many causes of glossitis, both local and systemic. Bacterial and viral infections can be a local cause of glossitis. Trauma or mechanical irritation from burns, teeth, and dental appliances are other local causes. Local irritants such as tobacco, alcohol, and hot or spicy foods can also cause glossitis. An allergic reaction from toothpaste, mouthwash, or other materials put in the mouth can be a local cause. Systemic glossitis can result from nutritional causes, skin diseases, and systemic infections. If an individual is malnourished or lacks iron or the B vitamins in the diet, glossitis can develop. Skin diseases such as oral lichen planus, erythema multiforme, aphthous ulcers, and pemphigus vulgaris can cause glossitis. Infections such as syphilis and human immunodeficiency virus (HIV) may have glossitis as their first symptom. Occasionally, the cause of glossitis is inherited.

An examination is the best way to detect glossitis. Occasionally if the cause is not clear or there is no improvement with treatment, a biopsy is done. In most cases, glossitis will resolve with outpatient treatment. Occasionally hospitalization will be required if the swelling is severe and blocks the airway.

Living With Your Diagnosis

The signs and symptoms of glossitis are variable because of the various causes. The basic signs are that the tongue changes color and is painful. The color changes vary from a dark "beefy" red to fiery red to pale to white. The tongue may be painful enough to cause difficulty chewing, swallowing, or talking. The fingerlike projections on the tongue surface are lost. This gives the tongue a smooth appearance. Ulcerations on the tongue occur with some cases of glossitis.

Treatment

The treatment of glossitis depends on the cause. Antibiotics are used for the treatment of bacterial infections. For a nutritional deficiency, supplementation with vitamins or iron is the treatment. The swelling and discomfort is treated with various over-the-counter and prescription drugs that are used locally. Mouth rinses with a half teaspoon of baking soda and 8 oz of warm water can provide relief. If the swelling is severe, corticosteriods taken by mouth may be necessary.

The DOs

- A bland or liquid diet may be needed while symptoms of glossitis are present.
- Good oral hygiene is necessary for prevention. Brush and floss teeth, and clean the tongue after each meal. See a dentist regularly.

The DON'Ts

- Avoid agents that may cause irritation or be sensitizing. This includes hot or spicy foods and alcohol.
- Stop smoking and avoid tobacco in all forms.

When to Call Your Doctor

- If you have breathing, speaking, chewing, or swallowing difficulties. This may mean the swollen tongue has blocked the airway. This is an emergency that needs immediate medical attention.
- If symptoms of glossitis persist for longer than 10 days.

For More Information
American Dental Association
211 E. Chicago Avenue
Chicago, Illinois 60611
312-440-2500
Fax: 312-440-2800

GONORRHEA

About Your Diagnosis

Gonorrhea is a contagious sexually transmitted disease. It is caused by the gonococcus bacteria. It affects the reproductive organs and may be passed from an infected mother to an infant during childbirth. In men the urethra is generally affected. In both sexes the eyes and joints can be affected. The disease is curable in 1–2 weeks with medical treatment. Testing for other sexually transmitted diseases should be done. Gonorrhea can be detected by a blood test or a culture of the discharge.

Living With Your Diagnosis

Symptoms usually will develop within 2 weeks after exposure. They include low-grade fever; green-yellow discharge from the vagina or penis; burning upon urination; tenderness in the lower abdomen; pain in the knees, ankles, or elbows; and rash on the palms of the hands. Females often have no symptoms.

Treatment

Antibiotics are needed to treat the infection, usually for 7 days. Thorough and frequent hand washing is needed after using the bathroom. Avoid touching your eyes. Sitz baths may be helpful to relieve discomfort, Notify sexual contacts so they may be tested. No special diet is needed, but caffeine and alcohol should be avoided. Follow-up cultures should be done. Complication can include blindness in children from gonococcal eye infections, infertility in women, impotence in men, and infectious arthritis.

The DOs

- Take antibiotics until finished.
- Notify your sexual contacts.
- Use sitz baths for discomfort.
- Wash hands frequently and thoroughly, especially after using the bathroom.
- Avoid drinking caffeine and alcohol.
- Use latex condoms during sexual intercourse.

The DON'Ts

- Don't skip doses or stop antibiotics until they are finished.
- Don't touch your eyes to prevent infecting them.
- Don't resume sexual activity until a follow-up culture shows that you are cured of the infection.

©1999, Mosby, Inc.

- Don't drink caffeinated beverages or alcohol because they irritate the urethra.

When to Call Your Doctor

- If fever, chills, and abdominal pain develop after treatment is started.
- If joint pain develops.
- If genital sores and swelling of the testicles develop.
- If you have been notified that a sexual contact has the disease.

For More Information
The CDC National STD Hotline
800-227-8922, Monday through Friday from 8 AM to 11 PM (EST).
American Social Health Association
800-972-8500, for pamphlets about sexual health and information about support groups.
Internet Sites
http://sunsite.unc.edu/ASHA/
www.healthfinder.gov (Choose SEARCH to search by topic)
www.healthanswers.com

GOUT

About Your Diagnosis

Gout is an abrupt and very painful form of arthritis. It usually affects only one joint at a time, typically the great toe, foot, ankle, knee, wrist, or elbows. Gout usually affects men older than 40 years. It is unusual in women until they have passed through menopause (the change of life).

Gout "attacks" are caused by the release of "crystals" into a joint, resulting in inflammation, pain, and swelling. These crystals are made of a substance in the blood called uric acid. In individuals with gout, either too much uric acid is made or not enough is eliminated by the kidney. Alcohol, aspirin, certain medicines, and rarely certain foods (liver and other organ meats, sardines, anchovies) may cause levels of uric acid to rise in individuals, making them more prone to developing gout. The only way to diagnose gout with certainty is to place a needle into the affected joint, remove the joint fluid and look for the gout crystals under a microscope.

Living With Your Diagnosis

Individuals who have an attack of gout notice rapidly developing pain, swelling, warmth, and redness in the affected joint. The pain can be so intense that even lightly touching the joint will cause severe pain. The pain is usually continuous and more painful if the joint is moved. Everyday activities such as walking, dressing, and lifting may be difficult.

Attacks may occur at any time; however, certain events can trigger attacks such as injuries, surgery, an acute illness, or ingestion of alcoholic beverages. Once the attacks are treated, the symptoms usually resolve within hours to a few days. If attacks are not treated, they may last several days. In between attacks the symptoms resolve completely. Individuals with higher uric acid levels in their blood are more prone to recurring attacks. Persistently elevated uric acid levels for many years can cause deposits of uric acid in nodules under the skin. These are called "tophi." Some individuals with gout are also prone to developing kidney stones.

Treatment

There are two ways to approach the therapy for gout: treatment of attacks and prevention of attacks.

Preventive treatment is necessary in individuals with tophi, kidney stones, and frequent attacks.

Attacks of gout are usually treated with nonsteroidal anti-inflammatory drugs (NSAIDs) such as indomethacin. Potential side effects of NSAIDs include stomach upset, ulcers, constipation, diarrhea, headaches, dizziness, difficulty hearing, and skin rash. Colchicine is another type of anti-inflammatory drug that is particularly effective early in the attack. Potential side effects of colchicine include stomach cramps, nausea, vomiting, and diarrhea. Occasionally, a more potent anti-inflammatory medicine such as prednisone, a cortisone-like medicine, is necessary. Potential side effects of cortisone-like medicines are increased appetite, weight gain, difficulty sleeping, easy bruising, and stomach upset. Removal of the joint fluid from the affected joint, followed by a cortisone injection is another common treatment for gout. Cortisone injections usually provide the most rapid and complete relief of pain and swelling. Aside from the discomfort of the injection, there are very few side effects from cortisone injections.

Prevention of gouty attacks is accomplished by lowering uric acid levels. Two common medicines that lower uric acid levels are allopurinol and probenecid. The specific medicine your doctor chooses will depend upon other medicines you are taking and other medical conditions you have. The most common side effects of allopurinol and probenecid are skin rash and upset stomach.

The DOs

- Rest the affected joint until the symptoms begin to improve.
- Take your medicines as prescribed.
- Ask your doctor which over-the-counter medications you may take with your prescription medications.
- Follow your doctor's advice by limiting your use of alcoholic beverages and avoiding certain foods or medications.

The DON'Ts

- Wait to see if side effects from the medications will go away.

When to Call Your Doctor

- You experience any medication side effects.
- The treatment is not decreasing your symptoms in a reasonable amount of time.

- You begin to lose more movement in the affected joint.
- You experience worsening warmth, redness, or pain after a cortisone injection.

For More Information

Contact the Arthritis Foundation in your area. If you do not know the location of the Arthritis Foundation, you may call the national office at 1-800-283-7800 or access the information on the Internet at www.arthritis.org.

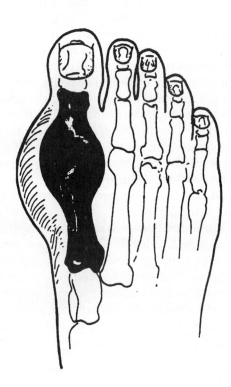

A common location of gout. (From LaFleur-Brooks ML: *Exploring Medical Language—A Student Directed Approach.* vol 3. St. Louis, Mosby–Year Book, 1993. Used by permission.)

GRANULOMA ANNULARE

For More Information
American Academy of Dermatology
930 N. Meacham Road
Schaumburg, IL 60173
847-330-0230

About Your Diagnosis

Granuloma annulare is a relatively uncommon skin disease. The cause is not known and it is not contagious. It is seen more commonly in children and young adults. It usually resolves on its own but recurrences are common. Treatment with medications applied to the skin may help speed up healing. Diagnosis is usually made by a doctor's visual inspection of the skin, and a minor skin biopsy is sometimes used to confirm the diagnosis. Although granuloma annulare tends to recur, it is not cancerous or life threatening.

Living With Your Diagnosis

Granuloma annulare may start as a small, red bump and develop into a ring of bumps or even multiple bumps. The bumps are red to tan, and the bump rings can grow up to a few inches but are usually smaller. Some bumps may go away within a few months, whereas others may persist for years. They usually occur on the arms, hands, legs, and feet.

Treatment

Treatment is usually not necessary. Steroid creams applied to skin may be prescribed. Apply a small amount of cream or lotion to the affected area and cover with Saran Wrap for 8 hours. It is best to do this just before bedtime and remove the Saran Wrap in the morning. For severe or extensive cases of granuloma annulare, medications by mouth may be prescribed. If given prescription medications, follow your doctor's directions.

The DOs

- Be patient. Granuloma annulare is not life threatening.
- Most cases eventually improve within years.
- Diet and exercise do not affect the condition.

The DON'Ts

- Patients with this disorder have no restrictions.

When to Call Your Doctor

- If itching or scaling occur.
- Any signs of infection occur such as fever, swelling, or pus drainage.

GRANULOMA INGUINALE

About Your Diagnosis

Granuloma inguinale is a sexually transmitted disease that is common in tropical areas and developing countries. It is a chronic infection affecting the genital and groin areas.

Living With Your Diagnosis

Signs and symptoms of the disease can take 1–2 weeks to appear after exposure. Large raised, red lesions appear on the penis, vulva, or vagina and may also appear in the groin area. The lesions are painless. As they ulcerate, the area becomes dark red and may have raised edges that heal with extensive scar formation.

Treatment

Antibiotics such as tetracycline or erythromycin must be taken for 3 weeks, until complete healing occurs. The areas should be kept clean and dry. Testing for other sexually transmitted diseases should be done. Activity restrictions are not needed. No special diet is needed. A follow-up examination with your doctor is important to make sure no other treatment is necessary.

The DOs

- Take the antibiotics until finished.
- Keep the lesions clean and dry.
- Keep follow-up appointments with your doctor to make sure the infection is cleared.
- Notify sexual contacts so they can be examined and treated if necessary.
- Get tested for other sexually transmitted diseases.

The DON'Ts

- Don't skip or stop the antibiotics until they are finished.
- Don't skip your follow-up appointments with your doctor. If not completely cleared the infection can recur.
- Don't apply creams or lotions to the lesions unless ordered by your doctor.
- Don't have sexual relations until cleared by your doctor.

When to Call Your Doctor

- If any lesions appear infected.
- If the lesions become painful or have increased drainage.
- If a fever develops during treatment.
- If you cannot tolerate the antibiotics.

For More Information:
The CDC National STD Hotline
800-227-8922, Monday through Friday from 8 AM to 11 PM (EST).
American Social Health Association
800-972-8500
Internet Site
http://sunsite.unc.edu/ASHA/

GRAVES' DISEASE

About Your Diagnosis

Graves' disease is an autoimmune disease caused by antibodies produced in your blood that stimulate thyroid activity and also cause eye disease. It is not contagious but may in some cases "run in families." Often, patients with Graves' disease have relatives with other thyroid disorders. Graves' disease is detected by blood tests for thyroid function and antibody levels against thyroid tissue. It is not completely curable, although both the high thyroid levels and eye problems can be treated. Graves' Disease affects primarily women.

Living With Your Diagnosis

Signs of Graves' disease may include problems with the thyroid, eyes, or both.

Eye problems include blurring vision, dryness, bulging of the eyeball (exophthalmos), or a persistent "staring" look. These can progress to cause double vision and blindness if not treated.

Thyroid problems include hyperactivity of the thyroid gland if left untreated. This results in heartbeat irregularities, high blood pressure, increased bowel function, and nervousness. Long- term complications include heart failure, bone loss (osteoporosis), and stroke.

Treatment

Eye problems must be assessed individually by an ophthalmologist (eye doctor) at least once a year. Treatments for eye disease include laser therapy and surgery, as well as eye drops and ointments.

Thyroid hyperactivity can be controlled by medicine, surgery, or radioactive iodine use; the choice is tailored to the patient's needs.

Medicines such as propylthiouracil (PTU) and methimazole (Tapazole) prevent the thyroid gland from producing thyroid hormone. They must be taken as directed without fail, because they are removed from the body very quickly. Side effects include decreased white blood cell counts, so your doctor will have your blood count checked periodically while on these medicines. Other medicines that may be useful are beta-blocking medicines, which decrease the excess thyroid's damaging effect on the heart, and warfarin (a blood thinner), which is used to prevent strokes from abnormal heart rhythms. Not all patients require beta-blocker or warfarin therapy. If your thyroid is well controlled,

you may not require either. Side effects of the beta-blockers include low blood pressure and depression, and these drugs often cannot be used in patients with asthma or diabetes. Side effects of warfarin include serious bleeding, especially if the dose is to high. Blood thinning levels (prothrombin or "pro" times) are checked periodically to minimize the risk of hemorrhage.

Other treatments for Graves' disease include radioactive iodine and surgery. Radioactive iodine generally has few side effects, is permanent, and very effective. It cannot be used during pregnancy. It can often be done as an outpatient or with a very short hospital stay. The long-term risk is hypothyroidism, because the thyroid function is reduced so effectively that supplemental thyroid may be needed to maintain normal levels.

Surgery is often reserved for patients who cannot have radiation therapy, or who are unable to use oral antithyroid medicines. Surgery carries less risk of long-term hypothyroidism but an increased risk of damage to the vocal cord nerves and the glands that regulate calcium. Voice changes, or the need for daily calcium tablets may result.

No matter which treatment method is chosen, your doctor will need to evaluate your thyroid function, blood pressure, and heart rhythm periodically.

The DOs

- Take your medicines exactly as prescribed. Antithyroid medicines do not have long-term effects, and skipping doses makes them useless. Beta-blockers are very effective when taken, but missed doses can result in higher blood pressure ("rebounding"), which can cause heart attack or stroke. Warfarin therapy may be dosed on an irregular basis because it has long-term effects, but be sure to follow your doctor's orders for dosage, and have your prothrombin times checked routinely. Blood thinners only work to prevent stroke when used consistently.
- Eat a healthful, low-fat diet. Minimize sources of vitamin K (leafy greens) if you are using warfarin.
- Exercise daily if approved by your doctor. Twenty minutes of moderate exercise (walking) can improve your sense of well-being and overall health.
- Visit your ophthalmologist (eye doctor) at least once each year to protect your vision. With advancing eye disease, more frequent visits may be necessary.

The DON'Ts
- Don't skip medication doses.
- Don't eat large amounts of leafy green vegetables.
- Don't miss your laboratory test appointments. They are essential to help you and your doctor properly treat your disease.

When to Call Your Doctor
- You have sudden worsening of nervousness or jitters.
- You have palpitations, shortness of breath, or chest pain.
- Eye pain or visual changes occur.
- A sore throat is present.
- You have fever, chills, nausea or vomiting.

For More Information
National Graves' Disease Foundation
320 Arlington Road
Jacksonville, FL 32211

HALITOSIS

About Your Diagnosis

Halitosis is the medical term for bad breath. More than 25 million Americans are affected with foul- or unpleasant-smelling breath. A number of factors and conditions cause bad breath. The most common cause of halitosis is the breakdown of food in the mouth by the bacteria that are always present there. Certain foods may make this condition worse. There are medical conditions that can cause bad breath. These include infected teeth, gums, or oral mucosa, oral cancers, the common cold, lung and sinus infections, postnasal drip, tonsillitis, untreated nasal polyps, diabetes, syphilis, and other diseases of the stomach, lungs, liver, and kidneys. Medications may also be a cause of halitosis. However, all of these medical problems taken together affect a very small percentage of individuals with halitosis.

Stress or nervous tension makes the bad breath worse. One of the major effects of stress is drying of the mouth. Saliva is the mouth's natural mouthwash; it has antibiotic elements in it that reduce the numbers of bacteria in the mouth.

Living With Your Diagnosis

An individual with bad breath is rarely aware of it. You generally cannot detect your own mouth odor even when you exhale into your hand, or lick it to smell the odor. You usually only become aware that you have halitosis when you notice that individuals are avoiding you or when someone tells you. All of us are more or less susceptible at one time or another to halitosis. Bad breath can come when you least expect it, and it tends to get worse and more frequent as you get older. The intensity of the odor is variable.

Treatment

The key to treatment is good oral hygiene. Daily brushing and flossing are essential. Using an over-the-counter mouthwash or a 50/50 mixture of hydrogen peroxide and water will help remove food particles and help neutralize odors. Regular dental checkups are a must to prevent, identify, and treat potential problems. Avoiding aggravating foods and tobacco can also help. If a medical condition or infection is the cause, proper treatment of the underlying condition is appropriate. Taking a vitamin C supplement may be of benefit, particularly in smokers. A vitamin C deficiency may make halitosis worse.

The DOs

- Brush with a baking soda toothpaste, floss between the teeth, and clean the tongue after each meal.
- Make sure your mouth is moist by drinking adequate water. Hold water in the mouth for as long as possible, swishing it vigorously to remove food particles.
- Increase saliva production by chewing sugarless gum or sugarless candy mints.
- Rinse mouth with 50/50 mixture of hydrogen peroxide and warm water for 1 minute.
- Snack on carrots, celery, or other vegetables to keep plaque from forming.
- Use an oral irrigation device to clean the teeth.

The DON'Ts

- Avoid foods and beverages that can cause bad breath, such as garlic, raw onions, cabbage, horseradish, eggs, broccoli, Brussels sprouts, fish, red meat, peppers, alcohol, and coffee.
- Avoid cigarettes and tobacco products.

When to Call Your Doctor

- You should consult your physician or dentist if bad breath becomes chronic and the simple treatments do not work.

For More Information
American Dental Association
211 E. Chicago Avenue
Chicago, Illinois 60611
312-440-2500
Fax: 312-440-2800

HAND-FOOT-AND-MOUTH DISEASE

About Your Diagnosis

Hand, foot, and mouth disease is a viral infection that starts in the throat. It is caused by coxsackievirus A16. It is spread from individual to individual. It usually affects children up to 3 years of age. The disease requires no specific treatment and usually resolves in 4 or 5 days.

Living With Your Diagnosis

Signs and symptoms of the disease include a sudden onset of fever; a sore throat with ulcers in the mouth and throat; a rash with blisters on the hands and feet and sometimes the groin area; loss of appetite; and headache.

Treatment

Tylenol or tepid sponge baths can be used to reduce the fever.

Children who are old enough should rinse their mouth with a mild salt water solution. To avoid spreading the disease, use separate eating utensils and boil them, or use disposable utensils. Boil bottle nipples separately from bottles for 20 minutes. Pacifiers should also be sterilized. Keep the child out of day care or pre-school to prevent spreading the infection to other children. Rest until the fever is gone. Encourage fluid intake by offering ice creams, custards, and jello, because solid foods may not be tolerated.

The DOs

- Keep the child home from preschool or day care for 4 or 5 days.
- Use Tylenol or tepid sponge baths for the fever. Don't give aspirin.
- Boil bottle nipples, pacifiers, and eating utensils after use.
- Use a mild salt water solution to rinse the mouth if the child is old enough (<cf1/2> teaspoon in 1 cup warm water).
- Rest until the fever is gone.
- Encourage liquids and soft foods.

The DON'Ts

- Don't give aspirin to a child with a viral infection because aspirin use has been associated with Reye's syndrome.
- Don't send a child to preschool or day care for 4 or 5 days.

- Don't share drinking cups or eating utensils.

When to Call Your Doctor

- If symptoms last longer than 4 or 5 days.
- If a high fever develops and does not respond to Tylenol or sponge baths.
- If the child has severe difficulty swallowing and can't maintain good fluid intake.

For More Information

The American Academy of Pediatrics
141 NW Point Blvd.
Elk Grove Village, IL 60007-1098
National Institute of Allergy and Infectious Diseases
9000 Rockville Pike
Bethesda, MD 20892
301-496-5717

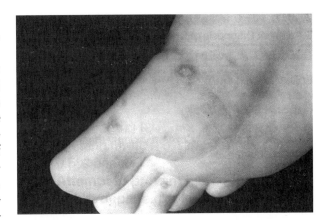

Hand, foot, and mouth disease. Note oval lesions on an erythematous base. (From Goldstein BG, Goldstein AO: *Practical Dermatology*, vol 1. St. Louis, Mosby–Year Book, 1992. Used by permission.)

HEADACHE, CLUSTER

About Your Diagnosis

Cluster headaches, although uncommon, are one of the more severe forms of head pain. They occur more commonly in men and are characterized by severe and constant pain deep in and around the eye on the affected side. The pain is generally intense and nonthrobbing, and often radiates into the forehead, temple, and cheek. The pain may leave as rapidly as it began or fade away gradually. Almost always the same eye is affected. The exact cause of cluster headaches is unknown.

Living With Your Diagnosis

These headaches occur in "clusters." The cluster usually begins in the spring or fall, and each cluster lasts approximately 2–3 months. The headaches usually occur nightly after 1–2 hours of sleep or several times during the day and night. Each attack lasts nearly an hour. Often a distinct pattern is detectable, with headaches recurring with remarkable accuracy at the same time each day for a period of 6–12 weeks, followed by complete freedom from headaches for many months or years. In addition to the headache, some individuals have watering eyes, drooping eyelids, or visual problems on the side of the headache.

Treatment

There are many treatment options for cluster headaches. Once the disorder is diagnosed, patients may be started on medication to prevent further headache attacks. Calcium channel blocking medications and ergotamine tartrate are often the first-line medications for prevention. Intranasal lidocaine or subcutaneous sumatriptan can be used to abort an attack. Methysergide or predisone may also be effective for cluster headaches.

For breakthrough headaches, headaches that occur despite being on a preventive medication, the most effective treatment is inhaling pure oxygen. If breakthrough headaches are frequent, your doctor may prescribe oxygen therapy for use at home. If attacks are less frequent, there are oral medications that are also effective and more convenient than pure oxygen.

The DOs

- Maintain an adequate and regular sleep schedule.
- Take your medications as prescribed.

- If you are taking a prescription drug, check with your doctor before using over-the-counter pain relief medications.
- Keep your follow-up appointments for reassessment.

The DON'Ts

- Don't use alcohol and tobacco.
- Avoid exposure to oil-based solvents, high altitude, and strenuous exercise because they may precipitate an attack.

When to Call Your Doctor

- If you have a fever with your headache.
- If you have a headache that is more severe than your usual headache and is resistant to the medication that is normally effective for you.
- If you have any weakness, numbness, or tingling in your arms or legs.
- If you have difficulty walking or talking.
- If you have severe vomiting that cannot be controlled with your medication.
- If you have any problems associated with your medication.

For More Information
American Association for the Study of Headache
and American Council for Headache Education
875 Kings Highway, Suite 200
Woodbury, NJ 08096
609-845-0322
National Headache Foundation
428 W. St. James Place, 2nd floor
Chicago, IL 60614-2750
312-388-6399
Health Partners–Neurologic Disorders Publications Program
Department of Neurology
2220 Riverside Ave. S.
Minneapolis, MN 55454-1478
612-371-1715
World Wide Web
http://www.healthpartners.com/group/neuro/ghineuro.htm
http://www.headaches.org

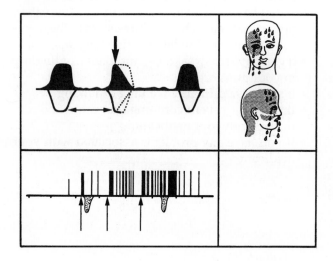

Profile of a cluster headache. (From Noble J: *Textbook Primary Care Medicine,* vol 2. St. Louis, Mosby–Year Book, Inc., 1995. Used by permission.)

HEADACHE, MIGRAINE

About Your Diagnosis

Migraine headaches are intense, recurrent headaches that may occur at any age but usually begin between the ages of 10 and 30 years. The precise cause is unknown, but it is hereditary in 60% to 80% of patients with migraine. The attacks occur less often with advancing years, and remission in patients older than 50 years is common.

Living With Your Diagnosis

Some individuals have a prodrome or a symptom that alerts them that a headache is developing. This may occur hours to days before a headache and may disappear shortly before the headache appears or may merge with it. Common prodromal symptoms include change in mood, hyperactivity, sluggishness, fatigue, changes in appetite, or nausea. In addition to the prodrome, many patients have an aura, a subjective sensation or motor phenomenon, before their headaches. Auras usually last 10–30 minutes, and the headache frequently follows within the hour. The most common type of aura is a visual disturbance such as flashes of light, flickering lights, or a blind spot.

Migraine headaches usually affect one side of the head and are throbbing. Typically, migraines last from 4 to 72 hours. Many individuals have nausea, vomiting, and hypersensitivity to light and sound during the headache. If you have a prodrome or aura that precedes your headaches, you should take your migraine medication as soon as possible. Early treatment is the key to faster relief of the headache.

Many patients link their migraine attacks to certain dietary items, particularly chocolate, red wine and port, cheese, onions, fatty foods, and acidic foods (oranges, tomatoes, etc.). Some of these foods are rich in tyramine, an amino acid, which has been incriminated as a provoking factor in migraine. Avoiding these items may reduce the chances of a migraine attack.

Treatment

There are many options for treating migraine headaches. Individuals who have frequent migraines may need to take preventive medication such as beta blockers, calcium channel blockers, antidepressants, anticonvulsants, nonsteroidal anti-inflammatory drugs, or hormones. If your migraines are infrequent, you may take medication only when needed. Your doctor will select the best therapy for you.

The DOs

- Keep a diary/calendar of your headaches and any events that seem to cause them.
- Take your medication as prescribed as soon as you feel a migraine developing.
- Get plenty of rest.

The DON'Ts

Many factors have been found to aggravate or precipitate migraine headaches. The following should be avoided:

- Stress.
- Changes in sleep habits.
- Fatigue.
- Certain dietary items such as alcohol (especially red wine), chocolate, cheese, Nutrasweet, and caffeine.
- Strong sensory stimuli (bright glare, loud noise, etc.).

When to Call Your Doctor

- If your headache lasts longer than usual, is more intense than usual, or is resistant to the medication that normally works for you.
- If you have severe vomiting that cannot be controlled with your medication.
- If you have a fever with your headache.
- If you have any problems associated with your medication.

For More Information

American Association for the Study of Headache and American
Council for Headache Education
875 Kings Highway
Suite 200
Woodbury, NJ 08096
609-845-0322
National Headache Foundation
428 W. St. James Place, 2nd floor
Chicago, IL 60614-2750
312-388-6399
World Wide Web
National Headache Foundation: http://www.headaches.org

Factors influencing the onset of migraine headaches from the external, physiologic, and psychologic environments. (From Noble J: *Textbook Primary Care Medicine,* vol 2. St. Louis, Mosby–Year Book, Inc., 1995. Used by permission.)

HEADACHE, TENSION-TYPE

About Your Diagnosis

Tension headaches are usually dull, aching, or throbbing headaches that are often associated with other sensations of fullness, tightness, or pressure (a feeling as if the head is going to burst, or as if it is bound or clamped in a vise). These sensations usually involve both sides of the head and neck, especially where the muscles of the neck attach to the skull. Tension headaches also involve the forehead and temples. This type of headache may last for weeks, months, or even years.

Living With Your Diagnosis

Patients with tension headaches may have nausea or increased sensitivity to light or sound. Avoiding these conditions may prevent the headache from worsening. Because stress and depression often play a role in perpetuating the headaches, counseling or stress reduction therapy is often worthwhile.

Treatment

Interestingly, patients who have tension headaches generally do not have increased muscle tension. For many years it has been taught that these headaches are caused by excessive muscular contraction and constriction of the scalp arteries. Neither of these speculations are supported by scientific studies. Nevertheless, despite these findings, tension headaches respond best to massage, relaxation, and the use of an antianxiety medication. Simple analgesics such as aspirin or acetaminophen are rarely helpful. In addition, biofeedback may be used to teach the patient how to reduce or prevent these headaches.

The DOs

- Learn effective strategies for reducing your stress.
- Sleep regularly.
- Keep a record of your headaches—time of day they occur, how long they last, associated stress, etc.
- Take your medications as prescribed.

The DON'Ts

- Avoid stimulants such as caffeine.
- Don't depend upon narcotic analgesics for relief; you may develop an addiction.
- If you feel a headache developing, avoid high-stimulation environments (e.g., loud noise or music, bright lights).

When to Call Your Doctor

- If your symptoms are more severe or last longer than usual, or if your headache is resistant to the medication that normally gives you relief.
- If you have a fever, vomiting, or change in vision.
- If you have any difficulty related to your medication.

For More Information

World Wide Web
National Headache Foundation: http://www.headaches.org
American Association for the Study of Headache
and American Council for Headache Education
875 Kings Highway, Suite 200
Woodbury, NJ 08096
609-845-0322
e-mail: lmgillicuddy@aash.ccmail.compuserve.com
National Headache Foundation
428 W. St. James Place, 2nd Floor
Chicago, IL 60614-2750
312-388-6399

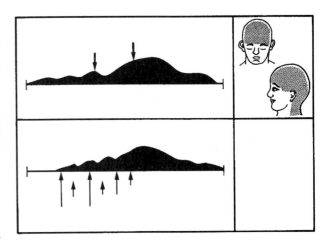

Profile of muscle contraction headache. (From Noble J: *Textbook Primary Care Medicine,* vol 2. St. Louis, Mosby–Year Book, Inc., 1995. Used by permission.)

HEART BLOCK, SECOND-DEGREE

About Your Diagnosis

Heart block refers to a delay of conduction of electrical signals from the atrium through the atrioventricular node (part of the electrical wiring of the heart). This node carries the electric signals from the atria that tell the ventricles to contract. The block can affect different parts of the conduction system of the heart. It is generically referred to as *heart block,* and there are many different types of blocks of electrical signals in the heart. Second-degree heart block affects the node (type I block) or conduction below the node (type II block). The atria contract normally, but because they do not receive the proper signal, the ventricles may not contract as often as they are supposed to.

Living With Your Diagnosis

Symptoms of heart block relate to insufficient pumping of blood from the heart. Heart block may produce no symptoms. Often it can cause extreme fatigue, lightheadedness, or syncope (fainting). Severe heart block can cause angina (chest pain) or stroke (not enough blood flow to the brain).

Heart block is relatively common. About one half of persons with heart block have no known cause. Most of the others have some form of heart disease. They may have had damage to the heart from a heart attack (myocardial infarction) or myocarditis (inflammation of the heart muscle). Heart block may come from overdosing of digitalis medications (digoxin). It may also be caused by some a congenital heart abnormality (one that one is present at birth). Heart block is detected with an electrocardiogram (ECG). Usually the patient has normal impulses from the atrium, but there is evidence that some of the impulses do not reach the ventricles.

A patient with type I second-degree heart block may have no symptoms. Type II block is usually the result of heart disease. Patients with type II block are at risk for complete heart block, cardiomyopathy (disease of the heart muscle), or death from asystole (the heart not beating). Medications that cause the condition have to be stopped or changed.

Treatment

If you have type I block and have no symptoms and no heart disease, no treatment is required. Patients with either type of heart block or those who have symptoms because the ventricle is not beating fast enough to meet blood demands may need a pacemaker (Fig 1). A pacemaker is an electrical device with a wire to the heart muscle that signals the ventricles to contract regularly (fixed-rate pacers) or to beat faster in response to increased activity (demand pacers). The pacemaker may be external with the wire entering through a vein, or it may be implanted in the patient with a minor operation. Older pacemakers were susceptible to damage from microwaves and strong electronic equipment. New pacemakers are safer and more reliable. You must still exercise caution around strong magnetic or ultrasonic forces such as those used in some physical therapy settings or in airport security screens. If you have a pacemaker, you will be given instructions by the cardiologist regarding maintenance and care of the pacemaker.

The DOs

- Make your diet one for a healthy heart, which means make it low in fat and cholesterol. Lose weight and stop smoking.
- Continue other medical treatments as directed.

The DON'Ts

- Do not exercise until you have clearance from your physician.

When to Call Your Doctor

- If you have worsening dizziness, fainting, chest pain, or shortness of breath.

For More Information

Contact the American Heart Association at 1-800-242-8721 and ask for the literature department.

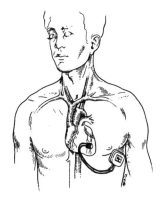

Cardiac pacemaker. (From LaFleur-Brooks ML: *Exploring Medical Language—A Student Directed Approach.* vol 3. St. Louis, Mosby–Year Book, 1993. Used by permission.)

HEAT EXHAUSTION AND HEAT STROKE

About Your Diagnosis

Heat exhaustion is a complex of symptoms caused by exposure of the body to excessive heat production or absorbtion. The end result of the excessive heat exposure is loss of body fluids and salt (sodium). Although heat exhaustion can make one look and feel quite ill, it is considered a minor illness and is easily treatable with replenishment of the body's fluids and sodium. Heat exhaustion is fairly common during "heat waves," or with vigorous exercise in warm environments. Heatstroke, on the other hand, is a rare but very serious and deadly illness. Heatstroke is caused by an inability of the body to regulate its temperature when faced with a heat challenge. Heatstroke requires intensive medical treatment if the individual is to survive.

Living With Your Diagnosis

Heat exhaustion should be suspected whenever someone has been sweating heavily in a warm or hot environment and begins to feel ill. The victim will usually appear pale and sweaty. The skin may feel cool and clammy or warm and moist. The victim's temperature may be normal or elevated. The pulse rate is usually fast. The victim often feels dizzy, lightheaded, achy, weak, and very tired. The victim may vomit. Standing or sitting upright usually makes the victim feel and look much worse. Fortunately, with treatment the symptoms usually resolve quickly. The victim may feel tired and "wrung out" for several hours, but complete recovery almost always occurs within a few hours.

Heatstroke usually is associated with very hot and dry skin. The victim is often unconscious or appears intoxicated. Heatstroke can affect many of the body's vital organs and systems. Recovery from heatstroke requires rapid treatment by trained rescuers, nurses, and physicians.

Treatment

The treatment for heat exhaustion should first be to provide a cooler environment for the victim. Simple measures would be moving to an area with shade, fans, or air conditioning. Excessive or tight-fitting clothing should be removed. The victim should be allowed to lie down. Fluids should be given. If the illness is mild, fluids can be given by

mouth. Sports drinks are preferred, but any nonalcoholic beverage can be substituted. At least one quart should be slowly consumed. If the illness is more severe, or if the victim is unable to drink or is vomiting, fluids may need to be given by vein by health professionals. Heatstroke victims require emergency medical care.

The DOs

- Do drink plenty of nonalcoholic fluids when perspiring or hot.
- Do wear light and loose-fitting clothing when in hot environments.
- Do avoid overexertion when the environment is hot.
- Do seek shade, fans, or air conditioning if you are hot and feel ill.
- Do watch the elderly for signs of heat exhaustion.
- Do start rehydration as soon as possible if signs of illness occur.
- Do seek emergency care if the victim appears unconscious or "drunk."

The DONT's

- Don't exercise during times of high heat and humidity.
- Don't plan activity in hot environments without plenty of fluids.
- Don't plan heavy activity during the hottest part of the day.
- Don't expose yourself to hot environments if you are feeling ill.
- Don't "overdo it." Plan plenty of rest, cooling, and water breaks.
- Don't restrict water to athletes during heavy exercise.

When to Call Your Doctor

- If the symptoms are more than mild.
- If the victim is unconscious or appears intoxicated.
- If chest pains or trouble breathing occur.

For More Information
Heatstroke Help
http://www.seas.smu.edu/~justin/inline_h.heat.html
First Aid Book
http://www.medaccess.com/first_aid/FA_TOC.htm
Your local American Red Cross chapter

HEMOCHROMATOSIS

About Your Diagnosis

Hemochromatosis is a condition in which the patient's body is overloaded with iron. The excess iron accumulates in various organs.

There are many causes of hemochromatosis. Some patients inherit a gene that causes them to absorb too much iron from their food. Others have the disease after taking iron pills for a long time. Red blood cells are very rich in iron, so patients who receive many blood transfusions may experience hemochromatosis. Hemochromatosis also may occur in association with certain types of anemia characterized by destruction of red blood cells (hemolytic anemia).

The most common form of hemochromatosis in the United States is the hereditary type. About one of ten persons in the United States carries the abnormal gene, and two to three per 1000 inherit a copy from both parents. Men have symptoms of hemochromatosis more frequently and at an earlier age than women, because women lose iron in their menstrual periods.

Hereditary hemochromatosis is transmitted genetically from parent to child. Only persons who inherit a copy of the gene from both parents are at risk for the disease. Some of the anemia that can predispose to hemochromatosis, either through destruction of red blood cells or through necessitating multiple blood transfusions, also are hereditary. Hemochromatosis is not contagious.

Hemochromatosis is detected with blood tests that measure the amount of iron stored in the body. Often a biopsy of the liver is needed to confirm the diagnosis. Computed tomography (CT) or magnetic resonance imaging (MRI) of the liver may be useful in the diagnosis of hemochromatosis.

Hemochromatosis is not curable, but treatment can prevent progression of the disease and in some instances reverse the symptoms.

Living With Your Diagnosis

The most common symptoms of hemochromatosis are darkening of the skin, arthritis, weakness, and loss of libido or impotence. The excess iron in the body of a patient with hemochromatosis accumulates in many organs. Patients may have diabetes, liver disease, heart disease, thyroid disease, or malfunction of the gonads. Patients with liver disease are at risk for liver cancer.

Treatment

The therapy of choice for hemochromatosis is removal of iron from the patient through drawing of blood once or twice a week (phlebotomy). Patients who have anemia (low red blood cell count) and cannot tolerate having their blood removed are treated with desferoxamine, a drug that binds iron. The medicine is pumped under the patient's skin over several hours each day.

There are little or no side effects of phlebotomy among patients who do not have anemia. Allergic reactions to desferoxamine can occur. Desferoxamine also can cause hearing loss. If given to very young children, it can cause poor growth.

The DOs
- Take your medication as prescribed.
- Eat a balanced diet.
- Restrict exercise if you have heart disease due to hemochromatosis. Otherwise exercise as tolerated.
- Ask your brothers and sisters to be tested for the disease, if you have hereditary hemochromatosis, so they can begin treatment before heart or liver disease develops.

The DON'Ts
- Do not take iron pills or vitamin C (especially if you are also taking desferoxamine), because it can increase the toxicity of iron. Do not take medication that may cause liver toxicity unless you have the express advice of your physician.
- Do not drink alcohol, because it increases your risk for liver disease.
- Avoid shellfish, unless it is very well cooked, because you are at risk for severe infection from several organisms that may occur in shellfish.
- Restrict exercise if you have heart disease due to hemochromatosis.

When to Call Your Doctor
- If you experience fever, chest pain, shortness of breath, or abdominal pain.

For More Information
National Heart, Lung, and Blood Institute Information Center
P.O. Box 30105
Bethesda, MD 20824-0105
301-251-1222
MedMark Hematology: http://medmark,bit.co.kr/hematol.html

HEMOPHILIA

About Your Diagnosis

Hemophilia is a genetically transmitted disease that predisposes to excessive bleeding. Hemophilia is hereditary. It is relatively rare, occurring among 1 per 10,000 to 30,000 newborn boys. It is usually transmitted to the male offspring by their mothers. Women usually have no symptoms. The reason is simple: Hemophilia is transmitted by the X chromosome. Women have two X chromosomes, and men have only one. Women can have one affected chromosome, but the other one compensates with normal genes. That does not occur among men, causing the disease.

Hemophilia predisposes to bleeding. This is caused by the lack of one of the important factors necessary for blood coagulation, factor VIII. The severity of this disease depends on how much of the factor is present in the circulation. Some patients can bleed from the time they are born, whereas others rarely bleed.

Living With Your Diagnosis

The most characteristic manifestation of hemophilia is bleeding into one of the large joints, such as the knee. This condition usually begins once a child reaches the toddler stage but can occur spontaneously at any time in more severe cases. With time this condition can develop into chronic joint contracture, especially if the patient is not treated. Other bleeding manifestations include blood in the urine or mouth or bleeding after trauma or a surgical procedure. Persons with milder hemophilia may not experience bleeding until an operation is performed or after a tooth extraction. With tooth extractions, the procedure usually is completed without problems, but within a few hours, the tooth socket begins to ooze, and healing is disrupted.

In the presence of any trauma, the patient should go to the hospital immediately. There the proper physical examination and tests help determine whether the patient needs blood factor replacement.

Whenever a patient with hemophilia needs a surgical procedure, factor VIII level must be brought to normal. The therapy may persist for many days once the operation is over.

Treatment

Once the diagnosis of hemophilia is established, the patient should be treated at a specialized center. When the bleeding starts, it is imperative that treatment be initiated promptly. To prevent further damage, any bleeding into a muscle or joint must be stopped as soon as possible. It is recommended that once the bleeding episode begins, so should the treatment, usually as self-infusion of factor VIII. Once started at home, supplementation can continue at the hospital, under a doctor's supervision.

How safe is the therapy? Factor VIII is a derivative of blood. As with every blood product, use of factor VIII carries risk for transmission of diseases such as hepatitis B and C as well as human immunodeficiency virus (HIV) infection. Lately these products have become safer, going through many purification processes. Disease transmission has decreased to almost zero.

Can hemophilia be prevented? Hemophilia is genetically transmitted. As such, it can be identified in the affected family. Consulting a physician may be important to determine whether one is at risk to transmit the disease to one's offspring. Some centers can provide detailed information through studying the patient's blood and that of family members.

The DOs

- Notify your physician before dental extractions or any type of operation.
- Notify your physician if you experience any excessive bleeding.
- Go immediately to the closest emergency room if you experience severe trauma.
- Participate in regular exercise, such as swimming.

The DON'Ts

- Do not participate in contact sports.
- Do not use aspirin, ibuprofen (eg, Motrin, Advil), naproxen (eg, Aleve), or other nonsteroidal anti-inflammatory drugs (NSAIDs).
- Avoid intramuscular injections.

When to Call Your Doctor

- If you are to undergo a tooth extraction.
- If you are to undergo any surgical procedure.

For More Information
MedWeb   Hematology:http://www.gen.emory.edu/

medweb.hematology.html
MedMark Hematology: http://medmark.bit.co.kr/hematol.html
National Heart, Lung, and Blood Institute Information Center
P.O. Box 30105
Bethesda, MD 20824-0105
301-251-1222
World Federation of Hemophilia: http://www.wfh.org/

HEPATITIS A

About Your Diagnosis

Hepatitis is an inflammation of the liver. There are at least five virus types that cause the disease. One of the types of viruses is the A virus. Hepatitis A infects about 150,000 individuals in the United States each year. The rate is much higher in underdeveloped countries.

The hepatitis A virus is usually transmitted by food or fecal contaminated water. Contaminated shellfish are a common source of infection. Outbreaks have been reported in day-care centers, the military, at institutions for the disabled, and because of infected restaurant workers. Transmission can also occur through direct contact with an infected individual. In more than 40% of the reported cases, it is not known how the individuals were infected.

Hepatitis A is detected by a blood test that is positive for the antibody to the virus. The antibody appears about 4 weeks after the infection. Liver function tests are abnormally elevated, often to very high levels. The vast majority of individuals who get hepatitis A recover within 6 months and do not have any serious health problems.

Living With Your Diagnosis

Not all individuals who have hepatitis A infection will have symptoms. This is particularly true if the patient is younger than 2 years. If a patient does have symptoms, they will normally appear during the first 4 weeks of infection. One of the main symptoms of hepatitis A is jaundice, a yellow color to the skin or whites of the eyes. The jaundice is caused by the excess bilirubin in the blood. The excess bilirubin can also lead to other symptoms such as pale or clay-colored stools, dark urine, and generalized itching. "Flulike" symptoms of fatigue, loss of appetite, nausea and vomiting, and low-grade fever, as well as pain in the liver area, may occur several days before the jaundice appears.

A very small percentage of individuals infected with hepatitis A are at risk for liver failure. This group includes those individuals with alcoholic hepatitis, chronic hepatitis with cirrhosis, and those individuals older than 60 years. These patients may improve in their symptoms and liver function tests only to have a relapse. This usually occurs after 4 weeks and can occur more than once. There is no way to predict who will sustain a relapse. It is rare for hepatitis A–infected pregnant women or their newborns to have serious complications.

Treatment

There is no specific treatment for hepatitis A. Most individuals can be cared for at home. Proper amounts of rest for 1–4 weeks after the diagnosis is made is important. During this time, intimate contact with other individuals should be avoided. The diet should include foods that are high in protein. Individuals who have come into contact with the patient should be given temporary immunization with immune serum globulin. This must be given within 2 weeks of exposure.

The DOs

- Bed rest may be necessary until the jaundice disappears and appetite returns.
- Eating a well-balanced diet with plenty of fluids is essential.
- Make sure you properly wash your hands if you have hepatitis or are caring for someone with the disease. This is particularly important after contact with fecal material.
- An individual with hepatitis A should use separate or disposable eating and drinking utensils.
- If you have multiple sexual partners, a latex condom should be used. It may prevent transmission of the virus.
- If exposed to blood, fecal material, and other body fluids on the job, use proper protective equipment such as gloves and eye protection to lessen the chance of accidental exposure.
- Day-care workers should use proper hand-washing techniques after changing a diaper and before doing anything else.
- Restaurant workers should use proper hand-washing techniques at all times.
- If traveling to areas that have a high incidence of hepatitis A, a vaccine is available.

The DON'Ts

- Avoid any substances that may be harmful to the liver. The avoidance of alcohol is key.
- Eating fatty foods may not be well tolerated in individuals with hepatitis A
- If you are an intravenous drug addict, do not share needles and other equipment because they can be contaminated with the hepatitis A virus.

When to Call Your Doctor
- If you have been exposed to someone who has hepatitis A or if you have symptoms of the disease.
- Call if hepatitis A symptoms do not resolve within 4 weeks.

For More Information
Hepatitis Foundation International
30 Sunrise Terrace
Cedar Grove, NJ 07009
800-891-0707

HEPATITIS, ALCOHOLIC

About Your Diagnosis

Alcoholic hepatitis is caused by excessive and chronic alcohol use. It is the first phase of alcoholic liver disease. It progresses to fatty liver and cirrhosis if alcohol abuse continues. A history of alcohol abuse is the key to diagnosis. Yet drunkenness is not needed for the development of the disease. To confirm the diagnosis a liver biopsy can be done. The disease usually affects those older than 30 years. The incidence is 3 cases per 10,000 individuals. The recovery is slow. It may take weeks to months for the liver to heal. If cirrhosis has developed, the liver may not be able to recover.

Living With Your Diagnosis

The symptoms of alcoholic hepatitis may not appear until the disease is severe. The symptoms are similar to those of viral hepatitis. The first symptoms may be a variety of rashes, joint pains, and other "flulike" symptoms. Finally jaundice, a yellow color to the skin or whites of the eyes, may be noted. The jaundice results from the excess bilirubin in the blood. The excess bilirubin can also lead to other symptoms such as pale or clay-colored stools, dark urine, and generalized itching. The symptoms of severe disease include high fever and enlargement of the liver, ascites (abdominal swelling caused by fluid), mental confusion, and coma. Because of the drinking of alcohol, the individual may be malnourished.

Treatment

The treatment of alcoholic hepatitis is supportive. The key to healing is to stop drinking alcohol. Working with an alcohol rehabilitation program is important in assisting with this. Dietary support is the treatment for malnurishment. The recommended diet is high in carbohydrates and calories. The nutritional status may be so severe that intravenous feedings are necessary. Salt (sodium) restriction may also be necessary to prevent ascites. Also needed is vitamin supplementation, especially B_1 and folic acid.

The DOs

- *Stop drinking.*
- Eat a well-balanced diet. Protein may need to be avoided in the diet because the liver may not be able to break it down.
- Modify activity according to the symptoms. A good fitness program may help with the fatigue.
- Seek treatment for your alcohol problem.

The DON'Ts

- *Avoid alcohol.*
- Avoid medications that can be harmful to the liver such as acetaminophen, sedatives, and tranquilizers.

When to Call Your Doctor

- If you need help stopping drinking.
- If symptoms suggestive of alcoholic hepatitis develop.
- If symptoms develop after prolonged or heavy drinking.

For More Information

Alcoholism

Alcoholics Anonymous World Services
P.O. Box 459
Grand Central Station
New York, NY 10163
212-686-1100

Liver Disease

American Liver Foundation
908 Pompton Ave.
Cedar Grove, NJ 07009
201-857-2626
800-223-0179

2 Information Way
Bethesda, MD 20892-3570
www.niddk.nih.gov
nddic@aerie.com
Crohn's and Colitis Foundation of America
386 Park Avenue South, 17th Floor
New York, NY 10016-7374
800-923-2423

HEPATITIS B

About Your Diagnosis

Hepatitis is an inflammation of the liver. There are at least five virus types that cause the disease. One of the types of viruses is the B virus. More than 1 million individuals are carriers of the hepatitis B virus in the United States. About 200,000 individuals contract this disease each year. Certain racial and ethnic groups have higher rates of infection, including blacks, Asians, Pacific Islanders, Hispanics, and Native Americans.

Hepatitis B is more infectious than the human immunodeficiency virus (HIV). The main ways the hepatitis B virus is transmitted is by sexual contact with an infected individual, receiving contaminated blood, or from using nonsterile needles or syringes. Hepatitis B can also be transmitted from an infected mother to her newborn. It is transmitted through infected blood and other body fluids (seminal fluid, vaginal secretions, breast milk, tears, saliva, and open sores). As with other types of hepatitis, the method of transmission in many patients is unknown.

Hepatitis B is detected by a blood test that is positive for the antibody to the virus. Liver function tests are abnormally elevated, often to very high levels. About 90% of the individuals who get hepatitis B recover within a few months, and they will never get hepatitis B again. However hepatitis B is a serious disease. Approximately 1% of patients die during the acute stage of the disease. Other individuals infected with hepatitis

B become carriers of the disease or become chronically infected. This occurs in about 10% of adults, 25% to 50% of young children, and 70% to 90% of infants.

Living With Your Diagnosis

Hepatitis B has a long incubation period, occasionally taking up to 6 months to become apparent. The first symptoms may be a variety of rashes, joint pains, and other "flulike" symptoms. Ultimately jaundice, a yellow color to the skin or whites of the eyes, may be noted. The jaundice is caused by the excess bilirubin in the blood. The excess bilirubin can also lead to other symptoms such as pale or clay-colored stools, dark urine, and generalized itching.

If the acute infection does not resolve, the symptoms can vary. Some individuals will remain well and just be a carrier of the virus. Others will have severe and persistent liver inflammation. This may eventually lead to cirrhosis and liver failure. Cirrhosis is scarring of the liver. The scarring does not allow the liver to do its job of removing toxic substances from the blood. Cirrhosis can lead to additional complications, including accumulation of fluid in the body (ascites) or bleeding from veins in the esophagus (varices). If the liver is chronically scarred, hepatocellular cancer can develop.

Treatment

There is no specific treatment for hepatitis B. Most individuals can be cared for at home. Proper amounts of rest for 1–4 weeks after the diagnosis of hepatitis B is made is important. Intimate contact with other individuals should be avoided during this time. The diet should include foods that are high in protein. Individuals who have come into contact with the patient should be given temporary immunization with hepatitis B immune globulin plus immunized with hepatitis B vaccine. This must be given within 2 weeks of exposure. This combination should also be given to newborns of infected mothers.

The DOs

- Bed rest may be necessary until the jaundice disappears and appetite returns.
- A well-balanced diet with plenty of fluids is essential.
- Make sure you properly wash your hands if you have hepatitis or are caring for someone with the disease. This is particularly important after contact with blood or other body fluid.
- An individual with hepatitis B should use separate or disposable eating and drinking utensils.
- A latex condom should be used. It may prevent transmission of the virus.
- If exposed to blood and body fluids on the job, use proper protective equipment such as gloves and eye protection to lessen the chance of accidental exposure.
- If you are in a high-risk group, you should receive the hepatitis B vaccine. High-risk groups are health workers, homosexual men, and household contacts of carriers.
- All newborns and children should be immunized with hepatitis B vaccine.

The DON'Ts
- Avoid any substances that may be harmful to the liver. The avoidance of alcohol is key.
- Fatty foods may not be well tolerated in individuals with hepatitis B and should be avoided.
- Avoid sexual contact with an individual infected with hepatitis B.
- Avoid contact with blood or blood products.
- If you have had hepatitis B, you should not donate blood. All blood is screened for the hepatitis B virus.
- Women who have had hepatitis B or have chronic hepatitis B should not breast-feed their babies.
- If you are an intravenous drug addict, do not share needles and other equipment because they can be contaminated with the hepatitis B virus or another virus.

When to Call Your Doctor
- If symptoms of hepatitis B develop.
- If hepatitis B symptoms do not resolve in 2 or 3 weeks, or if new symptoms develop.
- If you belong to a high-risk group for hepatitis B and have not yet been vaccinated against the disease.

For More Information
American Liver Foundation
1425 Pompton Avenue
Cedar Grove, NJ 07009
1-800-223-0179

HEPATITIS C

About Your Diagnosis

Hepatitis is an inflammation of the liver. It is caused by at least five different types of viruses. One of the types of viruses is the C virus. Hepatitis C has also been called non-A, non-B hepatitis. The incidence of hepatitis C is 1 case per 10,000 individuals. Hepatitis C is transmitted though exposure to infected blood or blood products. The hepatitis C virus causes most cases of hepatitis that occur after a blood transfusion. Hepatitis C can also be transmitted through intravenous drug use, and other exposures from contaminated blood or blood-containing products. In about 40% of cases, the exposure is not identified.

In general, individuals infected with hepatitis C are often identified because they are found to have elevated liver enzymes on a routine blood test. Others are identified because a hepatitis C antibody is found to be positive at the time of a blood donation. At least 50% of the cases of hepatitis C may become chronic. In these individuals, a liver biopsy may need to be done to determine the severity of liver damage.

Living With Your Diagnosis

One of main symptoms of hepatitis C is jaundice, a yellow color to the skin or whites of the eyes. The jaundice is caused by the excess bilirubin in the blood. The excess bilirubin can also lead to other symptoms such as pale or clay-colored stools, dark urine, and generalized itching. "Flulike" symptoms of fatigue, loss of appetite, nausea and vomiting, and low-grade fever may occur several days before the jaundice appears.

If chronic hepatitis C develops, the symptoms can vary. Some individuals may remain well. Others will have severe and persistent liver inflammation. This may eventually lead to cirrhosis and liver failure. Cirrhosis is scarring of the liver. The scarring does not allow the liver to do its job of removing toxic substances from the blood. Cirrhosis can lead to additional complications, including accumulation of fluid in the body (ascites) or bleeding from veins in the esophagus (varices). If the liver is chronically scarred, hepatocellular cancer can develop.

Treatment

There is no specific treatment for acute hepatitis C. Most individuals can be cared for at home. Rest and proper diet are recommended when the symptoms are most severe. Individuals with acute hepatitis should avoid alcohol and any substances that are toxic to the liver.

Individuals with chronic hepatitis C can be treated with the drug, interferon alpha-2b. However only 10% to 15% of patients treated with interferon have a long-lasting response. Patients can be treated a second time in hopes of inducing a remission. The goal of treatment with interferon is to improve or normalize the liver function tests and reduce the inflammation in the liver. This will in turn slow or interrupt the development of the complications of cirrhosis. Interferon frequently causes side effects, including "flulike" symptoms, depression, headache, and decreased appetite. In addition, interferon can cause problems with the bone marrow.

The DOs
• Bed rest may be necessary until the jaundice disappears and the appetite returns.
• A well-balanced diet with plenty of fluids is essential.
• Make sure you properly wash your hands if you have hepatitis or are caring for someone with the disease. This is particularly important after contact with blood or other body fluids.
• An individual with hepatitis C should use separate or disposable eating and drinking utensils.
• If you have multiple sexual partners, a latex condom should be used. It may prevent transmission of the virus.
• If exposed to blood and body fluid on the job, use proper protective equipment such as gloves and eye protection to lessen the chance of accidental exposure.

The DON'Ts
• Avoid any substances that may be harmful to the liver. The avoidance of alcohol is key.
• Fatty foods may not be well tolerated in individuals with hepatitis C
• If you have had hepatitis C, you should not donate blood. All blood is screened for the hepatitis C virus.
• Women who have had hepatitis C or have chronic hepatitis C should not breast-feed their babies.

- If you are an intravenous drug addict, do not share needles and other equipment because they can be contaminated.

When to Call Your Doctor
- If you have been exposed to someone who has hepatitis C or if you have symptoms of the disease.
- If hepatitis C symptoms do not resolve within 16 weeks.

For More Information
Hepatitis Foundation International
30 Sunrise Terrace
Cedar Grove, NJ 07009
800-891-0707
The Hepatitis C Foundation
1502 Russett Drive
Warminster, PA 18974
215-672-2606
Fax: 215-672-1518

HEPATITIS, CHRONIC

About Your Diagnosis

Chronic hepatitis occurs when there is persistent injury and inflammation to the liver cells that lasts for longer than 6 months. This condition can be divided into two classifications: chronic persistent and chronic active hepatitis. There are several causes: viruses, metabolic conditions, immunologic abnormalities, and medications. The most common causes are hepatitis B and C. Jointly these two viruses are the cause of more than 75% of the cases of chronic hepatitis. If you have chronic hepatitis B or C, you can be infectious to others. About 20% of the time autoimmune chronic hepatitis is the cause. In this condition, the body's immune system reacts to itself, causing damage to the liver. There are also some inherited disorders that can cause chronic hepatitis. These include Wilson's disease and alpha-1-antitrypsin deficiency. Long-term use of some medications can also cause a small number of cases of chronic hepatitis. These drugs include phenytoin, nitrofurantoin, and isoniazid.

Chronic hepatitis occurs in about 2 in 1,000 individuals. The condition is detected by a liver biopsy. Evaluation of infectious hepatitis blood markers are of use if the cause is infectious. The prognosis is generally good with chronic persistent hepatitis. About 40% to 50% of patients with chronic active hepatitis die within 5 years of the onset of symptoms. The cause of death is usually from liver failure and complications of portal hypertension (increased pressure in the liver veins).

Living With Your Diagnosis

The most common symptom of chronic hepatitis is fatigue. Other symptoms include mild upper abdominal discomfort, decreased appetite, and achy joints. Some patients may have signs of liver failure and cirrhosis. Signs of liver failure are jaundice (a yellow color to the skin or whites of the eyes), ascites (abdominal swelling caused by fluid), and coma. Depending on the cause, other organ systems can be affected. Those organs include the thyroid, intestines, eyes, joints, spleen, kidneys, and skin. Because of the chronic scarring of the liver, hepatocellular cancer can develop in some patients with chronic hepatitis.

Treatment

The treatment of chronic hepatitis depends on the cause. Prednisone or other corticosteroids help to reduce the inflammation. Azathioprine or mercaptopurine are drugs used to treat chronic hepatitis caused by immune disorders. Interferon is a drug used to treat chronic hepatitis caused by hepatitis B and C. However interferon is not effective in all cases. Relapses can occur in about half of those treated. In severe cases of liver failure, a liver transplantation is an option.

The DOs

- Modify physical activity according to the symptoms. A good fitness program may help with the fatigue.
- A well-balanced diet is necessary.
- Make sure you properly wash your hands if you have chronic hepatitis or are caring for someone with the disease. This is particularly important after contact with blood or other body fluid. It will help with prevention and transmission of the disease.
- An individual with chronic hepatitis B or C should use separate or disposable eating and drinking utensils.
- Use latex condoms. It may prevent transmission of the hepatitis B and C.
- If exposed to blood and body fluids on the job, use proper protective equipment such as gloves and eye protection to lessen the chance of accidental exposure.
- If you are in a high-risk group, you should receive hepatitis B vaccine. High-risk groups are health workers, homosexual men, and household contacts of carriers.
- All newborns and children should be immunized with Hepatitis B vaccine.

The DON'Ts

- Avoid alcohol
- Avoid medications that can be harmful to the liver such as acetaminophen, sedatives, and tranquilizers.
- Avoid salt in the diet.
- Avoid sexual contact with an individual infected with hepatitis B.
- Avoid contact with blood or blood products.
- If you have had chronic hepatitis B or C, you should not donate blood.

- Women who have chronic hepatitis B or C should not breast-feed their babies.
- If you are an intravenous drug addict, do not share needles and other equipment because of possible contamination.

When to Call Your Doctor
- If symptoms of chronic active hepatitis develop.
- If symptoms worsen or do not improve with treatment.
- If new symptoms develop, particularly worsening jaundice or abdominal pain.

For More Information
American Liver Foundation
1425 Pompton Avenue
Cedar Grove, NJ 07009
1-800-223-0179

HERPANGINA

About Your Diagnosis

Herpangina is an inflammation of the throat and mouth that is caused by a virus called coxsackievirus. It is spread from individual to individual through close contact, such as kissing or sharing food. It is more common in young children between the ages of 1 and 10 years. It may be confused with strep throat or canker sores. Recovery takes a few days to a week with little treatment required.

Living With Your Diagnosis

Symptoms usually appear 2–9 days after exposure. They include a temperature of 100°F to 104°F; a sore throat with a sudden onset, making swallowing painful; grayish white spots on the upper mouth; headache; loss of appetite; and fatigue.

Treatment

No specific treatment is needed. A nonaspirin medication such as Tylenol can be used for the fever and pain. Tepid sponge baths can be used to reduce fever. Careful hand washing is needed to prevent the spread of the disease. Avoid kissing and sharing food. Increase fluid intake to prevent dehydration. Rest until the fever is gone. A soft or liquid diet should be given until the throat discomfort has decreased. Ice pops, jello, and ice chips may ease mouth and throat pain. Avoid acidic fruit juices that may further irritate the throat.

The DOs

- Rest until the fever is gone.
- Give nonaspirin medication such as Tylenol for the pain and fever, or use tepid sponge baths to reduce the fever.
- Increase your fluid intake.
- Eat a liquid or soft diet until the inflammation subsides.
- Use ice pops or ice chips to decrease discomfort.

The DON'Ts

- Don't share food or kiss anyone.
- Don't give aspirin to a child younger than 16 years (because of the risk of Reye's syndrome).
- Don't give acidic fruit juices, which will irritate the mouth and throat.
- Avoid spicy foods that may irritate the mouth.

When to Call Your Doctor

- If symptoms are not gone in 1 week.
- If fluids cannot be tolerated.
- If there are signs of dehydration such as dry, wrinkled skin, dark urine, or a decrease in the need to urinate.
- If anyone else in the family shows signs of the disease.

For More Information

National Institute of Allergy and Infectious Diseases
9000 Rockville Pike
Bethesda, MD 20892
301-496-5717
Internet Sites
www.healthfinder.gov (Choose SEARCH to search by topic)
www.healthanswer.com

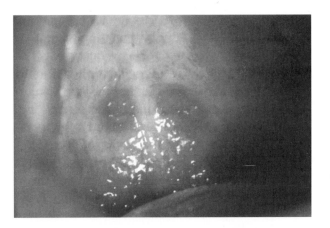

Herpangina with shallow ulcers in the roof of the mouth. (From Goldstein BG, Goldstein AO: *Practical Dermatology*, vol 1. St. Louis, Mosby–Year Book, 1992. Used by permission.)

HERPES SIMPLEX

About Your Diagnosis

Herpes simplex is a virus in the family of viruses that cause chickenpox, shingles, cold sores, and mononucleosis.

The principal cause is the herpes simplex virus type 1. This particular virus type is the primary cause of fever blisters and cold sores. The initial infection usually occurs in childhood.

It is estimated that about 80% of all adults have had exposure to the virus, but only a few can recall a specific first infection.

Herpes simplex is mainly transmitted by non-sexual intimate contact with saliva of an infected individual; for example, a child kissed by an adult relative who is shedding the virus but has no evidence of an infection. The virus from an infected individual can enter your body by passing through a break in your skin or through the tender skin of your mouth. It is extremely difficult to trace the transmission because a current outbreak may be the result of an infection acquired months or years in the past.

Herpes simplex is usually detected by inspection of the infected site. You may know when a recurrence is about to happen because you may feel itching, tingling, or pain in the places where you were first infected. The typical appearance is heralded by a tingling or discomfort at the site of the outbreak; then small blisters emerge and proceed to form ulcers and crusts. Healing occurs over 10–14 days. In special circumstances, specific laboratory tests can be used to verify the identity of the virus, but are not usually necessary in typical cases.

Herpes virus infections are not curable and may recur throughout life.

Living With Your Diagnosis

The typical appearance is heralded by a tingling or discomfort at the site of the outbreak; then small blisters emerge and proceed to ulceration and crusting. Healing occurs over 10–14 days.

This is a chronic infection that is impossible to eradicate, but millions of individuals are living a normal life with the disease.

Treatment

Although there is no cure, the drugs acyclovir, valacyclovir, and famciclovir can be very helpful.

The recommended treatment for primary episodes is 200 mg of acyclovir taken orally five times daily for 10 days, or 400 mg of acyclovir taken orally three times daily for 10 days. Treatment can significantly shorten the course. Acyclovir speeds up healing and can lessen the pain of herpes simplex infection for many individuals. It is used to treat infections and can also be used to lessen the number of recurrences. To soothe pain, take aspirin, acetaminophen, or ibuprofen. Penciclovir (Denavir) is an effective topical cream for treatment of recurrent herpes on the lips and face. Other topical antiviral agents have been popular but have not been shown to abort recurrent episodes. Many popular remedies are available including moisturizing or anesthetic lip balms, but there is no evidence that they are effective.

Common side effects of the antiviral medications include nausea, vomiting, and itching. Allergic reactions and side effects of the medication are possible.

The DOs

- Take medication as prescribed by your doctor.
- Avoid stress. Reactivation of the virus can occur with emotional or physical stress and menstruation. Therefore, stress reduction measures such as avoiding stressful situations or learning how to deal with them effectively are important.
- Apply sunscreen to susceptible areas. Sunlight is also a precipitating cause, and application of sunscreen may decrease recurrences.
- Learn to recognize the early symptoms of tingling or itching; then avoid kissing anyone until the sores have completely healed.
- Keep hands well washed.
- Keep the lesion clean and dry.
- Avoid shaving the affected area.
- Avoid sharing individual hygiene items.

The DON'Ts

- Do not scratch. Scratching can lead to a secondary infection.

When to Call Your Doctor

- For infections that recur more than four to six times per year.
- For infections that involve a sensitive organ or tissue such as the eye.

For More Information
Call the National Herpes Hotline at 919-361-8488, or send a self-addressed, stamped envelope to the Herpes Resource Center, PO Box 13827, Research Triangle Park, NC 27709.

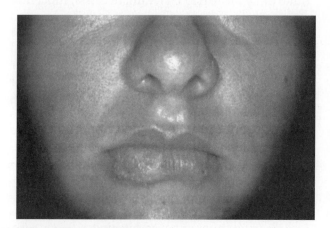

Herpes simplex. Note grouped vesicles on an erythematous base, and subsequent edema. (Courtesy of John Cook, M.D. From Goldstein BG, Goldstein AO: *Practical Dermatology,* vol 1. St. Louis, Mosby–Year Book, 1992. Used by permission.)

HERPES SIMPLEX, GENITAL

About Your Diagnosis

Genital herpes is an infection of the genitals that is caused by the herpes type 2 virus. It is transmitted by sexual contact, and generally affects the penis, vagina, and cervix. Diagnosis is made by culturing a lesion. This disease is considered to be incurable because symptoms recur when the virus is reactivated; however, symptoms can be controlled.

Living With Your Diagnosis

Painful blisters occur on the penis or vaginal area, and may extend into the vagina to the cervix. They are preceded by burning and itching. In several days the blisters rupture and leave shallow, painful ulcers, which take about 3 weeks to heal. There may be painful urination and occasionally fever.

Treatment

Your doctor may prescribe an antiviral medication called acyclovir. The most common side effects of this medication are nausea, vomiting, diarrhea, headache, and dizziness. Warm sitz baths may ease discomfort. Intercourse must be avoided until symptoms are gone. Condoms do not provide a safe barrier because the virus and lesions can also be on the thighs and buttocks. Careful hand washing is a must. Do no allow anyone to share towels or washcloths. Women must get a Pap smear yearly because herpes has been shown to be associated with the development of cervical cancer.

The DOs

- Continue to take the medication prescribed even if the symptoms are gone; the virus is still there.
- Use warm sitz baths or soaks with Epsom salts to ease the discomfort.
- Try pouring warm water over the genitals if urination is painful.
- Notify sexual partners if you have symptoms for the first time.
- Avoid contact with lesions.
- Wash hands well after using the toilet.
- Avoid sexual intercourse until symptoms are gone.
- Use latex condoms during intercourse after symptoms are gone.
- Women should wear underpants or pantyhose with a cotton crotch.
- Remind your doctor of your disease if you become pregnant so precautions can be taken to prevent the baby from becoming infected.
- Avoid situations that may trigger an outbreak: stress, sunbathing, other infections, and trauma.

The DON'Ts

- Don't skip doses or stop taking the medications if the symptoms are gone.
- Don't share towels or washcloths.
- Don't have intercourse until symptoms are gone, and then use latex condoms.

When to Call Your Doctor

- If during treatment you have unusual swelling or bleeding.
- If you have a fever and feel ill after treatment has begun.
- If your symptoms don't improve in a week after beginning treatment.

For More Information
Herpes Resource Hotline
415-328-7710
The CDC National STD Hotline
800-227-8922
Herpes Resource Center
800-230-6039
American Social Health Association
P.O. Box 13827
Research Triangle Park, NC 27709
National Womens Health Network
202-628-7814, Monday through Friday from 9 AM to 5 PM (EST).
National Institute of Allergy and Infectious Diseases
9000 Rockville Pike
Bethesda, MD 20892
301-496-5717
Internet Sites
www.healthfinder.gov (Choose SEARCH to search by topic.)
www.healthanswers.com

HERPES ZOSTER

About Your Diagnosis

Herpes zoster is also known as shingles. It is an uncomfortable and often very painful outbreak of skin blisters and sores. The condition is caused by the varicella-zoster virus, the same virus that causes chickenpox. After you recover from chickenpox (usually in childhood), the virus remains in your body doing no harm. When you become older, changes in your body allow the virus to become active again. This new disease is different from chickenpox and is called shingles. When you have had a case of chickenpox, you seldom if ever will have chickenpox again; however, 1 in every 10 individuals who have had chickenpox will have shingles.

The virus causing herpes zoster (shingles) is already in you from your earlier infection with chickenpox. Therefore, you do not catch shingles nor do you give shingles to someone. However, if you have active shingles and come in contact with an individual who has never had chickenpox, it is possible that the individual can catch chickenpox from your shingles. Remember, it is the same virus that causes chickenpox and herpes zoster (shingles).

Although anyone who has had chickenpox can subsequently have herpes zoster (shingles), it is much more common in individuals older than 50 years. Also certain diseases or drugs that lower your natural resistance, such as acquired immunodeficiency syndrome (AIDS), cancer, and steroids, can make you more likely to have shingles. It is rare, but possible, to have additional episodes of shingles during your lifetime.

The condition is not curable; anyone having had chickenpox probably has live varicella-zoster virus in their body. At present, we do not have any drugs that can cure this infection, but we do have medications that can shorten the course of the illness, its severity, and most importantly, prevent some of the complications of herpes zoster (shingles).

Living With Your Diagnosis

Herpes zoster or shingles virus lives in the nerves near your spine. When the virus becomes active, it travels along the nerves to the skin. It then breaks out on the skin in groups or bands where the nerve endings are. Thus the rash seldom crosses the midline of the body and is usually confined to a band going across part of the body. The rash can occur anywhere including the face.

Early signs of an outbreak are often vague, consisting of mild itching, tingling, pain, headache, fever, or a flulike syndrome. This is followed by the rash, which is made up of many small, fluid-filled blisters in groups that dry, scab over, and heal (much like chickenpox) within a few weeks.

The amount of pain and discomfort of shingles varies from individual to individual. The usual time from appearance of blisters to healing is usually 1–2 weeks. Healing in the majority of cases is complete and uneventful. Unfortunately in a significant number of individuals, especially those older than 50 years, the pain associated with these lesions can persist greater than 30 days. This is called postherpetic neuralgia and can be so severe that it interferes with daily activity. Another complication can be secondary bacterial infection of the rash. This occurs through contamination by scratching and can lead to possible infection and deep scarring.

Herpes zoster (shingles) infections that occur on the face are of particular concern. These infections can involve the eye and result in serious scarring of the eye and loss of vision. Shingles infections about the face and nose require immediate medical attention and possible referral to an eye doctor.

Treatment

The main goals of treatment are to decrease the duration of the infection, its discomfort, and to prevent complications such as postherpetic neuralgia and bacterial infection. Until relatively recently, treatment was only for symptoms; however, physicians now have antiviral drugs that actually kill the virus and shorten the infection. The use of these drugs must be started early. Once the infection has been present for 3 or 4 days, the antiviral medication is of little help. These medications include acyclovir, valacyclovir, and famciclovir. The antiviral drugs are effective at decreasing symptoms, but the infection may still be painful and irritating. Your doctor may wish to add other medications and lotions to help lessen the pain and itching. If secondary bacterial infection occurs, you will be given antibiotic medications as well.

The DOs

- Do seek medical attention as soon as you suspect you may have herpes zoster. The antiviral medication must be given within 2 or 3 days of the rash to be helpful.

- Do tell your doctor if you are pregnant; some antiviral medications may not be good for your unborn baby.
- Do take precautions to avoid contact with those who have never had chickenpox because they may become infected from you.
- Do keep the rash clean and notify your doctor if it appears to be infected (pus, increasing redness, not getting better).
- Do see your doctor immediately if the rash is on the face or nose.

The DON'Ts

- Don't scratch, contaminate, or break the blisters.
- Don't use home remedies that might make it worse such as detergents, kerosene, etc.
- Don't wait to see your doctor; the sooner you start antiviral medication, the better.

When to Call Your Doctor

- Anytime the rash is on the face or nose.
- If the pain is not getting better after the rash has healed.
- If the rash appears to have become secondarily infected, i.e., pus, increasing pain, increasing redness.

For More Information
American Academy of Dermatology
930 N. Meachum Road
Schaumburg, IL 60173
847-330-0230

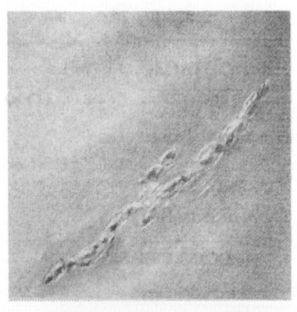

HERPES ZOSTER (SHINGLES)

Herpes zoster (shingles). (From LaFleur-Brooks ML: *Exploring Medical Language—A Student Directed Approach.* vol 3. St. Louis, Mosby–Year Book, 1993. Used by permission.)

HIATAL HERNIA

About Your Diagnosis

A hiatal hernia is a weakness or stretching of the opening where the esophagus passes through the diaphragm. The diaphragm is the muscle separating the chest from the abdomen. Because of the weakness or stretching, acid from the stomach may flow backward into the esophagus (the tube that connects the mouth and stomach) causing irritation. The stomach may also come through the opening into the lower chest. This condition can affect individuals of all ages, although it is more common in individuals older than 50 years. The cause of this condition is unknown; however, there are many factors that increase the risk including obesity, pregnancy, smoking, constant straining or lifting with tightened abdominal muscles, coughing, abdominal trauma, and chronic constipation or straining with bowel movements.

Endoscopy, using a small light tube with a tiny video camera on the end, or a barium swallow x-ray are used to detect a hiatal hernia. Pressure measurements (manometry) may be done to prove a reduced pressure at the esphagogastric junction.

Living With Your Diagnosis

Symptoms generally occur about an hour after meals. Symptoms include heartburn, chest pain, belching, and rarely swallowing difficulties. Bending over or lying down can make the heartburn worse. A possible complication of a hiatal hernia is bleeding, caused by irritation of the esophagus. However, frequently individuals with a hiatal hernia are symptom free.

Treatment

The treatment of a hiatal hernia is designed to control the symptoms and to prevent complications. The main treatment options are lifestyle and diet modifications along with antacids. To help keep stomach acid away from the hernia, raise the head of your bed 4–6 inches. Use wooden blocks or bricks to do this. You should not use 2 or 3 pillows to elevate your head. You should avoid foods and drinks that aggravate the symptoms. Antacids are most effective when taken on a regular schedule. Suggested dosing schedules for antacids are 1–2 hours after meals and at bedtime, or 1 hour before meals and at bedtime. If constipation is a problem, stool softeners can be taken.

If the symptoms cannot be controlled, or complications such as scarring, ulceration, or strangulation (twisting in a way that cuts off the blood supply) are occurring, surgery to correct the hernia may be necessary.

The DOs

- Lose weight if overweight.
- Eat slowly.
- Eat four or five small meals a day.

The DON'Ts

- Avoid alcoholic drinks and caffeine products (coffee, tea, cocoa, cola drinks).
- Avoid fried, spicy, and fatty foods, citrus juices, peppermint, and spices that aggravate the symptoms of hiatal hernia.
- Avoid large meals.
- Do not eat anything for at least 2 hours before bedtime.
- Do not bend over or lie down immediately after eating.
- Do not smoke.
- Avoid tight fitting pants, belts, and undergarments.
- Do not strain during bowel movements, urination, or lifting.

When to Call Your Doctor

- If you have the sensation that food stops beneath the breastbone.
- If you have pain that happens with shortness of breath, sweating, or nausea.
- If you vomit blood or have recurrent vomiting.
- Symptoms do not improve after 1 month of treatment.

For More Information

National Digestive Diseases Information Clearinghouse
2 Information Way
Bethesda, MD 20892-3570
www.niddk.nih.gov
nddic@aerie.com

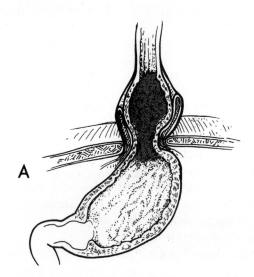

Hiatal Hernia. (From LaFleur-Brooks ML: *Exploring Medical Language—A Student Directed Approach.* vol 3. St. Louis, Mosby–Year Book, 1993. Used by permission.)

HIP PAIN

About Your Diagnosis
The hip is made up of the hip bone (greater trochanter) and the surrounding structures, such as the muscles, tendons, and ligaments. Hip pain can be caused by an injury, a fracture, a tumor, or a disease that affects the hip joint, such as osteoarthritis, rheumatoid arthritis, or ankylosing spondylitis. Hip pain also may be caused by tendinitis (inflammation of a tendon around the joint capsule) or bursitis (inflammation of the thin, fluid-filled sac that protects the joint). Problems in the sacroiliac joints or low back can cause pain in the hip area.

A physician diagnoses hip pain by taking a medical history, performing a physical examination, and possibly by taking a radiograph (x-ray) of the joint. Your doctor may order blood tests to determine whether your hip pain is caused by any diseases that may cause similar symptoms. Computed tomography (CT), magnetic resonance imaging (MRI), or a bone scan may be performed if the doctor needs a clearer picture of the bones and surrounding structures.

Living With Your Diagnosis
Hip pain may cause difficulty dressing, standing, bending, walking, and going up or down steps. The pain may keep you awake at night. If it becomes severe, it may be necessary to use a cane to decrease the hip pain.

Treatment
Management of hip pain depends on the cause of the pain. If the pain is due to osteoarthritis, your doctor may prescribe acetaminophen or a nonsteroidal anti-inflammatory drug (NSAID). If your hip pain is caused by bursitis or tendinitis, the doctor may prescribe an NSAID, recommend physical therapy, or do both. Physical therapy usually consists of application of deep heat or ultrasound or both. If bursitis is severe, your physician may inject a steroid-containing medication into the bursa. This medication is a powerful anti-inflammatory agent.

All medications can cause side effects. Acetaminophen may cause kidney or liver problems. The NSAIDs may cause stomach upset, diarrhea, constipation, ulcers, headache, dizziness, difficulty hearing, or a rash. There are few side effects of cortisone injection because most of the medicine stays in the hip area, although bleeding or bruising may occur after the injection.

The DOs
- Take your medications as prescribed.
- Call your doctor if you are experiencing side effects from medications
- Ask your doctor which over-the-counter pain medications you may take with your prescription medications.
- Perform prescribed hip exercises daily.

The DON'Ts
- Do not wait for a possible medication side effect to go away on its own.
- Do not continue an exercise program that causes pain. Pain that continues after exercise usually means the exercise has to be modified for you.
- Do not cross your legsthis can aggravate your hip pain.

When to Call Your Doctor
- If you experience side effects that you believe may be due to your medications.
- If medication and other treatments are not helping the pain.
- If you believe you need a referral to a physical therapist for exercise.

For More Information
Contact the Arthritis Foundation in your area. If you do not know the location of the Arthritis Foundation, call the national office at 1-800-283-7800 or access information on the Internet at www.arthritis.org.

HIRSUTISM

About Your Diagnosis

Hirsutism means excess male-pattern body hair growth in women. Hirsutism is caused by increased secretion of androgens or increased sensitivity of hair follicles to androgens. Androgens, usually thought of as male hormones, are produced by the adrenals and ovaries in women as well. Androgens are important for normal pubertal development in women.

Excess circulating androgens may arise from either an adrenal, an ovarian, or an outside source. Adrenal causes of excess androgens include an adrenal tumor or congenital adrenal hyperplasia (CAH). Congenital adrenal hyperplasia is an inherited enzymatic defect that interrupts the normal production of cortisol. The body shunts the extra cortisol precursors to a different metabolic pathway, producing extra androgens.

Ovarian sources include an ovarian tumor or polycystic ovarian syndrome (PCOS). Polycystic ovarian syndrome is associated with irregular menstrual periods, obesity, and insulin resistance in the form of diabetes.

Outside sources of androgens include anabolic steroids taken for muscle development, or other medications with androgen effects such as phenytoin, oral steroids, diazoxide, progestins, cyclosporine, and minoxidil.

Increased sensitivity of hair follicles may also occur in certain endocrine disorders such as Cushing's syndrome or acromegaly. Idiopathic hirsutism is a diagnosis for individuals who have excess body hair from an unknown cause.

Excess body hair is extremely common, occurring in 5% to 10% of all women. Very few seek medical attention. Only a small minority have a tumor. Increased body hair is a normal hereditary trait in many Caucasian women of Mediterranean origin.

Hirsutism is detected by examination of excess hair. Next, androgens levels are measured in the blood. Two important hormones are testosterone and dehydroepiandrosterone sulfate (DHEAS). A suppression test with dexamethasone is administered for 5–8 days if these hormones are elevated. Elevated DHEAS levels arise from the adrenals. If DHEAS remains elevated after this test, an adrenal tumor is the most likely cause of the hirsutism.

Increased testosterone may arise from either the adrenals or the ovaries. If the testosterone remains elevated after dexamethasone suppression, an ovarian disorder is the culprit. Very high levels of testosterone are suggestive of a tumor. An ultrasound of the ovaries is performed to determine whether a tumor is present. Usually, the cause is not a tumor, but PCOS.

Initially elevated DHEAS or testosterone levels that are suppressed with dexamethasone suggest CAH as the cause of the hirsutism. Although present since birth, this enzymatic defect may not become clinically apparent until young adulthood in some cases.

Most hirsutism may be improved with therapy; however, it may take months to be effective.

Living With the Diagnosis

Symptoms include new, thick, dark, curly hair in a male pattern on the face or beard, anterior chest, upper back, or lower abdomen spreading up to the umbilicus. Some hair on legs, arms, upper lip, or around the breast is normal. Rapid growth of hairs associated with balding or deepening of the voice requires careful medical evaluation.

Hirsutism may be associated with muscle development, a change in sexual desire, frontal balding, deepening of voice, or infertility.

Treatment

Treatment depends upon the cause of the hirsutism. Patients with normal androgen levels are treated with bleaching, shaving, or electrolysis. Many of these patients may also benefit from birth control pills. If an adrenal or ovarian tumor is diagnosed, surgery is performed. Polycystic ovarian syndrome is best treated with birth control pills to decrease ovarian androgen production. Congenital adrenal hyperplasia is best treated by dexamethasone, usually given as a single dose at bedtime, which decreases adrenal androgen secretion. Medications causing hair growth should be stopped. Cushing's syndrome or acromegaly should be treated. Antiandrogen medications such as cimetidine, cyproterone acetate, or spironolactone may also be prescribed. Spironolactone may cause nausea, fatigue, headache, or high potassium levels. It must not be used in pregnant women because it can interfere with normal testicle and penis development in male fetuses.

The DOs
- Discuss your goals for treatment with your doctor at your first visit.
- Have blood androgen levels measured.
- Tell your doctor if you have shaved, plucked, or bleached your hair, or if you have received electrolysis.
- Tell your doctor if you desire to become pregnant.
- Consider bleaching, shaving, and electrolysis.

The DON'Ts
- Don't forget, hirsutism is a common condition.
- Don't expect complete or immediate resolution of your hirsutism.
- Don't take spironolactone if you plan to become pregnant.

When to Call Your Doctor

- You notice male-pattern hair growth.
- You have hirsutism and desire contraception or want to become pregnant.
- You have nausea, fatigue, or headache associated with spironolactone therapy.

For More Information
National Adrenal Diseases Foundation
505 Northern Boulevard, Suite 200
Great Neck, NY 11021
516-487-4992
Endocrine Society
4350 East West Highway, Suite 500
Bethesda, MD 20814-4410
1-888-ENDOCRINE

HIV (HUMAN IMMUNODEFICIENCY VIRUS) INFECTION

About Your Diagnosis

Human immunodeficiency virus infection causes the body's immune system to fail, resulting in a decrease in the body's ability to fight infections. The HIV virus accomplishes this by invading and destroying the cells of the immune system. Acquired immunodeficiency syndrome (AIDS) results from HIV infection. You can be infected with HIV but not show signs of AIDS. The virus is transmitted by sexual contact with an infected individual, by sharing contaminated needles, by blood or blood products transfused from an infected individual, or from an infected mother to her unborn child. Diagnosis of the infection is done by a blood test. The infection is considered incurable; however, with new treatment to control symptoms, survival rates are increasing. With continued research, it is hoped that the prognosis for patients with HIV infection will improve.

Living With Your Diagnosis

The initial phase of the infection may have no signs or symptoms. As the infection progresses to AIDS, the following signs and symptoms may be present: fever, night sweats, diarrhea, fatigue, unexplained weight loss, frequent recurring respiratory and skin infections, swollen glands, and mouth sores. A cancer frequently present in men who have AIDS may develop. It is called Kaposi's sarcoma and appears as raised dark lesions on the skin.

Treatment

A complete medical evaluation is needed to determine the stage of infection. Medications will be prescribed accordingly. It is important to avoid exposure to other infections. Support groups are available in most communities. Activities are not restricted; however, it is important to get adequate rest and maintain good nutrition. Prevent exposing others to the infection by using condoms during intercourse, and by not donating blood or sperm. Human immunodeficiency virus infection cannot be transmitted through casual contact. Medications that may be included in the treatment regimen for HIV infection are AZT and the new protease inhibitors. Side effects of these medications include anemia, loss of appetite, abdominal pain, nausea and vomiting, headache, confusion, insomnia, nervousness, rash, and muscle pain. Blood tests must be done frequently to determine the effectiveness of the medications.

The DOs

- Contact local support groups.
- Avoid getting pregnant if you have the virus.
- Use condoms during sexual intercourse.
- Avoid exposure to other infections.
- Take the antiviral medications prescribed by your doctor. Maintain the scheduled times for the doses.
- Schedule rest periods.
- Maintain a well-balanced diet. Vitamin supplements may be helpful.
- Avoid eating possibly contaminated foods, such as raw eggs or unpasteurized milk.
- Avoid alcohol and drugs.
- Keep appointments for medical follow-up and blood tests.
- Inform sexual contacts of your infection so they can be tested.

The DON'Ts

- Don't have unprotected sex.
- Don't skip doses of your antiviral medications. Proper blood levels need to be maintained to help keep the infection under control.
- Don't skip doctor's appointments. Frequent medical attention is needed to monitor the condition.
- Don't expose yourself to known infections (avoid contact with anyone who has a cold, the "flu," or chickenpox, for example, and avoid consuming possibly contaminated food or water).
- Don't drink alcohol or use drugs.
- Don't share needles.
- Don't donate blood or sperm.

When to Call Your Doctor

- If there are signs of a secondary infection: fever, cough, severe diarrhea, or skin lesions.
- If you cannot tolerate the antiviral medications because of the side effects.
- If you have weakness, nausea, or vomiting that interferes with maintaining good nutrition or fluid intake.

For More Information

The CDC National AIDS Hotline:
800-342-AIDS
800-SIDA (Spanish)
800-AIDS TTY (Hearing impaired)
National Native American AIDS Prevention Center
Indian AIDS Hotline
2100 Lake Shore Avenue, Suite A
Oakland, CA 94606
800-283-AIDS
National Pediatrics HIV Resource Center
15 South 9th St.
Newark, NJ 07107
800-362-0071
Internet Web Sites
www.healthfinder.gov (Choose SEARCH to search by topic)
www.healthanswers.com
www.cc.emory.edu/WHSCL/medweb.aids.html
http://cornelius.ucsf. edu/~troyer/safesex

HODGKIN'S DISEASE

About Your Diagnosis

Hodgkin's disease is a cancer of the lymph nodes. Lymph nodes and lymph vessels are part of your immune system that filter off infection from the rest of the body. The cause of Hodgkin's disease is not known, but many scientists believe a virus transforms normal lymph cells to cancer cells (Reed-Sternberg cell). Nearly 7500 new cases of Hodgkin's disease are diagnosed each year in the United States, usually among persons in their 20s or 30s and persons older than 50 years.

The only sure way to diagnose Hodgkin's disease is for a physician to obtain tissue, generally from a swollen lymph gland, and look at it under a microscope (biopsy). Hodgkin's disease if detected early can be cured in most patients.

Living With Your Diagnosis

The first sign is swelling of lymph glands in your neck, groin, or armpits. Other symptoms associated with the swollen glands are weight loss, night sweats, itching, and fatigue. Hodgkin's disease spreads in a predictable way, usually to adjacent lymph nodes and ultimately to the organs. Shortness of breath, wheezing, and coughing can occur with spread to the lungs. Abdominal pain, jaundice (yellow skin), nausea, and loss of appetite can occur with involvement of the liver. Bone pain occurs with involvement of the bone marrow.

Treatment

Hodgkin's disease is confirmed at biopsy and is classified into one of four types. Treatment depends on the stage, or extent of disease. The extent of the disease tells what parts of the body the cancer has involved. The physician performs an examination and orders blood tests, chest radiographs (x-rays), and computed tomography (CT) of the abdomen and pelvis to exclude involvement of the lungs, liver, and abdominal lymph nodes. A lymphangiogram (examination with dye injected into the lymphatic vessels of the feet) is obtained to look for lymph nodes in the abdomen and pelvis. A bone marrow biopsy (placing a needle into the back of the pelvic bone and drawing marrow to be analyzed for cancer cells) is performed.

In certain circumstances, staging laparotomy (exploratory operation on the abdomen) is performed to obtain a biopsy specimen of the liver, remove the spleen (splenectomy), obtain a biopsy specimen of bone marrow, and remove suspicious lymph nodes.

Therapy for Hodgkin's disease consists of radiation therapy alone, radiation and chemotherapy, or chemotherapy alone. The decision depends on the stage of disease. Radiation alone is generally used to cure early stages of disease primarily located in one region.

Complications of radiation therapy depend on the site being irradiated. Underactive thyroid function can occur with radiation to the neck. Inflammation of the heart lining (pericarditis) and lung (pneumonitis) can occur with radiation to the chest. Sterility and suppression of the bone marrow can occur with radiation to the pelvis. Inflammation of the spinal cord can occur with radiation to that area.

Combination chemotherapy and radiation therapy is used in specific situations decided by a physician. Chemotherapy alone is used to manage advanced stages of Hodgkin's disease. Complications of chemotherapy are nausea, vomiting, easy bruising and bleeding, infection, hair loss, and numbness.

The DOs

- Remember the importance of nutrition after surgical therapy, chemotherapy, and radiation therapy. Ask for nutritional supplements to maintain your calorie intake.
- Ask for emotional support.
- Remember treatment is a team approach coordinated by your primary care physician and including an oncologist (cancer physician), radiation oncologist (physician with expertise in radiation treatment), surgeon, nutritionist, and social services.
- Ask about the effects of treatment on the sperm and female reproductive organs, especially if you are planning on having children.

The DON'Ts

- Do not ignore any swollen lymph glands.
- Do not miss follow-up appointments during or after treatment, because blood tests, radiographs, and scans are obtained to look for side effects of treatment and response to therapy.
- Do not be afraid to ask for medications for pain, nausea, or vomiting.

When to Call Your Doctor

- If you are having pain, fever, or drainage from the incision after surgical treatment.
- If you have shortness of breath, chest pain, or coughing with a fever after radiation.
- If you have bleeding, bruising, fevers, nausea, or vomiting after chemotherapy.
- If you are feeling depressed.
- If you feel any swollen glands.

For More Information
National Cancer Institute (NCI)
9000 Rockville Pike
Bethesda, MD 20892
Cancer Information Service
1-800-422-6237 (1-800-4-CANCER)

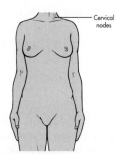

Stage I
Involvement of a single lymph node or a single extranodal site

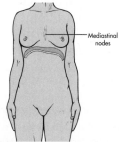

Stage II
Involvement of two or more lymph node regions on the same side of the diaphragm or localized involvement of an extranodal site and one or more lymph node regions of the same side of diaphragm

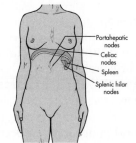

Stage III
Involvement of lymph node regions on both sides of the diaphragm. May include a single extranodal site, the spleen, or both; now subdivided into lymphatic involvement of the upper abdomen in the spleen (splenic, celiac, and portal nodes) (*Stage III$_1$*) and the lower abdominal nodes in the periaortic, mesenteric, and iliac regions (*Stage III$_2$*)

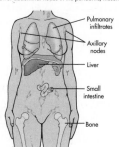

Stage IV
Diffuse or disseminated disease of one or more extralymphatic organs or tissues with or without associated lymph node involvement; the extranodal site is identified as *H*, hepatic; *L*, lung; *P*, pleura; *M*, marrow; *D*, dermal; *O*, osseous

Staging system for Hodgkin's disease and non-Hodgkin's lymphoma. (From Lewis SM, Collier IC, Heitkemper MM: *Medical-Surgical Nursing: Assessment and Management of Clinical Problem,* vol. 4. St. Louis, Mosby–Year Book, 1995. Used by permission.)

HOOKWORM

About Your Diagnosis

Hookworm infestation is a parasitic disease that is common in the tropic and subtropics. It affects the skin, lungs, and intestines. Contact with moist soil where the larvae of the hookworm lives is needed for the infection. The larvae enter through the skin and migrate through the bloodstream to the lungs and intestines. It is possible to ingest them in contaminated food and water. Hookworm is detected by laboratory examination of a stool specimen.

Living With Your Diagnosis

Signs and symptoms include itching and redness of the skin where the larvae penetrated (commonly the feet). A skin infection caused by scratching may also be present. When the larvae are migrating through the lungs, there may be a dry cough, blood-tinged sputum, wheezing and a low-grade fever. After 2 weeks they make their way to the upper small bowel where the mature worm attaches itself to the lining of the bowel and sucks blood. At this point there may be a loss of appetite, diarrhea, abdominal pain, and anemia.

Treatment

Medication to kill the parasite usually will be given twice a day for 3 days. If anemia is present, iron pills will be prescribed. After the anemia is corrected, a high-protein diet and vitamin supplements may be needed for about 3 months. Patients should rest until their strength returns and their anemia resolves.

The DOs

- Rest until the symptoms subside.
- Take the medication as prescribed.
- Maintain a high-protein diet for 3 months.
- Take vitamin supplements as directed by your doctor.
- Wash hands well after using the bathroom and before eating.
- Wear shoes when visiting tropical areas.

The DON'Ts

- Don't skip doses or stop the medication before finished.
- Don't walk barefoot when visiting tropical areas.

©1999, Mosby, Inc.

When to Call Your Doctor

- If the skin at the area of entry appears infected, red, swollen, and warm.
- If a fever develops.
- If chest pain or shortness of breath develops.
- If you cannot tolerate food or fluids.

For More Information

National Institute of Allergy and Infectious Disease
9000 Rockville Pike
Bethesda, MD 20892
301-496-5717
National Heart, Lung and Blood Institute
800-575-WELL
Internet Sites
www.healthfinder.gov (Choose SEARCH to search by topic.)
www.healthanswers.com

HYPERCHOLESTEROLEMIA

About Your Diagnosis

Hypercholesterolemia is a high cholesterol level in the blood. High blood cholesterol is one of the risk factors for atherosclerosis (hardening of the arteries) and heart disease. Heart disease from atherosclerosis and coronary artery disease is the leading cause of death in the United States.

Cholesterol is a lipid, a type of fat. It performs many normal functions in the body. Cholesterol is made in the liver for involvement in the formation of hormones. It is also part of the cell structure. It transports fats in the blood stream. Cholesterol is part of fat-protein structures in the blood called *lipoproteins*. Lipoproteins are classified on the basis of their density from very low-density lipoproteins (VLDLs) to high-density lipoproteins (HDLs). The more cholesterol in the lipoprotein, the denser is the cell. VLDLs are mostly fat and can clog the arteries. Denser lipoproteins, the HDLs, can help remove fats (lipids) from the bloodstream. That is why HDLs are considered the good cholesterol.

Living With Your Diagnosis

Cholesterol levels are determined by means of analysis of blood samples. Most persons with high blood cholesterol have no symptoms. The fat deposits in their blood vessels do not produce symptoms until the vessels are nearly closed or become clogged. Some persons with high cholesterol have xanthomas, which are small fatty deposits under the skin.

A desirable cholesterol level is less than 200 milligrams per deciliter (mg/dl). If your cholesterol level is less than 200 mg/dl, have your level checked every 3 to 5 years.

A borderline high cholesterol level is 200 to 239 mg/dl. A borderline high cholesterol level is especially important if you have two or more other risk factors for cardiac disease (male sex, female sex after menopause without estrogen replacement, age older than 55 years, family history of heart disease, smoking, obesity, diabetes, high blood pressure, lack of activity, and high fat and cholesterol intake). You need to try to lower your blood cholesterol to a desirable level.

A cholesterol levels greater than 240 mg/dl is considered high, and this by itself is a risk factor for heart disease. You need to lower your cholesterol level.

Some genetic conditions can cause high or low cholesterol and high or low levels of HDLs. Women tend to have higher HDL levels because of the influence of the female hormone estrogen. HDL levels can be increased with endurance exercise, low body fat (leanness), consumption of moderate amounts of alcohol (particularly those with high flavinoids such as red wine), and with insulin and lipid-lowering drugs. HDL levels are made decreased by male hormones, menopause (lack of the female hormone estrogen), obesity, a sedentary lifestyle, a high triglyceride level, diabetes, and cigarette smoking.

Because it is produced in the body by the liver, no one needs to consume cholesterol. The best way to lower cholesterol level is to decrease intake and promote removal by raising levels of HDLs. Diseases such as diabetes must be carefully monitored and managed.

Treatment

Lipid-lowering drugs are used to treat persons who are unsuccessful at reducing blood cholesterol levels. Continuation of the measures discussed earlier is important even after starting the lipid-lowering medicines. The main classes of medicines for management of hypercholesterolemia include bile acid–binding resins, nicotinic acid, statins (HMG CoA reductase inhibitors), and fibric acid (gemfibrozil).

Bile acid–binding resins are the primary treatment of most patients who need drugs; they include cholestyramine and colestipol. These drugs increase the passage of cholesterol into the intestines for removal through the colon (large bowel). Nicotinic acid (niacin) helps lower VLDL levels and increase HDL levels. The statins (atovarstatin, fluvastatin, lovastatin, pravastatin, simvastatin) decrease production of cholesterol and LDLs. Gemfibrozil helps increase the removal of VLDL.

These medicines each can have an unpleasant taste and can cause nausea, abdominal pain, and diarrhea or constipation. Niacin can cause facial flushing and itching. It cannot be used by persons with liver disease, diabetes, or gout.

The DOs

• Lower your cholesterol and raise your HDLs as follows by eating a diet low in cholesterol and saturated fats.

- Eat fruits and vegetables and high-fiber foods such as oat bran.
- Cook with oils high in polyunsaturated fats such as safflower oil, sunflower oil, and corn oil (omega-6 fatty acids).
- Eat fish, because fish oils contain omega-3 fatty acids, which may help lower cholesterol.
- Stop smoking.
- Lose weight to lower body fat. This is best accomplished through dietary changes (reducing calories and fat) and participating in regular aerobic exercise such as walking, jogging, bicycling, or swimming. The exercise should be done for at least 30 minutes a day 3 to 4 days per week. Exercise helps lower your body weight and body fat, helps control your blood pressure, strengthens the heart, and helps most persons with diabetes control the disease.
- Ask your physician if you should take estrogen replacement therapy. Postmenopausal women can obtain cardiac protective benefits from estrogen replacement (if they do not smoke and have no history of clotting disorders or breast or gynecologic cancer).
- Consume moderate amounts of alcohol (usually a glass or two of red wine a day). Not everyone should consume alcohol. Discuss this with your physician.
- Take your medications as directed.

The DON'Ts
- Do not forget to treat any other medical conditions and take your regular medications as directed.

When to Call Your Doctor
- If you have hypercholesterolemia, have regular follow-up visits with your doctor to monitor your blood cholesterol and heart disease. Discuss the progress of your diet and exercise and any side effects of your medications.

For More Information
The American Heart Association has information on healthy-heart diets. Call 1-800-242-8721 and ask for the literature department.

HYPERHIDROSIS

About Your Diagnosis

Hyperhidrosis or excessive sweat production is a relatively common problem that can also be associated with abnormal sweat odor called bromhidrosis. Hyperhidrosis frequently affects the feet but can also involve the hands and armpits. The cause of hyperhidrosis is not known but may be related to stress in some individuals. Other less common causes include certain types of arthritis, nervous system diseases and trauma to the spinal cord, disorders of the blood system, and certain medications. Diagnosis is made based on the history and physical examination. It is usually not curable but it is treatable.

Living With Your Diagnosis

Patients with hyperhidrosis have excess sweating of the feet, hands, or armpits, or sometimes a combination of all three. Occasionally other areas of the body are affected. The sweating can cause embarrassment and sometimes foul odor. Shirt, socks, and shoes can become stained.

Treatment

Hyperhidrosis of the feet, hands, and armpits is frequently treated with Drysol (20% aluminum chloride hexahydrate). Before bedtime, wash and dry affected areas and apply a small amount of Drysol. Wash off in the morning. Repeat nightly for 1–2 weeks, then once per week or as needed. For sensitive skin apply less frequently. Once symptoms are under control, apply Drysol as infrequently as possible, especially in the armpit area to keep symptoms under control. Other medications to apply to the affected areas may also be prescribed if Drysol is not effective. Occasionally oral medications called anticholinergics are prescribed, but these may cause side effects such as dry mouth, blurred vision, and dizziness.

Iontophoresis–application of a mild electric current in tap water–is used in some cases for about 30 minutes a day.

The DOs

- During initial use of Drysol for armpit sweating, do not use other commercial deodorants or antiperspirants. Dry the armpit with a hairdryer first, apply Drysol, then dry with hairdryer immediately after application. Once you decrease Drysol treatments to once or twice a week, it is O.K. to use other antiperspirants and deodorants during the day.
- Drink plenty of water to avoid dehydration. Increase fluid intake during hot summer months to 8–10 glasses (8 ounces per glass) of water per day. Drink more if in hot sun.
- Wear cotton clothing that absorbs sweat, and change clothing and socks frequently.
- Take a bath or shower every day, more often if necessary.
- If stress is a major cause of sweating, consider stress reduction counseling.
- It is O.K. to shave armpit hair.

The DON'Ts

- Don't wear nylon or man-made fabrics.
- Avoid applying deodorants and antiperspirants to the armpits during the initial 1–2 weeks of Drysol therapy. Baking soda can be used instead. Avoid stressful situations that worsen the sweating.

When to Call Your Doctor

- If redness, swelling, or any pus drainage occurs.
- If symptoms are not improved in 3–4 weeks of treatment.

For More Information
American Academy of Dermatology
930 N. Meacham Road
Schaumburg, IL 60173
847-330-0230

HYPERLIPOPROTEINEMIA, PRIMARY

About Your Diagnosis

Hyperlipoproteinemia is high lipoprotein levels in the blood. A high blood lipoprotein level is one of the risk factors for atherosclerosis (hardening of the arteries) and heart disease. Heart disease from atherosclerosis and coronary artery disease is the leading cause of death in the United States.

Cholesterol is a lipid, a type of fat. It performs many normal functions in the body. Cholesterol is made in the liver for involvement in the formation of hormones. It is part of the cell structure. It transports fats in the blood stream. Cholesterol is part of fat-protein structures in the blood called *lipoproteins*. Lipoproteins are classified on the basis of their density from very low-density lipoproteins (VLDLs) to low-density lipoproteins (LDLs) to high-density lipoproteins (HDLs). The more cholesterol in the lipoprotein, the denser is the cell. VLDLs are mostly fat and can clog the arteries. Denser lipoproteins, the HDLs, can help remove fats (lipids) from the bloodstream. That is why HDLs are considered the good cholesterol.

The desirable level of LDL is less than 130 mg/dl. Borderline high levels are 130 to 159 mg/dl. High levels are 160 mg/dl or higher. Desirable levels of HDL are greater than 35 mg/dl; A level greater than 45 mg/dl may help protect from cardiovascular disease.

Living With Your Diagnosis

You cannot feel high cholesterol in your blood. Some genetic conditions can cause high or low cholesterol and high or low levels of HDLs. Primary hyperlipoproteinemia is a genetically inherited disorder of metabolism of fats that causes high blood lipoprotein levels. Secondary disorders are associated with a disease or condition that causes the disorder. Persons with this genetic predisposition to high blood lipoproteins are at increased risk for early heart disease and stroke.

Women tend to have higher HDL levels than men because of the influence of the female hormone estrogen. HDL levels can be increased with endurance exercise, low body fat (leanness), moderate amounts of alcohol (particularly those with high flavinoids such as red wine), and insulin and lipid-lowering drugs. HDL levels are decreased with male hormones, menopause (lack of the female hormone estrogen), obesity, sedentary lifestyle, high triglyceride levels, diabetes, and cigarette smoking.

Cholesterol levels are determined by means of analysis of blood samples. Specific types of lipoproteins can be calculated with these blood tests. Most persons with high blood lipoprotein or cholesterol have no symptoms. The fats deposited in the blood vessels do not produce symptoms until the vessels are nearly closed or become clogged. Some patients with hyperlipoproteinemia have pancreatitis (inflammation of the pancreas) or xanthomas, which are small fatty deposits under the skin.

Because it is produced in the body by the liver, cholesterol does not have to be consumed. The best way to lower lipoprotein and cholesterol levels is to decrease fat and cholesterol intake and to promote lipoprotein removal by raising HDLs. Diseases such as diabetes must be carefully monitored and managed.

Treatment

Lipid-lowering drugs may be used to treat persons who are unsuccessful at reducing blood lipoprotein and cholesterol levels. Continuation of the measures described earlier is important even after starting lipid-lowering medicines.

The main classes of medicines for management of hyperlipoproteinemia and hypercholesterolemia include: bile acid–binding resins, nicotinic acid, statins (HMG CoA reductase inhibitors), and fibric acid (gemfibrozil). Bile acid–binding resins are the primary treatment of most patients who need drugs; they include cholestyramine and colestipol. These agents increase the passage of cholesterol into the intestines for removal through the colon (large bowel). Nicotinic acid (niacin) helps lower VLDL and increase HDL. The statins (lovastatin, pravastatin, simvastatin) decreases production of cholesterol and LDL. Gemfibrozil helps increase removal of VLDL.

The medicines can have an unpleasant taste and can cause nausea, abdominal pain, and diarrhea or constipation. Niacin can cause facial flushing and itching. It cannot be used by persons with liver disease, diabetes, or gout.

The DOs

- Eat a diet low in cholesterol and saturated fats.
- Eat fruits and vegetables and high-fiber foods such as oat bran.

- Cook with oils high in polyunsaturated fats such as safflower oil, sunflower oil, and corn oil (omega-6 fatty acids).
- Eating fish, because the fish oils contain omega-3 fatty acids that may help lower cholesterol.
- Stop smoking.
- Lose weight to lower body fat. This is best accomplished with dietary changes (reducing calories and fat) and performing regular aerobic exercise such as walking, jogging, bicycling, or swimming.
- Exercise. The aerobic exercises should be done for at least 30 minutes a day at least 3 or 4 days per week. Exercise helps lower your body weight and body fat, helps control your blood pressure, helps most persons with diabetes control the disease, and strengthens the heart.
- Discuss estrogen replacement therapy with your physician. Postmenopausal women can obtain cardiac protective benefits from hormone replacement (if they do not smoke and have no history of clotting disorders or breast or gynecological cancers).
- Consume moderate amounts of alcohol (usually a glass or two of red wine a day). Not everyone should consume alcohol. Discuss this with your physician.

The DON'Ts
- Do not forget to take your medications as directed.

When to Call Your Doctor
- If you have hyperlipoproteinemia, have regular follow-up visits with your doctor to monitor your blood lipoprotein and cholesterol and heart disease. Discuss the progress of your diet and exercise and any side effects of medications.

For More Information
The American Heart Association has pamphlets on healthy-heart diets. Call 1-800-242-8721 and ask for the literature department.

HYPERPARATHYROIDISM

About Your Diagnosis

Hyperparathyroidism simply means overactivity of the parathyroid glands. These four tiny glands are normally located in the neck next to the thyroid gland. Occasionally they may be found in the chest or within the thyroid itself. Wherever they are located, the parathyroids control normal calcium balance in the body. If blood calcium levels fall too low, the parathyroid secretes a hormone into the bloodstream to restore normal calcium levels. This hormone is aptly named parathyroid hormone (PTH). Parathyroid hormone works by increasing calcium absorption from the gut and bone, and by decreasing calcium excretion from the kidneys.

Individuals with hyperparathyroidism have a disruption in the finely tuned mechanism of calcium balance, with increased blood calcium levels. The large majority of individuals with hyperparathyroidism (85%) have a benign tumor (adenoma) of one of their parathyroid glands. Most others have an enlargement of two or more glands (hyperplasia). Rarely, hyperparathyroidism may be caused by cancer of the parathyroid gland. Hyperparathyroidism is diagnosed in 100,000 individuals per year, and there is a female-to-male ratio of 2:1. There is increased risk with increasing age. Five percent of patients have familial disorders associated with other endocrine conditions.

Hyperparathyroidism is diagnosed by simultaneously elevated blood calcium levels and PTH levels. Surgery will cure 95% of individuals.

Living With Your Diagnosis

Patients may have no signs or symptoms of their disease. It often is discovered incidentally on routine blood tests. Some patients may feel weak, fatigued, and depressed, or complain of muscle aches and joint pains. They may have a decreased appetite, nausea, vomiting, constipation, confusion, or frequent urination and thirst.

Hyperparathyroidism left untreated can lead to osteoporosis, kidney stones, high blood pressure, inflammation of the pancreas, or stomach ulcers.

Treatment

The best treatment for hyperparathyroidism is surgical removal of the tumor. This is only necessary for individuals with high calcium levels, both-ersome symptoms, or when cancer is suspected. Many individuals may simply be monitored closely by their doctor. In an emergency, intravenous fluids, diuretics, and bisphosphonates may be given to abruptly lower dangerously high calcium levels.

Complications of surgery include bleeding and infection. A low calcium level occurs, which may be temporary or permanent. Many surgeons recommend patients take calcium and vitamin D supplements postoperatively until the first outpatient visit to prevent a low calcium. Voice changes may be temporary when caused by anesthesia or permanent when caused by nerve damage at surgery.

The DOs

- Tell your doctor if you have a family history of parathyroid or other endocrine tumors.
- Provide old records for your doctor so he can determine when your blood calcium first became elevated.
- Drink plenty of water to prevent high blood calcium levels.
- Find an experienced surgeon to perform the operation. The likelihood of the success of surgery depends greatly upon the experience and skill of the surgeon.
- See your doctor regularly if no surgery is planned. It is recommended that blood work, urine, bone density testing, and kidney function testing should be performed on a regular basis for those who elect not to have surgery.

The DON'Ts

- Don't allow yourself to become dehydrated.
- Don't take calcium supplements unless approved by your doctor. This can lead to kidney stone formation and high calcium levels in the blood.

When to Call Your Doctor

- You become dehydrated or immobilized because of trauma or illness.
- You have symptoms suggestive of a kidney stone, including severe pain on your side or back and blood in your urine.
- You notice muscle spasms, face twitching, or numbness around the lips after your operation. These are symptoms of an underactive parathyroid glands and require immediate attention.

For More Information

The National Institutes of Diabetes and Digestive and Kidney Diseases
http://www.niddk.nih.gov/hyperparathyroidism
The Paget Foundation for Paget's Disease of the Bone and Related Disorders
200 Varix Street, Suite 1004
New York, NY 10014-4810
1-800-23-PAGET

HYPERTENSION

About Your Diagnosis

Hypertension is high blood pressure. Blood pressure is the force at which blood flows through the large blood vessels (the arteries) from the heart. Blood pressure readings, in millimeters of mercury (mm Hg), are divided into two numbers, for example, 110/70. The top number is the systolic pressure, which is the pressure generated when the left ventricle of the heart contracts. The bottom number is the diastolic pressure, the pressure that remains when the ventricle is relaxed to allow filling with blood. A systolic reading greater than 140 at rest or a diastolic reading greater than 90 at rest constitutes hypertension. Hypertension is diagnosed with blood pressure readings. Usually, high readings have to be recorded on at least three separate occasions to be considered accurate. The higher the readings, the more severe is the condition. Readings near these high values, for example, 135/85, might be considered borderline (at risk for developing) hypertension.

Living With Your Diagnosis

Hypertension develops among nearly 2 million persons in the United States each year. Risk for hypertension increases with aging. Approximately 20% of white and 30% of black persons are affected in adulthood. Hypertension is the single greatest risk factor for atherosclerotic (hardening of the arteries) heart disease. Heart disease is the leading cause of death in the United States. Nearly 90% of persons with hypertension have no known cause of the high blood pressure. The other persons may have kidney disease, adrenal or endocrine disorders, or one of a variety of unusual diseases.

Systolic blood pressure normally increases to a high level when someone exercises to help get blood to the exercising muscles. When those muscles stop exercising and do not require as much blood, blood pressure returns to normal. Regular exercise helps train the blood vessels to respond better to changes in pressure and keeps the walls of the vessels elastic (stretchable) and healthy.

Hypertension has been called a silent killer because it usually has no symptoms. Why is it dangerous? High blood pressure causes the heart to work harder to maintain high pumping pressures, and the heart muscle eventually weakens. The higher pressure can damage blood vessels. Imagine a garden hose with water flowing from it onto some dirt. Now imagine what happens to the dirt if you put a narrow nozzle on the end of the hose without changing the flow. The water squirts out with more pressure and tears up the dirt a lot more. A similar thing happens to the inside walls of your blood vessels. After a while they are damaged by the higher pressure. The damage affects smaller arteries most frequently, leading to scarring, which stiffens the vessels. Stiff vessels do not transport blood efficiently and are weaker than normal vessels. Eventually these stiff, weakened vessels may break. If they harden too much and become clogged with scar tissue and fatty deposits (such as cholesterol), they fail to deliver blood. Decreased blood flow causes those areas to die. If this happens to the brain, it causes a stroke; in the heart muscle, it causes a heart attack.

After hypertension is diagnosed, any evidence of damage to the small vessels is explored. The retinas of the eye are examined, laboratory tests are performed to check kidney function, and the heart is studied with an electrocardiogram (ECG) and chest radiograph (x-ray). Additional testing is done depending on the findings.

Treatment

If a cause for the condition is known, it should be managed. Most often, however, no cause is found. Hypertension is managed initially with lifestyle changes. If these measures do not successfully correct the blood pressure, antihypertensive medications may be needed. Classification of blood pressure medications includes diuretics, sympathetic nervous system agents (to reduce the nervous system response that tries to keep blood pressure high), receptor blockers (primarily beta-blockers and calcium channel blockers), vasodilators, and angiotensin-converting enzyme (ACE) inhibitors. Each of these drugs functions to reduce the blood volume, decrease the nervous system blood pressure response, or decrease resistance to blood flow. Different persons have different responses to these medications, and combinations are sometimes needed. Changes may be made in medications early in treatment to find what works best for the patient.

The DOs

- Stop smoking. This is most important, because it lowers blood pressure and helps prevent further damage to the arteries, heart, and lungs.

- Reduce saturated fats in the diet. This lowers blood pressure and helps weight loss.
- Reduce sodium in your diet. This decreases fluid retention in the blood. Less fluid to pump lowers the pressure.
- Decrease your alcohol consumption. Heavy alcohol consumption raises blood pressure.
- Decrease your caffeine intake. Caffeine is a stimulant that affects the heart.
- Relax. Reduce stress. Meditation, biofeedback, psychotherapy, and exercise all may be beneficial in reducing stress levels and blood pressure.
- Lose weight. This is extremely important. Weight loss reduces the workload of the heart by lowering resistance to blood flow. This is best accomplished through dietary changes (reducing calories and fat) and doing regular aerobic exercises such as walking, jogging, bicycling, or swimming.
- Exercise regularly. Aerobic exercise should be performed for at least 30 minutes a day at least 3 to 4 days per week. Exercise helps lower body weight and body fat, helps control blood pressure, helps reduce stress, helps most persons with diabetics control their disease, and strengthens the heart.

The DON'Ts
- Do not forget to carefully monitor and manage other conditions such as diabetes or hyperthyroidism.

When to Call Your Doctor
- If you notice chest pain, shortness of breath, or changes in vision, urination, ability to speak, swallow, walk, or use your limbs. The danger of hypertension is the damage it can do to other tissues.
- If you have side effects of your medications, including nausea, vomiting, diarrhea, persistent cough, unusual swelling, or symptoms, such as lightheadedness, of dehydration or blood pressure that is too low.

For More Information
The American Heart Association has information on healthy-heart diets. Call 1-800-242-8721 and ask for the literature department.

HYPOPITUITARISM

About Your Diagnosis

Hypopituitarism literally means an underactive pituitary gland. The pituitary gland, sometimes called the master gland, is a small gland that sits beneath the brain and regulates normal thyroid, adrenal, and gonadal function. It is important for regulating water balance, blood pressure, sexual function, stress response, and basic metabolism. One or more of these hormone systems may be dysfunctional in a patient with hypopituitarism.

There are many causes of hypopituitarism such as pituitary or hypothalamic tumors or infections, hemorrhage of the pituitary, trauma, pituitary surgery, stroke, congenital malformations, familial syndromes, or radiation therapy for malignant disease.

Some degree of hypopituitarism is common in individuals with predisposing conditions as outlined above. However, in the general population it is relatively uncommon.

Hypopituitarism is detected by performing a complete medical history and physical examination, followed by blood tests. Tests are now readily available to check anterior pituitary control of thyroid function (thyroid-stimulating hormone [TSH]), gonadal function (follicle-stimulating hormone [FSH] and luteinizing hormone [LH]), adrenal function (adrenocorticotropin hormone [ACTH]), and growth (growth hormone [GH]). Lack of posterior pituitary vasopressin, or antidiuretic hormone (ADH), is detected by excess water excretion (diabetes insipidus) and low ADH levels.

Tumors of the hypothalamus and pituitary that cause compression may be removed by surgery. This may relieve some symptoms of hypopituitarism, although permanent deficits may remain. Replacement of each missing hormone is currently possible, which can alleviate symptoms and prevent complications.

Living With Your Diagnosis

Some individuals may have no symptoms whatsoever until in a stressful situation. Others may have a sudden onset of headache, pain, blurry vision, and increased light sensitivity with neck stiffness. Most, however, have symptoms related to the specific hormonal disorders. Patients with abnormal thyroid function will notice weakness, tiredness, constipation, bloating, and weight gain. Women with abnormal gonadal function will notice a change in their menstrual periods, whereas men will have impotence. Women may also notice vaginal dryness and painful intercourse. Abnormal ACTH levels lead to weakness, especially under conditions of exertion or stress, dizziness upon standing, nausea, and increased abdominal pain. Absent growth hormone leads to poor growth in childhood.

Treatment

Treatment is based on treating the underlying tumor or process causing the hypopituitarism, followed by hormone replacement. Patients with underactive thyroids are treated with levothyroxine. Such hormone replacement may result in palpitations or unmasking of underlying coronary artery disease. Patients with gonadal dysfunction can receive exogenous testosterone or estrogen. Patients with underactive ACTH production will receive cortisol. Excess cortisol replacement may result in the Cushing's syndrome, leading to weight gain, easy bruising, high blood pressure, or diabetes. Patients with low ACTH levels must learn to use Solu-Cortef for injection in the case of emergency. Family members should also be trained. Children with short stature caused by growth hormone deficiency may be treated with growth hormone injections. Improper treatment may result in early fusion of bones, resulting in a decrease in final height.

The DOs

- Check the entire pituitary if there is one system that is malfunctioning. Often these malfunctions travel in groups.
- Take extra hydrocortisone if you are sick, injured, or stressed. The dose should be doubled or tripled for minor illnesses. Injection of Solu-Cortef should be taken for severe trauma or life-threatening emergencies.
- Wear a Medic Alert bracelet indicating that you have hypopituitarism.
- Take your medicines as prescribed and have regular blood work performed to ensure that hormone levels are optimal.

The DON'Ts

- Don't skip your medicines, especially when you are sick.
- Don't take growth hormone except under the direction of a board-certified pediatric endocrinologist or other specialist.

- Don't leave home without your emergency treatment kit.

When to Call Your Doctor

- You are scheduled for surgery.
- You have a fever, nausea, or vomiting.
- You feel weak or dizzy.

For More Information
The Pituitary Tumor Network
16350 Ventura Boulevard, Suite 231
Encino, CA 91436
1-800-642-9211
Endocrine Society
4350 East West Highway, Suite 500
Bethesda, MD 20814-4410
1-888-ENDOCRINE

HYPOTHERMIA

About Your Diagnosis

Hypothermia is a condition of low body temperature. The "normal" temperature in humans is 98.6°F. Hypothermia victims have temperatures below 95°F. There are many causes of hypothermia. The most common cause is prolonged exposure to low temperatures without adequate clothing. In this setting, alcohol consumption often is involved. Wet clothes or skin, windy conditions, and exposed skin contribute to temperature loss. Cold water immersion is the fastest way to become hypothermic. A number of medical conditions and drugs can contribute to hypothermia. Very small children and the elderly are especially at risk.

Living With Your Diagnosis

The early signs of hypothermia are feeling cold, shivering, "goosebumps," blue discoloration of the lips, cold hands and feet, and the discomfort of the inability to get warm. As the body temperature falls below 90°F, shivering stops and the victim becomes confused. The heart rate slows and may become irregular. Alcohol and drugs may change the signs and symptoms. Alcohol may actually cause the victim to feel warm while the body temperature is falling. Fortunately, most victims respond to rewarming and recover fully.

Treatment

The treatment for hypothermia is to remove the victim from the cold and rewarm. Wet clothes should be removed and replaced with dry clothes. Warm, noncaffeinated beverages can be given. The victim should be placed near a safe heat source. Wind and draft exposure should be avoided. The confused or unconscious hypothermia victim should receive emergency medical care.

The DOs

- Do dress appropriately for cold weather.
- Do consider the wind chill effect for prolonged cold weather exposure.
- Do take extra care with the elderly and small children.
- Do maintain adequate calorie and fluid intake.
- Do stay alert for dangerous weather situations and plan accordingly.
- Do replace wet clothing with dry as soon as possible.
- Do get out of cold water immediately. A few minutes can be deadly!

The DON'Ts

- Don't drink alcoholic beverages before or during cold exposure.
- Don't underestimate the effect of wind and weather conditions.
- Don't go boating alone on cold water.
- Don't ignore your body's signals that you are getting cold.
- Don't travel in remote areas during cold weather without notification.

When to Call Your Doctor

- If the victim seems hypothermic and confused.
- Someone with medical conditions (such as diabetes) is hypothermic.
- If the very young or elderly become even mildly hypothermic.
- If the victim was ill before becoming hypothermic.

For More Information
First Aid Book
http://www.medaccess.com/first_aid/FA_TOC.htm
Cold Injuries
http://www.nols.edu/School/Pubs/FirstAid/EX9Cold#HYPO
Your local American Red Cross chapter

HYPOTHYROIDISM

About Your Diagnosis

Hypothyroidism is the lack of normal thyroid hormone production. It may occur at any age and is screened for in all newborns. Hypothyroidism may be caused by birth defects, viruses, or autoimmune diseases. Often hypothyroidism results from the treatment of hyperthyroidism after the abnormal thyroid gland is removed by surgery, or after it is treated with radioactive iodine (especially for Graves' disease). It is not contagious but may affect an unborn child if the pregnant mother does not produce adequate thyroid hormone. It is very easily treated by the use of synthetic thyroid tablets, and the effectiveness of these tablets can be easily checked by blood tests.

Living With Your Diagnosis

Because thyroid hormone controls the energy use and general activity of all the body's organs, low thyroid has many signs and symptoms. Patients may feel tired, sluggish, depressed, weak, and gain weight. They may retain fluid, have slowed heartbeats, and even slowing of the bowel movements. Skin and hair may be coarse. In infancy and childhood, slow growth and poor mental development occur. Prolonged hypothyroidism can result in heart failure, poor growth, mental retardation (in infants), and severe swelling of the hands and feet.

All of these symptoms can be prevented and treated if proper thyroid replacement therapy is used.

Treatment

The best, and only, treatment for hypothyroidism is replacement of thyroid hormone. Many years ago, animal thyroid was used for this purpose; however, synthetic thyroid hormone is now available. It is inexpensive, very effective, and available in a wide range of doses to allow accurate dosing for each patient. The dose should be taken daily because the body needs a new supply each day. Your doctor can test your blood to determine the right dose for you. With the proper dosage, there are no side effects from synthetic thyroid hormone. At doses that are too high, you may have palpitations, nervousness, shakiness, bone loss, and increased bowel movements. These symptoms should prompt blood tests to check the need for a change in dose.

The DOs

- Take your medication daily because it is used and removed from the bloodstream daily.
- Follow a low-fat, low-cholesterol diet with close attention to maintaining a reasonable weight. One complication of hypothyroidism is increased cholesterol in the blood. In some cases, this may be completely corrected with the proper diet and an adequate thyroid replacement dose. Your doctor will check a fasting cholesterol level periodically to monitor your need for other cholesterol therapy.
- See your doctor as recommended. Remember, if you have Graves' disease, you will still need to see your ophthalmologist (eye doctor) on a regular basis, even though your thyroid has been controlled.
- Exercise daily; 20–30 minutes per day of moderate exercise, if approved by your doctor, will help to control your weight and your cholesterol levels. If you have not previously exercised, your doctor may have you undergo a stress treadmill test first, to see how much exercise you can safely undertake.

The DON'Ts

- Don't skip your thyroid medicine because you feel well. Serious, life-threatening complications such as heart failure may begin slowly and without warning.
- Don't increase your dose unless told to by your doctor, because you may cause bone loss, heart rhythm disturbances, or other side effects.
- Don't forget to have your thyroid hormone levels checked periodically, even if you are feeling fine. Your needs may change over time with changes in weight and age, and your doctor will change your thyroid dose accordingly.

When to Call Your Doctor

- You gain weight, retain fluid, or feel depressed.
- You have palpitations, tremor, or nervousness.
- Your vision is blurred or you have eye pain.
- You are short of breath.

For More Information
The American Thyroid Association
1-800-542-6687
The Thyroid Foundation of American
Ruth Sleeper Hall, RSL 350
40 Parkman Street
Boston, MA 02114-2698
The Thyroid Society for Education and Research
1-800-THYROID

IDIOPATHIC THROMBOCYTOPENIC PURPURA

About Your Diagnosis

Idiopathic thrombocytopenic purpura (ITP) is a disorder of the immune system that affects the platelets. Platelets are small cellular particles the function of which is to help form blood clots. Platelets are formed in the bone marrow and then circulate in the peripheral blood. In ITP, platelets are made normally, but while circulating in the blood, they become coated by antibodies or immune complexes and are destroyed by the patient's spleen. This causes patients with ITP to have too few platelets in their blood, and their blood may not clot normally.

ITP may be associated with other autoimmune disorders, such as systemic lupus erythematosus or immune thyroid disease, with malignant disease of the lymphocytes, or with human immunodeficiency virus (HIV) infection. However, many patients with ITP have no associated predisposing disease, and for these patients, the cause is unknown. ITP among children usually is caused by a viral infection.

ITP is diagnosed among 66 adults per 1,000,000 population per year and 10 to 40 children per 1,000,000 population per year. Childhood ITP affects boys and girls equally, but ITP is more common among adult women than men.

ITP is not contagious. There are very rare reports of ITP occurring in families, and some patients with ITP have family members with autoimmune disease. However, ITP is not considered a hereditary disease.

The diagnosis of ITP is made by means of finding a low platelet count in a blood test and normal to increased platelet precursors (megakaryocytes) at bone marrow biopsy. After the diagnosis is made, some patients may be undergo tests for conditions that are associated with ITP, such as autoimmune disorders and HIV infection.

ITP among children usually resolves on its own within 6 months. ITP among adults almost never resolves without treatment. Many adult patients with ITP can be cured with available medical and surgical therapies. Most patients who are not cured can have a platelet count maintained at a high enough level to allow a normal lifestyle.

Living With Your Diagnosis

Patients with ITP have too few platelets in their blood. If your platelet count is very low, your blood may not clot normally. You may bruise easily or bleed from the nose and gums. You may have very heavy menstrual flow. You also may have "blood blisters" and tiny red spots on your skin (petechiae), which are caused by bleeding into the skin or mucous membranes. You also may have serious bleeding in the gastrointestinal tract or brain, but this is rare.

Treatment

Patients with ITP whose platelets are low enough to place them at risk for spontaneous bleeding need treatment. First-line therapy for ITP is prednisone, a steroid, in the form of daily pills. Prednisone suppresses the immune destruction of platelets. More than half of patients with ITP respond to prednisone. However, because of the many side effects of prednisone, permanent treatment is not desirable, and about half of persons who respond have relapses as the drug is tapered.

Side effects of prednisone include weight gain, fluid retention, stomach irritation, mood swings, and insomnia. Patients with diabetes or high blood pressure may have worsening of these conditions, necessitating an increase in medication. Some patients who do not have preexisting diabetes or high blood pressure may have them while taking prednisone. Prednisone pills suppress the body's normal production of steroids. Therefore, patients receiving prednisone cannot simply stop taking it; the drug must be tapered slowly to allow the body time to adjust.

The suppression of the immune system caused by prednisone can make patients susceptible to infection. Prednisone also masks fevers, making infections more difficult to detect. Long-term use of steroids can lead to many complications, including ulcers, cataracts, glaucoma, muscle weakness, osteoporosis, and development of a moon-shaped face.

The most commonly used treatment option for patients who have relapses after taking prednisone is surgical removal of the spleen (splenectomy), which eliminates the site of platelet destruction. About two thirds of patients who undergo splenectomy respond, and responses usually occur within 1 week of the operation. Patients who have undergone splenectomy are at increased risk for infection with certain types of bacteria. Therefore they should receive a pneumococcal vaccine before the operation.

A new treatment option for patients with ITP is intravenous administration of Rho (D) immune globulin (eg, WinRho D). This drug, an antibody to the Rh antigen on red blood cells, binds to the patient's red blood cells. The patient's immune system becomes occupied with destroying the antibody-coated red blood cells and leaves the platelets alone. The drug is given intravenously over a half hour or less. Its effects last for 3 to 6 weeks. Rho (D) is effective only for Rh-positive patients who have not undergone splenectomy. Its main side effect is anemia, a decrease in red blood cells.

The DOs
- Undertake therapy for ITP as prescribed.
- Take only acetaminophen (eg, Tylenol) for pain or fever. Other over-the-counter pain and fever medications can damage platelet function.
- Eat a healthful, balanced diet.
- Brush your teeth with a soft toothbrush and shave only with an electric razor.
- Inform your surgeon or dentist that you have ITP before undergoing any surgical procedure or tooth extraction.

The DON'Ts
- Do not take aspirin or nonsteroidal anti-inflammatory drugs (NSAIDs; eg, Motrin) because these can damage platelet function.
- Do not play contact sports if your platelet count is low enough to place you at increased risk for bleeding. If your platelet count is only slightly below normal, you may not have to restrict your activities.

When to Call Your Doctor
- If you have bleeding that does not resolve after application of pressure to the area for 5 minutes.

For More Information
National Heart, Lung, and Blood Information Center
P.O. Box 30105
Bethesda, MD 20824-0105
301-251-1222
MedMark Hematology: http://medmark.bit.co.kr/hematol.html

IMPETIGO

About Your Diagnosis

Impetigo is a very common and mild skin infection. It is seen most frequently in children. It is caused by common skin bacteria, usually staph (staphylococci) or strep (streptococci). Impetigo is contagious and is frequently seen in brothers and sisters. It is curable with medication applied to the skin or with medication taken by mouth.

Living With Your Diagnosis

Impetigo usually starts as small red bumps or blisters. These can become large, especially in children. Drainage that appears honey crusted is common. If left untreated, impetigo can continue for weeks. Rarely kidney inflammation occurs after impetigo, causing blood or protein in the urine. (Seek medical attention if this occurs.)

Treatment

Antibiotics applied to the skin or taken by mouth are used to treat impetigo. You can expect improvement in 5–10 days. Bactroban is an antibiotic ointment effective against impetigo. Wash the affected area and gently scrub off crusting and loose dead skin with a cloth. Dry off and apply a small amount of Bactroban. Do this three times per day. If you are given an antibiotic by mouth, take the entire prescription as directed by your doctor.

The DOs

- Maintain good hygiene. Bathe or shower at least once per day while infected with impetigo. Wash entire body with an antibacterial soap.
- Wash bedding, clothing, and towels frequently.
- Maintain good individual hygiene.
- Trim children's nails if scratching is a problem.

The DON'Ts

- Over-the-counter medications are usually not helpful.
- Do not shave infected areas or anywhere that is red and inflamed.
- Don't share washcloths, towels, or beds while infected with impetigo.
- Don't break the blisters, and avoid scratching.

When to Call Your Doctor

- If not better in 7–10 days.
- If temperature of 101°F occurs in spite of treatment.
- If other family members become infected.
- If urine is discolored or there is blood in the urine.

For More Information
American Academy of Dermatology
930 N. Meacham Road
Schaumburg, IL 60173
847-330-0230

INFLAMMATORY MYOPATHY (MYOSITIS)

About Your Diagnosis

Myositis is a condition that causes inflammation in muscles. Two types of myositis are "polymyositis" and "dermatomyositis." They are uncommon conditions that cause muscle weakness in children and adults. Although muscle inflammation is the most common feature of these types of myositis, other organs in the body can be affected such as the skin, lungs, esophagus (food pipe), and joints. No one knows what causes these types of myositis, but it is not an infectious illness (like colds); therefore you cannot "catch" it from another individuals.

Myositis is diagnosed by a medical history, physical examination, and blood tests that detect muscle inflammation. In individuals who appear to have myositis, further studies of the nerve and muscle, as well as a muscle biopsy specimen, are used to confirm the diagnosis. Treatment of myositis usually improves the symptoms, but most individuals need to stay on therapy for several years.

Living With Your Diagnosis

Myositis causes weakness, especially in muscles around the shoulder and hip. Individuals therefore have difficulty carrying heavy objects, combing their hair, reaching overhead, getting out of bed or chairs, walking up stairs, and standing for long periods. Some individuals have muscle pain. Fatigue, fever, and poor appetite are common. Arthritis causing pain, swelling, and stiffness in joints can make day-to-day activities difficult. Occasionally, individuals with myositis have an associated lung condition that causes a cough or difficulty breathing. Because the esophagus is made of muscle, some individuals with myositis have difficulty swallowing or have problems with heartburn. Dermatomyositis differs from polymyositis by its typical skin rash, which appears on the chest, shoulders, face, and hands. Many of the symptoms of myositis improve with treatment.

Treatment

Myositis is most commonly treated with corticosteroids (cortisone-like medicines such as prednisone). Potential side effects of corticosteroids are increased appetite, weight gain, difficulty sleeping, easy bruising, and stomach upset. Longer term use of corticosteroids can lower your resistance to infection, as well as cause stomach ulcers, muscle weakness, and bone thinning (osteoporosis). Corticosteroids should always be taken with food to prevent stomach upset. In addition, patients should receive adequate amounts of calcium and vitamin D to help prevent osteoporosis.

Despite corticosteroid therapy, some individuals continue to have symptoms and require more potent medications such as methotrexate or azathioprine (Imuran). Methotrexate can cause poor appetite, nausea, headaches, mouth sores, and diarrhea. Imuran can cause nausea, vomiting, and diarrhea. Routine blood cell counts and liver function tests are necessary to monitor for abnormalities with both methotrexate and azathioprine.

Treatment may continue for several years. All individuals with myositis should rest their muscles during the early part of the treatment. After the muscle inflammation is improved, special exercises to strengthen muscles should be started.

The DOs

- Rest your muscles until the muscle inflammation improves.
- Take your medicines as prescribed.
- Ask your doctor which over-the-counter medications you may take with your prescription medications.
- Eat a well balanced diet low in carbohydrates and fat to prevent excessive weight gain.

The DON'Ts

- Wait to see if side effects from medications will go away.
- Begin a rigorous exercise program without your doctor's advice.
- Stop taking the corticosteroid medicine unless your physician instructs you to do so.
- Forget to inform your doctor and dentist that you are taking a corticosteroid (prednisone).
- Overeat, because corticosteroids may increase your appetite.

When to Call Your Doctor

- You experience any medication side effects.
- The treatment is not decreasing your symptoms in a reasonable amount of time.
- You begin to notice the return of muscle weakness.

For More Information

Contact the Arthritis Foundation in your area. If you do not know the location of the Arthritis Foundation, you may call the national office at 1-800-283-7800 or access the information on the Internet at www.arthritis.org.

The Myositis Association of America, Inc. will also provide information about these conditions by calling 1-540-433-7686 or writing the Myositis Association of America, 1420 Huron Court, Harrisonburg, Virginia 22801.

INFLUENZA

About Your Diagnosis

Influenza is a common, acute, and highly contagious respiratory tract infection caused by a virus. Symptoms usually appear 24–48 hours after exposure. It is spread by contact with infected individuals. It affects individuals of all ages, but is especially dangerous for the very young, the elderly, and anyone with a chronic illness. The entire respiratory tract is affected. Influenza cannot be cured, but symptoms can be controlled with medications. It can be prevented by obtaining the flu vaccine offered in the fall.

Living With Your Diagnosis

Signs and symptoms include sudden onset of chills and fever (a temperature of 101°F to 104°F), muscle aches, cough, sore throat, runny nose, headache, fatigue, and weakness. These usually last 3–5 days, with the cough and fatigue lasting longer.

Possible complications include middle ear infections, sinus infection, bronchitis, pneumonia, and Reye's syndrome.

Treatment

The best treatment is rest. For discomfort use nonaspirin medications, such as Tylenol or Advil, as well as cough syrups and decongestants. Do not give aspirin to a child younger than 16 years because research has shown a link between using aspirin for a viral infection and the development of Reye's syndrome. Some cough medications and decongestants may cause drowsiness.

Warm baths or a heating pad can help relieve the muscle aches. A cool-mist vaporizer may help thin secretions, but remember to change the water and clean the unit daily. Gargling with warm salt water or mouthwash may ease the sore throat.

The DOs

- Rest in bed as much as possible. Continue to rest for 2 or 3 days after the fever subsides.
- Increase fluid intake to at least 8 glasses a day. Fluids help to thin lung secretions. In small children, avoid milk because it sometimes thickens secretions.
- Limit visitors and close contact with other family members.
- Wash hands frequently. Dispose of all tissue in a paper or plastic bag at the bedside.

- Encourage those who have contact with you to wash their hands well.

The DON'Ts

- Don't go to work or school if you think you have the flu. You need to rest, and you would only be spreading the virus to others.
- Don't allow anyone with a chronic illness or suppressed immune system (such as a patient with AIDS or someone receiving chemotherapy) to come in contact with the infected individual.
- Don't share glasses or eating utensils.
- Don't give aspirin to a child younger than 16 years.
- Don't give a young child milk because it thickens secretions.

When to Call Your Doctor

- If your fever or cough worsens.
- If shortness of breath or chest pain occurs.
- If there is a thick discharge from the ears or sinuses along with pain.
- If you have neck pain or stiffness.
- If you cough up bloody sputum.

For More Information

Center for Disease Control and Prevention
Voice Information System
404-332-4555
National Jewish Center for Immunology and Respiratory Medicine
1400 Jackson Street
Denver, CO 80206
800-222-5864, Monday through Friday from 8 AM to 5 PM (MST), to reach a nurse who will answer questions and send information; or 800-552-5864, for recorded information 24 hours per day.
National Heart, Lung and Blood Institute
Information Line 800-575-WELL
Internet Sites
www.healthanswers.com
www.healthfinder.gov

INSOMNIA

About Your Diagnosis

Insomnia is a very common condition. Studies show that 36% or about 80 million American adults currently have problems with sleep. About a third of those individuals complain that their sleep problems are chronic or recur frequently. Disturbed sleep is particularly frequent in the elderly and in patients who have other psychiatric disorders such as depression and anxiety. About half of all patients with schizophrenia have insomnia, as well as 75% of those who have a mood disorder such as depression. Adults in the United States are currently getting less sleep than was typical 100 years ago. The average adult sleeps 7<cf1/2> hours per night during the work week, but earlier figures suggest that 9 hours per night was more common in the past. It is believed that the decrease in average sleep time is related to many factors, including late night television watching, high-pressure lifestyles, and family and work stresses.

Living With Your Diagnosis

Primary insomnia can involve less sleep, less restful sleep, interrupted sleep, and delayed onset of sleep. Some individuals report lying in bed for hours trying to sleep and being unable to do so. They may be reliving the events of the day, or they may have a number of worries that they cannot stop thinking about. This type of trouble falling asleep is much more common with anxiety. In depression, the usual sleep disturbance is that of early morning awakening. The patient will be awake at 2 AM or 3 AM for no apparent reason, and then will be unable to fall back asleep. Restless sleep is often unnoticed by the patient initially. The patient may actually have slept 7 or 8 hours, but the sleep was tormented. Often someone who sleeps with the patient may describe how much he thrashed around during the night or how distressed he seemed to be during sleep. Therefore, measuring the total amount of sleep is not enough to detect insomnia; the quality of sleep also has to be assessed.

Primary insomnia includes those sleep disturbances in which no other known sleep disorder, such as narcolepsy or sleep apnea, is present. Psychiatric criteria for the diagnosis of insomnia are that insomnia must be present for at least 1 month, and that it must have a negative impact on the individual's social functioning, work functioning, or both.

Secondary insomnia is usually related to either a psychiatric disorder such as depression or anxiety, a medical condition affecting sleep, or the use of alcohol, caffeine, or illicit drugs such as amphetamines and cocaine. In secondary insomnia, treating the condition that is causing the sleep problem will improve the sleep, and no additional medication is required.

One of the most common cause of sleep disruption is a nightmare. A nightmare often occurs in the early phases of sleep, usually about 60–90 minutes after sleep has begun, and is usually remembered by the patient. This is different from night terrors, which occur often in children. Terrors occur later in sleep and are not remembered. Frequently a child experiencing night terrors will suddenly sit straight up in bed, be sweaty, have a fast heart rate, and be extremely frightened, but will not remember what they were dreaming about.

Other conditions that can affect sleep include nocturnal enuresis (bed-wetting) and sleepwalking. Sleepwalking can be of concern because patients may harm themselves while sleepwalking; for example, they may fall downstairs or even leave the house. Sleepwalking also occurs during the later stages of sleep. Although elderly patients tend to spend more time in bed, their sleep is often interrupted and they are more easily aroused than are younger individuals. The elderly also complain of more trouble falling asleep.

Treatment

A number of herbal, over-the-counter, and prescription medications are used to treat insomnia. Some of the popular over-the-counter medications include Sominex, Nytol, and different cough/cold preparations (e.g., Tylenol PM, Nyquil) that may have a sleep inducer in them. In addition, there has been a marked increase in the use of natural herbal agents for sleep. Perhaps the ones that are most commonly used are melatonin and Valerian Root, which are available in most pharmacies or health food stores. Many patients will try some of these medications before consulting a physician about their sleep disturbance. Unfortunately, the most frequently used self-prescribed sleep inducer is alcohol. However, what most individuals don't recognize is that although alcohol may cause them to fall asleep, alcohol-induced sleep is fragmented and not restful. In fact, many individuals who consume alcohol at bedtime sleep very deeply initially, then awaken and are unable to fall back to sleep. Consequently, sleep is actually made worse by the use of alcohol. A variety of prescription medications are used for sleep. These drugs generally belong to the sedative/hypnotic category of medications. Perhaps the most commonly used medications are the benzodiazepines. These include drugs such as Restoril and Halcion. The main thing to remember about these drugs is that they are to be used temporarily because there is potential for drug addiction with the use of these agents. That implies that there is some withdrawal upon stopping them. Other drugs that are commonly used for sleep include Ambien, chloral hydrate (Noctec), and in some cases the barbiturates. If depression is also a problem, some of the more sedating antidepressants, such as Sinequan, Elavil, or Trazodone, are often used for sleep.

There are some important side effects associated with medications used to treat insomnia. These include daytime drowsiness, potential difficulty operating motor vehicles and dangerous equipment, respiratory problems (especially if another condition such as asthma, bronchitis, or emphysema is present), some rebound insomnia once the medication is stopped, memory problems (especially with agents such as Halcion), and as mentioned previously, interactions with alcohol. Some reminders, if you are taking sleep medication:

1. Sleep medications are to be used only temporarily. Sleep problems that last longer than a couple of weeks may be caused by a more serious condition.
2. It is a good idea to leave no more than one night's dose by your bedside to avoid the temptation of taking extra medication.
3. The medication should be taken on an empty stomach with ample fluids to promote rapid entry of the drug into your bloodstream.
4. If you use the medication for more than a few nights, then it should be tapered and not discontinued all at once.
5. Remember that over-the-counter sleep aids such as Sominex and Nytol, and some herbal agents, although available without prescription, may have serious interactions with other medication you may be taking.
6. Remember that diet is important. Any caffeine or other stimulants should not be taken late in the evening, nor should you drink a lot of fluids toward bedtime. This will certainly interrupt sleep.
7. When considering the use of medication, consider some natural aids to sleep, such as warm milk (without cocoa), melatonin, and valerian root.

The DOs

- If possible, take a medication for any pain you may be having. Pain interferes with sleep.
- Engage in exercise two or three times a week, but avoid exercising just before bedtime.
- Try to get on a consistent schedule so you go to bed about the same time every night.
- Try to avoid excessive stress or tension in the bedroom.
- If you find yourself lying in bed unable to sleep, get up, find a relaxing chair, and read or knit, or do something else until you become more drowsy. Lying in bed when you are unable to sleep will only increase the insomnia.

The DON'Ts

- Do not go to bed to try to sleep when you are not tired.
- Avoid napping during the day, even when you are tired. Also avoid early evening naps.
- Try not to consume food or drugs that are high in caffeine, especially later in the evening. These will adversely affect your sleep.

When to Call Your Doctor

- If you are sleepwalking, having night terrors, or are snoring excessively.
- If you have any side effects from prescribed medications, such as respiratory problems, amnesia, or daytime drowsiness.
- If you feel your insomnia is caused by depression, anxiety, or mania.

For More Information

Contact your physician, a local sleep disorders clinic, or check out these Web sites:
http://www.cloud9.net/~thorpy
http://www.sleepnet.com
sleep docs @ http://www.cloud9.net/~thorpy/sleepdoc.htm/
Note that the sleep doc site is a fee-based (you will be charged) site, where you can E-mail sleep professionals for personal responses to your questions.

IRRITABLE BOWEL SYNDROME

About Your Diagnosis

Irritable bowel syndrome (IBS) is a disease affecting the intestine. It is also called spastic colon or colitis. The cause of IBS is not known, but stress and emotions are thought to play a role. Irritable bowel syndrome is a common disorder, affecting up to 15% of the population. Most individuals generally begin having symptoms in their early 20s. Many of these individuals never see a doctor about their complaints.

The diagnosis of IBS is made by eliminating other causes. Other causes of abdominal pain and changing bowel habits must be ruled out before making the diagnosis of IBS. This means laboratory studies must be done. Procedures such as a barium enema x-ray or flexible sigmoidoscopy (a lighted flexible instrument used to examine the lower part of the colon) are sometimes done to exclude other causes. This disease is not curable. It is usually recurrent throughout life. The symptoms can be managed with diet, medications, and lifestyle changes. It does not appear that IBS causes other conditions such as cancer.

Living With Your Diagnosis

The main symptoms of IBS are episodes of abdominal pain and changing bowel habits. These episodes can last for days to months. The abdominal pain is described as crampy and does not occur in any particular location. Other symptoms such as indigestion, heartburn, and bloating occur less frequently. Rarely nausea and vomiting occur. The pain generally begins after meals and is relieved by bowel movements. The changing bowel habits may involve diarrhea, constipation, or periods of both. With constipation, the bowel movement may be "pelletlike" or in small balls. The diarrhea may have mucus in it.

Treatment

The treatment of IBS focuses on lifestyle and dietary changes. A high fiber diet is the mainstay of treatment. Fiber supplements are helpful if used on a regular basis. Increased gas and bloating may occur for the initial 2 weeks of fiber supplements and generally resolve with time. Constipating agents such as loperamide (Imodium) will relieve diarrhea symptoms. Antispasmodics will help with abdominal cramping.

The DOs

- See your physician; the symptoms may be from another condition.
- Maintain proper eating habits, and select foods carefully.
- Stop smoking.
- Increase fiber in the diet. Fresh fruits and vegetables are good sources, but be careful because they can cause gas and bloating. Psyllium-containing products are also good sources of fiber.
- Heat to the abdomen may help the pain and cramping.
- Try to reduce stress. Biofeedback might help.
- Maintain proper physical fitness.

The DON'Ts

- Avoid large meals.
- Avoid spicy, fried, and fatty foods.
- Avoid milk products.
- Avoid alcohol.

When to Call Your Doctor

- If fever develops.
- If there is blood in the stool or the stool is black and tarry.
- If vomiting develops.
- If unexplained weight loss occurs.
- If symptoms do not improve with treatment.

For More Information
National Digestive Diseases Information Clearinghouse
2 Information Way
Bethesda, MD 20892-3570
www.niddk.nih.gov
nddic@aerie.com
International Foundation for Bowel Dysfunction
P.O. Box 17864
Milwaukee, WI 53217
414-241-9479

KAPOSI'S SARCOMA

About Your Diagnosis

Kaposi's sarcoma is a rare cancer believed to start from the cells that line the blood vessels. The following four types of Kaposi's sarcoma have been described:

1. Classic Kaposi's sarcoma, which was first described in the 1870s and usually was found among Jewish and Mediterranean men. Most persons survived more than 10 years with this cancer and usually died of something other than the Kaposi's sarcoma.
2. African Kaposi's sarcoma, which was discovered among young black men in Africa. This lesion had either a slow, benign course (indolent) or an aggressive, lethal course (florid).
3. Immunosuppression-related Kaposi's sarcoma, which was found among recipients of kidney transplants. Transplantation necessitated use of strong medications to suppress the immune system and prevent it from rejecting the kidney. This type of Kaposi's sarcoma can have a slow, inactive course or an aggressive course.
4. Epidemic Kaposi's sarcoma, which is associated with acquired immunodeficiency syndrome (AIDS). In the 1980s this lesion started being found among homosexual men and a few heterosexual users of intravenous drugs. Most patients with AIDS and no rare infection survive 2 years. However, less than 20% of patients with AIDS and a rare infection survive 2 years. This cancer is believed to be transmitted sexually.

The only sure way to diagnose Kaposi's sarcoma is means of biopsy of the area in question and examination of the tissue with a microscope.

Living With Your Diagnosis

A skin rash (lesion) is the usual presentation. The lesion looks like a small node that can be reddish purple in color. The lower legs are the most common place to find the lesion, but Kaposi's sarcoma can be found on the nose and the rest of the face. The cancer can spread and involve the lymph nodes, stomach, and lungs. If the cancer involves the stomach, bleeding or abdominal pain can occur. With involvement of the lungs, shortness of breath occurs.

Treatment

Treatment depends on the extent of disease and generally consists of observation, supportive therapy, radiation therapy, or chemotherapy. The decision to undergo treatment must be made with a specialist who has experience with Kaposi's sarcoma. Information concerning the extent of disease (whether it is local in the skin or lymph nodes or has it spread to the stomach or lungs), blood tests for patients AIDS (CD4 count), and symptoms all weigh heavily in the need for treatment.

Generally inactive forms of the classic, African, and immunosuppressive types of Kaposi's sarcoma necessitate only observation and follow-up visits to look for symptoms or for plastic surgical repair.

Radiation therapy is effective therapy for single lesions that cause symptoms. Complications of radiation therapy depend on which part of the body is irradiated. Fatigue and dry, red, itchy skin can occur. Dryness and irritation of the eyes, nose, and mouth can occur if the radiation is given for Kaposi's lesions on the face.

Chemotherapy can be given directly into the lesion or intravenously for one lesion, multiple lesions, or advanced disease. Side effects of chemotherapy are nausea, vomiting, hair loss, easy bruising and bleeding, and infections.

The DOs

- Seek an expert's opinion. The cancer is rare and treatment has side effects.
- Remember there are four types of Kaposi's sarcoma and that the way the disease acts (indolent or aggressive) varies with each type.

The DON'Ts

- Do not forget that among the homosexual population, Kaposi's sarcoma is believed to be transmitted sexually through anal sex.
- Do not think that if you are not homosexual, you will not get the disease. Women can contract Kaposi's sarcoma after having sex with bisexual men. Safe sex cannot be overemphasized.
- Do not use illicit drugs. Abusers of intravenous drugs can contract Kaposi's sarcoma.

When to Call Your Doctor

- If you find a lesion on your face, nose, or legs that is discolored.
- If you are in pain.
- If you are short of breath.

- If you are vomiting blood.
- If a skin lesion breaks down.
- If you feel any swollen lymph glands.

For More Information
National Cancer Institute (NCI)
9000 Rockville Pike
Bethesda, MD 20892.
Cancer Information Service
1-800-4-CANCER
American Cancer Society
1599 Clifton Road, N.E.
Atlanta, GA 30329
1-800-ACS-2345
Reference: Murphy G, Lawrence W, Lenhard R: *American Cancer Society Textbook of Clinical Oncology.* 2nd ed. Washington, Pan American Health Organization, 1995, p 619.

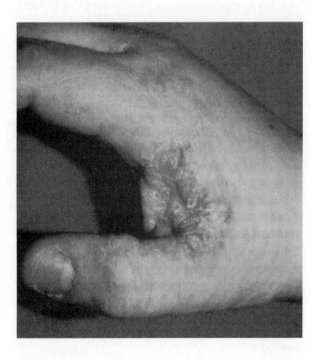

Kaposi's sarcoma. Note multiple violescent lesions in a patient with AIDS. (Photo courtesy of Beverly Sanders, M.D., Macon, Georgia. From Goldstein BG, Goldstein AO: *Practical Dermatology*, vol 1, St Louis, Mosby–Year Book, 1992. Used by permission.)

KELOIDS

About Your Diagnosis

Keloids are an overgrowth of scar tissue on the skin most often seen on the shoulders and chest. They can appear anywhere and usually arise in an area of injury, such as after a burn or severe acne, or from a minor scratch. Keloids are more frequent in blacks than in whites and are not transmitted from individual to individual.

Keloids are detected by observing the formation of firm, hard, and raised scars. Keloids are generally considered harmless and noncancerous.

Living With Your Diagnosis

Keloids may itch, cause pain, or be tender. Scars may continue to grow. There are usually no adverse effects.

Treatment

There is no routinely effective treatment for all keloids. A variety of treatment methods exist, including steroid injections into the keloid. Drugs, lasers, topical medications, and compression treatments are currently undergoing study for effectiveness. Keloids may recur in the same areas despite adequate treatment.

The DOs

- Do continue to lead a normal, healthy lifestyle. There are no restrictions associated with keloids.

The DON'Ts

- Do not injure the skin.
- Those individuals who have a known tendency to form keloids should avoid elective surgery.

When to Call Your Doctor

- When you observe the signs of keloid formation.

For More Information
American Academy of Dermatology
930 N. Meachum Road
Schaumburg, IL 60173
847-330-0230

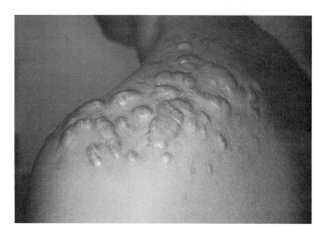

Keloids. Raised, flesh-colored lesions in typical area (shoulder). (From Noble J: *Textbook Primary Care Medicine,* vol 2. St. Louis, Mosby–Year Book, Inc., 1995. Used by permission.)

KLINEFELTER'S SYNDROME

About Your Diagnosis

Klinefelter's syndrome is an inherited disorder of men that results in characteristically long arms and legs, and a failure of the development of normal male secondary sexual characteristics of puberty.

Klinefelter's syndrome is caused by a chromosomal defect from birth in the sex chromosomes. Normal females have a chromosomal pattern of 46,XX, whereas normal males have a 46,XY pattern. In Klinefelter's syndrome, the chromosomal pattern is 47,XXY. This extra X chromosome interferes with normal male sexual development as a fetus and at puberty. Other related hormonal patterns may also be classified under Klinefelter's syndrome.

Klinefelter's syndrome has been estimated to affect from 1 in 400 to 1 in 1,000 males.

Klinefelter's is usually detected by a physical examination of a boy who fails to undergo normal pubertal development. Occasionally, an adult male initially is seen because of complaints of impotence (or the inability to get an erection) or infertility (or the inability to bear children). Blood tests reveal a low testosterone level and an increased follicle-stimulating hormone (FSH) level, indicating the primary problem lies in the gonads. Classically, the diagnosis was established by the identification of Barr bodies on a smear taken from the buccal mucosa of the mouth. Today, Klinefelter's is usually diagnosed by performing a karyotype, which identifies the exact chromosomal number and type.

There is no cure for Klinefelter's syndrome. The infertility (inability to father a child) is generally not reversible. However, other symptoms such as impotence (inability to obtain an erection) are treatable with medicine.

Living With Your Diagnosis

Most men have long arms and legs relative to their trunks, and a low or absent sperm count associated with infertility. The testicles are small and firm, and men may have breasts (gynecomastia). There may be difficulty with erections, a small penis, a poor beard, and slight underarm or pubic hair growth. Symptoms vary greatly among individuals.

The effects of Klinefelter's are that of poor secondary sexual development with resulting infertility, osteoporosis, an increased risk for breast cancer, and occasionally personality disorders.

Treatment

There is no treatment for the infertility because the testes have not developed normally and there is no sperm that can be produced. The treatment of the underdeveloped male secondary sexual characteristics is testosterone replacement. This may be provided as an injection or a skin patch. Testosterone leads to normal male muscle development and hair growth on the beard, underarms, and genitals. It may, however, cause mood changes, aggressive behavior, abnormal prostate growth, or high blood pressure. In addition, the patch may cause a localized skin reaction.

The gynecomastia or male breast development can be treated surgically with breast reduction. Complications are rare but would include bleeding, bruising, infection, or abnormal scar formation. Any lump noted in the breast should be evaluated for the possibility of breast cancer, which is more common in patients with Klinefelter's syndrome than in other males.

The osteoporosis (decreased bone density) may be treated with hormone replacement of testosterone to prevent fractures. Patients should also have adequate calcium and vitamin D intake and maintain a regular weight-bearing exercise program.

The DOs

- Consult an endocrinologist if you have concerns about male sexual development or function.
- Obtain a testosterone and an FSH test to confirm that the gonads are the source of the sexual dysfunction.
- Obtain a karyotype of the chromosomes to establish a diagnosis of Klinefelter's syndrome.
- Begin testosterone replacement for secondary sexual development, normal bone growth, and a sense of well-being.
- Consult a surgeon if gynecomastia is troubling or if a lump is noted.

The DON'Ts

- Don't assume your child has Klinefelter's just because he is behind his peers in pubertal development. Consult a pediatric endocrinologist.
- Don't forget that help is available if you are having difficulty adjusting emotionally to your diagnosis.
- Don't put the testosterone patch on the same spot of skin every time. It must be rotated to prevent rash or skin breakdown from occurring.

When to Call Your Doctor

- You notice a breast lump.
- You are having severe mood swings with testosterone replacement.
- You notice sudden bone pain in the back, hip, wrist, or rib.
- You have a persistent rash while using the testosterone patch.

For More Information

The American Association of Clinical Endocrinologists
701 Fisk Street, Suite 100
Jacksonville, FL 32204
904-353-7878
http://www.aace.com/guidelines/hypogonadism
The Endocrine Society
4350 East West Highway, Suite 500
Bethesda, MD 20814-4410
1-888-ENDOCRINE
http:\\www.endo-society.org

KNEE PAIN

About Your Diagnosis

Knee pain is a relatively vague diagnosis. If you are referred to an orthopedic surgeon, he or she attempts to define whether the pain is located in the anterior (front) part of the knee just beneath the kneecap or is deep within the knee joint itself. The many causes of knee pain include a sprained or torn ligament, torn cartilage, or arthritis of the kneecap or entire joint. Inflammatory conditions such as rheumatoid arthritis or osteoarthritis also may manifest themselves with knee pain. Knee pain is extremely common and is usually self-limiting. In other words, when the offending activity is discovered and discontinued, the knee pain usually resolves. Depending on the particular cause of knee pain, it is often curable.

Living With Your Diagnosis

Knee pain is usually accompanied by swelling and sometimes by a clicking or popping sensation. Sometimes the knee can actually catch and lock. In that situation, a torn piece of cartilage has become trapped within the joint and is preventing bending or straightening of the knee.

Treatment

Initially, with knee pain, the most important aspect is to determine the cause, particularly if the a activity has been initiated recently, such as aggressive walking or jogging. Many persons who participate in court sports that require lateral movement experience knee symptoms, and when these activities are eliminated for 2 to 6 weeks, the symptoms gradually subside.

The use of nonsteroidal anti-inflammatory drugs (NSAIDs), such as ibuprofen or naproxen, which can be obtained over the counter, helps to decrease inflammation and pain. These medications should be used with caution; they can cause stomach problems and should be taken with meals. Patients with a history of ulcers or bleeding ulcers should consult their physician before initiating the use of these medications.

Kneecap pain usually can be managed with physical therapy to aggressively strengthen the quadriceps muscles in the front of the thigh and stretch the hamstring and calf muscles on the back of the thigh and lower leg. Sprained ligaments often heal with rest and time. However, torn liga-

ments around the knee sometimes necessitate immobilization followed by aggressive physical therapy for rehabilitation. A surgeon may recommend surgical reconstruction. As with any surgical procedure, there can be risks and complications, which are usually discussed with you before the actual surgical procedure.

Once the symptoms have subsided, activities can be resumed gradually, beginning with straight-ahead activities such as walking or cycling. Working back into the preferred activity can be attempted with caution.

The DOs

- Take your medications as prescribed.
- Consult your primary care physician when beginning a new medication if you take other prescription medications.
- Eliminate the activity that causes the pain.
- Resume activity gradually; resume the offending activity with extreme caution.

The DON'Ts

- Do not use nonsteroidal anti-inflammatory medications if you have a history of bleeding ulcers.
- Do not continue the offending activity, such as running, in the belief that you can "run it off." This can cause additional injury to the knee, which may worsen or damage the joint itself.

When to Call Your Doctor

- If you have attempted conservative measures on your own and the symptoms persist.
- If you are undergoing a prescribed physical therapy or rehabilitation program and your symptoms worsen. Physical therapists usually offer to contact the physician, but do not hesitate to ask if you notice that the therapy seems to be worsening the symptoms.
- If you have side effects from the medication.

For More Information
http://www.mayo.ivi.com/mayo/9312/htm/kneepain.htm

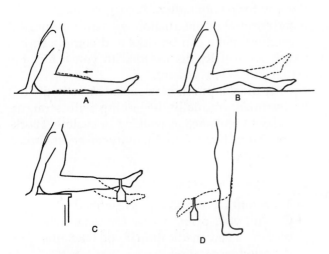

Knee exercises. A, Isometric quadsetting. The muscle is tightened and the knee stiffened and relaxed several times. B and C, Isotonic short-arc knee extension. The knee is straightened through the last 30 degrees (to prevent peripatellar pain). Weights are gradually added beginning with 2 kg and progressing to 10 kg. D, Isotonic knee curls for hamstring strengthening. Weight is increased as with quad strengthening. All exercises are performed as five sets of ten lifts each, three times a day. Exercises should not cause pain or swelling. (From Mercier LR: *Practical Orthopedics*, vol 4. St. Louis, Mosby–Year Book, 1995. Used by permission.)

LABYRINTHITIS

About Your Diagnosis

Labrynthitis may be caused by a viral or bacterial infection, but most episodes have no known cause. Labyrinthitis results in a functional disturbance of the balance mechanism in your inner ear. It is often associated with hearing loss, vertigo (a subjective impression of movement in space or a sense of objects moving around the individual), loss of balance, and nausea.

Living With Your Diagnosis

The symptoms of labyrinthitis usually do not include vomiting; however, if the symptoms are particularly severe or prolonged, vomiting may occur. The symptoms may develop suddenly and last for several days. After most acute attacks, the vertigo usually subsides in several days. Hearing returns to normal in most patients. Partial recovery of hearing may occur in others; however, if hearing is likely to return, it generally returns slowly within 10–14 days.

Labyrinthitis may follow a middle ear infection. Bacteria may enter the inner ear and, although rare, the infection may even spread to the space surrounding the brain, resulting in meningitis. Bacterial labyrinthitis may result in complete and permanent hearing loss.

Treatment

The treatment of labyrinthitis depends upon determining the source of the problem, if possible. Bacterial labyrinthitis is treated with antibiotic medications and sometimes requires surgical drainage of the infection. All cases of labyrinthitis are also treated with medications to alleviate symptoms. These may include an anti-inflammatory agent and a medication to minimize the vertigo. In addition, your doctor may prescribe medications to reduce or stop the nausea and vomiting that may be associated with labyrinthitis.

The DOs

- Rest in bed to reduce the symptoms associated with motion.
- Take your medications as prescribed. If you are prescribed an antibiotic, be certain to complete the entire prescription to effectively clear up the infection.

The DON'Ts

- Avoid activities that require good balance.
- Do not drive until you are entirely symptom free off of medication.
- Avoid using alcohol, tobacco, and caffeine because they may worsen your symptoms

When to Call Your Doctor

- If your symptoms suddenly worsen.
- If you have a severe headache or a stiff, sore neck associated with your symptoms, call your doctor immediately.
- If you have a fever in addition to your other symptoms, call immediately.
- If your vomiting is not controlled by the medications you were given.
- If you have any problems associated with your medication.

For More Information

World Wide Web: http://www.teleport.com/~veda
Vestibular Disorders Association
P.O. Box 4467
Portland, OR 97208-4467
Phone: 503-229-7705
800-837-8428
Fax: 503-229-8064

LACTOSE INTOLERANCE

About Your Diagnosis

If you have difficulty digesting cow's milk, you have lactose intolerance. Lactose is the main sugar in cow's milk. This inability to digest lactose is caused by a shortage of the enzyme lactase.

Lactase is normally made by the cells that line the small intestine. If these cells are damaged by injury or certain diseases, the production of lactase can be decreased or absent. In rare cases a child is born with the condition and is unable to produce lactase. The lactase breaks down milk sugar into simpler forms that can then be absorbed into the bloodstream. When there is not enough lactase to digest the amount of lactose consumed, you may have symptoms.

Lactose intolerance is a common condition. Between 30 and 50 million Americans have the condition. It occurs more commonly as you age. It also occurs more commonly in certain racial and ethnic groups. As many as 90% of Asian Americans and 75% of African Americans and Native Americans are lactose intolerant. This condition is least common in individuals of Northern European descent.

The condition is detected by tests used to measure the absorption of lactose from the digestive tract. These tests are the lactose tolerance test, the hydrogen breath test, and the stool acidity test. The stool acidity test should be used in children. All of these tests can be done as an outpatient. Rarely a small tissue sample (biopsy) may need to be taken from the small bowel.

This condition is not curable but the symptoms are controllable with diet modification and treatment.

Living With Your Diagnosis

Common symptoms of lactose intolerance usually begin 30 minutes to 2 hours after eating or drinking foods containing lactose. Symptoms include nausea, abdominal cramps, bloating, gas, and diarrhea. In children the symptoms are slightly different. Children tend to have foamy diarrhea and diaper rash and sometimes vomiting. Children also have slowed growth and development.

Treatment

Lactose intolerance is easy to treat. Infants and young children with lactose intolerance should not have foods containing lactose. Older children and adults generally do not have to avoid lactose products completely but should identify the amounts they can tolerate. If an older child or adult can only tolerate small amounts of lactose, lactase enzymes in drop and chewable forms are available over-the-counter. The drops can be put in milk before drinking. The chewable tablets are used to help individuals digest solid foods that contain lactose.

The DOs

- Read food labels carefully to avoid foods that may contain lactose.
- Talk to your physician or a dietitian about a proper balanced diet.
- Ensure adequate calcium intake through either diet or supplementation. Foods that are high in calcium include broccoli, kale, greens, oysters, and fish with soft bones (salmon and sardines).
- Yogurt and hard cheeses may be better tolerated and are high in calcium.
- Ensure adequate vitamin D intake to help with calcium metabolism. Exposure to sunlight will help with this. Eggs and liver are also good sources of vitamin D.
- If you have a family history of lactose intolerance, consider breast-feeding your baby.
- Infants with lactose intolerance should be given a soy-based formula.

The DON'Ts

- Avoid foods that may contain hidden lactose. These include bread and other baked goods, processed breakfast cereals, instant potatoes, soups, breakfast drinks, margarine, lunch meats (other than kosher), salad dressings, candies, and mixes for pancakes, biscuits, and cookies.
- Avoid prescription and over-the-counter medications that contain lactose as a base if you have severe lactose intolerance. Ask your pharmacist about specific medications.

When to Call Your Doctor

- If you or your child has symptoms of lactose intolerance.
- If a milk-free diet does not improve symptoms.
- If your child fails to gain weight.
- If your child refuses food or formula.

For More Information
Lactose Intolerance: A Resource Including Recipes, Food Sensitiv-

ity Series (1991).
American Dietetic Association
216 West Jackson Blvd.
Chicago, IL 60606
312-899-0040
800-366-1655 (Consumer Nutrition Hot Line)
Resource book provides recipes and information about food products.
National Digestive Diseases Information Clearinghouse
2 Information Way
Bethesda, MD 20892-3570
www.niddk.nih.gov
nddic@aerie.com

LARYNGITIS

About Your Diagnosis

Laryngitis is a minor inflammation of the vocal cords and surrounding area that results in hoarseness. It can be caused by a viral or bacterial infection, excessive use of the voice, and allergies. Recovery usually takes 7–10 days.

Living With Your Diagnosis

Signs and symptoms include a sore throat with hoarseness or loss of voice, slight fever, difficulty swallowing, and a dry cough.

Treatment

For minor discomfort a nonaspirin preparation can be used. Cough syrups and lozenges can help relieve discomfort. Resting the voice by whispering or writing notes is usually all that is needed. If the cause is a bacterial infection, antibiotics will be prescribed and should be taken until finished. No special diet is needed, although liquids may be better tolerated. No activity restrictions are necessary.

The DOs

- Rest your voice. Write notes or whisper for a few days.
- If antibiotics are needed, finish all of them.
- Use a cool-mist humidifier to soothe the airway. Remember to change the water and clean it daily.
- Increase fluid intake.

The DON'Ts

- Don't use your voice unless absolutely necessary.
- Don't skip doses or stop taking any prescribed antibiotic.

When to Call Your Doctor

- If a high fever or breathing difficulty occurs.
- If symptoms last longer than 2 weeks.

For More Information

National Institute on Deafness and Other Communication Disorders Information Clearinghouse
800-241-1044, Monday through Friday from 8 AM to 5:30 PM (EST).
Internet Site
www.healthanswers.com

LARYNGOTRACHEOBRONCHITIS (CROUP)

About Your Diagnosis

Croup is an inflammation and obstruction of the upper airway usually caused by a viral infection. It affects the vocal cords and surrounding tissue, resulting in labored breathing and a "barking cough." Children younger than 6 years are the most frequently affected. Croup is more common in children with allergies and those with a family history of croup. It generally occurs in the fall and winter months. Recovery takes a few days.

Living With Your Diagnosis

Signs and symptoms of the disease include hoarseness, throat pain, fever, and a barking cough with difficulty breathing. These may worsen at night.

Treatment

Tylenol can be given for the pain and fever. During an attack, steam from a hot shower can help soothe the air passages and make breathing easier. Hold a young child on your lap in the bathroom while the shower runs. A cool-mist vaporizer at the child's bedside can also be helpful. Remember to change the water and clean it daily. Keep the child calm because breathing becomes more difficult with anxiety. Prop the child in a semiupright position.

The DOs

- Keep the child calm, playing quietly in bed.
- Give plenty of fluids such as ice pops, fruit juices, or ginger ale.
- Use a cool-mist vaporizer at the bedside. Remember to change the water and clean it daily.
- Prop the child in a comfortable semiupright position.
- Give Tylenol for pain and fever.

The DON'Ts

- Don't give a young child aspirin because it has been associated with Reye's syndrome.
- Don't give solid foods until the child can breathe easily.
- Don't worry if the child doesn't eat much; loss of appetite is common. However, make sure he takes fluids.

When to Call Your Doctor

- If your child has trouble breathing, cannot swallow water or saliva, or his lips become darker or blue—GO TO THE NEAREST EMERGENCY DEPARTMENT.
- If your child develops an earache, productive cough, another fever, or shortness of breath a few days after the attack is over.

For More Information

American Lung Association
(provides information on respiratory diseases)
800-LUNG-USA (800-586-4872)
National Jewish Center for Immunology and Respiratory Medicine
1400 Jackson Street
Denver, CO 80206
800-222-5864, Monday through Friday from 8 AM to 5 PM (MST), to reach a nurse who will answer questions and send information; or 800-552-5864, for recorded information 24 hours per day.
National Institute of Child Health and Human Development of the NIH
31 Center Drive
MSC 2725
Building 31/2A32
Bethesda, MD 20892
301-496-5133

LEAD POISONING

About Your Diagnosis

Lead poisoning defines a state in which there is an excessive amount of lead in the blood. Lead is a metal. When ingested in excess it inhibits one of the crucial steps in blood formation. This may cause severe anemia, especially among children, who are more susceptible than adults. Acute intoxication may become apparent with severe abdominal pain and neurologic symptoms such as confusion. Children are more sensitive than adults to lead poisoning and can have subtle symptoms such as speech and language deficits and learning problems. Adults whose professions involve exposure to lead, such as construction workers and painters, are at risk.

Living With Your Diagnosis

If lead poisoning is highly likely, the results of simple blood and urine tests are diagnostic. Lead-poisoning anemia is characterized by the presence of small blood cells with small spots (basophilic stippling). Lead blocks an enzyme essential for red blood cell formation; other products accumulate in these cells and are excreted in the urine. Therefore, a urine test is part of the diagnosis. Another test is to measure the level of lead itself in the blood. This is used as a screening tool and provides a measurement of the severity of exposure.

The first and most important step in managing lead poisoning is to identify and eradicate the source. You should always be careful with your children's toys, including those in public areas, such as swings. Newspapers and magazines are a source of lead, and children should not be allowed to touch or play with them. Most pediatricians obtain a lead level in the infants blood as a screening test. Lead poisoning can cause chronic damage but can be fully managed if correctly diagnosed in the early stages.

Treatment

For very sick patients, admission to a hospital is advised. The doctor may administer drugs that bind to lead in the circulation and help excrete it faster. The patient may have to continue the medication after discharge to make sure that the body is free of the metal.

The DOs

- Make sure toys are lead free and that children avoid contact with newspapers and magazines.
- Let water run for 20 to 30 seconds before using it for cooking or drinking if your water supply has been found to contain lead.

The DON'Ts

- Avoid overexertion.
- Do not allow children to eat paint chips or mouth newspapers and magazines.
- Do not work around lead without taking proper precautions.
- Do not drink or cook with water that has just come out of the faucet if your water supply is found to contain lead. Also avoid using hot water directly from the faucet, because hot water leaches more lead from pipes. Boiling water does not remove lead.

When to Call Your Doctor

- If you or your child experiences severe abdominal pain, shortness of breath, fatigue, or chest pain.
- If you believe you or your child has been exposed to lead.

For More Information

MedWeb Hematology: http://www.gen.emory.edu/medweb.hematology.html
MedMark Hematology: http://medmark.bit.co.kr/hematol.html
National Heart, Lung, and Blood Institute Information Center
P. O. Box 30105
Bethesda, MD 20824-0105
301-251-1222
National Lead Information Center: http://www.nsc.org/ehc/lead.htm
Housing and Urban Development Office of Lead Hazard Control: http://www.hud.gov/lea/leahome.html
Environmental Protection Agency Office of Pollution Prevention and Toxics-Lead Program: http;//www.epa.gov/opptintr/lead/index.html

LEGG-CALVÉ PERTHES DISEASE

About Your Diagnosis

Legg-Calvé Perthes disease is a cause of hip pain among children. Legg-Calvé Perthes disease is a loss of the blood supply to the ball portion of the ball-and-socket hip joint. It usually occurs among children between the ages of 5 and 12 years. The disease is not extremely common, and if it is detected early enough, can be successfully treated. Although symptoms are usually limited to one hip, sometimes they can occur in both hips.

Living With Your Diagnosis

Legg-Calvé Perthes disease usually begins with hip pain, although some children report pain in the thigh or near the knee. A physical examination shows marked tenderness with rotation of the hip, and the child has a limp. The diagnosis is suggested by the patient's age and history and the findings at physical examination, but radiographs (x-rays) are needed to confirm the diagnosis. Magnetic resonance imaging (MRI) provides additional information about how much of the femoral head (ball of the hip joint) is involved. The loss of blood supply to the femoral head can lead to collapse and early arthritis and stiffness of the hip joint.

Treatment

There are no medications, diets, or exercise programs that adequately manage this condition. It has to be evaluated and managed by an orthopedic surgeon who has experience with pediatric patients. The use of body casts or long-leg braces can be inconvenient and uncomfortable for patient and family but is essential to ensure the best possible outcome. The best treatment is early detection. Once the diagnosis has been confirmed by an orthopedic surgeon, several treatment options are available. Depending on the age of the child and the appearance of the joint on radiographs, the patient may be treated with casting, bracing, and sometimes a surgical procedure. Again, there can be side effects and potential complications with each of these forms of treatment. An operation carries with it the risks of anesthesia and surgical manipulation. Risk for infection is always a concern with surgical treatment; however, among children surgical infection is extremely rare.

The DOs

• To relieve itching, use a hair dryer on a cool setting to blow air into the cast or tap on the cast directly over the itch rather than inserting an object into the cast.

The DON'Ts

• Do not insert anything inside the cast to scratch. This can cause a skin sore, which can become infected.

When to Call Your Doctor

• If your child consistently feels pain well localized to a single area beneath the cast. This may be a pressure sore. The physician determines whether inspection of the skin beneath the cast is warranted.
• If redness, swelling, or a foul odor emanates from the cast.
• If after the appropriate treatment regimen has been chosen, there are any deviations from the treatment program.

For More Information
http://www.icondata.com/health/pedbase/files/LEGG-CAL.HTM

LEGIONNAIRE'S DISEASE

About Your Diagnosis

Legionnaire's disease is a type of pneumonia usually caused by the bacteria, *Legionella pneumophilia*. The disease is named as such because it was first recognized as a type of illness when it affected many individuals attending an American Legion Convention in the 1970s. Legionella can cause both epidemics and isolated episodes of infection.

The bacteria normally lives in water. Man-made water reservoirs such as evaporative units of commercial air conditioning cooling towers seem to be prone to contamination, explaining why many individuals can be affected in one location. Exposure is thought to occur when droplets containing *Legionella* are inhaled. The organism is not spread from person to person. There is no vaccine.

Legionnaire's disease typically occurs in middle-aged men, although women and children have been affected. Smoking, cancer, chronic illnesses (such as diabetes, kidney failure, and lung disease), and use of drugs that decrease the body's immune system increase one's risk for developing *Legionella* pneumonia.

Living With Your Diagnosis

The illness begins with headache, fever, muscle aches, fatigue, and weakness. Cough, phlegm production, shortness of breath, and chest pain follow. Nausea, vomiting, and diarrhea are other common symptoms. Legionnaire's disease may be life threatening, and hospitalization is required in severe cases. Diagnosis may be difficult because the symptoms are not specific, and the bacteria is not always identified in the sputum or blood.

Treatment

Antibiotics are given for 14–21 days. Hospitalized patients begin therapy with intravenous antibiotics, then switch to oral antibiotics before discharge. The drug of first choice is usually erythromycin. Intravenous erythromycin may cause burning at the intravenous site. Oral erythromycin may cause nausea. Symptoms generally begin to improve within 48–72 hours of starting antibiotic therapy.

The DOs
- Take your antibiotics as prescribed. If you miss a dose, simply resume with the next dose and continue to take the pills as scheduled until they are gone. Rest until you feel better. Some symptoms may persist for several months, but all should eventually resolve.
- Tell your doctor if you are allergic to erythromycin.
- Take acetaminophen or aspirin for relief of fever and pain.
- Drink plenty of fluids (six to eight glasses a day) and/or breath moist air to help raise phlegm.

The DON'Ts
- Home treatment of *Legionella* pneumonia with antibiotics should be avoided if the home environment is not stable and conducive to rest and recovery.

When to Call Your Doctor
- If you suspect pneumonia because of a generalized sense of not feeling well, fever, shortness of breath, green or bloody phlegm production, or chest pain.
- If you fail to improve or become more ill after 48 hours of antibiotic therapy.
- If nausea prevents you from taking the erythromycin.

For More Information
American Lung Association
1118 Hampton Avenue
St. Louis, MO 63139
800-LUNG-USA
www.lungusa.org

LEUKEMIA, CHRONIC LYMPHOCYTIC

About Your Diagnosis

Chronic lymphocytic leukemia (CLL) is a malignant disease that results in abnormal collection of relatively mature lymphocytes in the bone marrow, lymph nodes, liver, spleen, and other organs, resulting in their enlargement. As the disease progresses, the accumulation of abnormal lymphocytes in the bone marrow decreases production of normal blood cells, causing anemia (low red blood cell count), leukopenia (low white blood cell count), and thrombocytopenia (low platelet count).

Genetic factors play an important role in causing CLL. There is an increased rate of CLL in some families. Relatives of patients with CLL are at higher risk for this disease than is the general population. The normal genotype for humans is 23 pairs of chromosomes. One third of patients with CLL have an extra chromosome 13, resulting in trisomy 13. Other common chromosome abnormalities include 14q+, 13q+, and 12q+. Radiation does not increase risk for CLL.

CLL is the most common type of leukemia in western countries. The disease typically occurs among patients older than 50 years and is unusual among persons younger than 30 years. The disease effects men twice as frequently as women. CLL is a malignant not an infectious disease, so it is not transmitted by means of casual contact.

Approximately 25% of patients have no symptoms at the time of diagnosis. These patients have blood lymphocytosis (increased number of lymphocytes), enlarged lymph nodes, or an enlarged spleen found during a routine examination or evaluation of an apparently unrelated disease. The most common symptom that causes a patient to consult a physician is fatigue or a vague sense of ill-being. Sometimes enlarged lymph nodes or the development of an infection is the initial symptom. Some patients describe easy bruising or other bleeding problems.

Living With Your Diagnosis

Patients have normal life expectancy in the early stages of the disease. Approximately 25% of patients have no symptoms at the time of the diagnosis. As the disease progresses, however, patients may experience discomfort because of large lymph nodes and splenomegaly. Anemia and thrombocytopenia can give rise to symptoms of fatigue, generalized weakness, easy bruising, and bleeding. Immune system disturbances in CLL give rise to the formation of antibodies against one's own red blood cells and platelets, causing what is called *autoimmune hemolytic anemia* and *autoimmune thrombocytopenia*. In these conditions growth of malignant lymphocytes suppresses production of normal blood cells and results in anemia and thrombocytopenia.

Immune dysfunction and hypogammaglobulinemia increase risk for bacterial, fungal, and atypical viral infections. Most patients with CLL die of either severe infections or unrelated causes.

Treatment

Patients are treated if they have aggressive CLL, defined by generalized symptoms, anemia, thrombocytopenia, painful enlargement of the lymph nodes and spleen, or frequent infections. Treatment is with chemotherapy. Single agents or combinations of alkylating agents, purine analogs, and steroids are used. Chlorambucil and cyclophosphamide with or without prednisone are effective in controlling CLL. Fludarabine and cladribine (2-CDA) also are effective in the management of new and refractory cases of CLL.

In addition to chemotherapy, radiation therapy to the spleen and lymphoid tissue can control the symptoms. Bone marrow transplantation is potentially curative treatment of younger patients with CLL.

Common side effects of chemotherapy include nausea, vomiting, diarrhea, and mouth sores. Chemotherapy lowers normal blood counts, and patients can contract infections, including pneumonia and blood infections. Patients who have increased weakness and lack of energy because of low red blood cell counts need blood transfusions. Platelet counts also can drop, increasing risk for bleeding. Chemotherapy can cause abnormalities in the genetic material of cells, which increases risk for cancer of the organs.

The DOs

- Participate in your chemotherapeutic regimen as directed.
- Take antibiotics as directed if you have an infection.
- Avoid dairy products, fresh fruits, and vegetables during the periods of myelosuppression that follow chemotherapy.

The DON'Ts
- Do not use medications more frequently than recommended.
- Avoid eating uncooked vegetables, fruits, and milk products, because these products harbor bacteria that are not harmful for healthy persons but can cause severe infections among patients with low white blood cell counts.
- Avoid strenuous exercise if you have low blood cell counts.
- Stop exercising if you have any chest pain or shortness of breath. Your red blood cell count may be very low, and ischemia (lack of blood) of the vital organs can develop.

When to Call Your Doctor
- If you have a fever, abdominal pain, rapid increase in size of your spleen or lymph glands, or bleeding from the gums or any other orifices.

For More Information
American Cacer Society
1599 Clifton Road, NE
Atlanta, CA30329-4251
1-800-ACS-2345
Leukemia Society of America
600 Third Ave., 4th Floor
New York, NY 10016
1-800-955-4LSA (1-800-955-4572)

LEUKEMIA, CHRONIC MYELOGENOUS

About Your Diagnosis

Chronic myelogenous leukemia (CML) is cancer of the white blood cells. The cause of CML is unknown, but it has been linked to exposure to benzene and high doses of radiation. CML cells contain an abnormal shift of DNA between two chromosomes (BCR-ABL translocation). In most patients, this rearrangement takes the form of an abnormal chromosome called the *Philadelphia chromosome*.

About 20% of cases of leukemia among adults are CML. CML occurs among persons of all ages, but is most common in middle age. CML is not contagious and usually is not hereditary.

Both the BCR-ABL translocation and the Philadelphia chromosome can be detected with special tests performed on the blood or bone marrow. These tests are used to diagnose CML.

The only cure for CML is replacing the patient's abnormal bone marrow with marrow from a healthy donor (allogeneic bone marrow transplantation). Other treatment options exist that can improve symptoms and prolong the life of patients with CML.

Living With Your Diagnosis

Patients with chronic phase CML usually have no restrictions on their lifestyle.

CML originates in the bone marrow, where blood cells are formed. Three types of blood cells normally are formed in the marrowred blood cells, which carry oxygen; white blood cells, which fight infection; and platelets, which assist in clotting. CML cells multiply in the marrow, slowly crowd out the normal cells, and then enter the peripheral blood. The blood of a patient with CML usually contains an increased number of abnormal, immature white blood cells, which are affected by CML.

There are three stages of CMLa chronic phase, an accelerated phase, and an advanced phase known as blast crisis. With CML in the *chronic phase*, which may persist for years, patients have relatively few symptoms. The disease is diagnosed when a routine blood test reveals a high white blood cell count. The platelet count also may be elevated in chronic-phase CML. Some patients with chronic-phase CML may feel abdominal fullness because of growth of the spleen in the left upper abdomen.

Rare patients may have fatigue, weight loss, fever, night sweats, or bone pain.

The foregoing symptoms generally become more prominent in the *accelerated phase* of CML. As CML accelerates, the malignant cells overgrow the normal blood cells in the bone marrow, leading to anemia (low red blood cell count) and thrombocytopenia (low platelet count). Symptoms of anemia include fatigue, dizziness, and shortness of breath; symptoms of thrombocytopenia include increased bleeding. As the disease progresses, the white blood cells in the blood and marrow become progressively more immature. These immature white blood cells cannot fight infections properly, making some patients with CML highly susceptible to infections.

The most immature type of white blood cell is called a *myeloblast*. When most of the white blood cells in the blood or marrow of a patient with CML are myeloblasts, the patient is said to have *advanced CML* or *blast crisis*. Patients with advanced CML may have very high numbers of immature white blood cells in their blood. If the number of these cells does not decrease (usually with medication), the cells may become stuck in various parts of the body, most notably the lungs, brain, or penis. Patients with advanced CML who experience sudden, severe headaches, shortness of breath, or an erection unassociated with sexual arousal should call their physicians immediately.

Treatment

The only cure for CML is replacing the patient's abnormal bone marrow with marrow from a healthy donor (allogeneic bone marrow transplantation). In most cases, the donor is a close relative, usually a brother or sister, whose marrow is genetically similar to the patient's. Patients who do not have a relative whose marrow matches theirs can sometimes find a match from a national list of voluntary bone marrow donors.

Bone marrow transplantation is a long process that takes place in a hospital. First the patient's marrow is destroyed with high doses of chemotherapy or radiation. After a few days, the patient receives the healthy marrow through an intravenous catheter. The marrow finds its way into the bones and begins making normal blood cells. The patient remains in the hospital until the new marrow has made enough cells to perform most of the functions of the blood, usually about 4 weeks.

Bone marrow transplantation is most effective performed soon after the diagnosis of CML is made. More than half of patients who undergo transplantation while the disease is in the chronic phase are alive and disease-free 5 years after transplantation. The results are poorer for patients who undergo transplantation while the disease is in the accelerated phase or blast crisis. Results also are better for patients who undergo transplantation early in the chronic phase than for patients who have had CML for more than 1 year.

There are many side effects of bone marrow transplantation. The chemotherapy or radiation therapy causes hair loss and mouth sores. Patients need transfusions of red blood cells and platelets for the first few weeks after bone marrow transplantation, because the new marrow has not yet made enough of these cells. Patients also are at increased risk for infection for the first few months after bone marrow transplantation, and most patients need medications to prevent or manage these infections.

The most common complication of bone marrow transplantation is infection. Another complication is graft-versus-host disease. In graft-versus-host disease, the new marrow recognizes the patient's body as foreign and attacks it. Patients who undergo bone marrow transplantation take medications to prevent graft-versus-host disease; new medications are added if graft-versus-host disease still occurs. The number and severity of complications of bone marrow transplantation usually increase as the patient's age increases. Many hospitals do not perform bone marrow transplantation on patients older than 50 years.

Although bone marrow transplantation is the only cure for CML, many patients with CML cannot undergo this treatment, either because of their age or because of inability to obtain matched bone marrow. These patients receive treatments to improve the symptoms of the disease and increase the length of the chronic phase. The most commonly used treatment is interferon-alfa (IFNα), which is given by means of daily injection under the skin. Most patients who receive IFNα normalize their blood counts and spleen size. Some patients actually decrease or eliminate CML cells in their bone marrow, measured by means of determining the percentage of cells with the Philadelphia chromosome. Patients who eliminate CML cells from their marrow live longer than patients who do not.

All patients who take IFNα experience a flu-like syndrome immediately after beginning treatment. This improves after a few weeks. The most serious complication of taking IFN α is impairment of concentration and memory. Patients with these symptoms should inform their physician and stop IFNα therapy immediately.

The DOs
- Participate in your chemotherapy regimen as determined by your physician.
- Eat a healthy balanced diet, unless you have neutropenia.
- Use caution in exercise.
- Receive a vaccination against the influenza virus every fall.
- Brush your teeth with a soft toothbrush and shave only with an electric razor if you have accelerated or advanced CML.
- Stop exercise at once if you experience dizziness, pain, or shortness of breath.

The DON'Ts
- Avoid uncooked fruits, vegetables, and milk products if you have neutropenia (low white blood cell count). These foods can harbor bacteria that are not dangerous to healthy persons but can cause an infection if you have neutropenia.
- Avoid contact sports if your platelet count us so low you are at increased risk for bleeding.

When to Call Your Doctor
- If you experience unexplained fatigue, weight loss, or left upper abdominal pain; these symptoms may indicate progression to the accelerated phase.
- If you have a fever. Fever can indicate either infection or progression of CML.
- If you have any bleeding that does not resolve after pressure is applied to the area for 5 minutes.
- If you have sudden severe headaches, shortness of breath, or an erection unassociated with sexual arousal.

For More Information

American Cancer Society
1599 Clifton Road, NE
Atlanta, GA 30329-4251
1-800-ACS-2345
Leukemia Society of America
600 Third Ave.
New York, NY 10016
1-800-955 4LSA
Cancer Information Service of National Cancer Institute
1-800-4-CANCER

LEUKEMIA, HAIRY CELL

About Your Diagnosis

Hairy cell leukemia is a malignant disease of the lymphocytes, a type of white blood cell. The name *hairy cell leukemia* refers to the hair-like projections that can be seen on the malignant cells under a microscope.

The cause of hairy cell leukemia is unknown. No chemical or radiation exposure has been definitively linked to development of the disease, although one study found a weak association between hairy cell leukemia and employment in woodworking and farming. Only 600 new cases are diagnosed every year in the United States. Hairy cell leukemia is more common among men than women, and it usually develops around middle age.

Hairy cell leukemia is not contagious. It rarely occurs in two or more members of the same family. However, it is usually not hereditary.

The diagnosis of hairy cell leukemia is made by means of finding the characteristic hairy cells. This usually necessitates biopsy of the bone marrow. Sometimes the diagnosis is be made by means of examination of the blood. Sometimes the diagnosis may necessitate removal of the spleen (splenectomy). Chemotherapy often leads to long-lasting complete remission of hairy cell leukemia.

Living With Your Diagnosis

The hairy cells infiltrate the spleen and bone marrow, leading to the signs and symptoms of the disease. Many patients with hairy cell leukemia have abdominal fullness or discomfort due to expansion of the spleen in the left upper abdomen. Others have low blood counts, because the hairy cells crowd out the normal blood cells formed in the bone marrow (red blood cells, white blood cells, and platelets). A low red blood cell count (anemia) can cause fatigue or shortness of breath. A low white blood cell count (neutropenia) can increase susceptibility to infection. A low platelet count (thrombocytopenia) can lead to easy bruising or bleeding.

Patients with hairy cell leukemia have extremely low white blood cell counts, either because of the crowding out of normal white blood cells or as a side effect of chemotherapy for hairy cell leukemia. Patients with neutropenia are at high risk for bacterial infections and should avoid eating uncooked fruits, vegetables, and milk products. These foods can harbor bacteria that are not dangerous to healthy persons but might cause an infection in a person with neutropenia. Patients with hairy cell leukemia who do not have neutropenia should simply eat a healthful, balanced diet.

Many patients with hairy cell leukemia have a low tolerance for exercise because of anemia. They should stop exercise at once if they experience dizziness, pain, or shortness of breath.

Patients with hairy cell leukemia may have a thrombocytopenia, either because of the hairy cell leukemia itself or as a side effect of chemotherapy. Patients with hairy cell leukemia with platelet counts low enough to place them at increased risk for bleeding should brush their teeth with a soft toothbrush and shave only with an electric razor.

Treatment

Not all patients with hairy cell leukemia need immediate treatment. The most common reasons for treatment are low blood counts or symptoms caused by an enlarged spleen. New drugs have been found to be effective in hairy cell leukemia. The most commonly used of these is called 2-chlorodeoxyadenosine(2-CDA, cladribine). Patients receive the drug as a week-long intravenous infusion, and about three fourths of patients have a complete response. Side effects of 2-CDA include a temporary decrease in blood counts and numbness and tingling in the fingers and toes. A low white blood cell counts may lead to increased susceptibility to infection. Decreased platelets may lead to increased risk for bleeding.

The DOs
- Participate in your chemotherapy regimen as determined by your physician.
- Eat a healthful diet if you do not have neutropenia.
- Be vaccinated against the influenza virus every fall. Also consider being vaccinated to protect yourself against several types of pneumonia.
- Brush your teeth with a soft toothbrush and shave only with an electric razor.

The DON'Ts
- Avoid uncooked fruits, vegetables, and milk products if you have neutropenia.
- Avoid contact sports if your platelet count is so low you are at increased risk for bleeding.
- Stop exercise at once if you experience dizziness, pain, or shortness of breath.

When to Call Your Doctor
- If you have a fever.
- If you have any bleeding that does not resolve after pressure is applied to the area for 5 minutes.

For More Information
American Cancer Society
1599 Clifton Road, NE
Atlanta, GA 30329-4251
1-800-ACS-2345
Leukemia Society of America
600 Third Ave.
New York, NY 10016
1-800-955 4LSA
Cancer Information Service of National Cancer Institute
1-800-4-CANCER

LEUKOPLAKIA

About Your Diagnosis

Leukoplakia is a term used to describe white spots that occur on the inner lining of the mouth, lips, tongue, or vaginal area. Smoking is the most common cause of leukoplakia of the mouth. Sun exposure and chronic irritation are also associated with leukoplakia. Ill–fitting dental appliances can be a source of chronic irritation. If untreated, up to 20% can become cancer. Leukoplakia is not contagious. A doctor can sometimes diagnose leukoplakia upon examination of the involved area. A biopsy (removal of a sample of involved area) is required to determine the presence or absence of cancer or precancerous lesions. In most cases, leukoplakia can be cured with treatment, but recurrences are common and require retreatment.

Living With Your Diagnosis

The most common sign of leukoplakia is a small white patch inside the mouth or on the tongue or lips. The patch is slightly raised and well defined. There can be multiple patches.

Treatment

A biopsy is performed by first deadening the area with an anesthetic such as lidocaine. A sharp sterile knife or biopsy tool is used to remove a sample of the leukoplakia. This is sent to a special laboratory for microscopic analysis. Subsequent treatment depends on the location and the results of the biopsy.

All patients should stop smoking. Small areas of leukoplakia will sometimes disappear after you stop smoking.

Complete removal of a suspicious-looking area is sometimes performed instead of biopsy at the initial visit. Electrosurgery (using an electric needle) and cryosurgery (freezing) can be used to treat small areas of leukoplakia.

Beta-carotene (a form of vitamin A) and isotretinoin (Accutane) are two medications taken by mouth that can cure some types of leukoplakia. These usually have to be taken daily for up to a few months. Isotretinoin can cause birth defects and should not be taken by pregnant women.

Leukoplakia of the lip and outer vaginal area can sometimes be treated with application of 5-FU (Efudex) cream, applied two times per day for 2–3 weeks. This causes redness, soreness, and inflammation and actually destroys the involved area.

The DOs

- Report any suspicious-looking or unusual areas to your doctor, including anything on the skin, inside the mouth, on the tongue, or in the vaginal area.
- Follow your doctor's advice until the leukoplakia is completely gone.

The DON'Ts

- If you smoke, stop immediately. Smoking is the major risk factor for leukoplakia of the mouth and tongue.
- If you chew or use any tobacco products, stop immediately.
- Remove any chronic irritation caused by teeth or dentures or sharp dental appliances.

When to Call Your Doctor

- If the leukoplakia does not go away after treatment.
- If any new white patches occur.
- If any fever or bleeding occur after treatment.

For More Information
American Academy of Dermatology
930 N. Meacham Road
Schaumburg, IL 60173
847-330-0230

LICHEN PLANUS

About Your Diagnosis

Lichen planus is a skin condition that has no known cause. It usually occurs in the middle decades of life (30–60 years of age). Lichen planus has no known racial or sexual preference. It consists of small, raised, many-sided lesions that are red or purple and have white lines on the top of them. The lesions are typically itchy and occur most frequently on the wrists, arms, ankles, male genitals, the back of the hands, and the front of the lower legs. They may also occur in the mouth and the female genital area, but they have a different appearance in these areas. New lesions may occur in areas in which the skin has been scratched or traumatized. This is not caused by spreading any germ or toxic substance but by the way the skin reacts in this disorder. Nails may also be involved in some cases; they are frequently thin and have ridges.

Living With Your Diagnosis

The disorder is not very common but is seen in about 1% of all the patients seen by skin specialists. There is no known cure, although some treatments may bring about a remission. The disease tends to resolve after 6–18 months, but in some patients it will recur. You cannot give this disease to others by contact or by the spread of germs. It is also not known to be inherited or to run in families. There are some drugs that tend to cause lichen planus–like reactions, including gold, antimalarials, penicillamine, tetracycline, diuretics, quinidine, quinine, propranolol, captopril, and methyldopa. Photographic developers can also cause this type of rash. You should review all your medications and chemical exposures with your physician.

The diagnosis of lichen planus can be made by its appearance and by a biopsy (taking a small piece of skin to look at under the microscope). No other laboratory tests are useful. However, your doctor may ask you to discontinue a medication that is known to be related to the disorder. Check with the physician that prescribed the medication if the medication is for a chronic condition, such as high blood pressure. You may need a substitute medication.

Treatment

There are multiple treatments of this disorder. Because the cause of the disorder is not known, there is no single treatment that controls the problem in all patients. Some of these treatments are to control the symptoms, and some may decrease the number of lesions. Antihistamines are given for the itching. Cortisone-like medications are the most frequent drugs used. They are applied as creams, injected into the lesions, or taken by mouth. Griseofulvin, dapsone, phototherapy, and systemic retinoids are other types of therapy that may be used.

Because of the various treatments for the disorder, the problems and side effects of each treatment are also diverse. Cortisone-like (steroids) creams can cause thining and pigment changes of the skin when used for a long period. These same effects can be seen when the drugs are injected into the lesions. When steroids are taken by mouth and in fairly large doses for a long period, multiple side effects can occur including weight gain, elevated blood sugar, high blood pressure, susceptibility to infections, and cataract formation. The side effects of all the various treatments are beyond the scope of this chapter. Be sure and discuss these with your doctor if other treatments are used.

The DOs

There is no specific diet, exercise, or other medications that will improve this condition. Because it is a condition caused by inflammation, and trauma can cause further lesions, gentle treatment of the skin is indicated.

The DONT'S

- Avoid over-the-counter medications, perfumes in creams or lotions, or anything that can irritate the skin.
- Avoid excessive sun exposure because sunburn is traumatic to the skin. (Sun exposure itself is not known to make this condition worse.)

When to Call Your Doctor

- If the lesions in the mouth become so painful that you cannot eat.
- If the lesions on the other parts of the skin are scratched and become infected and drain pus.
- If irritation of the eye develops when you have this condition, you should see an eye doctor (ophthalmologist).

For More Information

The Internet Dermatology Society
http://netaxis.com/rdrugge/work/html
The PDR Family Guide to Prescription Drugs, 3rd edition, 1995.
American Medical Association Family Medical Guide, 3rd edition.
Also available on CD-ROM.
American Family Physician's Family Health and Medical Guide
Word Publishing, 1997

LOW BACK PAIN

About Your Diagnosis

Acute back pain usually results from an injury or an accident and lasts 1 to 7 days. *Chronic* low back pain may last for more than 3 months. Management of low back pain depends on the cause and duration of pain.

The back is made up of vertebrae, disks between the vertebrae, the spinal cord, which contains the nerves, and surrounding structures, such as muscles and ligaments. The muscles in the back and abdomen help support the spine. If the muscles, nerves, or vertebrae are injured, pain can result.

Approximately 80% of persons in the United States experience some type of low back pain during their lifetimes. Some persons have low back pain after sitting for a prolonged length of time or after reaching for an object that is out of reach. Many low back injuries are caused by twisting or other sudden movement. Some persons experience low back pain after an accident or fall. Obesity, poor posture, and weak back and abdominal muscles all contribute to low back pain. Low back pain may occur in association with diseases such as osteoarthritis, ankylosing spondylitis, Reiter's syndrome, or fibromyalgia.

A physician diagnoses low back pain by taking a medical history, performing a physical examination, and possibly ordering radiographs (x-rays). The doctor may order blood tests to determine whether the low back pain is caused by another disorder that may cause similar symptoms. Computed tomography (CT), magnetic resonance imaging (MRI), or a bone scan may be performed if the doctor needs a clearer picture of the bones or nerves, the disks between the vertebrae, and other soft tissue. Sometimes an electromyogram (EMG), which helps identify muscle and nerve problems, may be obtained if the physician believes the back is causing numbness or tingling in the legs because of pressure on the nerves. Most of the time radiographs are not needed.

Living With Your Diagnosis

You may experience difficulty bending at the waist, lifting, walking, and standing. Sometimes the pain may keep you awake at night. If the low back pain lasts for months, it may affect your ability to do your job.

Treatment

Management of low back pain depends on the cause of the pain. If the pain is due to an injury, the physician may recommend a short period of bed rest and application of heat or cold to the affected area. Sometimes the physician may prescribe acetaminophen or nonsteroidal anti-inflammatory drugs (NSAIDs) to decrease the pain. If the pain is particularly severe, stronger narcotic-containing pain medicines may be needed for a short time. If you are having muscle spasms, a doctor may prescribe a muscle relaxant. All medications have side effects. The NSAIDs may cause stomach upset, diarrhea, ulcers, headache, dizziness, difficulty hearing or a rash. Side effects of muscle relaxants includes drowsiness, dizziness and a rash.

Physical therapy may be helpful to decrease low back pain. If you are experiencing chronic low back pain, low back and abdominal exercises are helpful.

The DOs
- Take your medications as prescribed.
- Call your doctor if you are experiencing side effects from medications.
- Develop a weight loss plan with your physician if you are overweight.
- Participate in daily back stretching and strengthening exercises.
- Practice good posture when sitting, standing, or lifting.

The DON'Ts
- Do not wait for a possible medication side effect to go away on its own.
- Do not give up. If your back pain does not decrease, ask your physician about participating in a multidisciplinary low back management program.
- Do not stop exercising.

When to Call Your Doctor
- If you have side effects of medications.
- If you continue to have low back pain.
- If you need a referral to a physical therapist or counselor.
- If you have new pain that runs down the side of your legs.
- If you have new numbness or tingling in your legs.
- If you have difficulty urinating or have loss of control of your bowels or bladder.

For More Information

Contact the National Arthritis Foundation in your area. If you do not know the location of the Arthritis Foundation, call the national office at 1-800-283-7800 or access information via the Internet at www.arthritis.org.

LUMBAR DISC SYNDROMES

About Your Diagnosis

Your lumbar spine (low back) is made of five vertebrae separated by cartilaginous discs that serve as the "shock absorbers" of the spine. They act as a cushion between the bones and allow some flexibility of the lower back. Degenerative changes or trauma may rupture the annulus fibrosus, the tough band of cartilage surrounding each disc, and disc material may bulge or herniate into the spinal canal or nerve root canal. The herniated or bulging piece of the disc or degenerative bone spur may compress the spinal cord or nerve root, causing pain in the back or "tingling and numbness" that may radiate to the buttocks, hips, groin, or legs. The pain from a bulging or herniated disc is worse on movement and may be worsened by coughing, laughing, or straining while having a bowel movement. Some patients also have weakness, clumsiness, drop foot, or walking intolerance.

Living With Your Diagnosis

Degenerative changes in the discs are a normal process as we age. Tobacco abuse, poor posture, and strenuous work with poor lifting technique may accelerate the degenerative changes. The discs gradually become worn, less plump, and eventually flattened. When the disc space becomes narrow enough that the vertebrae rub one another, then wear and tear changes develop at the edges of the vertebrae. This wear and tear causes bone spurs to develop that may begin to press on the end of the spinal cord and/or one of its nerve roots. As the nerve becomes irritated, it may cause back and leg pain, tingling and numbness, or weakness in the legs or feet. Rarely, with extremely large, acute disc herniations, a loss of bladder and bowel control may occur.

Treatment

If your physician suspects that you have a lumbar disc that is causing a problem, one or more of the following tests may be ordered: computed tomography (CT) scan (special x-ray pictures of the neck); magnetic resonance imaging (MRI: special non–x-ray pictures of the neck); myelogram/CT (x-ray of the spinal canal and nerve roots); or an electromyogram/nerve conduction velocity test (EMG/NCV: an electrical test of the nerves and muscles). Conservative treatments such as physical therapy, ultrasound, localized heat, and special exercises are usually performed by a trained physical therapist. Injection of steroids and an anesthetic medication into the spinal canal may provide some relief in patients with chronic pain. Generally, surgery is the final option if conservative treatments have failed to relieve the symptoms. Your surgeon will discuss the risks and benefits of surgery.

The DOs

- Maintain good posture while sitting and walking.
- Always wear a seat belt when traveling in a motor vehicle.
- If you must sit for long periods, make a lumbar support by placing a small pillow or rolled towel between your low back and the seat. Stand and walk about frequently (about every hour) to reduce low back fatigue and strain.
- Always lift heavy objects with proper straight spine posture. Hold the object close to your body and use your thigh and leg muscles to lift.
- Participate in a regular exercise program approved by your physician.

The DON'Ts

- Avoid sitting for long periods. If you must sit or drive for long periods, stop in a safe place and walk for 10 minutes.
- Avoid lifting and twisting, pushing or pulling heavy objects; always use your leg muscles to lift.
- Don't use tobacco. This causes cumulative injury to your spine by damaging the normal repair process in the discs and vertebrae.
- Don't return to work without clearance from your physician.
- Don't engage in any strenuous activities until cleared with your physician.
- Don't resume driving until you are pain free or your pain is tolerable without pain medications.

When to Call Your Doctor

- If you have any problems associated with your medications.
- If your symptoms become much worse or if you have new signs of weakness.
- If you have difficulty walking, develop weakness or inability to move your limbs, or have loss of control of your bowels or bladder.

For More Information
North American Spine Society
6300 North River Road, Suite 500
Rosemount, IL 60018-4231
847-698-1630
e-mail: nassman@aol.com
World Wide Web
http://www.webd.alink.net/nass/

LUNG NEOPLASM, PRIMARY

About Your Diagnosis

Cancer of the lung is the most common cancer among both men and women. Every year more than 170,000 new cases are diagnosed. Nearly 90% of lung cancers originate from the lining of the tubes in the lung called *bronchi* and *bronchioles* or from the air sacs called *alveoli*. Lung cancer is usually divided into two types: non–small-cell lung cancer and small-cell lung cancer. Therapy is different for each type. Nearly 90% of all lung cancers occur among persons who smoke or are former smokers. This makes use of cigarettes, cigars, or pipes the main cause of lung cancer. Other possible causes include asbestos exposure, especially for smokers, radon and radiation exposure, and secondhand smoke.

The only sure way to diagnose lung cancer is by means of tissue biopsy. This procedure is performed in different ways depending on the location of the suspected area in the lung. Bronchoscopy (examination with a lighted scope that passes through the mouth into the breathing passages) is the procedure of choice to obtain the biopsy specimen. If this procedure is unsuccessful, needle aspiration (placing a needle through the chest into the tumor to retrieve cells) is performed. Sometimes there is fluid in the space that surrounds the lung. This fluid can be removed with a needle to check for cancer cells (thoracentesis). If none of these procedures leads to a definite diagnosis, an operation can be performed to open the chest (thoracotomy).

Some lung cancers can be cured but only if detected very early, before any spread (metastasis) occurs.

Living With Your Diagnosis

The signs and symptoms of lung cancer include a persistent cough, coughing up blood-tinged phlegm, wheezing, shortness of breath, recurrent pneumonia, loss of appetite, and weight loss. Sometimes the tumor can press on a large vessel, which causes swelling of the face and neck. If the tumor is pressing on nerves near the lung, this can lead to pain in the shoulder, arm, and hand. Lung cancer also can produce hormones that lead to various syndromes.

Treatment

Once lung cancer has been diagnosed, staging is performed to determine whether the tumor has spread. For non–small-cell lung cancer, staging helps determine whether the tumor can be removed and whether surgical treatment is possible. Computed tomography (CT) of the chest and abdomen is ordered to help detect the spread of lung cancer to the lymph nodes or liver. Mediastinoscopy or mediastinotomy (operations to obtain biopsy specimens of lymph nodes in the chest) is performed, and a bone scan is ordered to look for spread to bone. Breathing tests (pulmonary function tests) help determine whether you can tolerate an operation.

For small-cell lung cancer, CT of the head and a bone marrow biopsy are performed to look for spread into the brain or involvement of the marrow.

For patients with non–small-cell lung cancer that is localized, an operation is the treatment of choice and provides the best hope for cure. For patients with more advanced disease or those who cannot tolerate an operation, radiation therapy alone or radiation and chemotherapy are recommended.

For patients with small-cell lung cancer, chemotherapy or combined chemotherapy with radiation therapy is recommended according to the findings at staging.

The types of treatment and common complications are as follows:

1. Surgical treatment. The main complication is pain, especially with turning, coughing, and deep breathing. Patients may feel short of breath, but this may gradually improve as the remaining lung tissue expands, making it easier to breath.
2. Radiation therapy. Fatigue is a common complication. The skin over the treated area may become red, dry, tender, and itchy. A dry sore throat may occur. Scarring of the lungs may occur, which can lead to shortness of breath.
3. Chemotherapy. Complications depend on the drugs used. Anticancer drugs affect cells that divide rapidly, including blood cells, which fight infection and help the blood to clot. Therefore easy bruising and bleeding may occur. Hair cells and digestive tract cells become affected, leading to nausea, vomiting, and hair loss.

The DOs

- Understand the consequences of smoking.
- Seek the advise of an oncologist (cancer specialist) regarding therapy for lung cancer.

- Understand the importance of nutrition before and after therapy for lung cancer.

The DON'Ts
- Do not be afraid to ask questions.
- Do not smoke.
- Do not be afraid to ask for a second opinion. Therapy for lung cancer is complex, and many decisions have to be made before you feel comfortable with the type of treatment you receive.
- Do not be afraid to ask about support groups.

When to Call Your Doctor
- If you have a persistent cough or are coughing up blood.
- If you are more short of breath.
- If you have no appetite and are losing weight.
- If you have a fever while undergoing chemotherapy.
- If you are having pain.

For More Information
National Cancer Institute (NCI)
9000 Rockville Pike
Bethesda, MD 20892
Cancer Information Service
1-800-422-6237 (1-800-4-CANCER)
American Cancer Society
1599 Clifton Road, N.E.
Atlanta, GA 30329
1-800-ACS-2345
American Lung Association
740 Broadway
New York, NY 10019
212-315-8700

LUPUS ERYTHEMATOSUS, DISCOID (DLE)

About Your Diagnosis

Discoid lupus erythematosus (DLE) is a chronic skin disorder characterized by red, raised plaques with sharply defined margins. The lesions usually occur on sun-exposed areas, especially the face, scalp, and neck.

The exact cause is unknown, although DLE is likely autoimmune (i.e., a condition in which your immune system mistakenly attacks normal parts of the body, resulting in tissue injury and disease).

Discoid lupus erythematosus affects women more frequently than men, typically occurring in adults between 20 and 50 years of age. The condition can be more severe in Afro-Americans.

This condition is hereditary but is not infectious or cancerous. Other members of your family may have DLE. Exposure to sunlight increases your risk of developing the condition. Avoiding sunlight exposure and using sunscreen to protect your skin from the effects of sunlight decreases the severity.

Diagnosis is usually based upon the appearance of the skin lesions. Your doctor may perform blood tests and a skin biopsy (removal of a small piece of skin or other tissue) for laboratory evaluation to assist in diagnosis.

Discoid lupus erythematosus is a chronic condition with periods of remissions occurring between episodes. Treatment aims to control symptoms and to lessen the severity of disease, but does not cure the condition.

Living With Your Diagnosis

Skin lesions are typically red, raised papules (smaller than 1 centimeter) and plaques (larger than 1 centimeter) that have clearly defined borders. Lesions may also have scaling and atrophy. Lesions early in the disease are typically bright red and are raised. Later lesions tend to be flat and are faint pink or white. In Afro-Americans, lesions may be hyperpigmented (darker than the normal skin). Lesions tend to be round or oval with irregular borders. They typically involve the face, scalp, and neck, and may also occur on the nose, forearms, hands, fingers, and toes. Occasionally, the trunk and the lining of the mucous membranes are involved. Scalp lesions are frequently associated with hair loss.

Late lesions tend to show atrophy and depression in the central aspect, with slightly raised borders. Scarring is common, particularly in untreated DLE. Lesions scar as they heal and scarring may be extensive. The condition usually burns out in 10–20 years. More than 95% of individuals with DLE live a normal lifespan. However, 1% to 5% percent of patients progress to systemic lupus erythematosus (SLE), an inflammatory disease of connective tissue. This condition involves multiple body organ systems, including the skin, joints, kidneys, heart, brain, liver, and lungs. Life expectancy in individuals with SLE is shortened, although the symptoms can be controlled for many years in most individuals.

Treatment

Specific treatment depends upon the location and severity of your DLE, its impact on the quality of your life, and your response to therapy. Treatment does not cure DLE, but it lessens the severity of your condition and reduces scarring. Treatment includes the avoidance of precipitating factors, general measures, and medications.

Avoid or decrease exposure to sunlight to lessen the severity of the disease. Remain indoors between 10 AM and 2 PM, when the sun's ultraviolet rays are strongest. Use maximum-protection sunscreens and wear protective clothing to minimize the harmful effects of sunlight to your skin. Avoid fluorescent lights whenever possible.

Your doctor may prescribe a variety of medications to reduce inflammation, scarring, and to lessen the severity of DLE. These medications include:
1. Topical sunscreens (SPF 30).
2. Topical steroid creams, lotions, or ointments are effective in reducing the severity of DLE. Your doctor may recommend placing occlusive dressings over the topical medications to increase their effects. Side effects include skin atrophy, formation of abnormal, small blood vessels, and absorption of medication through the skin into the bloodstream, which can cause toxic effects. To decrease the risk of side effects, do not exceed the recommended dose prescribed by your doctor.
3. Hydroxychloroquine (Plaquenil) inhibits your immune system, thereby lessening the severity of disease. It is effective in treating DLE. Side effects include inflammation of the liver and potential toxicity to the eyes. Your doctor will

recommend evaluation by an ophthalmologist (an eye specialist) before starting, and at routine intervals while you are taking this medication. Your doctor will also periodically check laboratory tests to monitor for toxic effects of this medication. 4. Steroid medication injected into skin lesions reduces the severity of your condition and helps to reduce scarring.

The DOs
- Take medications as prescribed by your doctor.
- Inform your doctor of all other medications, including over-the-counter medicines, that you are taking. Continue these medications unless your doctor instructs you to stop them.
- Read the labels of medicines and follow all instructions. Consult your doctor if you have any concerns or if you have possible side effects caused by the medication.
- Avoiding exposure to sunlight lessens the severity of your disease.
- Keep scheduled follow-up appointments with your doctor; they are essential to monitor your condition, your response to therapy, and to screen for possible side effects of treatment. Regular checkups are important, even when your disease is in remission.

The DON'Ts
- Do not stop your medicine or change the prescribed dose without consulting your doctor.
- Do not exceed recommended doses of medicines, because higher doses can increase your risk of toxic effects.
- Do not use potent topical steroids on the skin of the face or genitals, because these areas are most prone to skin atrophy (thinning and wasting of the skin associated with wrinkling and abnormal, small blood vessels).
- Do not abruptly stop steroids or immunosuppressive therapy because you may experience a rebound worsening of your condition. In particular, do not suddenly stop steroid medication, because severe fatigue, weakness, and low blood pressure may result. Consult your doctor before stopping these medications.
- Avoid exposure to sunlight and indoor fluorescent lighting to reduce the severity of your disease.

<#4>When to Call Your Doctor
- If you notice that lesions are becoming worse or if new lesions appear despite appropriate therapy.
- If you have new or unexplained symptoms, which may indicate a complication of your condition or side effects from medications.

For More Information
Lupus Foundation of America
1717 Massachusetts Avenue, N.W.
Suite 203
Washington, DC 20036
800-558-0121

LYME DISEASE

About Your Diagnosis

Lyme disease (LD) can affect many parts of the body including the skin, nerves, brain, heart and joints.

Lyme disease is a curable infection caused by a microorganism called *Borrelia burgdorferi*. This organism is carried and spread to individuals by certain types of ticks. However, only half of the individuals who have LD actually remember being bitten by a tick. Lyme disease is mainly present in certain regions of the United States including the Northeast, the Midwest (mainly in Wisconsin and Minnesota), and along the West Coast. Although LD is an infection, you cannot catch it from an individual who already has it.

Lyme disease is usually diagnosed by the types of symptoms it causes. A blood test may help confirm the diagnosis, but it is not 100% accurate. Therefore, Lyme tests should not be relied upon to make the diagnosis unless you have symptoms that are very likely caused by LD.

Living With Your Diagnosis

Lyme disease often occurs in stages, and individuals may only have one or a few of the symptoms before it is diagnosed and treated. Treatment of LD cures the infection and prevents progression of the disease. Some of the earliest symptoms of LD are a rash and flulike symptoms such as fever, chills, muscle and joint aches, fatigue, headache, and enlarged lymph glands. The rash occurs at the site of the tick bite (often on the armpit, groin, or thigh) and is usually raised or flat, and red with a white area in the center. A later stage of LD affects the brain, nerves, and heart. The infection can cause meningitis, headache, weakness in the face, arm, and legs, or nerve pain in the arms and legs. Infections in the heart can cause inflammation and heart rhythm changes, causing fluttering in the chest, chest pain, shortness of breath, lightheadedness, or fainting. The last stage of LD occurs months after the infection. In this stage arthritis develops, causing attacks of pain, swelling, and stiffness in joints, especially the knee. Fatigue may persist throughout the stages of LD.

Treatment

Because LD is an infection, it is treated with antibiotics. Depending on the stage of the disease or the types of symptoms being treated, the antibiotics may be given by mouth or by vein. Unfortunately, despite treatment, some individuals with LD have persistent fatigue, headaches, muscle aches, and joint pain. These symptoms are not caused by an ongoing infection and do not improve with further antibiotic therapy. While the infection is being treated with antibiotics, symptoms such as pain can be treated with acetaminophen or nonsteroidal anti-inflammatory drugs (NSAIDs). Potential side effects of NSAIDs include stomach upset, ulcers, constipation, diarrhea, headaches, dizziness, difficulty hearing, and rash.

Prevention of LD can be accomplished by reducing your risk of exposure to ticks when you are in areas where LD is known to occur. Precautions include using good insect repellents (containing "DEET"), wearing long sleeves and pants, tucking pant legs into socks, wearing closed shoes rather than sandals or loafers, brushing off clothes, and inspecting for ticks. If a tick becomes attached, it should be removed with a tweezers by grasping the tick close to the skin and gently pulling it out.

The DOs
- Take your medicines as prescribed.
- Ask your doctor which over-the-counter medications you may take with your prescription medications.
- Take preventive measures to avoid tick exposure.

The DON'Ts
- Wait to see whether side effects from medications will go away.

When to Call Your Doctor
- You experience any medication side effects.
- The treatment is not decreasing your symptoms in a reasonable amount of time.
- You have new or unexplained symptoms.

For More Information
Contact the Arthritis Foundation in your area. If you do not know the location of the Arthritis Foundation, you may call the national office at 1-800-283-7800 or access the information on the Internet at www.arthritis.org.

LYMPHANGITIS

About Your Diagnosis

Lymphangitis is an inflammation of the lymphatic vessels. It is generally a complication of a wound that becomes infected by the staph or strep bacteria. The infection may progress rapidly and lead to septicemia ("blood poisoning"). It is curable with treatment.

Living With Your Diagnosis

Signs and symptoms include red streaks appearing near the wound and running toward the nearest area of lymph nodes. For example, if the infection is in the arm, the nodes in the armpit will be affected; if in the leg, the nodes in the groin will be affected. Fatigue, throbbing pain at the wound site, loss of appetite, chills, and fever also occur.

Treatment

Antibiotics and pain medications will be needed. Hot moist compresses or a heating pad applied to the site several times a day will help ease the inflammation. The affected area should be elevated and immobilized if possible. Wound care, including drainage of the wound if needed, should be done only after antibiotics are started.

The DOs

- Take antibiotics until finished.
- Use nonprescription medications such as Tylenol or Advil to relieve pain.
- Notify your doctor if the nonprescription medications don't relieve the pain.
- Increase fluid intake and maintain good nutrition to promote healing.
- Immobilize and elevate the affected area.
- Apply hot moist compresses to the area to relieve inflammation and increase blood flow to the area.
- Have any wound treated promptly if it shows signs of infection.

The DON'Ts

- Don't skip doses or stop antibiotics until finished.
- Don't use the affected limb. Keep it elevated.
- Don't neglect a wound if it appears infected.

When to Call Your Doctor

- If you continue to have a high fever after antibiotics are started.
- If red streaks continue to appear near the wound and "travel" toward the nearest area of lymph nodes after treatment is started.
- If pain increases or is not controlled by nonprescription medications.

For More Information

National Heart, Lung and Blood Institute
Information Line
800-575-WELL
Internet Site
www.healthanswers.com

LYMPHOGRANULOMA VENEREUM

About Your Diagnosis

Lymphogranuloma venereum is a venereal disease that involves the lymph glands and genitals. It is contagious. It is found mostly in subtropical and tropical locations, and generally affects men aged 20–40 years. It is caused by a bacteria called *Chlamydia*. Symptoms occur 1–4 weeks after exposure. Complications that can occur are chronic infection, impotence, and bowel and bladder dysfunction. If treatment is successful, a cure is usually seen in 6 months; otherwise lymphogranuloma venereum becomes a chronic problem.

Living With Your Diagnosis

Signs and symptoms of the disease occur in the following order. A blister forms on the genitals and ulcerates but heals quickly. Then the lymph glands in the groin area become large, red, and tender. Abscesses form and drain thick pus and bloody fluid. Fever, muscle aches, headache, loss of appetite, nausea, vomiting, and joint pain also occur.

Treatment

Antibiotics are needed to fight the infection and must be continued for 3 weeks. Nonprescription pain medications such as Tylenol or Advil can be used for minor discomfort. No special diet is needed, but good nutrition should be maintained to promote healing. Surgery may be necessary to drain the affected glands or remove the abscesses.

The DOs

- Take medications as directed by your doctor and until they are finished.
- Rest during the acute phase of the infection, then resume your normal activities gradually.
- Use condoms during sexual activity with new partners.
- Keep follow-up appointments with your doctor.
- Notify your sexual contacts so they can be examined for signs of infection and treated if necessary.

The DON'Ts

- Don't have unprotected sexual intercourse.
- Don't touch your eyes without washing your hands first, to prevent spreading the infection to your eyes.
- Don't skip doses or stop the antibiotics.
- Don't resume sexual activity until completely healed.

When to Call Your Doctor

- If a high fever occurs during the treatment.
- If pain is severe and is not relieved with nonprescription medications.
- If diarrhea develops.
- If for any reason you cannot tolerate the medication.

For More Information

American Social Health Association
800-972-8500, for pamphlets about sexual health and information about support groups.
National Institute of Allergy and Infectious Diseases
9000 Rockville Pike
Bethesda, MD 20892
301-496-5717

LYMPHOMA, NON-HODGKIN'S

About Your Diagnosis

Lymphoma or non-Hodgkin's lymphoma is cancer of the white blood cells called *lymphocytes*. Lymphocytes are produced in the bone marrow, lymph nodes, and spleen. Lymphocytes are part of the immune system, which fights off infections. The cause of lymphoma is unknown. Some persons are at higher risk for lymphoma than are others. Weakened of the immune system by viruses such as the human immunodeficiency virus (HIV) and Epstein-Barr virus (EBV), use of medications connected with organ transplantation, and excessive amounts of radiation all increase the risk for lymphoma. More than 50,000 new cases of lymphoma were diagnosed last year.

The only sure way to detect lymphoma is by obtaining tissue, usually from a swollen lymph node, and examining it with a microscope (biopsy). Non-Hodgkin's lymphoma is usually classified as low grade, intermediate grade, or high grade. There is no cure for low-grade lymphomas, but the usual survival time is more than 10 years. With aggressive treatment, some intermediate and high-grade lymphomas can be cured.

Living With Your Diagnosis

The symptoms of lymphoma are swollen lymph glands in the neck, groin, or armpits. Some patients notice a lump in the abdomen. Non-Hodgkin's lymphoma, unlike Hodgkin's disease, does not spread in an orderly way. Therefore other organs can be involved even if a few lymph glands are swollen. Non-Hodgkin's lymphoma can involve the abdomen, liver, bone, brain, testis, thyroid, skin, sinus, tonsils, and gastrointestinal tract. Other symptoms include weight loss, nausea, vomiting, abdominal pain, fever, night sweats, loss of appetite, headache, double vision, and itching.

Treatment

When a biopsy of the tissue is performed, the pathologist tells the physician the specific type of cell causing the lymphoma. Once the diagnosis is confirmed, the physician determines the extent (stage) of the cancer. The stages are classified I through IV depending on how many areas of lymph nodes are involved, whether the involvement is above or below the diaphragm (muscle that sepa-rates the chest from the abdomen), and whether one or more organs are involved.

To determine the stage of lymphoma, the physician orders blood tests; radiographs (x-rays) of the chest; computed tomographic (CT) scans of the abdomen, pelvis, and possibly the head; and a bone marrow biopsy (drawing the blood-forming substance from the center of the pelvis or sternum). The physician also may order a lymphangiogram (injection of dye into the lymph vessels in the foot to look for abnormal lymph glands in the abdomen and pelvis). In some situations, a laparotomy (exploratory abdominal operation) is performed to remove the spleen (splenectomy) and lymph nodes and to obtain a biopsy specimen of the liver.

Non-Hodgkin's lymphoma is usually managed with chemotherapy, radiation therapy, or combined radiation and chemotherapy. Unlike Hodgkin's disease, non-Hodgkin's lymphoma spreads early and not in an orderly way. Therefore chemotherapy is usually used first. Radiation therapy plays a role in the management of local disease in its early stage, radiation therapy is used to assist the chemotherapy.

Different combinations of chemotherapy drugs are used. An oncologist (physician specializing in cancer) decides which combination to use. The management of lymphoma is complex and depends on the stage of disease (I to IV) and the grade of disease (low, intermediate, or high).

Side effects of radiation therapy depends on which part of the body is being irradiated. An underactive thyroid, dry mouth, and sore throat can occur if the neck is being irradiated. Inflammation of the lining of the heart (pericarditis) or lungs (pleurisy) can occur if the chest is being irradiated. Nausea, vomiting, diarrhea, sterility, and suppression of the bone marrow can occur if the abdomen and pelvis are being irradiated.

Side effects of chemotherapy are nausea, vomiting, loss of appetite, easy bruising and bleeding, numbness, hair loss, and infections.

The DOs

- Remember that management of non-Hodgkin's lymphoma is complex and involves a team of physicians and healthcare providers. An oncologist, radiation oncologist (physician specializing in radiation therapy), surgeon, nutritionist, social worker, rehabilitation physician, and psychiatrist all can help with difficult decisions.

- Continue with daily exercise and activities before, during, and after treatment.
- Ask for emotional support if needed.
- Discuss the option of bone marrow transplantation and investigational studies if treatment has not been successful.

The DON'Ts
- Do not ignore any swollen lymph nodes.
- Do not miss follow-up appointments during and after treatments. It is important to monitor side effects of treatment and to see whether the cancer returns after treatment.
- Do not be afraid to ask questions about infertility, stress, fear, life insurance, job discrimination, and limitations.

When to Call Your Doctor
- If you feel a swollen lymph node.
- If you have cough, nausea, vomiting, shortness of breath, diarrhea, bloody stools, fever, or bruising after radiation.
- If you have fevers after chemotherapy.
- If you have low back pain with numbness or pain shooting down your legs.
- If you feel depressed.

For More Information
National Cancer Institute (NCI)
9000 Rockville Pike
Bethesda, MD 20892
Cancer Information Service
1-800-4-CANCER
American Cancer Society
1599 Clifton Road, N.E.
Atlanta, GA 30329
1-800-ACS-2345

MALARIA

About Your Diagnosis

Malaria is an infection caused by a parasite that involves the blood cells, liver, and nervous system. It is transmitted from one individual to another by a specific type of mosquito common to tropical and subtropical areas. The parasite multiplies in the mosquito, then enters the human bloodstream during a bite. The parasite then travels to the liver and multiplies rapidly. It then reenters the bloodstream where it destroys the red blood cells. Some parasites stay in the liver and are released at a later time, causing intermittent attacks. Malaria can be diagnosed by examining a blood sample under the microscope. Complications include anemia and clumping of the blood cells, which can cause kidney damage.

Living With Your Diagnosis

Signs and symptoms of the disease can occur 10–35 days after being bitten by an infected mosquito. During the first 2 or 3 days, there may be an irregular low-grade fever, fatigue, headache, muscle aches, and a chilly sensation. Then there is the "cold stage"—hard shaking chills that last 1 or 2 hours—followed by the "hot stage." The hot stage includes a high fever for 12–24 hours with rapid breathing and heavy sweating. These attacks can come and go every 2 or 3 days. Without treatment they can last for years.

Treatment

Prevention of a secondary infection is necessary, so washing your hands frequently is essential. Your doctor will prescribe an antimalarial drug to kill the parasite. You must take the medication as directed and have frequent follow-up blood tests to make sure the parasite doesn't recur. Side effects of the medication include stomach upset and headaches. You should rest in bed during the period of fever and chills. Normal activities should be resumed gradually. No special diet is needed, but fluid intake should be increased because of the fever and sweating. A multivitamin supplement will be helpful during recovery.

The DOs

- Protect others by making your environment mosquito free.
- Rest in bed during the attacks of fever and chills.
- Take the antimalarial medication as prescribed and until finished.
- Increase fluid intake during the attacks.
- Resume normal activities gradually.
- Wash your hands and bathe frequently to prevent secondary infections.
- Maintain adequate nutrition.
- Take a vitamin supplement during recovery.
- Take preventive medications when traveling in a country in which malaria occurs. To find out which countries pose a risk for exposure to malaria, call the Traveler's Hot Line at 404-332-4559.

The DON'Ts

- Don't skip any doses of the medication or stop taking it because symptoms have gone.
- Don't donate blood until cleared by your doctor.

When to Call Your Doctor

- If you are weak for a long period after an attack.
- If you can't tolerate fluids.
- If you have any recurring symptoms, such as fever and chills, after treatment.
- If new symptoms develop.
- If you have severe side effects from the medications.

For More Information
National Institute of Allergy and Infectious Diseases
9000 Rockville Pike
Bethesda, MD 20892
301-496-5717
National Heart, Lung and Blood Institute
Information Center
P.O. Box 30105
Bethesda, MD 20924-0105
800-575-WELL
Internet Sites
www.healthfinder.gov (Choose SEARCH to search by topic.)
www. healthanswers.com

MARFAN'S SYNDROME

About Your Diagnosis

Marfan's syndrome is a rare inherited disorder involving the body's connective tissue. It primarily affects the eyes, heart, blood vessels, and skeleton. It is caused by a genetic chromosome defect affecting men and women of all races equally.

This condition is rare, affecting only 4–6 individuals per 100,000. Marfan's syndrome is transmitted genetically in 85% of cases and is present from birth. Each child has a 50% chance of inheriting the disorder from an affected parent.

Marfan's syndrome is not curable, but diagnosis and appropriate treatments prolong life. Without treatment, the average life expectancy is about 35 years. The major cause of death is dilation and rupture of the aorta.

Living With Your Diagnosis

Usually there are no major symptoms associated with Marfan's syndrome. It is usually detected by a physical examination but generally not until early adulthood. Diagnosis requires three of four of the following features: positive family history; eye conditions such as dislocation of the lens and nearsightedness; skeletal conditions such as tall stature with long spidery fingers, an arm span greater than height, and chest deformities; and heart valve abnormalities.

Treatment

Annual heart and eye examinations are essential to both identify problems and follow progression. Antibiotic treatment before certain surgical and dental procedures is necessary. Valve surgery may be necessary for severe progression of disease. Heart and vessel complications can be life threatening.

With surgery, most patients can live a normal life span. There is a slightly increased risk of death with heart surgery. Some heart drugs have been used to attempt prevention of certain complications.

The DOs

- Participate in low and moderate impact activities, such as golf, bowling, billiards, and archery. Vigorous exercise may lead to serious complications.
- Get genetic counseling if there is a family history of Marfan's syndrome.

The DON'Ts

- Don't participate in physically or aerobically demanding sports or activities without permission from your doctor. Avoid contact sports.

When to Call Your Doctor

- When you suspect you or your family has signs or symptoms of Marfan syndrome.

For More Information
National Marfan Foundation
800-862-7326

MASTOIDITIS

About Your Diagnosis

Mastoiditis is an infection of the mastoid process behind the ear. It is caused by bacteria, most commonly *Haemophilus influenzae*, *Staphylococcus*, or *Streptococcus*. Mastoiditis results in the destruction of the bony portion of the mastoid process. It can be a complication of an untreated middle ear infection. Mastoiditis is curable with antibiotic therapy, but advanced cases may require surgery to remove the infected bone and surrounding area. The major complication of the disease is hearing loss.

Living With Your Diagnosis

Symptoms can appear 2 weeks or more after the onset of an untreated middle ear infection. They include pain, redness, tenderness, and swelling behind the ear; increased pain in the affected ear; fever; dizziness; nausea; drainage from the affected ear; and decreased hearing in the affected ear.

Treatment

Identification of the bacteria causing the infection must first be done. A culture of the ear drainage will accomplish this. Antibiotics will be prescribed accordingly. The antibiotics must be continued for at least 2 weeks. If an abscess occurs, surgical drainage of the infected bone may be needed.

The DOs

- Take antibiotics until finished.
- Use nonaspirin products for fever and pain.
- Keep the ear clean and dry. A light cotton ball placed on the outer canal may be helpful to absorb drainage.
- Rest until symptoms subside, especially dizziness.
- Increase fluid intake during the fever.

The DON'Ts

- Don't skip doses or stop taking antibiotics until finished.
- Don't miss follow-up appointments with your doctor. It is important to make sure the infection is cleared.

When to Call Your Doctor

- If you continue to have a fever while taking antibiotics.
- If you have a severe headache, dizziness, weakness, or increased pain.
- If you have nausea, vomiting, or diarrhea.
- If a rash develops.

For More Information
American Academy of Otolaryngology
One Prince Street
Alexandria, VA 22314
703-836-4444, Monday through Friday from 8:30 AM to 5 PM (EST).
American Speech-Language-Hearing Association
800-638-8255, Monday through Friday from 8:30 AM to 5 PM, for an information specialist to answer questions and provide written material.
Internet Sites
www.healthfinder.gov (Choose SEARCH to search by topic.)
www.healthanswers.com

MEASLES (RUBEOLA)

About Your Diagnosis

Measles is an infectious disease caused by a virus. It is highly contagious and is spread by direct contact or by airborne respiratory droplets. Infection usually occurs 7–14 days after exposure to the virus. Outbreaks were common 20–30 years ago but have decreased since vaccinations have become routine. Anyone can be affected, but it is more common in children. Complications can include ear infections, pneumonia, strep throat, and meningitis. The course of the disease is usually 4–10 days.

Living With Your Diagnosis

The first symptom to appear is fever, followed by fatigue and loss of appetite. Later a runny nose, sneezing, a dry hacking cough, and sensitivity to light will develop. Tiny, bluish gray spots appear in the mouth, opposite the molars, and in the throat, followed by a reddish rash that starts on the forehead and around the ears and then spreads to the rest of the body. When the rash reaches the feet, it starts to fade. The rash can leave a brownish discoloration that disappears in 7–10 days.

Treatment

The patient with measles should be isolated for 4 days after the onset of the rash, and should rest in bed until the fever and rash are gone. Saline eye drops can be used for the eye irritation, and sunglasses can be use when light sensitivity is severe. Use nonaspirin products for the fever. Never give aspirin to a child younger than 16 years who has a viral infection because of the risk of Reye's syndrome. Antibiotics will not be necessary unless complications occur, such as an ear infection or pneumonia. No special diet is needed, but fluid intake should be increased.

The DOs

- Avoid contact with others for at least 4 days after the rash develops.
- Rest in bed until the fever subsides.
- Wash hands frequently.
- Dispose of tissues in a paper or plastic bag at the bedside.
- Use only nonaspirin products for fever and pain.
- Use a cool-mist vaporizer to soothe the cough and thin secretions. Remember to change the mater and clean the unit daily.

- Drink extra fluids including tea, cola, and fruit juices.
- Use saline eye drops for irritation and sunglasses for light sensitivity.

The DON'Ts

- Don't give aspirin to a child younger than 16 years during a viral infection because aspirin use has been associated with Reye's syndrome.
- Don't send a child to school for 7–10 days after the fever and rash subside.

When to Call Your Doctor

- If a sore throat and high fever develop during the infection.
- If an earache develops.
- If there is an increase in drowsiness or weakness.
- If breathing becomes difficult, or there is chest pain and a cough that produces thick yellow sputum.
- If a severe headache develops.

For More Information
Center for Disease Control and Prevention
Voice Information System
404-332-4555
National Institute for Allergy and Infectious Diseases
301-496-5717
Internet Sites
www.healthfinder.gov (Choose SEARCH to search by topic.)
www. healthanswers.com

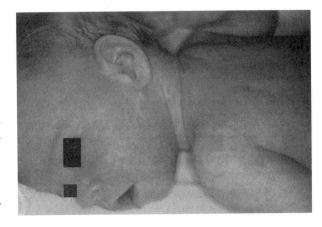

Measles. Note diffuse macules and fine papules with erythema. (From Goldstein BG, Goldstein AO: *Practical Dermatology,* vol 1. St. Louis, Mosby–Year Book, 1992. Used by permission.)

MELANOMA

About Your Diagnosis

Melanoma is a skin cancer that begins from melanocytes. Melanocytes are the cells that produce pigment. The number of new cases diagnosed in the United States has increased dramatically in the last 25 years. It is believed that the increase in melanoma is related to the increase in the amount of time people spend in the sun. Ultraviolet radiation damages the skin and leads to melanoma. Persons at risk for melanoma are those who have fair skin, blue eyes, blond hair, and freckles and burn easily. The risk increases if a close family member has the disease or if one has many abnormal moles (atypical nevi).

The best way to detect melanoma is to examine your skin from head to toe. You are looking for any new moles or for changes in any existing moles. When examining a mole, follow the rule of ABCD. Is the mole *a*symmetric? Does the mole have an irregular *b*order? Does the mole have variations in *c*olor? Is the *d*iameter of the mole increasing? The only sure way to diagnose melanoma is by means of biopsy. If detected early, approximately 85% of all melanomas are curable.

Living With Your Diagnosis

Most melanomas appear as new moles; however, some arise from an existing mole. The way melanoma grows and spreads is that at first the cells of the mole spread locally without penetrating deep into the layers of the skin. As the cancer continues to grow and goes undetected, the cells start to invade and penetrate deep into the skin, eventually spreading into the veins and lymph nodes. (fig 1) Melanoma commonly spreads to the liver, brain, lung, and bone. Signs and symptoms include the ABCD changes in a mole, swollen lymph nodes, shortness of breath with lung involvement, bone pain with spread to bone, and headache, seizures, visual disturbance with brain involvement.

Treatment

When a suspicious mole is found, a biopsy is performed. The biopsy is essential for determining the extent of the cancer (staging). The biopsy must show how thick the melanoma is and how deep the cancer has penetrated the skin (thickness and level of invasion). Once the diagnosis is confirmed with a biopsy, the physician looks for areas of swollen lymph nodes by means of an examination and orders blood tests, chest radiographs (x-ray), computed tomography (CT) of the head, and a bone scan to determine whether the cancer has spread. Treatment depends on the thickness and depth of the cancer, whether lymph nodes are affected, and whether there is spread to other organs.

An operation is performed for all stages of melanoma. For early stages without spread to organs such as the liver, lung, or brain, a surgeon cuts a wide margin of skin to make sure all the cancer is removed. The decision to remove nearby lymph nodes depends on the stage of the cancer, and the patient discusses this with the surgeon. If there is spread to other organs, surgical therapy helps to alleviate symptoms but does not cure the disease.

Radiation therapy is used primarily to relieve symptoms for patients whose melanoma has spread to other organs. Chemotherapy has not been very successful in the management of metastatic (spreading) melanoma. It is used primarily to alleviate symptoms. Immunotherapy with agents to stimulate the immune system to kill cancer cells can be tried, but it also has limited success.

The cure for melanoma that has spread has not been found; this emphasizes the importance of early detection.

The DOs

- Perform a skin self-examination at least once a month. Look at all moles on your body or any new moles that have developed.
- Use sunscreen that blocks the effects of the sun's rays. Sunscreens with a sun protection factor (SPF) greater than 15 provide the best protection from the sun.
- Remember that therapy for malignant melanoma involves a team effort coordinated by a primary care physician working alongside a dermatologist (skin physician), oncologist (cancer physician), and surgeon. Many decisions have to be made, including how much skin tissue should be removed, whether the nearby lymph nodes should be removed, and how to conduct follow-up care after surgical treatment.

The DON'Ts

- Do not forget the ABCD rule (asymmetry, border, color, and diameter).
- Do not stay out in the sun for long periods of time, especially if you burn easily.

- Do not delay if you see a mole that has changed or one that looks different.

When to Call Your Doctor

- If you are suspicious of any moles.
- If you feel any swollen lymph glands.
- If you have pain, fever, or drainage after surgical treatment.

For More Information
Cancer Information Service
1-800-4-CANCER
American Cancer Society
1599 Clifton Road, N.E.
Atlanta, GA 30329
1-800-ACS-2345
Skin Cancer Foundation
245 Fifth Ave., Suite 2402
New York, NY 10016
212-725-5176

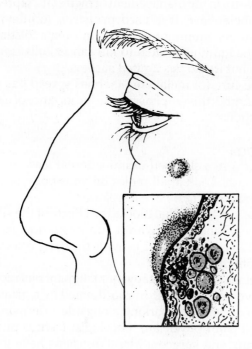

Types of cancer. (From LaFleur-Brooks ML: *Exploring Medical Language; A Student Directed Approach*, vol 3. St. Louis, Mosby–Year Book, 1993. Used by permission.)

MENIERE'S DISEASE

About Your Diagnosis

Meniere's disease is a disorder affecting the inner ear. The disorder results from increased pressure in the inner ear, usually on one side. Although the underlying cause of the increased pressure is not well understood, there are treatments available. Most individuals with Meniere's disease are affected in only one ear, but rarely, some patients have symptoms on both sides.

Living With Your Diagnosis

Meniere's disease is characterized by recurrent attacks of a feeling of fullness in one ear, with tinnitus (ringing, buzzing, roaring, or clicking in the ear), vertigo (sensation of movement), and hearing loss. The vertigo is the most disabling symptom. It can be an incapacitating illusion of movement or a sensation as if the external world were revolving around the patient or as if he were revolving in space. The attacks of vertigo appear suddenly, last from a few to 24 hours, and subside gradually, leaving you feeling dizzy or unsteady for a few days. The hearing loss and tinnitus associated with an acute attack are usually fully reversible early in the disease; your hearing should return to normal between attacks and the tinnitus should go away. In the later stages of the disease, the hearing loss becomes permanent and the tinnitus may be constant.

Treatment

During an attack of Meniere's disease, rest in bed is the most effective treatment, because the patient can usually find a position in which vertigo is minimal.

The treatment of Meniere's disease has two parts: treatment of symptoms during an attack and prevention of attacks. There are a variety of medications that may effectively treat an attack. Often it is difficult to predict which of these medications will be most effective. It may be necessary for your doctor to prescribe more than one to find the one that is best for you. In some patients these medications cause sedation; it will be important to know how the medication will affect you before you attempt resuming your normal activities.

For many years a low-salt diet, ammonium chloride, and diuretics (water pills) have been used in treating Meniere's disease, but their value has never been established. The same is true for mild dehydrating agents such as glycerol.

If the attacks are frequent and disabling, permanent relief can be obtained by surgical means. The decision to undertake a surgical procedure must be tempered by the fact that most patients with Meniere's disease recover spontaneously within a few years.

The DOs
- Take your medication as prescribed by your doctor.
- Rest in bed during an attack.
- Consult your doctor for a surgical opinion if symptoms are disabling.

The DON'Ts
- Avoid food or alcohol binges, particularly foods high in salt or sugar.
- Avoid alcohol, caffeine, and chocolate because they may increase the frequency of attacks.
- Avoid driving or any activity in which a sudden dizzy spell may put you in danger.

When to Call Your Doctor
- If your attacks become more frequent or last longer than usual.
- If you have any symptoms that are unlike your usual attack (such as fever or headache).
- If you become injured as a result of a fall.
- If your prescribed medication is ineffective.
- If you have any other problems associated with your medication.

For More Information

National Institute of Neurological Disorders and Stroke
9000 Rockville Pike
Building 31, Room 8A16
Bethesda, MD 20892
301-496-5751
World Wide Web
http://www.ninds.nih.gov
Vestibular Disorders Association
PO Box 4467
Portland, OR 97208-4467
503-229-7705
800-837-8428
Fax: 503-229-8064

MENINGIOMA

About Your Diagnosis

A meningioma is a tumor generally located along the surface of the brain, spinal cord, or along a spinal nerve root. It is caused by an abnormal growth of cells located on the surface coverings (meninges) of these structures. These tumors comprise approximately one fifth of all brain tumors. In approximately 80% of the cases, the patient will be cured if the tumor can be completely removed. Meningiomas are typically slow-growing tumors that occur nearly twice as commonly in women. The most common age at time of diagnosis is 45 years. Rarely, these tumors occur in children and adolescents.

Living With Your Diagnosis.

The majority of patients with meningiomas are cured with complete surgical removal. However, rarely these tumors can be cancerous (malignant) and may return rapidly, causing destructive changes in the normal surrounding tissues. Symptoms of brain tumors include morning headaches, visual changes, hearing changes, nausea and vomiting, weakness especially on one side of the body, numbness or tingling sensations, and loss of memory and the ability to think clearly. These tumors can recur within the first year after removal. Occasionally, meningiomas may irritate the surface of the brain, and patients may have epilepsy (seizure disorder) before or after surgical removal.

Treatment

The treatment of meningioma is surgery. However, before surgery, your physician may want to get a computed tomography (CT) scan, a magnetic resonance imaging (MRI) study, and/or an angiogram of the region containing the tumor. When the tumor is removed, it will be studied under a microscope to determine whether it is cancer. If cancer is discovered, then you may require additional treatment with radiation. Drug therapies currently being tested may be used for treating these tumors in the future. In some very select cases, noninvasive radiosurgery (focused radiation) may be used to treat deep tumors that are difficult to approach surgically. If you have seizures before or after your surgery, you may need to take an antiseizure medication to prevent further seizure activity.

The DOs
- Follow treatment as prescribed by your doctor.
- Keep all follow-up appointments for surveillance of your tumor.
- Return to activity as prescribed by your doctor.
- Take medications as prescribed by your doctor.

The DON'Ts
- DON'T PANIC. In most cases your illness can be cured with surgery.
- If you have had a seizure, don't drive unless you have been cleared by your physician.

When to Call Your Doctor
- If you have new or recurrent symptoms as noted above, or if they become markedly worse.
- If you have any problems associated with your medications.

For More Information…
World Wide Web
http://www.stepstn.com/nord/rdb sum/301.htm
http://www.brain-surgery.com/mening.html
http://pubweb.acns.now.edu./~lberko/abta_html/abta1.htm
http://www.childrensneuronet.org
American Brain Tumor Association
2720 River Road, Suite 146
Des Plaines, IL 60018
847-827-9910
e-mail: abta@aol.com
Children's Brain Tumor Foundation
274 Madison Avenue, Suite 1301
New York, NY 10016
212-448-9494

MENOPAUSE

About Your Diagnosis

Menopause is the phase of a woman's life when her ovaries stop producing hormones. This event occurs because the ovaries run out of eggs. Most women will go through menopause at an average age of 50 or 51 years. However, some women will go through menopause earlier, as early as 40 years, and others later, as late as 60 years. (Occasionally, women can go through menopause at even younger or older ages, but this is less common.)

Usually the diagnosis is made by the presence of "hot flashes" and the cessation of periods for approximately 6 months. If it is unclear whether a woman is going through menopause, a blood test can be done to determine whether the ovaries are slowing down or no longer working.

Living With Your Diagnosis

The most common symptoms are hot flashes and the periods stopping. Hot flashes can be very mild, just feeling a little warm in the face, to very severe, appearing red in the face and sweating profusely. But the key characteristic of a hot flash that makes it different from other temperature-regulating problems, such as thyroid problems, is that a hot flash only lasts a few minutes. Often women may feel a slight chill after the hot flash stops. Hot flashes can wake a woman up from sleeping, and so some women may feel very fatigued during the day.

Other symptoms include vaginal dryness, vaginal sensitivity, discomfort with intercourse, exacerbation of bladder control problems, weight gain, loss of libido (sex drive), and possibly, increased emotional lability.

Treatment

The most effective treatment for the symptoms of menopause is hormone replacement therapy (HRT). If you still have a uterus, you will need to take estrogen and progesterone. Both of these hormones were produced by your ovaries, so taking the hormones is simply supplying your body with hormones your ovaries no longer produce. Estrogen relieves the symptoms and will decrease your risk of developing coronary artery disease (clogged blood vessels) and heart attack. Taking HRT will also decrease your risk of developing osteoporosis (fragile bones). Progesterone decreases the risk of developing uterine cancer while taking estrogen. If you do not have a uterus, you do not have to take progesterone.

Because taking hormones may increase the risk of developing breast cancer slightly, prescribing HRT should be individualized. Women who may benefit from HRT are those who may be at increased risk of coronary artery disease (i.e., those women who smoke, have hypertension, have high cholesterol levels, or a family history of coronary artery disease), and women who may be at increased risk for developing osteoporosis (i.e., those women who have a history of low calcium intake, who are small boned or have a small frame, who have a family history of osteoporosis, or are smokers).

There are several ways to take HRT. The two most commonly prescribed regimens are:
1. Cyclical: estrogen on days 1 through 25 of each month; progesterone on days 14 through 25 of each month.
2. Continuous: estrogen and progesterone are taken every day.

With cyclical HRT, periods will usually occur every month, whereas with continuous HRT, all bleeding will usually stop after 3–4 months. At first the bleeding may be very irregular but generally not heavy.

After starting HRT, breast or nipple tenderness may occur and may last 3–4 months. After this period, the tenderness will usually decrease and not be bothersome. Some women may feel mildly bloated, irritable, or depressed when taking progesterone. Sometimes adjusting the dose or trying a different regimen or different type of progesterone can help.

If your doctor prescribes HRT, he may recommend that an endometrial biopsy be performed if you start to bleed irregularly while receiving cyclical HRT, or if you start to bleed while receiving continuous HRT, especially if you continue to bleed beyond the expected 3–4 months.

An endometrial biopsy is an office procedure in which a small plastic tube is placed into the uterus to obtain a sample of endometrium, the lining of the uterus. This procedure only takes a few minutes to do and can be done under local anesthesia or without any anesthesia. The biopsy is performed to make sure there is no precancerous tissue ("hyperplasia with atypia") or cancer.

The DOs

Do take your HRT as directed if it is prescribed. It can be taken anytime, i.e., in the morning or before bedtime. If you are experiencing more hot flashes during the day, you may want to take the HRT in the morning. If you are experiencing more hot flashes during the night, you may want to take the HRT before bedtime.

If you miss a dose, you can take it as soon as you remember. If you do not remember until the time of your next dose, do not take the missed medication and the usual medication at the same time. It would not be harmful, but it will not do much good either. Missed doses of HRT will only result in bleeding or hot flashes.

To slow down the development of osteoporosis (fragile bones), you should make sure you are taking in enough calcium. Women receiving HRT should take in 1,000 milligrams of elemental calcium; women not receiving HRT should take in 1,500 milligrams. Calcium can be taken in either through the diet or by taking a calcium supplement. It is usually very difficult to get enough calcium in the diet, so most women need to take some type of calcium supplement. The best absorbed and usually the best tolerated calcium supplements are calcium citrate (Citracal D) and calcium phosphate (Posture D). (The "D" in the brand names means it includes vitamin D.) Vitamin D is also necessary for the body to maintain bone strength. You cannot get vitamin D through any type of food, only by exposure to sunshine. Postmenopausal women should make sure they take in 400 IU of vitamin D daily. If you are older than 65 years, you should take in 800 IU daily.

Because the metabolism slows down with menopause, many women gain weight during this time, so it becomes increasingly important to eat healthy, low-fat foods and exercise. Exercise is very important because it helps to maintain bone strength and muscle mass (in menopause, muscle tends to turn into fat), and it helps to burn up calories during exercise. In addition, exercise will boost the body's metabolism for several hours, which will help to keep the weight off or help with weight loss.

The DON'Ts

Don't stop your HRT without letting your doctor know. If you are having side effects from the HRT, an adjustment or a change in the type of HRT can usually be made so that you can continue to take the HRT comfortably.

If you have a uterus, don't take estrogen without progesterone because it may significantly increase your risk of uterine cancer, unless you have specifically discussed this with your doctor.

When to Call Your Doctor

- If you have irregular or unexpected bleeding while receiving HRT.
- If your menopausal symptoms do not resolve with HRT.
- If you have persistent bothersome side effects.

For More Information

Understanding Your Body: Every Woman's Guide to Gynecology and Health. Felicia Stewart, M.D., Felicia Guest, M.D., Gary Stewart, M.D., and Robert Hatcher, M.D., Bantam Books, 1987.

MESOTHELIOMA OF THE LUNG

About Your Diagnosis

Your lungs have an outer layer called the *pleura*. The pleura is made of cells called *mesothelium*. Mesothelioma is cancer of these cells. The main cause of mesothelioma is asbestos exposure. Asbestos is resistant to heat and was used in products such as insulation, heat protectors, filters, materials for roofing, spackling, floor and ceiling tiles, boilers, and heating equipment in ships, cars, and homes.

Mesothelioma is rare. Approximately 2000 new cases are diagnosed each year in the United States. The cancer is difficult to diagnose, and the only sure way is by means of biopsy and examination of the tissue with a microscope. Even with tissue examination, the diagnosis can be inaccurate, so the tissue specimens should be reviewed by different pathologists. Malignant mesotheliomas usually is not curable.

Living With Your Diagnosis

Most patients with mesothelioma have shortness of breath and chest wall pain. The cancer tends to spread locally to nearby structures. Mesothelioma can involve the ribs, spinal column, esophagus, and heart. As the disease advances, patients report increasing shortness of breath, fatigue, and fevers with cough and pneumonia. Most patients die of pneumonia and breathing problems. Survival time ranges anywhere from 4 months to slightly longer than 1 year.

Treatment

A definite diagnosis must be made to exclude other, possibly curable forms of cancer with a similar presentation. If the biopsy tissue does not allow a definite diagnosis, a second biopsy or open lung biopsy can be performed by a surgeon. Bronchoscopy (examination with a lighted scope passed into the breathing tubes) is performed to look for possible lung cancer (not mesothelioma) as the diagnosis. Magnetic resonance imaging (MRI) or computed tomography (CT) of the chest can be performed to determine the extent of the cancer. This helps in staging of the disease and determining whether the cancer has spread. Stage I means the cancer is on one side of the chest and involves only the lining of lung, not the lung itself. Stage II means the cancer has invaded the esophagus, heart, or opposite lung. Stage III means the cancer has penetrated below the diaphragm (the muscle that separates the chest from the abdomen). Stage IV means the cancer has spread to distant parts of the body.

Treatment options include surgical, radiation, and chemotherapy. Surgical treatment is limited to stage I disease and involves removing the lining of the lung (pleurectomy). In a more radical operation, the surgeon removes the lining of the lung, the lung, the lining of the heart, and the diaphragm (extrapleural pneumonectomy). Some reports show that about 25% of patients survive 2 years after this treatment.

The effectiveness of radiation and chemotherapy is not well known. The decision to use these therapies should be made between you and your oncologist (physician specializing in cancer).

The DOs

- Seek advice from large cancer referral centers concerning the treatment of mesotheliomas. Mesotheliomas usually are not curable, but certain treatment options have enabled people to live longer than if they had no treatment.
- Understand the difficulty in diagnosing this form of cancer. You must be sure of the diagnosis before proceeding with risky treatment.
- Ask for a second opinion on the pathologic interpretation of your biopsy specimen. The difficulty in diagnosing mesothelioma cannot be overemphasized.

The DON'Ts

- Do not forget the cause of mesothelioma in most cases is exposure to asbestos. Avoid working with asbestos and take proper precautions.
- Do not forget that asbestos can cause scarring of the lung (pulmonary fibrosis). Fifteen percent of patients with asbestos involvement of the lung eventually have lung cancer, which is different from mesothelioma.
- Do not forget that the combination of asbestos and tobacco smoking markedly increases your risk for lung cancer.

When to Call Your Doctor

- If you notice blood in your phlegm.
- If you have a persistent cough.
- If you have shortness of breath.
- If you have chest pain.
- If you need emotional support.

- If you need referral to in-state or out-of-state cancer centers.

For More Information
National Cancer Institute (NCI)
9000 Rockville Pike
Bethesda, MD 20892.
Cancer Information Service
1-800-4-CANCER
American Cancer Society
1599 Clifton Road, N.E.
Atlanta, GA 30329
1-800-ACS-2345

METATARSALGIA

About Your Diagnosis

Metatarsalgia is a term used to describe pain in the ball of the foot. This type of forefoot pain can be confused with many other causes of forefoot pain, so it is important to ensure the diagnosis is correct. Specifically, metatarsalgia refers to inflammation or pain of the metatarsal heads. Or in other words, "bone pain." This pain usually is due to increased forces through the forefoot, such as when wearing high heels or when the normal fat pad has shrunk. Increased pressure through the ball of the foot results in inflammation of one or more of the metatarsal bones. Diagnoses that can be confused with metatarsalgia include Morton's neuroma (nerve pain), sesamoiditis, and synovitis.

Living With Your Diagnosis

Metatarsalgia usually can be managed without surgical intervention, but it may persist for several months or even years. Only after all nonsurgical treatments have failed should you consider surgical intervention. Many times a simple pad or soft shoe insert makes a dramatic difference. You must stop wearing the offending shoe to prevent a recurrence. Appropriate shoes are necessary to provide adequate cushioning for the painful foot.

Treatment

Metatarsalgia is managed with appropriate footwear such as running shoes, soft shoe inserts, and sometimes custom soft orthotic devices. All are designed to reduce friction and pressure through the forefoot. The soles of shoes can be modified to further reduce pressure by means of placement of a metatarsal bar or rigid rocker on the sole. When callouses are present, regular trimming may provide dramatic relief. Medications and diet are not as effective as local care and do not seem to alter the course of this painful condition. Surgical intervention before adequate attempts at conservative therapy may result in unpredictable results and actually worsen the condition.

The DOs

- Eliminate as much pressure and friction as possible by changing the type and style of shoes you wear.
- Switch to non-weight-bearing forms of exercise, such as cycling or swimming.

The DON'Ts

- Avoid wearing fashionable but impractical shoes.

When To Call Your Doctor

- If the pain becomes constant or does not respond to conservative therapy.

For More Information
http://www.countryliving.com/rb/health/07acheb9.htm

MITRAL REGURGITATION

About Your Diagnosis

The mitral valve is the valve in the heart between the left atrium and left ventricle. It opens when the atrium pumps blood into the ventricle. It closes when the ventricle pumps blood out of the ventricles to the body. This prevents the blood from going back into the atrium. If blood leaks back into the atrium from the ventricle this is called *regurgitation*. Sometimes it is called *mitral insufficiency* or *mitral incompetence*. If blood regurgitates back into the atrium, it is not pumped out of the heart efficiently, and the atrium cannot fill with the next cycle. Blood may become backed up in the right heart system (to the lungs) causing fluid to accumulate in the lungs. This means the left ventricle has to do more work to move the blood. After a while, the extra work may cause the heart to fail in its function.

Living With Your Diagnosis

Mitral regurgitation is caused by damage that happens to the mitral valve. The damage may be from a congenital abnormality (one that is present at birth). It may come from a heart attack (myocardial infarction, in which parts of the heart muscle or valve die because they do not have enough blood supply). An infection such as rheumatic fever (from streptococcal infections such as strep throat) also can cause damage to the valve. Connective tissue disorders such as lupus and inherited conditions such as Marfan syndrome may affect the mitral valve. Mitral valve prolapse also can lead to mitral regurgitation.

Blood moves abnormally through the valve in mitral regurgitation, producing an abnormal sound called a *murmur*. The murmur is heard when the heart is examined with a stethoscope. The timing of the murmur in the cardiac cycle and the location of the murmur help determine which valve is affected.

Often patients live for years without ever knowing of this condition. Most patients have no symptoms if the defect is small. Symptoms may develop after a few years and usually include fatigue and difficulty breathing. Chest radiographs (x-rays) often show the left atrium enlarged (from overfilling) and fluid leaking into the lungs. Arrhythmias (such as atrial fibrillation) occur if the changes in the atrium affect the electrical system of the heart. This may cause palpitations or a rapid heartbeat.

Treatment

Management of mitral regurgitation varies with severity. If the condition is mild, attempts are made to prevent possible complications. Abnormally functioning valves may be a target for an infection called *endocarditis*. Antibiotics are routinely given to patients with known mitral regurgitation for dental or surgical procedures and for bacterial infections to prevent spread of infection to the valve. Digitalis (digoxin) may be given for atrial fibrillation and heart failure. Some patients with atrial fibrillation are given anticoagulant medications to prevent a blood clot from forming in the atrium. If there is evidence of heart failure, diuretics may be used to reduce the fluid volume in the blood. Vasodilators such as nitrates, hydralazine, captopril, or enalapril may be used if heart failure becomes more prominent. These drugs decrease the workload on the heart. If heart failure becomes unmanageable with medication or the ability of the heart to keep working is threatened, heart valve replacement may be needed.

Side effects of the medications vary depending on the drug and choice of therapy. Allergies to antibiotics or the other drugs may exist. Digoxin levels in the blood must be checked periodically to limit side effects. Diuretics cause frequent urination and can cause dehydration and electrolyte (salt) abnormalities in the blood. Extra potassium pills may be needed if diuretics are used, and these can cause nausea, vomiting, or diarrhea. Nitrate medications may cause headaches or dizziness, and the other vasodilators can cause lightheadedness, fatigue, and intestinal problems.

The DOs
- Take your medications as directed.
- Restrict fluid and salt in your diet if you have symptoms of heart failure.
- Take antibiotics as prescribed before and after dental or surgical treatments, including tooth cleanings.
- Exercise as tolerated.

The DON'Ts
- Do not ignore worsening symptoms.

When to Call Your Doctor
- If you have side effects from your medications.
- If you have new or worsening symptoms, specifically chest pain, shortness of breath, difficulty

breathing at rest, lightheadedness, palpitations (rapid heartbeat), or new swelling in your feet or legs.

For More Information

Contact the American Heart Association about heart murmurs and valvular heart disease. Call 1-800-242-8721 and ask for the literature department.

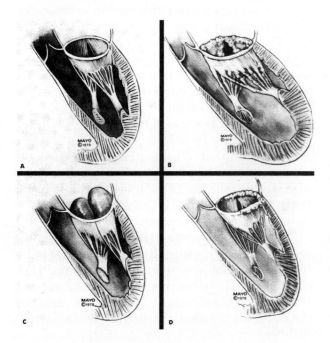

A stenosed valve leads to decreased blood flow through the valve and gradual hypertrophy of the preceding chamber (e.g., a stenosed mitral valve leads to a hypertrophied left atrium). An insufficient valve leads to backward flow through the valve and dilation of the preceding chamber (e.g., aortic insufficiency leads to a dilated left ventricle). (From Lewis SM, Collier IC, Heitkemper MM: *Medical-Surgical Nursing: Assessment and Management of Clinical Problem*, vol. 4. St. Louis, Mosby–Year Book, 1995. Used by permission.)

MITRAL STENOSIS

About Your Diagnosis

Mitral stenosis is abnormal narrowing of the mitral valve. The mitral valve is located between the left atrium and left ventricle. If this valve is narrow, the left atrium must pump harder to move its blood into the left ventricle. If the left atrium cannot empty itself properly, blood backs up into the right heart system and fluid leaks into the lungs. Mitral stenosis is most often caused by scarring of the valve from previous rheumatic fever. Rheumatic fever comes from a bacterial infection. Mitral stenosis occurs two to four times more often among women than among men.

Living With Your Diagnosis

Symptoms usually begin many years after the rheumatic fever. Symptoms of right heart failure in mitral stenosis include difficulty with breathing (especially when lying down) or edema (swelling in the legs or abdomen). Other symptoms include irregular heartbeat, coughing up blood, and abdominal or chest pain. Atrial fibrillation may develop, and the atrium does not contract normally causing blood to pool in the atrium. Clots may form and can travel out of the heart when normal contractions resume. Because of this, some patients undergo an operation to have their mitral valve widened or replaced.

Treatment

Treatment with antibiotics before and after dental and surgical procedures is required to prevent infection in the heart muscle (endocarditis). Digitalis helps manage atrial fibrillation. Anticoagulant drugs prevent clots from forming. Diuretics reduce the fluid in the blood. Other heart and lung conditions must be managed. Side effects of these medications include allergic reactions, nausea, vomiting, diarrhea, and dehydration from diuretics. Anticoagulants may cause easy bruising and prolonged bleeding from cuts.

The DOs

- Take your medications as directed.
- Change your diet to moderate salt restriction (do not add salt to your food).
- Exercise as tolerated.
- Seek the care of a cardiologist for monitoring if you are pregnant or planning pregnancy.

The DON'Ts

- Do not ignore worsening symptoms.
- Do not forget to ask your doctor about antibiotics for dental and surgical procedures.

When to Call Your Doctor

- If you have side effects of medications.
- If you have new or worsening symptoms such as chest pain, shortness of breath, or swelling in the legs or abdomen.
- If you are taking anticoagulants and have a cut that does not stop bleeding or if you sustain a head injury.

For More Information

The American Heart Association has more information on heart murmurs and valvular heart disease. Call 1-800-242-8721 and ask for the literature department.

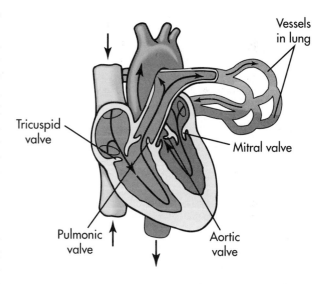

Cross section of valves of the heart.(From Lewis SM, Collier IC, Heitkemper MM: *Medical-Surgical Nursing: Assessment and Management of Clinical Problem,* vol. 4. St. Louis, Mosby–Year Book, 1995. Used by permission.)

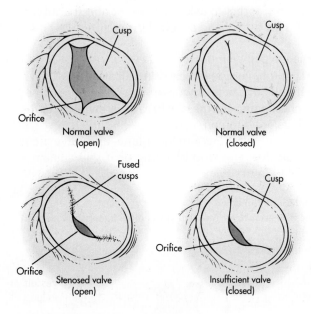

A stenosed valve leads to decreased blood flow through the valve and gradual hypertrophy of the preceding chamber (e.g., a stenosed mitral valve leads to a hypertrophied left atrium). An insufficient valve leads to backward flow through the valve and dilation of the preceding chamber (e.g., aortic insufficiency leads to a dilated left ventricle). (From Lewis SM, Collier IC, Heitkemper MM: *Medical-Surgical Nursing: Assessment and Management of Clinical Problem,* vol. 4. St. Louis, Mosby–Year Book, 1995. Used by permission.)

MITRAL VALVE PROLAPSE

About Your Diagnosis

The mitral valve is in the heart between the left atrium and left ventricle. *Prolapse* refers to a slight abnormality in the valve that makes it floppy. The mitral valve opens normally when the left atrium pumps blood into the ventricle. It closes to prevent the blood from going back into the atrium as the ventricle pumps blood out of the heart. If blood leaks back into the atrium from the ventricle, this is called *regurgitation*. If the valve bulges back into the atrium this is called *prolapse*. Prolapse can cause some degree of regurgitation. Severe regurgitation occurs among about 15% of persons with prolapse. This means the left ventricle must do more work to move the blood, and over time the heart may fail in its function.

Mitral valve prolapse is relatively common, affecting about 5% of the population. It affects women more than men. It may be caused by any damage to the mitral valve. This may be a congenital abnormality (one that is present at birth) or may come from a heart attack (myocardial infarction, in which parts of the heart muscle or valve die because they do not have enough blood supply). Other causes include infections such as rheumatic fever (from streptococcal infections such as strep throat), connective tissue disorders, and inherited conditions such as Marfan syndrome.

Blood moving against the valve in mitral valve prolapse produces an abnormal sound called a *murmur*. The murmur is best heard when the heart is examined with a stethoscope. The timing of the murmur in the cardiac cycle and the location of the murmur help determine which valve is affected.

Living With Your Diagnosis

Often patients live for years without ever knowing they have this condition. They generally do well and never have symptoms if the defect is small. Symptoms may develop after a few years and usually include palpitations (rapid heartbeat), fatigue, chest pain, or difficulty breathing. Arrhythmias (such as atrial fibrillation) may occur if the changes in the atrium affect the electrical system of the heart.

Treatment

Management of mitral valve prolapse varies depending on severity. If there are no symptoms and no evidence of mitral regurgitation, no treatment is needed. If there is regurgitation, attempts are made to prevent possible complications. An abnormally functioning valve may be a target for infection in the heart called *endocarditis*. Antibiotics are routinely given to patients with known mitral regurgitation for dental or surgical procedures and for bacterial infections.

Digitalis (digoxin) may be given for atrial fibrillation and heart failure. Some patients with atrial fibrillation take anticoagulant medications to try to prevent a blood clot from forming in the atrium. If there is evidence of heart failure, diuretics are sometimes used to reduce the fluid volume in the blood so the heart does not have to work as hard. Vasodilators such as nitrates, hydralazine, captopril, and enalapril may be used when heart failure becomes prominent. If heart failure becomes unmanageable with medication or the ability of the heart to keep working is threatened, heart valve replacement may be needed.

Side effects of the medications include allergies to antibiotics or other drugs. Digoxin levels in the blood are checked periodically. Diuretics cause frequent urination and can cause dehydration and electrolyte (salt) abnormalities. You may have to take extra potassium pills if you are taking diuretics, and the potassium may cause nausea, vomiting, or diarrhea. Nitrate medications may cause headaches or dizziness, and the other vasodilators may cause lightheadedness, fatigue, and intestinal problems.

The DOs

- Restrict fluid and salt in your diet if symptoms of heart failure have begun.
- Take antibiotics as prescribed before and after dental or surgical treatments, including tooth cleanings.
- Exercise as tolerated.

The DON'Ts

- Do not forget to take your medications as scheduled.
- Do not use too much caffeine, because excess caffeine may worsen your symptoms.

When to Call Your Doctor

- If you have side effects from your medications.
- If you experience new or worsening symptoms, especially chest pain, shortness of breath or difficulty breathing at rest, lightheadedness, palpi-

tations or rapid heartbeat, or new swelling in your feet or legs.

For More Information

The American Heart Association pamphlet *Mitral Valve Prolapse* explains this condition in detail. Call 1-800-242-8721 and ask for the literature department.

MONONUCLEOSIS

About Your Diagnosis

Mononucleosis is an acute infectious disease that affects the respiratory system, the liver, and the lymphatic system. It is caused by the Epstein-Barr virus. It is common in children and young adults. It is spread by close contact such as kissing, sharing food or utensils, and by coughing. Symptoms can appear from 10 to 30 days after exposure. It is easily detected with a blood test.

Living With Your Diagnosis

Signs and symptoms include sore throat (sometimes severe); fever, usually higher in the evening; loss of appetite; fatigue; swollen lymph glands in the neck, underarms, or groin; abdominal pain; headache; and general body aches. The liver and spleen enlarge and sometimes jaundice occurs. A ruptured spleen is a rare complication.

Treatment

Bed rest and good nutrition are the best treatment. For muscle aches and minor discomfort, use nonaspirin drugs such as Tylenol or Advil. Aspirin should not be given to children younger than 16 years because its use increases the risk of a type of encephalitis called Reye's syndrome. If the throat inflammation is severe, your doctor may prescribe a short course of steroids. Recovery takes from 10 days to months. Generally the fatigue last for 3–6 weeks after the other symptoms are gone.

The DOs

- Rest in bed until fever subsides.
- Maintain proper nutrition. Because of loss of appetite and sore throat, a diet of soups, juices, milkshakes, and bland foods may be better tolerated.
- Resume normal activity gradually after symptoms subside.
- Increase fluid intake to at least 8 glasses a day.
- Gargle with warm salt water to help ease sore throat.
- Because the occurrence of mononucleosis is greater in high school and college students, it may be necessary to arrange for schoolwork to be done at home.

The DON'Ts

- Don't use aspirin if younger than 16 years. Research has shown a link with Reye's syndrome when aspirin is used during a viral infection.
- Don't lift heavy objects.
- Don't strain hard for a bowel movement to prevent injury to an enlarged spleen.
- Don't participate in contact sports until after complete recovery or after your doctor's approval.

When to Call Your Doctor

- If your temperature is more than 102°F.
- If swallowing or breathing becomes difficult.
- If constipation is causing straining.
- If sudden severe abdominal pain occurs, especially in the left upper abdomen, and lasts longer than 5 minutes.
- If severe headache, neck pain, or stiffness occurs.

For More Information

National Institute of Allergy and Infectious Diseases of the NIH
9000 Rockville Pike
Bethesda, MD 20892
301-496-5717
Internet Sites
www.healthfinder.gov (Choose SEARCH to search by topic.)
www.healthanswers.com

MOTION SICKNESS

About Your Diagnosis

Motion sickness is an ill feeling caused by repetitive angular, linear, or vertical motion and is primarily characterized by nausea and vomiting. Seasickness, air-sickness, car-sickness, train-sickness, and swing-sickness are common forms. There are direct connections from the balance mechanism to the nausea/vomiting center in the brain, and with repetitive motion, fluid changes occur in your inner ear that may excessively stimulate your balance mechanism, causing a sensation of motion and nausea. This sensation generally resolves with or without treatment in 1–2 days.

Living With Your Diagnosis

Some individuals are more susceptible to motion sickness than others. Those individuals should minimize their exposure by choosing positions on ships or planes where there is the least motion (e.g., amidships, or in airplanes over the wings). A semireclined position with your head braced is best.

The sensation of motion and symptoms of nausea and vomiting generally go away within 48 hours.

Treatment

As with many medical problems, prevention is easier than treatment. However, there are several over-the-counter and prescription medications that may be used for motion sickness. Some medications help to prevent motion sickness from occurring, and others are for treating the symptoms of nausea and vomiting. Consult your pharmacist and/or physician.

The DOs

- Take frequent sips of fluids. Stay with simple fluids such as water, clear soda, or simple sports drinks.
- If you are having repeated vomiting, only consume liquids.
- Take your medication as instructed while the symptoms are present.
- While in a vehicle (car, boat, or plane), lie back in the seat and take slow deep breaths.
- While in a boat or airplane, try to sit in an area with the least motion.
- Keep line of vision at 45 degrees above horizontal.

The DON'Ts

- Avoid alcoholic beverages and overeating.
- Avoid areas where individuals are smoking.
- While in the vehicle do not read or watch the horizon.

When to Call Your Doctor

- The symptoms do not improve after resting 48 hours.
- You continue to have vomiting and notice that you become faint or dizzy when you change positions suddenly.

For More Information
Vestibular Disorders Association
P.O. Box 4467
Portland, OR 97208-4467
800-837-8428
503-229-7705
Fax: 503-229-8064

MULTIFOCAL ATRIAL TACHYCARDIA

About Your Diagnosis

Multifocal atrial tachycardia means the atrium of the heart beats too fast (tachycardia). This phenomenon is caused by abnormal electrical signals that come from different places in the heart (multifocal). It causes the heart to beat rapidly for no apparent reason. This abnormal heart rhythm is called an *arrhythmia*. It is often caused by heart or lung disease such as chronic obstructive pulmonary disease (COPD, or emphysema). It may occur off and on and rarely causes problems by itself. It is detected when a specific pattern is found on an electrocardiogram (ECG).

Living With Your Diagnosis

The symptoms of multifocal atrial tachycardia are related to rapid beating of the heart. They may be accompanied by shortness of breath or chest pain if you have lung or heart disease. A rapid heartbeat by itself can sometimes be slowed with one of the following maneuvers: straining as if lifting a heavy object, gently massaging the carotid artery for a few seconds, or placing a cold, wet towel on the face for a few minutes. If these maneuvers are unsuccessful, therapy for this condition focuses on the disease causing the tachycardia, particularly if it is associated with low oxygen levels (hypoxia). Medications may be used to slow the response of the ventricle to the arrhythmia. The medications generally used are calcium-channel blockers, such as verapamil and diltiazem. Propranolol and quinidine also may be used. Each of these medications may cause nausea, vomiting, or diarrhea. Propranolol slows the heartbeat and may make exercise difficult. Quinidine may cause fever, rash, or cinchonism (ringing in the ears, dizziness, and headache).

Treatment

The best treatment is one that manages the disease causing the multifocal atrial tachycardia. The usual medications for heart or lung disease should be taken as directed.

The DOs

- Make your diet one that is healthful for your heart (low fat and low cholesterol).
- Stop smoking.
- Exercise as tolerated unless your other medical problems prevent it.

The DON'Ts

- Do not forget to take your usual medications.
- Do not ignore worsening chest pain. Seek medical attention immediately.

When to Call Your Doctor

- If you have side effects of your medication.
- If you have new or worsening symptoms such as shortness of breath, chest pain, or fainting.

For More Information

Consult a textbook on cardiology at your local library or at a medical school in your region. Contact the American Heart Association at 1-800-242-8721 and ask for the literature department.

MULTIPLE MYELOMA

About Your Diagnosis

Multiple myeloma is cancer of the mature lymphocytes (plasma cells). A lymphocyte is a white blood cell involved in the immune system. Lymphocytes are produced in the bone marrow (the soft substance in the center of bones). They produce antibodies that attack any foreign substance (eg, virus, bacteria) in the body. The cause of multiple myeloma is not known. Many different theories exists, including genetic, viral, and radiation-related causes. More than 14,000 new cases of multiple myeloma were diagnosed last year in the United States. The disease is not contagious.

Multiple myeloma is diagnosed when a patient has the following findings: (1) an abnormal protein in the blood, (2) characteristic findings on bone radiographs (x-rays), and (3) an abnormal bone marrow biopsy (marrow removed from the bone and examined under a microscope). There is no cure for multiple myeloma.

Living With Your Diagnosis

Symptoms of multiple myeloma are caused by (1) expansion and invasion of the bone marrow, which prevents formation of blood cells and (2) production of substances by the cancer cells. Bone pain is the most common symptom of multiple myeloma. The back is most often affected. Myeloma cells destroy the bone and release calcium into the blood system, leading to other complications, such as nerve compression, lower leg weakness, and kidney failure. Elevated calcium levels in the blood can cause increased urination, weakness, and confusion. Anemia and infections are common among patients with multiple myeloma.

Treatment

Once the diagnosis is confirmed, multiple myeloma is classified into one of three stages. To determine this, the physician orders blood tests and radiographs of the bones. The staging of the cancer gives a prognosis. Many people live longer than 5 years if they have disease in stage I; patients with stage III disease have an average survival time of 15 months.

Management of multiple myeloma may involve no treatment at all unless signs and symptoms of bone pain, elevated calcium level, kidney failure, anemia, or compression of the spinal cord are present. Decisions about starting chemotherapy, the choice of chemotherapeutic drugs, the duration of treatment, and monitoring response are made by an oncologist (physician specializing in cancer). Side effects of chemotherapy are nausea, vomiting, loss of appetite, weight loss, hair loss, easy bruising and bleeding, and infections.

Radiation therapy is used to relieve bone pain and medical emergencies such as compression of the spinal cord. Side effects of radiation depend on which part of the body is irradiated. If the pelvic area is irradiated, nausea, vomiting, diarrhea, urinary difficulties, and fatigue may occur.

Orthopedic operations are needed for bone fractures. Supportive treatment such as use of antibiotics for infections, diuretics (water pills) for elevated blood calcium levels, and narcotic pain medications for relief of pain improve well-being.

The DOs

- Stay active. This helps keep calcium in your bones.
- Drink lots of fluid. This is the first line of management of elevated calcium blood levels.
- Take your medications as prescribed. A diuretic may be prescribed to help keep your calcium level down. Medicines for pain and infections may be prescribed in the appropriate situations.
- Use back support if needed.

The DON'Ts

- Do not be immobile. This can lead to a rise in calcium level.
- Do not do heavy lifting.
- Do not be afraid to ask for pain medication. Multiple myeloma can be painful because it involves the bone.
- Do not miss follow-up appointments. Your physician needs to repeat blood tests, radiographs, and urine collections to monitor response to treatment or to decide to start treatment.

When to Call Your Doctor

- If you are having pain.
- If you are having fevers.
- If you are having back pain, leg numbness or weakness, stool or urinary incontinence (leaking or loss of control). These can be caused by compression on the spinal cord.

- If you notice blood in stool, urine, phlegm, or vomit.
- If you feel depressed.

For More Information

National Cancer Institute (NCI)
9000 Rockville Pike
Bethesda, MD 20892
Cancer Information Service
1-800-4-CANCER
American Cancer Society
1599 Clifton Road, N.E.
Atlanta, GA 30329
1-800-ACS-2345

MULTIPLE SCLEROSIS

About Your Diagnosis

Multiple sclerosis is a slowly progressive disease of the central nervous system affecting at least 300,000 young Americans. This results from multiple areas of damage or destruction of the protective covering (demyelination) of nerve fibers. Each nerve is covered by a protective myelin coating. The myelin is much like the insulation covering of an electrical wire. If it is damaged or partially stripped away, an electrical signal cannot be transmitted without being interrupted. With nerves, the interruption of the impulse causes symptoms such as numbness, tingling, or weakness in the extremities, dizziness, unsteady gait, changes in vision, and difficulty with speech. Symptoms vary among individuals. Some individuals may have only one mild symptom, whereas others may have numerous severe symptoms. Although there are many theories about the cause, no cause is definitively known. Multiple sclerosis is more common in women than men, and in temperate climates as compared with the tropics. In most cases, patients are seen between the ages of 20 and 40 years with one or more symptoms, depending on the sites of initial demyelination.

Most patients have symptoms that develop slowly and improve with treatment. They may be without symptoms for a long period (remission) and later have a recurrence (exacerbation). The remissions and exacerbations are unpredictable. Some individuals have a more severe form of multiple sclerosis that progresses despite treatment. Multiple sclerosis is most often diagnosed by obtaining a medical history and performing a physical examination; results of a magnetic resonance imaging (MRI) scan of the brain can assist in establishing the diagnosis. Talk with your physician about what you should expect with remissions and exacerbations.

Living With Your Diagnosis

Living with multiple sclerosis can be a challenge because the symptoms are unpredictable and variable. It is important to practice a healthy lifestyle and make the most of the periods of remission. Although there are no dietary restrictions for patients with multiple sclerosis, it is advisable to maintain a normal weight for your height. Adequate rest and a regular exercise program, such as daily walking, will help to maintain muscle strength, tone, and energy. Always check with your physician before beginning any exercise program.

Treatment

Although currently there is no known cure for multiple sclerosis, there are many treatments available. Exacerbations are often treated with steroid medications. These medications are often given through an intravenous line, which may require a hospital stay. Other medications, such as a hormone (ACTH) and beta-interferon have also been used for both the remission and exacerbation phase. Many centers are currently researching new medications and treatments for multiple sclerosis.

The DOs
- Get plenty of rest.
- Participate in a regular exercise program approved by your physician.
- Maintain a healthy diet.
- Tell your physician about any new or worsening symptoms.
- Continue to work and participate in activities you enjoy.
- Contact local or regional support groups.
- Keep all follow-up appointments with your physician for reassessment.
- Take all medications as prescribed.

The DON'Ts
- Don't ignore worsening changes in your symptoms, especially visual changes, because these sometimes can be arrested if medication is begun promptly.
- Don't begin any new medications without your physician's approval.

When to Call Your Doctor
- If you have any problems associated with your medication.
- If you have facial weakness or weakness of a limb, partial blindness, and/or pain in one eye.

For More Information

Center for Neurologic Study
11211 Sorrento Valley Road, Suite H
San Diego, CA 92121
619-455-5463
National Multiple Sclerosis Society
733 Third Avenue
New York, NY 10017-3288
212-986-3240
e-mail: info@nmss.org
Multiple Sclerosis Association of America
706 Haddonfield Road
Cherry Hill, NJ 08002
800-833-4672
609-488-4500
World Wide Web
http://www.cnsonline.org
http://www.nmss.org

MUMPS

About Your Diagnosis

Mumps is a contagious viral infection that causes painful swelling of the salivary glands on both or either side of the jaw. Mumps had been a common childhood illness before the mumps vaccine became available. Since then, the incidence of mumps has decreased dramatically. Mumps is transmitted by airborne droplets or direct contact. Individuals with mumps are contagious 48 hours before the swelling begins and up to 6 days after it begins. It can take up to 3 weeks for symptoms to occur after exposure to the virus.

Living With Your Diagnosis

Signs and symptoms include fever, loss of appetite, fatigue, headache, sore throat, and painful swelling of the glands on either side of the jaw. The pain increases with chewing, swallowing, and drinking sour or acidic liquids. Recovery usually takes 10 days and leaves you with a lifetime immunity to the disease.

Treatment

Warm or cool compresses to the jaw can be applied to help ease the discomfort. Nonaspirin products such as Tylenol or Advil can be used for pain and fever. Don't use aspirin in children younger than 16 years with a viral infection. If fever is high, you can also use tepid sponge baths to reduce it. Increase fluid intake, but avoid acidic or sour liquids. Avoid spicy foods or foods that trigger salivation or require a lot of chewing. Rest until the fever disappears and strength returns. A child must be kept home from school until no longer contagious—about 8–9 days after swelling occurs.

The DOs
- Rest during the period of fever and until strength returns.
- Apply warm or cool compresses several times a day to the jaw to help ease the discomfort.
- Give Tylenol for fever and pain.
- Use tepid sponge baths to help reduce the fever.
- Increase the intake of fluids.
- Avoid sour or acidic liquids, which may cause more pain.
- Eat a soft diet without spicy irritating foods that may trigger salivation or require a lot of chewing.
- Keep a child home from school until no longer contagious—approximately 8 or 9 days.

The DON'Ts
- Don't give aspirin to a child younger than 16 years. The use of aspirin has been shown to increase the risk of developing Reye's syndrome when a viral infection is present.
- Don't drink sour or acidic liquids.
- Don't eat foods that require a lot of chewing or that are spicy.
- Don't send a child to school until the contagious period has lapsed—approximately 8 or 9 days.

When to Call Your Doctor
- If vomiting and diarrhea occur.
- If the temperature rises to more than 101°F.
- If a severe headache develops that is not relieved by Tylenol.
- If pain or swelling develops in the testicles.
- If a child becomes drowsy and cannot be kept awake.

For More Information
Write to request information
The American Academy of Pediatrics
141 NW Point Blvd.
Elk Grove Village, IL 60007-1098
National Institute of Allergy and Infectious Disease
301-496-5717
Internet Sites
www.healthfinder.gov (Choose SEARCH to search by topic.)
www.healthanswers.com

MYASTHENIA GRAVIS

About Your Diagnosis

Myasthenia gravis is a disease of the central nervous system that affects individuals of any age or ethnic group. It is characterized by sporadic muscular fatigue and weakness, occurring chiefly in the muscles of swallowing and chewing as well as the muscles of the eyes, face, and neck. The exact cause of myasthenia gravis not well understood, although it is believed to be a defect where the nerve meets the muscle. Also, the muscles of the arms and legs may become weak or easily fatigued. One of the first symptoms that many patients notice is double or blurred vision, and/or drooping of the eyelids. The muscles that control breathing may also be affected, which may result in shortness of breath. The symptoms of myasthenia gravis may get better (remission) for a period, then may worsen (exacerbation) for a period. The amount of time between remission and exacerbation is unpredictable. Unlike other disorders of the central nervous system, the progression of myasthenia gravis is exceedingly slow.

Myasthenia gravis is diagnosed by obtaining a medical history, performing a physical examination, and administering the "tensilon test." This test is performed in the hospital. The medication (tensilon) is injected through an intravenous line, and the physician observes the effect of the medication on the symptoms. The test usually takes about 30 minutes, but the patient is often observed for an hour or longer. Your physician will discuss the risks and benefits of this test with you. You may also need a computed tomography (CT) scan of your neck and upper chest to look for enlargement of the thymus gland.

Living With Your Diagnosis

Myasthenia gravis may affect your vision. If you are having double or blurred vision, you should avoid driving or operating heavy equipment and you should consult your eye doctor. There may be times when your ability to swallow will be affected. During those times, try foods of different consistency to determine what is easiest. Often thin liquids such as juice and water are more difficult to swallow than thick liquids. If you take medications regularly, ask your physician about liquid formulations instead of tablets.

One of the most frightening symptoms of myasthenia gravis is shortness of breath. This may occur at any time and may require medical attention. Your physician may request a test called a pulmonary function test. This is an office test that measures how well your lungs are working. It is usually done during a remission phase to determine a baseline so that testing during an exacerbation can be compared. If you have had shortness of breath, it is best to avoid smoke and dust. Wear a medic-alert bracelet or necklace in the event you have a sudden attack and need to be taken to a hospital.

Fatigue is a common symptom of myasthenia gravis so get plenty of rest. You may need brief rest periods during the day (about 10–15 minutes). Avoid strenuous work that may increase fatigue. If you have a stressful job, learn ways to manage stress more effectively. Often, employers or local schools offer seminars on stress management. A regular exercise program will also help with stress management, but check with your physician before beginning any exercise program.

Treatment

A short hospital stay is recommended to perform the necessary tests for diagnosis. Once the diagnosis is confirmed, treatment should begin. The goal of therapy is to treat the symptoms and to induce a period of remission. The most common medications used to treat myasthenia gravis are steroids and anticholinesterase medications (e.g., Mestinon). Your physician will discuss the medications and regimen best for you.

Try to maintain a daily exercise program as advised by your physician and physical therapist. They will teach you the proper exercises to strengthen and tone your muscles.

The DOs

- Get plenty of rest.
- Wear a medic-alert bracelet or necklace at all times that has "myasthenia gravis" engraved on it.
- Take your medications as prescribed.

The DON'Ts

- Don't use tobacco because it may worsen your shortness of breath.
- Avoid smoke (woodstoves, campfires).
- Avoid situations that may cause or aggravate allergies (pets, pollen, and dust).

When to Call Your Doctor

- If you have shortness of breath.

- If your symptoms worsen to include double vision, blurred vision, or weakness.
- If you have any problems associated with your medications.

For More Information

Myasthenia Gravis Foundation of America
222 South Riverside Plaza, Suite 1540
Chicago, IL 60606
800-541-5454

MYELODYSPLASTIC SYNDROMES

About Your Diagnosis

Myelodysplastic syndrome is a proliferation of abnormal bone marrow cells that leads to acute leukemia. There are five subtypes of this condition. Type I and Type II are characterized by refractory anemia. The other three types have an excessive number of *blasts* (leukemia cells). The higher the percentage of blasts, the shorter is the interval to development of leukemia. The cause is unknown in most instances. Chemotherapy and radiation therapy can be causative for so-called secondary myelodysplastic syndrome.

Myelodysplastic syndrome is uncommon. Among persons older than 60 years the incidence is 0.75 per 1000 per year. Less than 7% of patients are younger than 50 years. The disease occurs randomly. Some families have a predisposition to myelodysplasia.

Patients with anemia and low blood counts need to undergo examination. A blood smear review and examination of the bone marrow are necessary for diagnosis. Increased numbers of early blood cell precursors (blasts) are predictors of advanced disease. Special genetic analysis of the bone marrow cells helps define who has a poor prognosis.

Some young patients with a good prognosis can be cured with bone marrow transplantation. Combinations of chemotherapy and growth factors can cause remissions and improve the symptoms.

Living With Your Diagnosis

About 50% of patients have no symptoms. The most frequent sign is anemia (low red blood cell count and hemoglobin). Two thirds of patients also have a low white blood cell count or platelet count. With time 30% of patients have acute leukemia.

Pallor, excessive fatigue, and shortness of breath with exertion can occur with severe anemia. A low platelet count can lead to bleeding. The main risk of a low white blood cell count is development of serious infections.

Treatment

Supportive care with regular transfusions and antibiotics for infections is the mainstay of therapy. Transfusions with red blood cell and platelet concentrates support patients with low blood cell counts. Chemotherapy regimens with cytarabine, azacitidine, and etoposide can produce remissions, but the remissions are only temporary. Use of growth factors, erythropoietin, and filgastrim (Neupogen) can decrease the number of transfusions and episodes of infections for some patients. Different agents, such as vitamin A and D analogs, interferon, steroids, and androgen hormones can be tried, but they have limited success. Supplements with folic acid and vitamin B_6 (pyridoxine) are beneficial. A small proportion of young patients benefit from bone marrow transplantation.

Chemotherapeutic drugs, which can decrease blood counts even more during treatment, cause nausea and vomiting. Special antinausea medications and blood cell growth factors can prevent these effects. Bone marrow transplantation can have toxic effects on the liver, lungs, and brain and predispose to infections. The most serious complication of transplantation is graft-versus-host disease, in which the bone marrow cells of the donor attack the patient. This can be prevented and treated with immunosuppressive drugs. Long-term use of transfusions can lead to iron overload. A special iron-excreting drug can be administered with the transfusions.

The DOs

- Consider the option of bone marrow transplantation, either from a close relative or a suitable unrelated donor. The risks and benefits of this procedure are different for individual patients.
- Obtain a vaccination for hepatitis if you are undergoing transfusions. Revaccination is needed after transplantation.
- Use medical alert identification.
- Discuss contraceptive measures with your physician.
- Inform household members not to be vaccinated with live viruses (eg, polio) if you have undergone bone marrow transplantation.

The DON'Ts

- Avoid use of aspirin and aspirin-like medications; they can worsen the bleeding. Discuss use of other medications with your physician. Some medicines can lower blood counts.
- Avoid fresh vegetables and fruit, cheese and yogurt if you have a low white blood cell count.
- Avoid moderate and strenuous exercise if you have severe anemia. • Avoid interactive and potentially traumatic activities if you have a low platelet count.
- Avoid large crowds and persons who have signs

of infections if you have a low white blood cell count.

When to Call Your Doctor
- If you experience fever, bleeding, chest pain, or dizziness.

For More Information
Leukemia Society of America
600 Third Ave.
New York, NY 10016
800-955-4LSA
American Cancer Society
http://www.cancer.org
MedMark Hematology: http://medmark.bit.co.kr/hematolo.html
Blood & Marrow Transplant Newsletter
http://nysernet.org/bcic/bmt.news.html

MYELOPROLIFERATIVE DISORDERS

About Your Diagnosis

Myeloproliferative disorders are abnormal proliferation of one or more bone marrow cell lines. Four types are recognized. Polycythemia vera is mostly a disease of increased red blood cells. Chronic myelogenous leukemia (CML) is a disease of the white blood cell series. Essential thrombocytosis presents itself with an abnormally elevated platelet count. Myelofibrosis frequently manifests itself with low blood cell counts secondary to bone marrow fibrosis from overgrowth of blood cell precursors. All these conditions originate from an abnormality in the early blood cell progenitors and may evolve into acute leukemia.

The cause of myeloproliferative disorders is unknown. Survivors of atomic bomb explosions and patients treated with radiation for some types of cancer have an increased incidence of CML.

Myeloproliferative disorders are uncommon. Polycythemia vera occurs among 5 per 1 million persons per year; the other subtypes are less frequent. The mean age of patients is 60 years. Myeloproliferative disorders occur sporadically. They are not contagious.

Patients with elevated blood cell counts should undergo examination of a blood smear and bone marrow, which help establish the diagnosis. Additional tests, such as red blood cell counts and measurement of plasma volumes for polycythemia vera and platelet function for essential thrombosis may be necessary. It is important to rule out elevation of blood cell counts due to other conditions, such as lung disease, smoking, congenital heart anomalies, infections, tumors, and iron deficiency. Analysis of the genetic material (chromosomes) is essential to detect Philadelphia chromosome, which is diagnostic of CML.

Patients with polycythemia vera, essential thrombosis, or myelofibrosis can be treated effectively with specific medications. However, these disorders cannot be eradicated. Patients with CML can undergo curative bone marrow transplantation.

Living With Your Diagnosis

An increase in red blood cells causes an increase in blood viscosity and clotting. Elevation of the platelet count in essential thrombosis can predispose a person to both thrombosis and bleeding.

Myelofibrosis can first present itself with elevated blood cell counts but uniformly leads to lowering of these counts. Anemia and low white blood cell and platelet counts follow. Breakdown of the increased number of blood cells leads to an increase in uric acid. Most patients have an enlarged spleen, and many have an enlarged liver.

Increased viscosity can manifest itself as ruddy complexion, headaches, visual disturbances, lightheadedness, and shortness of breath. Patients with myeloproliferative disorders are at risk for strokes, heart attacks, and impaired circulation in the legs. Pain and whitening in the fingers and toes can occur. Bleeding from the mouth or gastrointestinal tract and easy bruising may be noticed. Itching, especially after a hot bath, is characteristic of polycythemia vera. An enlarged spleen can cause pain, heaviness in the left side of the abdomen, and a feeling of early satiety. An increased uric acid level can cause kidney stones and swelling of the joints (gout). Low blood cell counts show as anemia, fatigue, and pallor. A low white blood cell count predisposes to infections and a low platelet count to bleeding.

Hydroxyurea is administered as a pill daily, depending on your blood cell counts. Your physician monitors the blood counts and adjusts the dose.

Treatment

The chemotherapeutic drug hydroxyurea controls elevated blood cell counts for most patients. Anagrelide is indicated for elevated platelet counts in essential thrombosis and other conditions. Patients with polycythemia vera need treatment with regular phlebotomies (blood letting). Radioactive phosphorus is rarely used, mostly for elderly patients with polycythemia vera and essential thrombosis. Patients with anemia of myelofibrosis can benefit from use of androgen hormones and may need transfusions. Splenectomy or radiation to the spleen may offer relief to patients with painfully enlarged spleens.

Patients with CML receive specific treatment with interferon-alfa and chemotherapeutic agents. Young patients may undergo bone marrow transplantation.

Hydroxyurea can lower the white blood cell count and cause a rash and abdominal discomfort. Androgenic hormones can cause abnormal liver function and hair growth in a male pattern. Interferon-alfa can cause fever, fatigue, and flu-like symptoms.

Use of radioactive phosphorus is associated with increased risk for leukemia. For this reason it is reserved for elderly patients who are intolerant of other therapies. Anagrelide can worsen symptoms among patients with congestive heart failure. Interferon-alfa can cause abnormal liver and kidney function.

The complications of bone marrow transplantation are infection, toxic effects on the internal organs, and graft-versus-host disease, in which donor cells attack the recipient.

Phlebotomies are the treatment of choice among younger patients with polycythemia vera. The procedures are performed every other day initially (more cautiously for patient with heart disease or who have had a stroke). When the red blood cell count stabilizes, phlebotomy can be performed monthly. Patients who undergo any surgical procedure may need additional phlebotomies before the operation.

Anagrelide is a pill taken daily. Platelet counts should be regularly checked. Interferon is given as an injection under the skin, every day or every other day. Dose adjustments are necessary, depending on the tolerance of the drug. Allopurinol lowers uric acid level and prevents kidney stones and gout. Antihistamines improve itching for patients with polycythemia vera. Aspirin improves tenderness of the toes and fingers.

The DOs
- Take your medications as prescribed.
- Keep appointments with your physician for blood counts and dosage adjustments.
- Keep your phlebotomy appointments.
- Have your platelet counts checked regularly if you are taking anagrelide.
- Discuss your other medications with a medical professional; the drugs may interfere with your treatment.

The DON'Ts
- Do not take aspirin without consulting your physician.
- Abstain from fresh leafy vegetables and fruit, cheeses and yogurt if you have a low white blood cell count.
- Avoid interactive, potentially traumatic sports, because of bleeding risk.

When to Call Your Doctor
- If you have fatigue, chest pain, or shortness of breath that does not resolve with rest.
- If you have severe headaches, sudden weakness in one arm or leg, difficulty speaking, fever, or bleeding.

For More Information
Chronic Myelogenous Leukemia Patient Guide
Polycythemia Vera Patient Guide
Leukemia Society of America
600 Third Ave.
New York, NY 10016
800-955-4LSA
National Heart, Lung, and Blood Institute Information Center
P.O. Box 30105
Bethesda MD 20824-0105
301-251-1222
MedMark Hematology: http://medmark.bit.co.kr/hematol.html

MYOCARDITIS

About Your Diagnosis

Myocarditis is inflammation of the heart muscle. It is caused by an inflammatory response to an injury or infection. It may be caused by radiation or side effects of some medications. Most commonly it is caused by a virus, even the virus that causes the common cold.

Chest pain, difficulty breathing, fever or chills, inability to exercise, or feeling fatigued and run down much of the time are some of the early symptoms of myocarditis. The chest pain is from fluid collection in the lining of the heart. Some patients have a rash or joint pain (arthritis) related to rheumatic fever (from previous streptococcal infection) or other infection that can cause the myocarditis. Abnormal rhythms in the electrical activity of the heart (arrhythmias) may result from irritation of the heart muscle. This may cause a rapid heartbeat (palpitations) or lead to heart failure (the heart does not pump blood efficiently).

Myocarditis is detected through findings at a physical examination or on an electrocardiogram (ECG). Laboratory tests may be performed to help find the cause. Biopsy of the heart muscle sometimes is needed to confirm the diagnosis.

Living With Your Diagnosis

Rarely are additional tests needed. Symptoms generally clear up with rest and time. Avoid strenuous exercise until the condition has completely cleared. Exercise increases the work of the heart, and this may cause the inflammatory reaction to worsen rapidly and may cause dangerous heart rhythm disturbances.

Treatment

Management of chest pain and arrhythmias is most important. If heart failure occurs, treatment of this disorder is needed. Nonsteroidal anti-inflammatory drugs (NSAIDs) may be used to manage the inflammation and ease the chest pain. In more severe instances, steroid-containing medications or immunosuppressive drugs are used. These medications can cause severe stomach and intestinal irritation and may cause nausea, vomiting, or diarrhea. These drugs must be taken with food. They are to be avoided by patients with a history of ulcers or reactions to these medicines. Aspirin is used to manage fevers and joint pain. Antibiotics are given for acute rheumatic fever or other infections.

The DOs

• Take your medications as prescribed to manage symptoms and infections.
• Rest.

The DON'Ts

• Avoid exercise until your ECG is normal and you have clearance from your doctor.

When to Call Your Doctor

• If you cannot tolerate your medicines or have a reaction to them.
• If you have new or worsening chest pain, shortness of breath, or fainting
• If you notice blood in your vomit or stools.

For More Information
Contact the American Heart Association at 1-800-242-8721 and ask for the literature department.

NARCOLEPSY

About Your Diagnosis

Narcolepsy is a sleep disorder caused by a generalized disorganization of the sleep-waking functions within the brain. It often causes excessive daytime sleepiness, regardless of the amount of sleep that you have had. The exact cause remains undetermined but rarely may follow brain trauma or accompany other types of neurologic disease. Tissue typing has shown that some individuals are more genetically susceptible to this disorder.

Living With Your Diagnosis

Generally, the symptoms of narcolepsy are first noticed in teenagers and young adults but may go undiagnosed for years.

Another common symptom of this disorder is cataplexy, a partial or complete weakness of the skeletal muscles brought on by intense emotions such as laughter, excitement, or anger. Other symptoms may include (1) sleep attacks—short unintentional periods of sleep during the day; or (2) sleep paralysis—the inability to move as one drifts into or out of sleep. Also, some patients have hypnagogic hallucinations or visual or auditory experiences that occur when going to sleep or waking, which are hard to differentiate from reality. Others have disturbed nighttime sleep including frequent tossing and turning and awakening.

Treatment

There is no known cure for narcolepsy. No single therapy will control all the symptoms. Some medical stimulants combined with strategically placed 15- to 20-minute naps may improve the otherwise disabling effects of this sleep disorder. The timing and frequency of the scheduled naps has to be determined for each individual according to the usual time of the sleep attacks.

The DOs

- Take your medications as prescribed.
- Get plenty of rest.
- Educate your friends and family about your disorder.

The DON'Ts

- Avoid operating machinery and power tools unless cleared by your physician.
- Do not drive unless approved by your physician.

- Avoid situations that may pose danger for you should you fall asleep or lose muscle control.

When to Call Your Doctor

- If you have any problems associated with your medications.
- If your symptoms increase in frequency or severity.

For More Information...
American Sleep Disorders Association (ASDA)
1610 14th St., N.W.
Rochester, MN 55901-2200
507-287-6006
e-mail: asda@millcomm.com
Narcolepsy Network
P.O. Box 42460
Cincinnati, OH 45242
513-891-3522
National Sleep Foundation
1367 Connecticut Ave.
Washington, DC 20036
e-mail: natsleep@haven.ios.com
World Wide Web
http://www.uic.edu/depts/cnr/facts.html
http://www.wisc.edu/asds
http://www.sleepfoundation.org

NECK PAIN

About Your Diagnosis

The neck is made up of the vertebrae (neck bones), spinal cord (which contains the nerves), disks between the vertebrae, and the surrounding soft tissue such as the muscles and ligaments. The vertebrae, or bony part of the spine, protects the spinal cord. Neck pain may be caused by an injury or disease that affects this area.

Neck pain commonly occurs after one lies in an uncomfortable position for a prolonged period or as the result of poor posture. It may occur in association with diseases such as osteoarthritis, rheumatoid arthritis, ankylosing spondylitis, and fibromyalgia. Neck pain may result from an injury to the neck. Stress which causes increased muscle tension may worsen neck pain.

A physician diagnoses neck pain by taking a medical history, performing a physical examination, and possibly ordering radiographs (x-rays). The physician may order blood tests to determine whether the neck pain is due to diseases that may cause similar symptoms. Computed tomography (CT), magnetic resonance imaging (MRI), or a bone scan may be performed if the physician needs a clearer picture of the bones, nerves, disks between the vertebrae, and other soft tissue. Sometimes an electromyogram (EMG), which helps identify muscle and nerve problems, may be obtained if the doctor believes the neck problem may be causing numbness or tingling in the arms due to pressure on the nerves.

Living With Your Diagnosis

You may experience difficulty looking from side to side, driving, and reading. Sometimes the pain may keep you awake at night. Neck pain can cause headaches. If the neck pain lasts for months, it may affect your ability to do your job.

Treatment

Management of neck pain depends on the cause of the pain. If the pain is due to an injury, your physician may recommend the use of heat or ice on the affected area. Sometimes the physician may prescribe acetaminophen or nonsteroidal anti-inflammatory drugs (NSAIDs) to decrease the pain. If the pain is particularly severe, stronger narcotic-containing pain medicines may be needed for a short time. If you ex-perience muscle spasms, your doctor may prescribe a muscle relaxant. Physical therapy may be helpful to decrease the neck pain by means of deep heat treatments, traction, or exercise.

All medications have side effects. NSAIDs may cause stomach upset, diarrhea, ulcers, headache, dizziness, difficulty hearing, or a rash. Some side effects of muscle relaxants are drowsiness, dizziness, and a rash.

The DOs

- Take your medications as prescribed.
- Call your doctor if you are experiencing side effects from medications.
- Practice good posture when sitting and standing.
- Ask your doctor about the use of a cervical pillow.
- Perform neck exercises every day.

The DON'Ts

- Do not wait to see whether a possible side effect of medication goes away on its own.

When to Call Your Doctor

- If you experience side effects of medications.
- If you continue to have neck pain or headaches.
- If you have numbness or tingling in your arms.
- If you need a referral to a physical therapist.

For More Information

Contact the National Arthritis Foundation in your area. If you do not know the location of the Arthritis Foundation, call the national office at 1-800-283-7800 or access information through the Internet at www.arthritis.org.

NEPHROTIC SYNDROME

About Your Diagnosis

Each kidney is composed of 1 million fine filters to cleanse the blood of poisons. They are designed to keep the desired components in the bloodstream and to excrete the harmful substances. Sometimes there is "leakiness" of the filter leading to the loss of proteins from the blood. The loss of these proteins can result in swelling (edema), seen initially in the ankles and face. This entity is termed nephrotic syndrome.

There are a variety of kidney problems that can lead to nephrotic syndrome: the most common are primary inflammatory states of the kidney (called glomerulonephritis), and there are other diseases that can damage the kidney as a consequence. The condition is not transmissible. Nephrotic syndrome is seen frequently in kidney practice, although it is unusual in a general practice. It can vary in severity from patient to patient.

Typically, most patients see their physician because of swollen ankles/legs, or even a swollen face observed at first rising in the morning. The doctor finds protein in the urine on testing. Subsequent blood tests will confirm the diagnosis of nephrotic syndrome. In order for a cause to be diagnosed, to direct therapy, you may see a nephrologist for a biopsy. This is where the physician takes a small piece of kidney tissue with a special needle (no surgery usually needed).

All patients with nephrotic syndrome will have a tendency to high cholesterol levels in the blood. Some patients have a progressive loss in kidney function after developing this condition.

Living With Your Diagnosis

Nephrotic syndrome is a painless condition under most circumstances. Patients may gain massive amounts of water weight, to their distress and discomfort. Pain may be a sign of an underlying new infection, a clot in the leg or pelvis (especially if accompanied by redness and local tenderness), or inflammation in the abdomen. There will be a tendency to hold on to the water and salt that you take with your diet; hence the need for diet modification.

You will have a high cholesterol level that might require medications to help improve it, in addition to the dietary recommendations your doctor will suggest.

Treatment

Initially, the doctor will begin "water pills" (diuretics) to remove excess water (e.g., furosemide [Lasix]). Occasionally you might need to rest in hospital so the Lasix can be given by vein to be more effective. It is ideal to weigh yourself daily to see how successful the diuretic therapy is. There are additional and alternative diuretics that may be used, depending on the severity of the nephrotic edema and its responsiveness. Depending on your biopsy results, you might be offered treatment with powerful drugs against inflammation: prednisone, cyclophosphamide, or chlorambucil, for example.

Your doctor will want you to remain as active as possible because nephrotic syndrome is associated with an increased tendency to develop clots in the legs.

There are side effects seen with these drugs. Lasix can cause a rash, low blood pressure, and low potassium and magnesium levels (these will be monitored closely by your physician). Prednisone can lead to hypertension, high blood glucose, stomach irritation, osteoporosis, and changes in the skin, to name a few (your physician can counsel you on the remainder of effects).

The DOs

- Do stay out of bed and mobile to encourage fluid loss and discourage clots.
- Do take the diuretic pills as often as they are prescribed. They may prove less effective because of poor absorption from the gut, so large doses might be needed.
- Do take the dietary and fluid intake to heart: the purpose of the therapy is to reduce the amount of salt and water in your system.
- Do avoid foods rich in cholesterol.
- Do eat plenty of calories to help keep your strength up while the treatment is underway.
- Do weigh yourself daily and keep a log to map your progress and halt a decline.

The DON'Ts

- Don't become sedentary.
- Don't smoke.
- Don't take over-the-counter pills (especially nonsteroidal drugs like ibuprofen or Naproxen) that will confound the medical management of nephrotic syndrome.

- Don't forget the diet and fluid restrictions to help you get better faster.
- Don't forget your medicines. Call the physician if there is a problem taking them.
- Don't forget to weigh yourself to monitor progress.

When to Call Your Doctor

Call your physician if you have shortness of breath, or pain in the chest, abdomen, or legs. Call if you have fevers or chills. Record your weights and let your doctor know how the treatment is going. Always tell your doctor if you have problems with the therapy. A simple, timely explanation may go a long way to reassure you and your family members.

For More Information

You can read the pamphlet on nephrotic syndrome available from the National Kidney Foundation (NKF). Your local office of the NKF may be reached at 1-800-622-9010 or by writing the Head Office at 30 East 33rd Street, New York, NY 10016.

OBESITY

About Your Diagnosis

Obesity is an increased percentage of total body fat compared to normal. Overweight is an increased body weight relative to height. Both factors have an important impact on overall health.

Obesity is caused by an excess of caloric intake in the diet relative to caloric output by physical activity. Both genetic and environmental factors appear to be important in obesity.

According to the National Center for Health Statistics, greater than 40% of men and women older than 35 years are obese. This percentage continues to increase every year.

Body mass index (BMI) is one measure to determine whether someone is overweight. Body mass index is derived as follows:

$$BMI = Weight (kg) / Height^2 (m^2).$$

Lowest mortality is associated with a BMI between 22 and 25 according to life insurance tables. The U.S. Department of Health and Human Services recommends that men and women aged 19–35 years maintain a BMI between 19 and 25. Individuals older than 35 years should maintain a BMI of 21–27. Treatment is indicated for those individuals with a BMI greater than 27 who have other diseases, such as high blood pressure, diabetes, pulmonary hypertension, or coronary artery disease. Treatment is indicated in all individuals with a BMI greater than 30.

To determine the relative obesity of an individual, estimates are made of body fat content using skinfold measurements. Body fat distribution is determined by measuring waist and hip size. Males with a body fat content greater than 25%, and females with a body fat content greater than 33% are considered obese. An increased waist-to-hip ratio is a risk factor for diabetes and heart disease. Other techniques to measure body fat content are available but mainly used for obesity research.

Numerous treatments are available to reduce body weight or fat and decrease the risk of medical complications from obesity.

Living With Your Diagnosis

Obesity is a risk factor for high blood pressure, diabetes, coronary artery disease, and pulmonary hypertension. It adds strain to arthritic joints.

Treatment

Diet, exercise, medications, and surgery have all been used to treat obesity. Individuals 20% to 40% above ideal body weight or with a BMI of 27–30 should follow a low-fat, low-calorie diet in the range of 1,200–1,800 kilocalories per day. This should be designed by a registered dietician. Those 41% to 100% over the ideal body weight or with a BMI between 30 and 40 may benefit from short-term, very low calorie diets in the range of 400–800 kilocalories per day to achieve rapid weight loss over the short-term. Medical supervision is required for such a restrictive diet.

Exercise is very effective in reducing weight over the long-term. An individualized, medically supervised exercise program is recommended to prevent complications.

Few medications are available for treating obesity. A careful trial of diet and exercise must be instituted before resorting to the use of medicines. Amphetamines may lead to weight loss, but their use is limited because they cause anxiety and tremulousness. Dietary fat absorption inhibitors such as orlistat are available to limit the amount of calories that enter the bloodstream. This medicine causes flatulence and diarrhea.

Surgery is an option for the morbidly obese who are greater than 100% above their ideal body weight or have a BMI over 40. Gastric bypass or vertical band gastroplasty are the procedures of choice. Surgery leads to rapid weight loss over 12–18 months, with successful long-term weight reduction maintained in many patients. These procedures should be reserved for patients who have failed all other therapy. Infection, poor wound healing, and dumping syndrome (abdominal cramping or diarrhea) are potential complications that must be considered before undergoing surgery.

The DOs

- Learn your current weight, body mass index, and body fat content.
- Understand your risk factors for diabetes and heart disease.
- Begin a medically supervised diet and exercise program before considering medicines for your obesity.
- Consider surgery if you are greater than 100% above your ideal body weight and no other treatment has been successful

The DON'Ts
- Don't smoke cigarettes to control body weight.
- Don't follow fad diets.
- Don't become discouraged if your weight stabilizes after an initial weight loss.

When to Call Your Doctor

- Your weight continues to increase despite diet and exercise.
- You have side effects from the medicines prescribed.
- You have severe diarrhea or low blood sugars after surgery.

For More Information

Weight Control Information Network (WIN) of the National Institute of Diabetes, Digestive, and Kidney Diseases
One Win Way
Bethesda, MD 20892
1-800-WIN-8098
http:\\www.niddk.nih.gov\NUTRITIONDOCS.html.
Food and Nutrition Information Center USDA/National Agricultural Library, Room 304
10301 Baltimore Boulevard
Beltsville, MD 20705-2531
Center for Nutrition Policy and Promotion USDA
1120 20th Street NW, Suite 200 North Lobby
Washington, DC 20036.
American Diabetes Association
1-800-342-2383.

OBSESSIVE COMPULSIVE DISORDER

About Your Diagnosis

Obsessive compulsive disorder (OCD) is a fascinating and occasionally very disabling syndrome characterized by two components: obsessions and compulsions. The obsessions are unwanted, frequently occurring thoughts that the person has no control over and is unable to block. Obsessions can also be thoughts or impulses that you may be unable to dismiss, despite finding them very disturbing. Compulsions are behaviors. They are often repetitive behaviors that are intended to decrease anxiety. To diagnose OCD, these intrusive thoughts and compulsive behaviors must lead to some problem in your social or work life. The underlying problem with OCD is usually anxiety, and OCD occurs slightly more frequently in women than in men.

Living With Your Diagnosis

OCD usually begins in the late teens to early 20s. In most cases, the disease, once diagnosed, is fairly persistent without treatment. The obsessions, or abnormal thoughts, can be in many forms. Some common obsessions include aggressive obsessions, such as seeing violent images, the fear that you might harm others, that you might harm yourself, the fear of doing something embarrassing, the fear of acting on other impulses, such as robbing a bank, the fear of being responsible for things going wrong, and the fear that something terrible might happen. There are also contamination obsessions, which are disgusts with body waste, with dirt or germs, an excessive concern with environmental contaminants, and a concern that you will become ill beyond a reasonable expectation of that happening. Sexual obsessions include the fear that sexual activity might involve children, animals, incest, or homosexuality. There are also hoarding or collecting obsessions and religious obsessions. As can be seen, many of these obsessions involve socially unacceptable behaviors, which leads to feelings of guilt and increases the feeling of anxiety in patients who have them.

There are also many different kinds of compulsions. These include cleaning or handwashing compulsions, where individuals may wash their hands 50–60 times a day; counting compulsions; and checking compulsions, where individuals may get up during the night several times to make sure that appliances have been turned off, the door has been locked, and the windows have been closed. Even though individuals may not want to carry out these compulsive behaviors, they often are unable to control them. Some individuals may return to their home several times to make sure the door was locked and feel some relief of anxiety upon doing so. There are also repeating rituals and ordering or arranging compulsions, whereby individuals must have clothes, shoes, or dishes, for example, in a certain order, pointing a certain direction, to get some relief from their anxiety. These compulsive behaviors can occupy a large part of an individual's day and make other more productive activity less likely.

The diagnosis of OCD is usually easy to make and is based on the feelings of distress associated with the behaviors mentioned above. It is important to keep in mind that some individuals, by the nature of their personality, are perfectionists and like things ordered and arranged in a specific way. However, they are able to function well at their jobs and in their social relationships. These patients would not meet the criteria for OCD. It is those individuals who feel that their obsessions and compulsions are taking up the majority of their time, and are disturbed by this, who merit treatment. Often family members or a co-worker point out to the individual the obsessiveness of his behavior. Individuals who have OCD usually are aware of their behavior and would like to stop it, but are unable to do so.

Treatment

The treatment of OCD involves both medication and social intervention. Clomipramine, an older drug, or more likely one of the newer serotonin antidepressants such as Prozac, Zoloft, or Luvox are used to treat OCD. These drugs have been very effective in treating both the obsessions and compulsions associated with this condition. Side effects of clomipramine include blurred vision, racing heartbeat, dry mouth, and constipation, whereas side effects of the serotonin drugs include jitteriness or agitation, insomnia, weight loss, anorexia, and gastrointestinal distress.

The goals of any treatment are to reduce the frequency and intensity of symptoms as much as possible, and to minimize the amount of interference the symptoms cause in the patient's life. It is important to note that few patients experience a cure or complete remission of symptoms, but symptoms are usually much worse during times of psychological and psychosocial stress.

Behavior therapy is designed at decreasing the compulsive aspect of the condition. Compulsions such as handwashing are often very responsive to behavior therapy, where the patient makes a conscious effort to decrease the frequency of a compulsive behavior. The intent behind behavioral treatment of OCD is to convince the patient that although compulsion behavior decreases anxiety, this anxiety reduction is only short-term. However, if the individual resists the anxiety and urge to engage in the ritual behavior, the anxiety will eventually decrease on its own and the need to perform the ritual will eventually disappear. Because many patients are extremely distressed by the behavior, they may become impatient with behavioral therapy alone, and a combination of medications and behavior treatment may have to be used.

The DOs
- As with any anxiety condition, exercise can often be very helpful in decreasing feelings of nervousness and providing an outlet for them.

The DON'Ts
- Because of the strong anxiety component to OCD, drugs that produce stimulation or nervousness should be avoided. These, of course, include such illicit drugs as phencyclidine (PCP) and cocaine.
- The intake of foods and beverages that are high in caffeine should also be avoided.

When to Call Your Doctor
- If the anxiety associated with OCD increases to a point where you are having physical symptoms.
- If you begin having suicidal or homicidal thoughts.
- If the obsessive thoughts that you are having become increasingly bizarre. There is a potential for psychosis with this condition.

For More Information
Contact your local mental health center or crisis center line. For online information about OCD, check out the following Web sites:
http://www./g/ou.com/fairlight/ocd
http://mtech.csd.uwm. edu/~fairlite/ocd/htm/

ONYCHOMYCOSIS

About Your Diagnosis

Onychomycosis is an infection of the nails with fungal organisms. It is seen more frequently as individuals age. It occurs very frequently in elderly individuals who have poor circulation and in diabetics. The disorder is also seen more frequently in the toenails than in the fingernails. Usually a fungal infection of the feet (athlete's foot) is present along with the fungal infection of the toenails.

The diagnosis of this infection is made by the appearance of the nails, and also by scraping the nail and looking at the scrapings under the microscope. Cultures can also be done but are not usually necessary.

The fungi that most frequently cause this infection are called dermatophytes. These fungi are present all around us. It is not possible to pinpoint the manner in which the infection was acquired. Trauma to the nail makes the nail more likely to become infected. Broken skin on the feet makes it easier to acquire the athlete's foot that often precedes the infection of the nails. The warm, moist conditions that the feet are exposed to may partly explain why the toenails are more frequently infected than the fingernails.

Living With Your Diagnosis

Onychomycosis can vary in severity and in the depth of the infection of the nail. One or many nails may be involved. A very superficial infection is called superficial white onychomycosis and can be treated with medication applied to the nails. Other types of infection involve the nail bed to various degrees. The nails are usually thickened and may appear white, yellow, or even brownish. They also grow more slowly. There is an infection of the nails from another type of fungus called a yeast or *Candida* organism. This infection causes more inflammation than the skin fungi (dermatophytes).

Treatment

Fortunately two new drugs have recently been released that make curing this condition more likely than it was a few years ago.

Except for the superficial white form of the disorder, treatment with creams and lotions applied to the nails have little effect. Older treatment of this infection was with griseofulvin and required treatment for a year, especially for the toenails. There were also frequent relapses. If griseofulvin was not effective, then ketoconazole (Nizoral) was used.

The two newly available drugs are terbinafine HCl (Lamisil) and itraconazole (Sporanox). Treatment with both of these drugs is usually for 12 weeks for toenail involvement, although it takes much longer for the damaged nail to be replaced with healthy nail. Treatment of the fingernails takes about 6 weeks.

There are several regimens for the use of these drugs, and you and your doctor will decide which is best for you.

The most common side effects with terbinafine HCl are headache, diarrhea, and heartburn or dyspepsia. Cimetadine (Tagamet) should not be taken with this drug.

The most common side effects with itraconazole are nausea, vomiting, and diarrhea. Liver function tests may also become abnormal, and your doctor will want to check these several times while you are taking the drug. This drug must be taken with a full meal to be fully absorbed. Your physician should know all the other drugs you are taking when this drug (itraconazole) is prescribed because there are potentially serious side effects, especially with heart drugs, blood thinners, cholesterol-lowering drugs, and some drugs taken for anxiety.

The DOs

There is no specific food or diet that will help this condition. If you are diabetic, good control of the diabetes can make a less favorable climate for the fungus to grow. You also should keep your feet dry. You should wear shoes and socks that will let the air circulate and absorb moisture.

If you are diabetic and/or elderly and have trouble with trimming your toenails, a podiatrist will be very helpful and could help prevent serious problems with your feet.

The DON'Ts

Your physician may recommend that toenail fungus not be treated, especially if you are taking multiple other drugs. The older treatments took so long and there were so many relapses with treatment of the toenails that it often wasn't worthwhile. However, these newer drugs make a cure much more likely.

When to Call Your Doctor

You should call your doctor if you seem to be having a reaction to the medication that your doctor prescribed for you. Your doctor may also want to do occasional laboratory tests to check your liver or kidney function if you are taking certain of the medicines long-term. If the toes or fingers crack around the nails, become red and tender, or drain, you also need to see your doctor. Sometimes you will lose your nail. It will regrow but it may be somewhat deformed.

For More Information
Your local podiatric association
The American Medical Association Family Medical Guide, 3rd edition.
The American Academy of Family Physician's Family Health and Medical Guide
Word Publishing, 1997.
The PDR Family Guide to Prescription Drugs, 3rd edition.

OSGOOD-SCHLATTER DISEASE

About Your Diagnosis

Osgood-Schlatter disease is a painful condition that usually affects the rapidly growing knee. The pain is located at the bony prominence just below the kneecap where the tendon attaches to the leg bone (tibia). Some physicians believe that the bony attachment actually tries to pull away from the leg bone, resulting in acute inflammation and tenderness. It is usually due to inflammation of a small growth plate in that area. Radiographs (x-rays) sometimes reveal a small piece of bone that is separated from the attachment site.

Living With Your Diagnosis

Osgood-Schlatter disease usually responds to a modification in activity level until the attachment site heals. Healing may be more difficult than first suspected, particularly for adolescents. The pain generally disappears when the attachment site finally fuses to the leg bone. Depending on the severity of the symptoms, you may have to suspend some or all athletic activity.

Treatment

Most cases of Osgood-Schlatter disease respond to a fairly brief period of inactivity during the most painful phase. However, some cases require more aggressive treatment. A cylinder cast may be necessary in particularly painful cases. Regular doses of aspirin may be needed. Anti-inflammatory medications may be helpful. Physical therapy can then be directed at proper stretching and strengthening. Aggressive stretching and strengthening exercises can be effective in preventing recurrences. Surgical treatment is not indicated unless the attachment site fractures from the leg.

The DOs
- Rest and immobilize the area as needed.
- Take your medications as prescribed.
- Exercise as directed.

The DON'Ts
- Do not insert anything inside the cast to scratch. This can cause a skin sore, which can become infected.

When to Call Your Doctor
- If the pain begins to limit your activities or if it has returned after treatment.

For More Information
http://www.mayo.ivi.com/mayo/askphys/qacurr_3.htm
http://www.vh.org/Patients/IHB/FamilyPractice/AFP/June1995/Knee.html

OSTEOARTHRITIS

About Your Diagnosis

Osteoarthritis (OA) is also called "wear and tear" arthritis or degenerative joint disease. Osteoarthritis commonly affects the weight-bearing joints of the body such as the hips, knees, and spine, but it may also affect the hands (Fig 1). In OA, the cushion on the end of the bone, the cartilage, begins to wear down resulting in pain.

Although the exact cause of OA is unknown, a variety of factors may increase an individual's risk of developing OA. In the past, it was believed that OA developed as an individual got older because the joints "just wore out." However, age is just one cause of OA. Obesity, repetitive movements, and a prior severe injury to a joint can lead to OA. Osteoarthritis of the fingers develops more frequently in women than in men. Osteoarthritis occurs more frequently in some families.

Osteoarthritis is not an infectious illness. In other words, you cannot "catch" OA from another individual. A physician can diagnose OA by obtaining a medical history, performing an examination of the joints, and ordering x-rays. An x-ray will show that the joint space (where the cartilage separates the two bones) is narrowed or absent. The x-ray may also show bone spurs that can be responsible for some of the pain. Blood tests are usually normal in osteoarthritis.

Living With Your Diagnosis

Most individuals begin to notice OA as gradual joint pain and stiffness, most commonly in the hands, knees, hips, and back. Pain and stiffness usually worsen with activity and toward the end of the day. Osteoarthritis may also affect the neck and feet. Pain and stiffness may make it more difficult to perform some daily activities such as bending at the waist, grasping or reaching for objects, turning the neck, and walking or climbing stairs. There is no cure for OA; however, medications, exercises, and assistive devices can decrease the pain and improve one's quality of life.

Treatment

The best management of OA is a combination of different treatments. Acetaminophen or nonsteroidal anti-inflammatory drugs (NSAIDs) are used to decrease the pain and stiffness. Potential side effects of NSAIDs include stomach upset, ulcers, constipation, diarrhea, headaches, dizziness, difficulty hearing, and a rash. The NSAIDs should be taken with food. A physical therapist can provide exercises to strengthen muscles that provide stability to the joints, which may help decrease pain. Water exercise programs may be particularly beneficial because the water decreases the stress on the joints. An occupational therapist provides hand exercises and may discuss ways to do certain activities differently or suggest an assistive device to avoid pain. Joint surgery such as a hip or knee replacement may be recommended if the pain is particularly severe and if an x-ray shows there is no space between the two bones of a joint.

The DOs

- Take your medication as prescribed.
- Ask your doctor what over-the-counter pain medications you may take with your prescription medications.
- Eat a well-balanced diet and lose those extra pounds if you are overweight.
- Perform a physician-prescribed exercise program, because exercise can decrease the pain of osteoarthritis.

The DON'Ts

- Wait to see whether a side effect from the medication will go away.
- Overeat and assume a gain of 2 or 3 pounds a year will not affect the pain of OA.
- Continue an exercise program that causes pain. If pain after exercise continues, it usually means the exercise needs to be modified specifically for you.

When to Call Your Doctor

- You experience any medication side effects.
- The medication and other treatments are not decreasing the pain.
- You believe you may need a referral to a physical therapist or an occupational therapist.

For More Information

Contact the Arthritis Foundation in your area. If you do not know the location of the Arthritis Foundation, you may call the national office at 1-800-283-7800 or access information on the Internet at www.arthritis.org.

OSTEOCHONDRITIS DISSECANS

About Your Diagnosis

Osteochondritis dissecans is a term used to describe a finding on a radiograph (x-ray). It occurs most frequently in the knee joint, followed by the ankle and the elbow. The radiographic appearance is an area within the joint that is either darker or lighter than the surrounding bone. This abnormality eventually may lead to pain symptoms, but not always. It seems to occur more frequently among younger patients and is more common among men than women. The cause remains unclear, but it appears to be related to loss of blood supply in the underlying bone. This causes a small area of the bone to die, which results in a small crater near or in the joint.

Pain may be vague and intermittent, making the lesion difficult to diagnose. If a portion of the joint loosens, the affected joint may lock and swell. Radiographs are obtained with the patient standing. Sometimes MRI is necessary to determine the extent of the lesion.

Living With Your Diagnosis

Osteochondritis dissecans may produce only intermittent symptoms and not require any formal treatment other than observation. Minor alterations in lifestyle may eliminate additional symptoms. When pain becomes constant or if the joint actually locks and does not bend or straighten, surgical treatment may be indicated.

Treatment

Pain in the knee, ankle, or elbow may occur for various reasons. The radiographic finding of an osteochondritis dissecans lesion does not necessarily explain the source of the pain, because many lesions do not become symptomatic. An evaluation is performed to determine whether the osteochondritis dissecans lesion is the true source of the pain. Rest, immobilization, and anti-inflammatory drugs can provide excellent results in most instances. No diets or exercise programs speed the healing process.

Surgical treatment rarely is necessary, particularly for young patients. When the joint is protected with a cast or brace, the lesion may heal uneventfully. If, however, the pain worsens or the lesion becomes unstable, surgical treatment may provide relief. Many lesions can be managed with arthroscopic techniques, but some may require open treatment.

The DOs

- Rest and immobilize the area as needed.
- Take your medications as prescribed.

The DON'Ts

- Do not continue to participate or compete in an activity that produces symptoms consistent with osteochondritis dissecans. Doing so may harm the affected joint.

When to Call Your Doctor

- If pain becomes consistent or suddenly changes.
- If the joint locks and does not bend or straighten. Your doctor may be able to gently manipulate it or may recommend surgical treatment.

OSTEOMYELITIS

About Your Diagnosis

Osteomyelitis is an infection of the bone, bone marrow, and soft tissue surrounding the bone. The infection is usually caused by a staphylococcal infection, but other bacteria can be responsible. The bacteria can obtain access to the bone through the bloodstream from a compound fracture or other trauma, a boil or any break in the skin, a middle ear infection, or pneumonia. Osteomyelitis is curable with prompt treatment.

Living With Your Diagnosis

Signs and symptoms include fever; pain, swelling, warmth, and redness over the infected bone or nearby joint; and pus draining through a skin abscess. Possible complications include the formation of an abscess that will not heal until the underlying bone heals, and permanent stiffness of the nearby joint.

Treatment

A doctor's treatment is necessary. Hospitalization may be needed to drain the abscess or to give high doses of antibiotics intravenously. Large doses of antibiotics will be needed, generally for a period of 8–10 weeks. Side effects of the antibiotics may include nausea, vomiting, diarrhea, headaches, and dizziness. Pain relievers may be needed, which may also cause stomach upset and constipation.

Keep the affected limb at rest, slightly elevated and immobilized with pillows. No weight-bearing should be placed on the lower limb if it is affected. If prolonged bed rest is needed, continue to actively exercise the other limbs and change position frequently.

The DOs

- Take the antibiotics until finished.
- Increase your fluid intake:
- Maintain a diet high in calories, protein, calcium, and vitamin C to promote bone healing.
- If you are on bedrest, change position frequently to prevent pressure sores. Check skin for any redness at the pressure points.
- Do frequent isometric exercises to prevent muscle weakness and maintain joint flexibility,
- Increase normal activities gradually after symptoms subside.

- Use sterile dressings if an open would is present. Wash hands before and after changing dressings. If family members are unsure of wound care, request a visiting nurse until comfortable with treatment.

The DON'Ts

- Don't skip doses or stop taking antibiotics until finished.
- Don't dangle the affected limb. Keep it slightly elevated.
- Don't bear weight if the affected area is your leg. Crutches may be of help for trips to the bathroom.

When to Call Your Doctor

- If fever increases during treatment.
- If pain becomes intolerable.
- If an abscess forms over the affected area.
- If drainage increases from an existing abscess.
- If side effects from the medications become severe.

For More Information

National Institute of Arthritis, Musculoskeletal and Skin Disorders of the NIH
301-495-4484
Internet Site
www.healthanswer.com

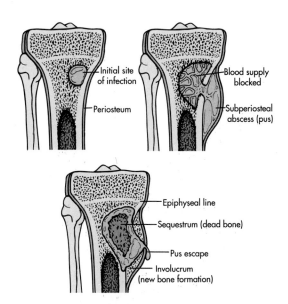

Development of osteomyelitis infection with involucrum and sequestrum. (From Lewis SM, Collier IC, Heitkemper MM: *Medical-Surgical Nursing: Assessment and Management of Clinical Problem*, vol. 4. St. Louis, Mosby–Year Book, 1995. Used by permission.)

OSTEOPOROSIS

About Your Diagnosis

Osteoporosis is a metabolic bone disease in which bones become brittle, predisposing them to fractures.

Decreased estrogen levels in postmenopausal women is one of the most common causes of osteoporosis. Oral steroids taken for asthma or arthritis may also cause osteoporosis. Osteoporosis may be caused by poor nutritional intake of vitamins and minerals, such as calcium and vitamin D. Cigarette smoking, alcohol consumption, and a sedentary lifestyle predispose individuals to osteoporosis. Small Caucasian women with a positive family history of osteoporosis are at high risk. Hyperthyroidism, hyperparathyroidism, or Cushing's syndrome can also lead to osteoporosis.

Osteoporosis has been diagnosed in 4–6 million individuals in the United States. It is four times more common in women than men. Risk increases with age. There are at least 275,000 osteoporotic fractures of the hip every year.

Osteoporosis may be detected on an x-ray of a bone. The osteoporosis must be advanced to be noticeable on x-ray. Dual- energy x-ray absorptiometry (DEXA) is a more sensitive measure of bone density and can be used to follow bone density over time. Osteoporosis is defined as a bone density of 2.5 standard deviations below the peak mean bone density of the general population. Patients with bone densities below this level are at high risk for having fractures. Patients with intermediate bone densities and a previous history of fracture also have osteoporosis.

Osteoporosis may be prevented or cured with proper medical therapy.

Living With Your Diagnosis

Many individuals with osteoporosis have no symptoms. Some have a loss of height and curvature of the spine. Others may have pain from a hip, spine, or wrist fracture.

Treatment

Regular weight-bearing exercise such as walking is excellent preventive therapy. Dietary calcium intake should be between 1,000 and 1,500 mg of elemental calcium a day. Vitamin D is necessary for the absorption of calcium from the diet; 400–800 international units (IU) of vitamin D is recommended daily. Postmenopausal women should also consider estrogen replacement therapy with 0.625 mg of conjugated equine estrogen per day. Alendronate, an oral bisphosphonate, in a dosage of 5–10 mg once a day has been approved for the prevention of osteoporosis. All of these preventive therapies may also be used in patients with established osteoporosis. In addition, calcitonin, available as a nasal spray or as an injection, is indicated for women who cannot take estrogen and who are postmenopausal by more than 5 years. Surgery is often required to repair fractured bones.

Side effects of treatment may include kidney stones caused by excess calcium replacement, vitamin D toxicity, or esophageal ulcers caused by alendronate therapy. Estrogen therapy has been associated in some studies with a mild increase in the risk for breast cancer, and a marked increase in endometrial uterine cancers. Women who have not had a hysterectomy must take estrogen in combination with a progestin to minimize the risk of endometrial cancer. Estrogen may also lead to breast tenderness and resumption of menses in postmenopausal women. Benefits of estrogen therapy include a markedly decreased risk of coronary artery disease and increased vaginal lubrication. Each woman with osteoporosis should discuss individual concerns about estrogen replacement therapy with a knowledgeable physician before beginning this therapy. Raloxifene (Evista) is a newer product recently approved for the prevention of osteoporosis. It shares some of the benefits of estrogens such as increased bone density and lowering of lipids and is without significant adverse effects on the endometrium and breasts. It can, however, cause hot flashes and increase the risk of thrombosis.

The DOs

- Minimize any risk factors for osteoporosis by quitting cigarette smoking, decreasing alcohol or caffeine intake, increasing exercise, and taking adequate calcium and vitamin D.
- Have a vitamin D level measured in your blood, especially if you live in a northern climate and have low sun exposure.
- Have regular breast examinations and mammograms if you take estrogen.

The DON'Ts
- Don't take alendronate with food; it will not be absorbed.
- Don't take alendronate when you lay down; it may cause esophageal ulcers. Instead, stand up and take it with a full glass of water.
- Don't take calcium without consulting your doctor if you have a history of kidney stones or hyperparathyroidism.
- Don't take more vitamin D than recommended by your physician.
- Don't take estrogen alone if you are postmenopausal and you have a uterus. Instead, take estrogen with a progestin.

When to Call Your Doctor
- You wish to have a bone density measured.
- You would like an assessment of your current calcium intake.
- You notice any new hip, back, wrist, or rib pain, especially if it occurs after falling, coughing, or sneezing.
- You wish to discuss the risks and benefits of estrogen replacement.
- You notice a new lump on your breast.
- You have heartburn while taking alendronate.

For More Information
National Osteoporosis Foundation
1150 17th Street, Suite 500 NW
Washington, DC 20036-4603
202-223-2226
http://www.nof.org/osteoporosis
NIH Consensus Development Conference Statement Online
http://text.nom.nih.gov/nih/cdc/www/43txt.html.
The Endocrine Society
4350 East West Highway, Suite 500
Bethesda, MD 20814-4410
1-888-ENDOCRINE
http:\\www.endo-society.org.

OTITIS EXTERNA

About Your Diagnosis

Otitis externa is an infection or inflammation of the outer ear canal (from the eardrum to the outer opening). It can be caused by bacteria or a fungus that infects the lining of the ear canal. The infection can come from swimming in contaminated water or from inflammation caused by an allergy to hair spray. It can also be caused by the regular use of earphones, which can trap moisture in the ear canal. It usually lasts 7–10 days with treatment.

Living With Your Diagnosis

Signs and symptoms include pain in the ear that worsens when the earlobe is pulled; itching of the ear canal; foul-smelling drainage from the ear; a slight fever; and temporary hearing loss on the affected side because of the swelling of the canal or drainage.

Treatment

Eardrops are prescribed that contain antibiotics and cortisone to control the inflammation and fight infection. Oral antibiotics may be needed if the infection is severe. Use nonprescription medications such as Tylenol or Advil for minor pain. Avoid getting the ear canal wet for 3 days after all symptoms disappear. Warm compresses may also help ease the pain.

The DOs

- Use eardrops as directed.
- Take a nonprescription medication for pain.
- Gently clean the outer ear daily to remove drainage.
- Keep water out of the ear.

The DON'Ts

- Don't irritate the ear by cleaning or scratching the ear with swabs, bobby pins, or other sharp objects.
- Don't swim in lakes that could be polluted. Lakes with large populations of duck or geese can be polluted from their droppings.
- Don't swim or get water in the ear for at least 3 days after the symptoms disappear.

When to Call Your Doctor

- If pain continues after treatment has begun.
- If pain become severe and is not relieved by non-prescription medications.
- If a high fever develops after treatment has started.

For More Information

Write for a brochure about swimmers ear:
American Academy of Otolaryngology
One Prince Street
Alexandria, VA 22314
703-836-4444, Monday through Friday from 8:30 AM to 5 PM (EST), or fax request to 703-683-5100.

OTITIS MEDIA

About Your Diagnosis

Otitis media is an infection involving the middle ear (the area between the eardrum and the eustachian tube). This area contains the nerves and small bones vital for hearing. Otitis media can affect individuals of any age, but is most common in infants and children. It can be caused by viruses or bacteria that travel to the middle ear through the eustachian tube, usually during an upper respiratory tract infection. It can also be caused by allergies, which cause the sinuses and eustachian tube to become blocked, or by the rupture of the eardrum. Otitis media is curable with treatment. Complications can occur if untreated, such as hearing loss, mastoiditis, or chronic infections.

Living With Your Diagnosis

Signs and symptoms include pain in the ear with a feeling of fullness or stuffiness, loss of hearing, fever, and drainage from the ear. These may occur along with a cold or shortly after. Your doctor will look in the ear to check for redness and protruding of the eardrum.

Treatment

Antibiotics will be needed. Eardrops or heat applied to the ear may help relieve the pain. Nonaspirin medications can be given to reduce fever and pain. Rest is recommended until the fever and pain subside. No special diet is needed, but fluid intake should be increased to help thin secretions.

The DOs

- Take antibiotics as prescribed. Finish all the medication because the infection can still be present even after the symptoms subside.
- Use nonaspirin medications to reduce fever and pain.
- Use heat (a heating pad or hot water bottle wrapped in a towel) to the ear to reduce pain.
- Increase fluid intake.
- Rest until the fever and pain are gone.

The DON'Ts

- Don't skip doses or stop taking the antibiotics.
- Don't swim until the infection clears.
- Avoid prolonged exposure to cigarette smoke.

In young children this can increase the chance of repeat infections.
- Don't put anything in the ear other than the drops prescribed by your doctor.

When to Call Your Doctor

- The earache lasts longer than 2 days after treatment starts.
- There is a severe headache or fever that continues after treatment starts.
- There is redness or swelling behind the ear.
- Dizziness is present.

For More Information

American Speech-Language and Hearing Association
800-638-8255, Monday through Friday from 8:30 AM to 5 PM EST); request pamphlet regarding otitis media.
National Institute on Deafness and Other Communication Disorders Information Clearinghouse
800-241-1044, Monday through Friday from 8:30 AM to 5 PM (EST); ask for ear infections information packet.
American Academy of Otolaryngology
One Prince Street
Alexandria, VA 22314
703-836-4444, Monday through Friday from 8:30 AM to 5 PM (EST), or 703-683-5100 to request information by fax.

OVARIAN CANCER

About Your Diagnosis

Ovarian cancer is a tumor of the female reproductive organs called *ovaries*. The ovaries produce the female hormones called *estrogen* and *progesterone*, which help regulate the menstrual cycle and pregnancy. The ovaries release eggs monthly in preparation for fertilization (when the sperm and egg unite). Nearly 27,000 cases of ovarian cancer are diagnosed each year, and about 1 in 70 women has this cancer in her lifetime.

The cause of ovarian cancer is unknown, but there are certain risk factors that increase one's risk for ovarian cancer. The risks include:

1. Family history. There is a 5% risk if a close relative has the disease. The risk increases to 50% if two family members have the disease.
2. Age. It is uncommon for ovarian cancer to occur before 40 years of age, but the risk increases with age, peaking in the 70s.
3. Breast cancer. Women who have breast cancer are at high risk for ovarian cancer.
4. Infertility, use of drugs to induce fertility (drugs used before in vitro fertilization), frequent miscarriages, and never being pregnant. Women who use birth control pills are less likely to have ovarian cancer than those who do not use the pill.

Ovarian cancer is difficult to detect in its early stages. This is because the tumor produces no symptoms in its initial stage to make the patient or physician aware anything is wrong. There is no effective early screening method. During pelvic examinations a physician attempts to feel for the ovaries and any abnormal lumps. Even with this method early ovarian cancer usually goes undetected. A Papanicolaou (Pap) smear is not reliable for ovarian cancer but is highly reliable for cancer of the cervix. Transvaginal ultrasonography (examination with an ultrasound probe placed in the vagina to look for ovarian tumors) has been tried as a screening tool, but it gives many false-positive results. A blood test to measure CA-125 (Cancer Antigen-125) has been tried as a screening test, but again there are many false-positive results. Unless there is are risk factors, screening is usually not performed on the general population. The best way to diagnose ovarian cancer is to obtain tissue by means of a surgical procedure and examine it with a microscope (biopsy).

Living With Your Diagnosis

In the early stages, ovarian cancer produces no symptoms. As the cancer grows and spreads, you may have lower abdominal discomfort, feel bloated and swollen, and have a loss of appetite. As the tumor presses on nearby organs such as the bladder and intestine (bowel), you may have frequent urination, constipation, and sometimes although not frequently, vaginal bleeding. Ovarian cancer can also produce fluid in the abdominal cavity called *ascites*.

Treatment

All women with suspected ovarian cancer undergo an abdominal operation (laparotomy). This allows the surgeon to diagnose and stage the disease. In the case of tumor that has spread, the surgeon removes as much of the cancer as possible. This is called *debulking* and reduces the amount of cancer to be treated with chemotherapy or radiation therapy. Complications are pain, menopausal effects such as hot flashes and vaginal dryness, and infection.

Depending on the stage of the disease (stage I, confined to the ovary; stage II, confined to the pelvis; stage III, spread into the abdomen; stage IV, spread outside the abdomen), the oncologist decides what chemotherapeutic drugs to use. Side effects depend on the drug used, but nausea, vomiting, hair loss, easy bruising and bleeding, and infections can occur.

The use of radiation therapy depends on the stage of the disease. Side effects include dry, itchy, red skin over the treated area. Radiation treatment to the lower abdomen can cause nausea, vomiting, diarrhea, pain with urination, vaginal dryness, and pain with intercourse.

The DOs

- Address symptoms with your primary care physician, especially if you are at high risk.
- Request second opinions about all types of treatment (surgical, radiation, and chemotherapy) if you are not sure what to do.
- Ask for pain medications after surgical treatment.
- Understand the importance of nutrition after treatment.
- Ask questions about prognosis of the tumor, survival times, and recurrence of the tumor.

The DON'Ts

- Do not miss follow-up appointments. When treatment is over, regular examinations are performed to look for recurrence of the tumor. This includes the examination, computed tomography (CT), and measurement of CA-125 in the blood. The blood level is often high before surgical treatment and returns to normal afterward. If CA-125 level begins to rise again, the cancer may have recurred.
- Do not be afraid to ask about emotional support groups.

When to Call Your Doctor

- If you have vaginal bleeding with abdominal swelling, bloating, or pain.
- If you have fever with chemotherapy.
- If you have drainage from the wound site, fever, or pain after your operation.
- If you have diarrhea, urinary frequency, or vaginal pain after radiation.

For More Information

National Cancer Institute (NCI)
9000 Rockville Pike
Bethesda, MD 20892
Cancer Information Service
1-800-422-6237 (1-800-4-CANCER)
American Cancer Society
1599 Clifton Road, N.E.
Atlanta, GA 30329
1-800-ACS-2345

OVARIAN CYSTS

About Your Diagnosis

Ovarian cysts are fluid filled structures that develop in the ovary. Ovarian cysts develop with every menstrual cycle. Fluid collects around developing eggs; one egg becomes "dominant" and that egg ovulates (leaves the ovary and goes into the fallopian tube). The ovulated egg leaves a cyst behind in the ovary. This cyst is usually 2–3 centimeters (1–2 inches) in diameter. This type of cyst is called a "physiologic cyst," "follicular cyst," or "simple cyst." If the cyst remains a normal size, it does not cause any symptoms. If the cyst grows larger, 4 centimeters or larger, it can cause pain. Symptomatic cysts are very common; in most cases, the cyst and symptoms will resolve without any treatment.

Occasionally, cysts can bleed into themselves. A very small blood vessel in the wall of the cyst breaks, and the blood goes into the cyst. These are called "hemorrhagic cysts" and sometimes are more painful. Hemorrhagic cysts are common as well. Occasionally, hemorrhagic cysts can rupture, and the blood goes into the abdominal cavity. No blood is seen out of the vagina. If a cyst ruptures, it is usually very painful. Hemorrhagic cysts that rupture are less common. Most hemorrhagic cysts are self-limiting; some need surgical intervention (see below). Even if the hemorrhagic cyst ruptures, in many cases it will resolve without surgery. Sometimes surgery is necessary.

Another condition that can occur with ovarian cysts is "torsion" or twisting of the ovary and fallopian tube. If the ovary and tube twist a little, this can cause pain, but it is not dangerous. If the ovary and tube twist completely around, this is very painful and immediate surgical treatment is necessary.

Cysts are usually diagnosed by pelvic ultrasound. This is a painless test in which the ovaries, fallopian tubes, and uterus can be seen so the cyst can be confirmed. If the cyst appears to be "clear" inside, the diagnosis of a physiologic cyst is made. If the cyst is not clear inside, then it is possible a hemorrhagic cyst is present.

Living With Your Diagnosis

Ovarian cysts can cause pelvic pain. The pain can be sharp, dull, or feel like pressure. It may be localized to one side of the abdomen, or it may be more diffuse across the lower abdomen. Activity such as walking, exercise, or intercourse will often make the pain worse. Usually bladder or bowel habits are not affected, although sometimes pelvic pain can cause urinary frequency (make you feel like you need to empty your bladder more often). Usually, the appetite is not affected unless the pain is severe.

If the pain is from a physiologic cyst or from a hemorrhagic cyst, it will usually resolve in a few days up to 10–14 days (by the next period).

If the pain is from a ruptured hemorrhagic cyst or an ovarian cyst that is twisting, the pain usually worsens until it is extremely severe, necessitating medical attention.

Treatment

If you have a physiologic cyst that grew larger than it should have, usually no treatment is necessary except to decrease the pain. Ibuprofen can be taken to decrease the pain: 400 milligrams every 4 hours or 600 milligrams every 6 hours or 800 milligrams every 8 hours. (Obviously, do not take ibuprofen if you have been told you should not take it because of a medical condition, an allergy to it, or because it is incompatible with another medication you are taking.) Sometimes a prescription pain medication will be prescribed if ibuprofen does not relieve the pain enough or cannot be taken. Sometimes a warm bath or heating pad can help lessen the discomfort. Often a follow-up pelvic ultrasound will be recommended to make sure the cyst has resolved.

If you have a ruptured or twisting cyst, you may need laparoscopic surgery. This is a procedure in which a telescope-like instrument and other instruments are placed into the abdominal cavity through very small incisions. The cyst can be seen and the bleeding stopped by cauterizing it. If the ovary and fallopian tube are twisting, sometimes the ovary and tube can be untwisted, or sometimes the ovary and tube have to be removed.

If you have recurrent ovarian cysts, birth control pills may be recommended. Birth control pills prevent most ovulation, so cysts do not develop.

The DOs

- Take ibuprofen 400 milligrams every 4 hours or 600 milligrams every 6 hours or 800 milligrams every 8 hours for pain. (Do not take ibuprofen if have been told you should not take it because of a medical condition, an allergy to it, or because

it is incompatible with another medication you are taking.)
- Sometimes a hot tub or heating pad can help relieve the discomfort.

The DON'Ts
- Refrain from strenuous activity (e.g., exercise, sexual activity). Activity will make the discomfort worse.

When to Call Your Doctor
- If the pain gets worse instead of gradually decreasing.
- If a fever, or nausea and vomiting develop.

For More Information
Understanding Your Body: Every Woman's Guide to Gynecology and Health. Felicia Stewart, M.D., Felicia Guest, M.D., Gary Stewart, M.D., and Robert Hatcher, M.D., Bantam Books, 1987.

PAGET'S DISEASE OF THE BONE

About Your Diagnosis

Paget's disease is a metabolic bone disease manifested by disorganized bone formation. Normally, bone cells called osteoblasts are constantly forming new bone in smooth even layers, like a bricklayer building a brick wall. At the same time, cells called osteoclasts are knocking down other older sections of this bony structure and hauling the pieces away in a process called resorption. This bony formation and resorption is delicately balanced, so that bones grow straight and strong. In Paget's disease, the process has gone awry. Giant osteoclasts are rapidly resorbing bone, and the busy osteoblasts are laying down new bone in a haphazard fashion. It's as if a brick wall was built with bricks facing in all directions, weakened by gaps and holes. The resulting bone is easily broken.

Researchers do not yet know what causes Paget's disease. Currently, researchers are testing whether a viral infection of the bone may be causing the cells to act in this unusual way.

Paget's disease is present in up to 4% of Caucasians of Anglo-Saxon descent who are older than 40 years. It is more common in males than females, but it is much less common in other ethnic groups. Only 5% of patients with Paget's disease have symptoms, however, and many of these patients have not been diagnosed.

Paget's disease may be detected by a patient's symptoms of bony pain. Blood tests reveal an elevated alkaline phosphatase level. Liver function tests, serum calcium, phosphorus, vitamin D, and parathyroid hormone (PTH) levels should also be checked to exclude liver disease, osteomalacia, or hyperparathyroidism. The diagnosis is supported by routine x-rays of the symptomatic bones, which reveal small fractures, abnormally thickened bone, or areas of bony resorption. A bone scan may also be performed to determine whether there are other areas of the body that are similarly affected. Some patients may require a bone biopsy to establish the diagnosis.

There is no cure for Paget's, but new medicines are now available to control the disease and prevent further progression.

Living With Your Diagnosis

Many patients have no symptoms. Others note bone pain, and warmth and swelling over the bone (especially the skull or the long bones of the legs). Numbness and tingling in the hands or feet, shortness of breath with exertion, or decreased hearing also occur.

Paget's disease can lead to bony fractures, curvature of the spine (kyphosis), and nerve compressions. Very susceptible areas include the ear and the spinal column. It may also cause congestive heart failure as a result of increased vascular growth in the pagetic bone. Less than 1% of patients may also have a bone cancer called a sarcoma.

Treatment

It is important to continue exercising whenever possible, because immobility may result in elevated calcium levels in the blood and urine, leading to formation of kidney stones. Patients without symptoms do not require treatment. Mild pain relievers such as acetaminophen or ibuprofen may suffice in many patients. Patients with advanced symptoms of bone pain or fracture should be treated with one of the new oral bisphosphenates, such as alendronate, 40 mg once a day. This has been shown to decrease bone pain in patients with Paget's. Nasal calcitonin may also be used to treat pain and prevent progression of bony changes. This appears particularly effective to prevent the deafness that may be associated with abnormal growth of the ear bones, which leads to compression of the nerves supplying the ear. Finally, surgery may be required when weight-bearing bones are fractured as a result of Paget's. It is important that medications be taken preoperatively to reduce the vascularity of the bone and to minimize the risk of bleeding.

The DOs

- Keep abreast of new treatments for Paget's, which will be available during the next few years.
- Take medicine before surgery to decrease the risk of bleeding.
- Medically supervised exercise should be done regularly because this will help prevent elevated calcium levels.

The DON'Ts

- Don't take alendronate with food. It is not well absorbed. Instead, take it on an empty stomach, 1 hour before eating.

- Don't lie down after taking alendronate. Instead, take it with a full glass of water after arising in the morning, then remain standing or sitting. This will prevent the possible side effect of esophageal ulcers.
- Don't take nasal calcitonin in the same nostril each time.

When to Call Your Doctor
- You have increased bone pain or nerve compression.
- Your hearing is decreased.
- You have shortness of breath on exertion or ankle swelling.
- You have severe heartburn while taking alendronate.

For More Information
The Paget's Foundation
200 Varick Street, Suite 1004
New York, NY 10014-4810
1-800-23-PAGET or 212-229-1582
The Endocrine Society
4350 East West Highway, Suite 500
Bethesda, MD 20814-4410
1-888-ENDOCRINE
http://www.endo-society.org

PAGET'S DISEASE OF THE BREAST

About Your Diagnosis

Paget's disease of the breast is a rare type of breast cancer. Breast cancer is the most common cancer among women; nearly 185,000 new cases were diagnosed in 1996. Of these breast cancers, approximately 1% are of the Paget's type. Paget's disease of the breast is not contagious, and the cause is not known. The cancer is curable if detected in its early stages, before it has had time to spread. The only sure way to detect Paget's disease of the breast is by means of biopsy and examination of the tissue with a microscope.

Living With Your Diagnosis

Paget's disease of the breast differs in presentation from breast cancer. You may have redness, scaling, and crusting of the nipple that is itchy and burning. Nipple drainage may occur. You may feel a lump just under the nipple. Paget's disease of the breast, like breast cancer, spreads to local lymph nodes and eventually in the blood stream to other parts of the body, such as the bone, lung, liver, and lymph nodes.

Treatment

Once the diagnosis is confirmed, a physician stages the cancer or determine the extent of the disease. Blood tests, radiographs (x-rays) of the breast and chest, computed tomography (CT) of the head, chest and abdomen, and bone scans may be ordered to look for spread of the tumor. If these studies do not provide any information, a surgical procedure is extremely important in staging. During the operation the surgeon determines the size of the tumor, whether the tumor spread to the lymph nodes, and whether the cancer has a specific hormone receptor. This information is vital in deciding what type of treatment is given.

Therapy for Paget's disease of the breast is similar to that of other forms of breast cancer. The exception is that the nipple and tissue just beneath the nipple must be removed. With other types of breast cancer the nipple is returned to its original location in reconstruction after surgical treatment. Therapy for Paget's disease can be surgical therapy (generally mastectomy), radiation therapy, chemotherapy, hormonal therapy or a combination of all of these treatments. Treatment involves many specialists working as a team. Treatment is coordinated by a primary care physician.

The side effects of surgical treatment depend on the type of operation. The degree of breast deformity depends on the amount of breast tissue the patient has and the type of procedure (mastectomy, breast-conserving operation). Because the lymph nodes under the armpit are removed, there may be arm swelling.

The side effects of radiation therapy include red, dry, itchy skin over the radiation site. Because irradiation is over the chest and armpit, shortness of breath, coughing, and arm swelling can occur.

The side effects of chemotherapy include nausea, vomiting, hair loss, easy bruising, bleeding, and infections.

The side effects of hormonal treatment include hot flashes, nausea, vomiting, irregular menstrual cycles, vaginal bleeding, and a skin rash.

The DOs

- Seek a team of physicians experienced in management of all aspects of breast cancer.
- Keep your appointments during and after treatment. This is important to monitor your response to treatment and to look for recurrence of the cancer. It is likely that many physicians and health care providers are involved in your care, including an oncologist (physician specializing in cancer), surgeon, radiation oncologist (physician specializing in treatments with radiation), nutritionist, and social worker.
- Remember the importance of exercise and nutrition during and after treatment.

The DON'Ts

- Do not ignore any lump, nipple discharge, or changes in the nipple skin.
- Do not forget that Paget's disease is a rare form of breast cancer but that as with breast cancer, the earlier it is detected, the better is the likelihood of a cure. Mammograms are important in screening for breast cancer. Ask your physician for the primary care teaching guide on breast cancer.

When to Call Your Doctor

- If you feel a lump.
- If you see any nipple drainage.
- If you feel any swollen lymph glands under your armpits.

- If you have fever, nausea, and vomiting after chemotherapy.
- If you have back pain, leg weakness, stool or urine incontinence (leaking), or bone pain.
- If you feel depressed.

For More Information
American Cancer Society
1599 Clifton Road, N.E.
Atlanta, GA 30329
1-800-ACS-2345
Cancer Information Service
1-800-4-CANCER

PANCREATITIS, CHRONIC

About Your Diagnosis

Chronic pancreatitis is a persistent inflammation of the pancreas. The pancreas is a gland located behind the stomach. It secretes digestive enzymes and the hormones insulin and glucagon. The persistent inflammation leads to the destruction of the functioning glandular tissue in the pancreas. The pancreatic digestive enzymes are not produced, resulting in an inability to properly digest and absorb fat in the diet. There is also a decrease in the production of insulin. Alcohol abuse is the most common cause of this condition. Hemochromatosis (a condition of excess iron in the blood) and cystic fibrosis are other know causes. The incidence of chronic pancreatitis is 2 cases per 10,000 individuals. Men are affected more often than women. Chronic pancreatitis is detected by reviewing the individual's history. Samples of blood are taken to look for the changes associated with this disease.

Living With Your Diagnosis

The most common symptom of chronic pancreatitis is pain. The pain is variable in its intensity. It may be a low-grade, persistent pain with recurring acute attacks. The pain may be constant and boring. The back and abdomen are the sites of pain. Weight loss is another symptom. This is due to the malabsorption of fat. Steatorrhea (large, foul bulky stools) will occur also because of the fat malabsorption in the gastrointestinal tract. There can be abdominal distention and fever also.

Treatment

There are two focuses of treatment. The first is the management of pain. The preferred treatment for the pain is nonnarcotic pain relievers. Long-term narcotic use can lead to dependence and addiction. Referral to a pain specialist may be helpful. The second focus is replacing the digestive enzymes and insulin that are normally made by the pancreas. Pancreatic enzymes are available in tablet form. These are taken with meals and snacks. Insulin injections are used to control the blood sugar level. It may be necessary to give vitamin supplements because of the malabsorption. Specifically, vitamins A, D, and K are replaced.

If the pain cannot be controlled, surgery is an option. The surgery involves draining the pancreatic duct. In advanced cases, removal of all or part of the pancreas is an option.

The DOs

- Eat a low-fat, well-balanced diet.
- Supplement with oral fat-soluble vitamins.
- Calcium supplementation is indicated to prevent bone problems.
- Take pancreatic enzyme supplements as prescribed.
- See a pain specialist if pain control is difficult.

The DON'Ts

- Avoid fatty foods.
- Avoid alcohol.
- Avoid caffeine.
- Avoid prolonged use of narcotics for pain control.

When to Call Your Doctor

- If symptoms of pancreatitis develop.
- If symptoms of pancreatitis worsen or do not improve with treatment.
- If pain is not controlled with the prescribed pain relievers.
- If fever develops.

For More Information
National Digestive Diseases Information Clearinghouse
2 Information Way
Bethesda, MD 20892-3570
www.niddk.nih.gov
nddic@aerie.com

PARKINSON'S DISEASE

About Your Diagnosis

Parkinson's disease is a chronic, neurologic disorder that generally affects individuals older than 60 years. It is slowly progressive and may not become incapacitating for years. Although the cause is still uncertain, environmental toxins are suspect. The early symptom of Parkinson's disease is a subtle tremor of the hand or fingers that is often first noticed when a patient has handwriting changes, or has difficulty with other fine motor movements such as buttoning clothes. Diagnosis is usually easy once the clinical picture is characteristic, but may be difficult in the early stages. Generally, the symptoms progress slowly over the course of 4–8 years.

Living With Your Diagnosis

The signs and symptoms are a result of degeneration of some of the cells in the brain that produce the neurochemical dopamine, causing tremor, muscle stiffness, gradual slowing and loss of motor function, and gait changes. As Parkinson's disease progresses, patients often require increasing assistance with activities of daily living. Consultation with an occupational therapist may be helpful to learn about creative solutions to address some of these changes.

Living with Parkinson's disease can be a challenge. It is important to continue participating in activities that you enjoy. Staying active is an important part of living with the disease. A daily exercise regimen, such as walking, will help keep your muscles limber and strong.

There are no dietary restrictions with Parkinson's disease. However, if swallowing becomes difficult, it may be easier to drink thick liquids (such as nectars or milk shakes) instead of thin liquids (apple juice or tea). Do not stop taking your medications abruptly, even if you think they are not helping. Always check with your physician before stopping or changing any medication.

Treatment

Treatment for Parkinson's disease usually involves treating the symptoms and preventing complications. There are many treatments for the symptoms, although currently there is no cure for Parkinson's disease. The best treatment will depend on the severity of the symptoms and the patient's response to medications. All the medications are used to treat the symptoms, or slow the progression of symptoms. These medications should be taken daily exactly as prescribed. If you have side effects related to the medications, you should notify your physician.

In some patients with Parkinson's disease, a form of surgery called stereotaxic surgery may be used to create a very precise lesion in the brain that will stop or markedly reduce the tremor.

The DOs

- Take your medications as prescribed.
- Keep all follow-up appointments so that your physician can monitor your response to medications.
- Consult your physician about an exercise program.

The DON'Ts

- Don't negotiate unfamiliar terrain without assistance if you are having gait difficulty.
- Don't drive unless you have been cleared by your physician.
- Don't operate machinery or otherwise dangerous equipment.
- Don't climb. A fall could result in injury or death.

When to Call Your Doctor

- If you have any problems associated with your medications.
- If you notice a change in the severity of your symptoms.
- If you begin having difficulty swallowing.
- If you fall or become injured.

For More Information
American Parkinson Disease Association, Inc.
1250 Hylan Blvd., Suite 4B
Staten Island, NY 10305
800-223-2732
718-981-8001
e-mail: apda@admin.con2.com
Parkinson's Disease Foundation (PDF)
William Black Medical Building
710 West 168th Street
New York, NY 10032
212-923-4700
Others:
National Parkinson Foundation, Inc.
The Parkinson's Institute
United Parkinson Foundation
Parkinson's Action Network

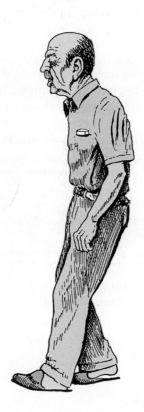

Parkinsonism. Parkinsonism is a syndrome typically found in individuals with Parkinson's disease. The signs include (but are not limited to) rigidity and trembling of the head and extremities, a forward tilt of the trunk, and a shuffling gait with short steps and reduced arm swinging. (From Thibodeau GA, Patton KT: *The Human Body in Health & Disease*, vol 2. St. Louis, Mosby–Year Book, 1996.Used by permission.)

PARONYCHIA

About Your Diagnosis

A paronychia is an abscess, or collection of pus, under the skin folds that surround the fingernails. It is a common condition that occurs when germs penetrate the area and grow. Common causes are nail biting, hangnail biting, thumb sucking, penetrating injury, and foreign bodies such as splinters. It is completely curable by draining the pus.

Living With Your Diagnosis

The signs of a paronychia are redness and swelling of the skin adjacent to the fingernails. As the problem progresses, fluid or pus may be seen under the nail. The area is usually very tender and feels puffy or fluid filled. As the paronychia progresses, throbbing pain often occurs. If treated, the pain resolves in a few hours, with the redness and swelling fading over a few days. If left untreated, the infection can spread to cause disabling or deforming injury to the hand.

Treatment

The treatment is to provide a way for the pus to drain. This may involve a small incision over the area or simply separating a small portion of the nail from the skin fold. The discomfort can be lessened by "blocking" the local nerves with an anesthetic. There is little risk from the procedure. A minute scar may form but is clearly preferable to the effects of untreated infection. In advanced cases, a small piece of the nail may be removed. The nail almost always regrows with a natural appearance. After the pus is drained, the doctor may leave a small "wick" in place for a few days for continued drainage.

The DOs

- Use any pain medication only as prescribed.
- Elevate the finger above the heart to decrease pain and swelling.
- Soak the finger in Epsom salts or soapy water several times a day.
- Remove adherent dressings by soaking in warm water.
- Keep the bandage clean and dry. Change the bandage at least twice a day.
- Take prescribed antibiotics as directed for the stated length of time.
- Keep your follow-up appointment for recheck

The DON'Ts

- Don't ignore or neglect a paronychia. Seek treatment early.
- Don't try to drain a paronychia with pins or pocketknives at home.
- Don't bite your nails.
- Don't remove a wick unless instructed to do so by the doctor.
- Don't allow the wound to become soiled until healed.

When to Call You Doctor

- If the pad of the finger becomes swollen or painful.
- If the finger becomes painful to bend or swollen.
- If a knuckle becomes painful or swollen.
- If you have red streaks from the area, fever, or chills.
- If your pain persists beyond 24 hours after treatment.
- If you have a reaction to a prescribed medication.

For More Information

Call your doctor or local emergency department.

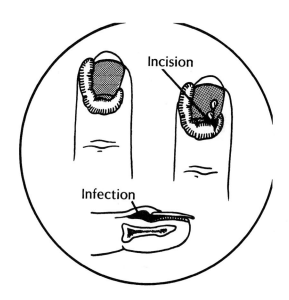

Paronychia. **A**, location of infection. **B**, incision and drainage with removal of a portion of the fingernail. (From Noble J: *Textbook Primary Care Medicine*, vol 2. St. Louis, Mosby–Year Book, Inc., 1995. Used by permission.)

PAROXYSMAL ATRIAL TACHYCARDIA

About Your Diagnosis

This condition often comes on suddenly (paroxysmal) and causes a rapid heartbeat (tachycardia) from abnormal electrical signals within the atria. The atria are above the ventricles, their position is often referred to as *supraventricular*; therefore, this condition may be called *paroxysmal supraventricular tachycardia* (PSVT). The abnormal signals produce an abnormal heart rhythm called an *arrhythmia*. These signals begin as the result of heart disease such as mitral valve disorders, problems with the walls of the atria, or preexcitation syndromes (when the ventricles are stimulated to contract too early and too often). About half of patients with PSVT have no heart disease and simply generate abnormal signals because of other conditions, such as thyroid disease. Nicotine from smoking, caffeine, or stress may cause this condition.

Living With Your Diagnosis

You may notice the rapid heartbeat because it often occurs at rest and may cause shortness of breath or chest pain. Attacks may last from a few seconds to several weeks. You may have to urinate frequently during prolonged attacks because the increased heart rate increases blood flow through the kidneys. Attacks may occur almost daily or may happen only a few times ever. You can try to stop the attack by gently massaging the carotid artery in the neck for a few seconds, straining as if lifting a heavy object, or placing a cold, wet towel on your face for a few minutes. Have your doctor show you how to do this before you try it on your own.

Treatment

The doctor can detect the rapid pulse and can read the rapid rate on an electrocardiogram (ECG). If the maneuvers used to slow the heart rate do not work, medications are used. Medications are often given in a hospital to allow monitoring of the heart. Digoxin helps control the rate and efficiency of contraction of the ventricles. Digoxin levels in the blood have to be measured periodically. Verapamil or beta-blocker medications may be used, especially by patients with hypertension (high blood pressure). These drugs may cause low blood pressure or a slowed heart rate and make exercise difficult.

They may cause fainting, lightheadedness, or fatigue. Hearts with PSVT not controlled with medicines may have to be electrically shocked back to normal (cardioversion).

The main complications of PSVT are related to the excess work done by the heart. This eventually puts a strain on the heart and cause it to work less efficiently (heart failure). For persons with heart disease, this may be a strain that the heart cannot handle. Prolonged symptoms of a rapid heartbeat, chest pain, shortness of breath, or feeling faint necessitate immediate attention.

The DOs

- Stop smoking.
- Reduce stress in your life.
- Exercise, but do not start unless advised by your doctor.
- Start a healthful diet for your heart that includes low-fat and low-cholesterol foods.

The DON'Ts

- Do not ignore worsening symptoms.

When to Call Your Doctor

- If you have any reactions to your medications.
- If you have chest pain, shortness of breath, fainting, or rapid heartbeat that affects your ability to rest.

For More Information

Consult your local library or medical school for a textbook on cardiology. Call the American Heart Association at 1-800-242-8721 and ask for the literature department.

PEDICULOSIS

About Your Diagnosis

Pediculosis is a skin inflammation caused by tiny parasites (lice) that live on the body or in clothing. There are three types: head lice, body lice, and pubic or crab lice.

Head lice are most common in children. More girls are affected than boys. There are 6–12 million cases per year in the United States.

Pediculosis is most commonly spread by direct person-to-person contact, usually occurring under crowded conditions. It can also be spread when combs, hats, or brushes are shared. Infestation does not indicate poor hygiene. Pubic or crab lice are transmitted by sexual contact.

Diagnosis can be made by observing the presence of nits (eggs) in the scalp along the hair shaft, in clothing, or on pubic hair. Symptoms of itching cause patients to scratch, resulting in crusting and scabbing of the skin.

Living With Your Diagnosis

Finding nits on the hair shafts or clothing makes the diagnosis. Itching and scratching are usual symptoms. Nits are eggs that appear as small, whitish flecks securely attached to the base of hairs. They cannot be easily brushed off.

Pediculosis is usually curable with medicated creams, shampoos, and lotions. Symptoms usually disappear in 5 days. Infection at sites of deep scratching is possible.

Treatment

Pediculosis is treated with anti-lice creams, lotions, or shampoos applied to affected body parts, according to instructions. Examples include:
1. Permethrin (Nix, Elimite): single application.
2. Pyrethrins (Rid, R and C, A-200): reapply in 7 days.
3. Lindane (Kwell, by prescription): reapply in 7 days.

Side effects of treatment, such as skin irritation or body absorption of the medication, can occur but are usually related to more frequent medication applications than recommended. All anti-lice preparations are toxic, but they are safe if used according to the directions. Keep all preparations out of the eyes and out of the reach of children.

The DOs

- Examine household members and close contacts for lice, and treated if infestation exists. Nits can be removed with a fine-tooth comb.
- Personal items such as combs or brushes should be soaked in hot water for 15 minutes.
- Clothes and bedding should be washed in hot water and dried in a dryer; or alternately, clothes and linen can be ironed, or sealed in a plastic bag for 10 days.

The DON'Ts

- Do not use medication more frequently than recommended.

When to Call Your Doctor

- When anyone in your household or a sexual partner has symptoms of lice or symptoms recur after treatment.

For More Information
National Pediculosis Association
PO Box 149
Newton, MA 02161
617-449-NITS

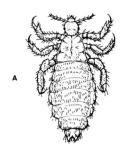
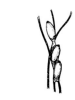

A, the female head louse (enlarged). B, enlargement of nits on hair shafts. C, life-sized louse. (From Ingalls AJ, Salerno MC: *Maternal and Child Health Nursing*, vol 7. St. Louis, Mosby–Year Book, 1990. Used by permission.)

PELVIC INFLAMMATORY DISEASE

About Your Diagnosis

Pelvic inflammatory disease (PID) is a bacterial infection of the pelvic organs. The infection usually comes from the bacteria in the vagina through the cervix. The infection may only include the fallopian tubes, or it may include all the pelvic organs, the uterus, ovaries, and fallopian tubes. Pelvic inflammatory disease is common, usually occurring in women of reproductive age who are sexually active.

Pelvic inflammatory disease may occur spontaneously (in sexually active women), but the presence of sexually transmitted diseases such as gonorrhea or chlamydia increases the risk of developing PID significantly. An intrauterine device (IUD), a birth control method, can increase the risk of developing PID during the first few months after the IUD is placed. Having multiple sexual partners increases the risk of developing PID. Having your partner use a condom or using a diaphragm can decrease your risk of developing PID.

Pelvic inflammatory disease is often diagnosed by the presence of pelvic pain, fever, and increased vaginal discharge. However, sometimes only pelvic pain is present, without fever or increased vaginal discharge. Gonorrhea and chlamydia are diagnosed by laboratory tests. If either sexually transmitted disease is diagnosed and either pelvic pain or fever are also present, the diagnosis of PID is made.

If PID is suspected or diagnosed, it should be treated promptly. Most cases of PID are cured with a 10- to 14-day course of oral antibiotics.

Living With Your Diagnosis

The most common symptoms are:

- Pelvic pain.
- Fever.
- Increased vaginal discharge.

However, in some cases, pelvic pain may be present without fever or increased vaginal discharge.

If PID is diagnosed early and treated promptly, in most cases there are no long-term complications. However, in some cases, even if it is diagnosed and treated promptly, the fallopian tubes can be damaged, leading to infertility. In other cases, patients may end up with chronic pelvic pain.

Treatment

You may be treated with an intramuscular injection of an antibiotic followed by an oral antibiotic for 10–14 days, or with just an oral antibiotic. As with any antibiotic therapy, an associated yeast infection may develop.

The DOs

- It is very important that you take all the medication as prescribed.
- To decrease your future risk of developing PID, have "safe sex," with your partner using a condom.

The DON'Ts

- Refrain from sexual activity until your symptoms have completely resolved or until your doctor okays sexual activity.
- To decrease your future risk of developing PID, avoid multiple partners.

When to Call Your Doctor

- If your symptoms have not improved within 48–72 hours.
- If your symptoms worsen despite treatment in the next 48 hours, i.e., fever is higher or pelvic pain is more severe.
- If you do not tolerate the antibiotic, i.e., are throwing up the medication.
- If you have any symptoms that may indicate an allergy to the medication.

For More Information
Understanding Your Body: Every Woman's Guide to Gynecology and Health. Felicia Stewart, M.D., Felicia Guest, M.D., Gary Stewart, M.D., and Robert Hatcher, M.D., Bantam Books, 1987.

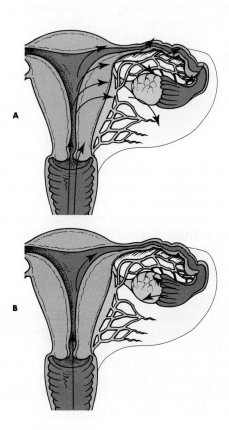

Common routes of the spread of pelvic inflammatory disease. **A,** direct spread of bacterial infection other than *Neisseria gonorrhoeae.* **B,** direct spread of *Neisseria gonorrhoeae.* (From Lewis SM, Collier IC, Heitkemper MM: *Medical-Surgical Nursing: Assessment and Management of Clinical Problem,* vol. 4. St. Louis, Mosby–Year Book, 1995. Used by permission.)

PELVIC ORGAN PROLAPSE

About Your Diagnosis

The uterus, bladder, and rectum are located around the vaginal canal and so are able to prolapse, or herniate, into the vaginal canal. If the uterus has prolapsed, it is called "uterine prolapse." If the bladder has prolapsed, it is called a "cystocele." If the rectum has prolapsed, it is called a "rectocele." The prolapsed organ can cause a bulge of tissue out of the vaginal opening. Often this is when the prolapse is first noticed, when the patient feels "something like a ball of tissue out of the vaginal opening." Sometimes the prolapse will be noticed by the physician when the Pap and pelvic examination are performed. If the organ has prolapsed, but it has not prolapsed out of the vaginal canal, usually the patient is unaware of it.

Childbirth is the most common cause of prolapse. The delivery of the baby stretches and may tear the muscles and connective tissue that support the pelvic organs. In addition to childbirth, aging and becoming postmenopausal contribute to the prolapse. Prolapse does not happen soon after childbirth; usually it occurs when women are postmenopausal, but it can occur in premenopausal women.

Living With Your Diagnosis

Women with mild or moderate prolapse may complain of pelvic pressure, low backache, or pain, or actually complain that they feel like "something is falling out." These symptoms may worsen at the end of the day, especially in women who have been on their feet all day. Sometimes urinary incontinence (leakage of urine) will accompany the other symptoms if there is loss of support to the bladder neck area. If a rectocele is present, difficulty evacuating the rectum may occur because the rectum is herniating into the vaginal canal.

With severe prolapse, a "bulge" is felt out of the vaginal canal. This bulge can be the uterus and cervix (the cervix is the opening to the uterus), the front wall of the vaginal canal with the bladder behind it, or the back wall of the vaginal canal with the rectum behind it. Sometimes the bulge can be felt intermittently because the prolapsed organ actually can go back up into the pelvis. Women with prolapse often notice that if they are on their feet a lot, they notice a lot of bulging. When they lie down, the bulge may disappear back into the vaginal ca-

nal. With severe prolapse of the bladder, some patients may experience difficulty emptying the bladder (voiding). This occurs because when the bladder has prolapsed very low, the prolapse can kink the urethra (the passage from the bladder to the outside). If the urethra is kinked, it can be difficult to empty the bladder, or patients notice a slow stream. (It is similar to a garden hose that is kinked and water will not run through it.)

Treatment

If the prolapse is mild or moderate (so no organs are actually bulging out of the vaginal canal) and the patient is not experiencing bothersome symptoms such as pelvic pressure, backache, urinary incontinence, or difficulty voiding, the prolapse can be observed and no treatment is needed. If the prolapse is severe and the pelvic organ is bulging out of the vaginal canal, most patients are extremely uncomfortable and want treatment to relieve their symptoms. Even if the pelvic organ is not prolapsed out, but the patient is experiencing bothersome pelvic pressure or backache, the patient may desire treatment.

If the prolapse is mild or moderate, sometimes properly performed "Kegel" exercises (tightening the pelvic floor muscles) can relieve the symptoms enough so no further treatment is necessary. Women with prolapse should perform 30–50 Kegels each day. To build up the muscles it is important to hold each Kegel for 5–10 seconds. Have your health care provider check to make sure you are doing your Kegel exercises correctly. It is also important to do a Kegel anytime you lift anything (a bag of groceries, baby, stack of books, luggage), or when you cough, sneeze, or laugh.

If Kegel exercises do not help, physical therapy may be an option. Physical therapy for the pelvic floor may include biofeedback and electrical stimulation. Sometimes, if Kegel exercises alone do not strengthen the pelvic floor muscles enough, physical therapy can further strengthen the muscles.

If Kegel exercises and/or physical therapy are not effective in relieving the symptoms, using a pessary or surgery are options. Pessaries are devices that are worn inside the vaginal canal to support the prolapsed organs. Pessaries come in many different shapes and sizes. Some pessaries can be removed by the patient, so the patient only has to visit the gynecologist once or twice each year. Some pessaries can only be removed by a health care provider, so the patient will have to come into the office every 3–4 months to have the pessary removed, cleaned, and replaced. If a pessary is used, estrogen cream should be used to prevent erosions of the vaginal walls and to prevent infection. If the pessary fits correctly, it should be very comfortable. However, not all women with prolapse can use a pessary because the pessary falls out with activity, i.e., with walking, bearing down to have a bowel movement.

Surgery is often recommended when a pessary cannot be fit to the patient (feels uncomfortable when it is in or falls out). Sometimes patients do not want to use a pessary and desire surgery to correct the prolapse. Usually the surgery is performed vaginally, but generally still requires a 2- or 3-day hospitalization and a 4- to 8-week recovery period. Occasionally, surgery will not correct all the symptoms, such as urinary incontinence or difficulty evacuating the rectum. Also, occasionally the prolapse can recur, although this usually happens years later.

The DOs
- Do the Kegel exercises (tightening the pelvic floor muscles—it should feel as though you are pulling in or up the rectum) as directed: 30–50 each day, holding each Kegel for 5–10 seconds.
- Do the Kegel when you lift anything (stack of books, luggage, bag of groceries, baby) or when you cough, sneeze, or laugh.

The DON'Ts
- Don't lift heavy objects (heavier than 20–25 lb).
- Don't miss your appointment if you are fit with a pessary. If you wait too long before being examined, vaginal wall erosions or vaginal infection may develop.

When to Call Your Doctor
- If you are having difficulty emptying your bladder. This usually only gets worse with time, and if you are unable to empty your bladder at all, you will need to have a catheter placed into the bladder (temporarily) to empty it.
- If you notice vaginal bleeding. This may indicate that there is an erosion from the pessary (if you have one) or an erosion on the prolapsed organ.
- If the pessary falls out or is uncomfortable.

For More Information
Understanding Your Body: Every Woman's Guide to Gynecology and Health. Felicia Stewart, M.D., Felicia Guest, M.D., Gary Stewart, M.D., and Robert Hatcher, M.D., Bantam Books, 1987.

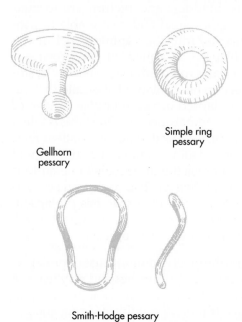

Gellhorn pessary

Simple ring pessary

Smith-Hodge pessary

A, examples of pessaries (Smith-Hodge, donut, inflatable types). **B,** pessary in place to hold cervix well backward and upward in pelvis. (From Willson JR, Carrington ER: *Obstetrics and Gynecology.* St Louis, Mosby, 1991. Used by permission.)

PEMPHIGOID, BULLOUS

About Your Diagnosis

Bullous pemphigoid is a chronic bullous disease of the skin and mucous membranes. It typically begins as an eruption of red wheals (urticarial lesions) and evolves over weeks to months to bullae (large blisters).

Bullous pemphigoid is an autoimmune disorder (i.e., a condition in which your immune system mistakenly attacks normal parts of the body, resulting in tissue injury or disease). It equally affects men and women and typically affects adults older than 60 years. It may occur in children. This condition may be hereditary but is not infectious or cancerous.

Diagnosis is usually based upon the appearance of skin lesions, evaluation of skin specimens, and blood tests. Your doctor may perform a skin biopsy (i.e., removal of a small piece of skin or other tissue) for laboratory evaluation to assist in diagnosis.

Medications that suppress your immune system have significantly improved symptoms and lessened the severity of the disease. However, bullous pemphigoid can persist for a long time, or it can recur.

Living With Your Diagnosis

Skin lesions typically begin as an eruption of red wheals (urticarial lesions) and evolve over weeks to months to bullae (large blisters). The bullae are typically tense and oval or round. They may arise from normal skin or from the red wheals. The bullae may rupture and cause erosions that may be painful. You may experience itching with the skin lesions. Bullous pemphigoid also can develop into erosions of the mouth, throat, anus, and vagina, which may also be mildly to moderately painful. The lesions can be generalized or localized to certain areas of the body. They typically involve the lower legs (often the first place that lesions develop), armpits, inner thighs, abdomen, and forearms.

You may have itching and pain, although these symptoms may be absent. Some bullae rupture, resulting in erosions of the skin and mucous linings. These erosions are prone to secondary bacterial infection, especially if you scratch the lesions. These infections often require antibiotic therapy. Significant pain and fever typically do not occur except in severe cases. You may also experience social embarrassment because of your skin's appearance.

Treatment

Specific treatment depends upon the location and severity of your bullous pemphigoid, its impact on the quality of your life, and your response to therapy. Treatment aims to lessen the severity of your condition and to prevent complications. Treatment consists of general measures and medications.

General measures are as follows:

1. Maintain good skin hygiene to reduce outbreaks and to decrease the risk of secondary bacterial infection.
2. Avoid skin injury, including scratching, which can aggravate bullous pemphigoid and contribute to secondary infections.
3. Individuals with bullous pemphigoid can become depressed or experience other psychological conditions. If you feel depressed or are having difficulty coping with your skin disorder, talk to your doctor about the best treatment options, including psychological counseling.

Your doctor may prescribe a variety of medications to reduce inflammation and symptoms and to lessen the severity and duration of bullous pemphigoid. These medications include:

1. Topical steroid creams, lotions, and ointments are effective in mild cases of bullous pemphigoid and as combination therapy for more severe cases. Your doctor may recommend placing occlusive dressings over the topical medications to increase their effects. Side effects of topical steroids include skin atrophy, formation of abnormal, small blood vessels, and absorption of medication through the skin into the bloodstream, which can cause toxic effects. To decrease the risk of side effects, do not exceed the recommended dosage prescribed by your doctor.
2. Corticosteroid tablets or injections are effective in treating bullous pemphigoid. Side effects are more likely with higher doses and include increased risk of infection, swelling, ulcers, diabetes mellitus, and osteoporosis (thinning of your bones). Do not stop steroid medications without first consulting your doctor because abrupt cessation of these medicines can result in severe weakness, fatigue, and low blood pressure.
3. Immunosuppressive medications such as azathioprine and cyclophosphamide are potent suppressors of your immune system and are effective in treating bullous pemphigoid. When these agents are combined with steroids, they allow less steroids to be used, thereby decreasing the

risk of side effects. Side effects of these agents include increased susceptibility to infection, and toxicity to your body's organs including the bone marrow (anemia, low values of white blood cells and platelets), liver, and kidneys. Your doctor will need to closely monitor your response to therapy and to perform laboratory tests to check for possible toxic effects.

4. Your doctor may prescribe dapsone to reduce skin eruptions and blistering and to lessen the severity of your condition. You will probably need to take this medication for an extended period. Your doctor will need to monitor for side effects by checking periodic laboratory tests. Side effects may include breakdown of red blood cells (hemolytic anemia), inflammation of the peripheral nerves (peripheral neuropathy), nausea, vomiting, and abdominal pains.

No specific dietary measures can prevent or treat bullous pemphigoid. In severe cases, lesions in the lining of your mouth or throat cause pain with eating or swallowing. You may need to follow a liquid or soft diet to ensure adequate nutrition.

You will need to aggressively cleanse and monitor your wounds to prevent complications such as infection. Your doctor may recommend one or more of the following measures to care for your bullous pemphigoid:

1. Cleansing baths.
2. Local cleansing of skin wounds.
3. Wound dressings including topical steroids and use of antibiotic ointments.

The DOs
- Take medications as prescribed by your doctor.
- Inform your doctor of all other medications, including over-the-counter medicines, that you are taking. Continue these medications unless your doctor instructs you to stop them.
- Read the labels of medicines and follow all instructions. Consult your doctor if you have any concerns, or if you have new or unexplained symptoms that may result from side effects of the medication.
- Eat a well-balanced, nutritious diet. If lesions in your mouth or throat are causing pain with eating or swallowing, follow a liquid or soft diet to ensure adequate nutrition.
- Avoid activities that cause overheating and excessive sweating or moisture. If you perform activities that result in excessive moisture, immediately shower and cleanse the skin lesions.
- Maintain good skin hygiene to reduce the risk of secondary bacterial infection.
- Keep scheduled follow-up appointments with your doctor. They are essential to monitor your condition, your response to therapy, and to screen for possible side effects of treatment.
- Monitor your skin for healing and for evidence of secondary bacterial infection. Signs and symptoms of infection include redness around the skin lesions, purulent discharge (pus), increased pain or swelling of the skin lesions or lymph nodes, and fever.
- Frequently wash clothing, towels, and linens when skin lesions are oozing, crusting, or infected. This action reduces the risk of transmission of infection.

The DON'Ts
- Do not stop your medicine or change the prescribed dose without consulting your doctor.
- Do not exceed recommended doses of medicines, because higher doses may increase your risk of toxic effects.
- Do not use potent topical steroids on the skin of the face or genitals because these areas are most prone to skin injury and atrophy (thinning and wasting of the skin associated with wrinkling, and abnormal, small blood vessels).
- Do not abruptly stop steroids or immunosuppressive therapy, because you may experience a rebound worsening of your condition. Suddenly stopping steroid medication may result in serious health consequences, including severe weakness, fatigue, and low blood pressure. Consult your doctor before stopping these medications.
- Do not drive or perform other potentially hazardous activities when taking medications that can cause drowsiness or sedation (antihistamines or pain medications).
- Avoid activities that can increase the risk of infection of skin lesions.

When To Call Your Doctor
- If you have any signs or symptoms of infection (see above).
- If you notice that lesions are becoming worse, or if new lesions appear despite appropriate therapy.

- If you have signs and symptoms of systemic illness, including fever, lethargy, confusion, or weakness.
- If you have new or unexplained symptoms that may indicate a complication of your condition or side effects from medications.

<#5>For More Information

Consult your primary care physician or your dematologist to learn more about bullous pemphigoid. You may also contact: American Academy of Dermatology
Attention: Communications Department
930 N. Meacham Road
Schaumberg, IL 60173
847-330-0230

PEMPHIGUS VULGARIS

About Your Diagnosis

Pemphigus vulgaris is a serious, bullous disease of the skin and mucous membranes. It may be acute or chronic and is characterized by bullae (large blisters) that burst. The lesions then become erosive and crusting. This disease can be fatal unless the patient is treated with immunosuppressive agents (i.e., medications that reduce inflammation).

The cause is likely autoimmune (i.e., a condition in which your immune system mistakenly attacks normal parts of the body, resulting in tissue injury or disease). Certain medications can trigger the disease.

Pemphigus vulgaris is rare. It equally affects men and women, and typically affects adults between 40 and 60 years of age. This condition is not infectious or cancerous.

Diagnosis is usually based upon the appearance of skin lesions, testing of skin specimens, and blood tests. Your doctor may perform a skin biopsy (i.e., removal of a small piece of skin or other tissue) for laboratory evaluation to assist in diagnosis.

Medications that suppress your immune system have significantly improved survival and recovery. Before immunosuppressive therapy, the disease was often fatal.

Living With Your Diagnosis

Pemphigus vulgaris typically starts as painful erosions of the mucous lining of the mouth, nose, throat, vagina, and anus. Many patients are unable to eat normally because of the pain associated with chewing and swallowing. As a result, patients can have weakness, fatigue, and weight loss caused by nutritional deficits. Your skin may not be affected for several months. The skin lesions are typically vesicles (i.e., small blisters) and bullae (i.e., large blisters) that are flabby, easily broken, and weeping. The blisters may be localized to certain areas of the skin for 6–12 months before becoming more generalized. As the bullae rupture, they develop extensive erosions that weep fluid, bleed easily, and crust. These erosions are prone to develop secondary bacterial infections. Irritation of the mucous linings can cause symptoms such as hoarseness, difficulty and/or painful swallowing, and bleeding.

Pemphigus vulgaris can be fatal if not aggressively treated with immunosuppressive therapy. Because of the extensive erosions, patients are highly susceptible to secondary bacterial infections, which may require debridement (aggressive local cleansing of the wounds) and antibiotic therapy. These infections are serious and have the potential to spread throughout the body. Individuals may have nutritional deficits because of the pain associated with eating and swallowing, resulting in weight loss, fatigue, and malnutrition. Dehydration and abnormalities of electrolytes (such as sodium and potassium) can occur as a result of nutritional deficits and extensive fluid loss from weeping of the ruptured bullae. Scarring can also occur, although scarring is markedly reduced if the bullae and erosions are allowed to heal spontaneously or to heal with appropriate immunosuppressive therapy.

Treatment

Treatment consists of various immunosuppressive medications. These agents lessen the effects of your immune system, reducing the formation of new blisters, decreasing inflammation and pain associated with the blisters, and promoting healing. In severe cases, patients require supportive measures including intravenous fluids, aggressive debridement of the wounds, antibiotic therapy to treat secondary bacterial infections, and intensive care of the wounds. These measures often require hospitalization.

Medications lessen the effects of your immune system, thereby reducing inflammation and suppressing the formation of new bullae. These agents are effective and have significantly improved the survival and recoverability for patients with pemphigus vulgaris. However, these medications may cause side effects.

Your doctor may prescribe one or more of the following agents:

1. Corticosteroids. High doses of these medications given as either tablet or injection are effective in treating pemphigus vulgaris. Side effects are more likely with higher doses, and include increased susceptibility to infection, swelling, ulcers, diabetes mellitus, and osteoporosis (thinning of your bones). Do not stop steroid medication without first consulting your doctor, because abrupt cessation of these medicines can result in severe fatigue, weakness, and low blood pressure. Topical steroid creams, lotions, and ointments are used for milder cases.

2. Immunosuppressive medications such as azathioprine, methotrexate, and cyclophosphamide. These medications are potent suppressors of your immune system and are effective in treating pemphigus vulgaris. When these agents are combined with steroids, they reduce the total steroid dose required to treat your condition, potentially decreasing side effects. Side effects of these agents include increased susceptibility to infection and toxicity to your body's organs, including the bone marrow (anemia and abnormally low values of white blood cells and platelets), liver, and kidneys. Your doctor will closely monitor your response to therapy and order laboratory tests to check for possible toxic effects.
3. Gold therapy for milder cases. These medicines are given as weekly injections. Your doctor will restrict the total dose of gold to reduce your risk of toxic effects to the liver and kidneys.

Your doctor may prescribe other medications to reduce symptoms and to treat complications of pemphigus vulgaris. These medications include:
1. Appropriate antibiotics to treat secondary bacterial infections.
2. Medications to control pain and discomfort.
3. Talc or powder to apply to the wounds and to bed linens. This can be used in combination with topical antibiotic ointments to help treat secondary bacterial infection.

No specific dietary measures can prevent or treat pemphigus vulgaris. However, malnutrition and imbalances of fluid and electrolytes are common. Therefore, your doctor will encourage you to eat and will closely monitor your nutritional status. If signs of malnutrition develop, your doctor may recommend hospitalization for more intensive fluid and nutritional care.

You will need to aggressively cleanse and monitor your wounds to prevent complications such as infections or imbalances of fluids and electrolytes.

Your doctor may recommend one or more of the following measures:
1. Cleansing baths.
2. Debridement and local cleansing of skin wounds.
3. Dressings including use of antibiotic ointments, topical steroids, and talc.
4. Correction of fluid and electrolyte imbalances.
5. Plasmapharesis. In severe cases, plasmapheresis is used in conjunction with medications. Plasmapheresis is a procedure performed by trained personnel in which some of your blood is removed from your body. The blood is then placed in a machine that can remove antibodies of your immune system which are causing your pemphigus vulgaris. Blood is then reinjected into your bloodstream. This treatment is effective in reducing the effects of your immune system.

The DOs
- Take medications as prescribed by your doctor.
- Inform your doctor of all other medications, including over-the-counter medicines, that you are taking. Continue these medications unless your doctor instructs you to stop them.
- Read the labels of medicines and follow all instructions.
- Consult your doctor if you have any concerns, or if you have new or unexplained symptoms that may be caused by side effects of the medication.
- Eat a well-balanced, nutritious diet. If lesions in your mouth or throat are causing pain with eating or swallowing, follow a liquid or soft diet to maintain nutrition.
- Keep follow-up appointments with your physician to evaluate your response to therapy, to monitor for complications of pemphigus vulgaris, and to assess for possible toxic effects of medications.
- Use general measures including cleansing baths, wound care, and dressings as instructed.
- Closely check your skin and mucosal lesions for healing. Contact your physician if you have any signs of secondary infection, including redness around the lesions, purulent discharge (pus), increased pain or swelling of the wounds or lymph nodes, and fever.
- Frequently clean towels, linens, and clothing to reduce your risk of secondary bacterial infection.

The DON'Ts
- Do not stop your medication or change the prescribed dose without first consulting your doctor. Do not exceed recommended doses of medications, because higher doses can increase your risk of toxic effects.
- Do not abruptly stop steroids or immunosuppressive therapy, because you may experience a rebound worsening of your condition. In particular, do not suddenly stop steroids, because this action can have serious effects to your health, including severe low blood pressure, fatigue, and

weakness. Consult your doctor before stopping these medications.

- Do not share towels, linens, or clothing with other individuals to reduce the spread of infection.
- Avoid swimming or using a Jacuzzi until cleared by your physician.
- To decrease your risk of infection, avoid activities that may result in contamination of your skin wounds and erosions.
- Do not drive or perform other potentially hazardous activities when taking medication that can cause drowsiness or sedation (e.g., pain medications).

When to Call Your Doctor

- If you have any signs or symptoms of infection (see above).
- If you notice that lesions are becoming worse or if new lesions appear, despite appropriate therapy.
- If you have signs and symptoms of systemic illness, including fever, lethargy, confusion, or weakness.
- If you have new or unexplained symptoms, which may indicate a complication of your condition or side effects from medications.

For More Information

Consult your primary care physician or your dematologist to learn more about pemphigus vulgaris. You may also contact: American Academy of Dermatology
Attention: Communications Department
930 N. Meacham Road
Schaumberg, IL 60173
847-330-0230

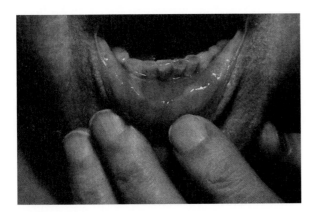

Pemphigus vulgaris with oral erosions and no intact bullae. (Courtesy of Department of Dermatology, University of North Carolina at Chapel Hill. From Goldstein BG, Goldstein AO: *Practical Dermatology*, vol 1. St. Louis, Mosby–Year Book, 1992. Used by permission.)

PEPTIC ULCER DISEASE

About Your Diagnosis

Peptic ulcers are erosions in the lining of the esophagus, stomach, or duodenum. Ulcers in the stomach are called gastric ulcers, and duodenal ulcers if in the duodenum. The cause of peptic ulcer disease (PUD) is not fully known. It is clear that Helicobacter pylori (H. pylori) does play a role in PUD.

Helicobacter pylori is a bacteria found in the stomach and duodenum. Drugs such as aspirin and non-steroidal anti-inflammatory drugs play a role in some cases of PUD, particularly with gastric ulcers.

Peptic ulcer disease is common; there is a 10% lifetime prevalence in men and 5% in women. Duodenal ulcers are four times more common than gastric ulcers. Peptic ulcer disease is detected by an upper gastrointestinal (GI) x-ray or endoscopy (a flexible lighted tube used to view the stomach and duodenum). Occasionally biopsy specimens are obtained during the endoscopy to make sure a more serious disease is not present. Testing is available to determine whether H. pylori is present in the stomach and duodenum.

With treatment, ulcers do heal within a few weeks. However ulcers do reoccur. Before treatments for H. pylori, reoccurrence was common. Many individuals required long-term maintenance treatment. Since the development of effective treatments for H. pylori, the reoccurrence rate is less than 10% in the first year.

Living With Your Diagnosis

The symptoms of a peptic ulcer do not vary depending on location. The most common symptom is pain, occurring in the epigastric (upper abdominal) area. It is described as a burning, gnawing, or boring pain. It generally occurs 1–3 hours after meals. It may awaken one from sleep. The pain is relieved by food or antacids. The pain appears in clusters. It may be present for a few weeks, then resolve for weeks to months only to return. Other symptoms of PUD include abdominal bloating, heartburn, nausea, and vomiting. Up to 25% of individuals with PUD will initially be seen with a complication of the disease. Internal bleeding is a common complication. Some individuals with PUD will have black, tarry stools indicating a bleeding ulcer. Others will have vomiting with blood or "coffee ground" material in it. The bleeding may be severe enough to cause shock. Others will initially be seen with a perforation. A perforation is a hole in the stomach or duodenum. The pain of a perforation happens suddenly and is severe. The pain starts in the epigastric area and moves to the right shoulder.

Treatment

The goal of treatment is to heal the ulcer, help the symptoms, stop relapses, and avoid complications. There are two treatment options: medication and surgery. Medications are used to decrease the acid production in the stomach and treat the H. pylori (when present). Antacids have been available for many years to treat ulcers. However, they can be inconvenient because of the frequency in which they have to be taken. To decrease acid production, a histamine-2 (H_2) blocker is frequently given. Another drug, sucralfate, coats the ulcer and protects the lining of the stomach from the acid. Proton pump inhibitors such as omeprazole can be used to suppress the acid secretion. Multiple drug combinations are used to treat the H. pylori infection. Antibiotics, proton pump inhibitors, and bismuth are used in various combinations. After the treatment is completed, many individuals are started on a lower dose of the medicine to prevent reoccurrence.

Surgery is an option when medications fail or there are serious complications. There are different options that the surgeon may choose depending on the type of ulcer and the complications that may be present. Because medications have improved in recent years, the frequency of surgery has declined.

The DOs
- Maintain proper eating habits.
- Take medications as prescribed.
- Antacids may help relieve the symptoms.
- Try to reduce the stress in your life. It can play a role in ulcer formation.

The DON'Ts
- Avoid smoking.
- Avoid excess alcohol consumption.
- Avoid aspirin and nonsteroidal anti-inflammatory drugs.
- Avoid caffeine and any food that makes the symptoms worse.

When to Call Your Doctor
- If you have symptoms of an ulcer.
- If you vomit blood or "coffee ground" material.

- If there is blood in the stool or stools are dark and tarry.
- If pain does not improve with treatment

For More Information
National Digestive Diseases Information Clearinghouse
2 Information Way
Bethesda, MD 20892-3570
www.niddk.nih.gov
nddic@aerie.com

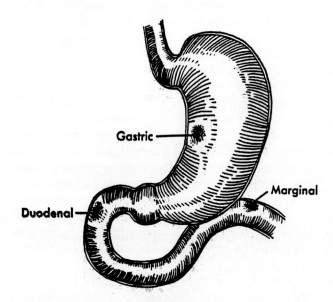

Common sites of peptic ulcers. (From LaFleur-Brooks ML: *Exploring Medical Language—A Student Directed Approach.* vol 3. St. Louis, Mosby–Year Book, 1993. Used by permission.)

PERICARDITIS

About Your Diagnosis

Pericarditis is inflammation of the pericardium. The pericardium is the fibrous, membranous sac that encases the heart. It helps hold the heart in place in the chest and helps lubricate the pumping of the heart. Inflammation in the pericardium can be caused by infection, myocardial infarction (heart attack), cancer, radiation, or allergic reactions. It may have no known cause. The inflammation may injure the membrane and cause scarring, which constricts the heart (constrictive pericarditis). It may also cause decreased blood flow from the heart. This decreased blood flow causes symptoms of heart failure (decreased pumping efficiency of the heart), including difficulty breathing and swelling in the tissues of the legs, feet, or abdomen (edema).

Living With Your Diagnosis

Symptoms include chest pain behind the sternum (breast bone) and pain with change in position or with deep breathing. You may have a fever if infection is the cause of pericarditis. Sometimes palpitations (rapid heartbeat) are felt. The diagnosis is made on the basis of clinical symptoms and findings at a physical examination. An electrocardiogram (ECG) and chest radiograph (x-ray) show evidence of the inflammation. An echocardiogram (ultrasound examination of the heart) may show fluid in the pericardial sac.

Treatment

Treatment focuses on the cause of the inflammation and the pain. Infections are managed with antibiotics. Pain is usually managed with nonsteroidal anti-inflammatory drugs (NSAIDs) such as aspirin or ibuprofen. Steroidal anti-inflammatory drugs may be used in more severe cases. If fluid in the pericardium affects the ability of the heart to function, an operation may be performed to cut a window in the membrane to allow the fluid to drain.

The DOs

• Take your medications as scheduled. Taking all prescribed antibiotics until completed is especially important to keep the infection from returning. The pain may last for several days after the antibiotics are completed, and repeat echocardiograms may be needed.

The DON'Ts

• Avoid strenuous exertion until after the symptoms have resolved.
• Do not drink alcohol if you are taking steroidal anti-inflammatory drugs.

When to Call Your Doctor

• If you have new or worsening chest pain or pain with deep breaths or changes in position.
• If you have severe stomach pain or vomiting of blood. You can take acetaminophen (eg, Tylenol) for pain even if you are already taking aspirin or anti-inflammatory drugs.

For More Information

Call the American Heart Association at 1-800-242-8721 and ask for the literature department.

PERTUSSIS

About Your Diagnosis

Pertussis or "whooping cough" is a highly contagious bacterial disease usually occurring in children younger than 4 years. The causative agent is *Bordetella pertussis*, which is usually transmitted by aerosol spread and inhalation. The incubation period is approximately 7–14 days, during which time the organism invades the upper and lower airways, resulting in increased mucus secretion.

Cultures of the nasopharynx, obtained by using a sterile cotton swab, as well as specific antibody testing are often diagnostic. Certain viral infections and tuberculosis can also mimic the pertussis syndrome.

Living With Your Diagnosis

There are usually three stages to the disease. The first stage has a relatively gradual onset and is associated with sneezing, runny nose, and fatigue, in addition to a hacking nighttime cough. After about 10–14 days, the cough becomes more frequent and more intense, followed by the whoop (a hurried, deep inspiration). During this second stage, lots of thick secretions may be produced, sometimes with vomiting and gagging. The recovery stage usually begins within 4 weeks, although recurrence of the coughing episodes may occur for several months in association with possible upper respiratory tract infections.

Treatment

The best treatment is prevention by active immunization. Starting oral antibiotic therapy during the incubation period, and continuing for 10–14 days may abort the infection. Isolation of affected individuals for at least 4 weeks or until symptoms have subsided is advised, although the use of antibiotic therapy may be helpful in diminishing infectivity to others. Hospitalization is recommended for seriously ill infants, in addition to use of small frequent meals and fluid replacement. Supplemental oxygen may be required, as well as close monitoring and aspiration precautions. Pertussis may be very serious in children younger than 2 years, with a mortality rate of approximately 1% to 2% in children younger than 1 year. Most frequent complications include bronchopneumonia, collapsed lung, convulsions, and hemorrhage. Ear infections are also common and may require further antibiotic therapy.

The DOs

Pertussis immunization has reduced the problems of this illness. Respiratory isolation and completion of antibiotic therapy as advised by your doctor is important. Careful hand washing and close attention to nutritional needs, especially fluid intake when vomiting occurs, are very important.

The DON'Ts

Don't stop medications unless advised by your doctor, even if the child is feeling well. Bed rest is not completely necessary for older children with mild disease. Do not force children to eat large quantities of food because this may only aggravate gagging and vomiting during coughing spells. Suction of excess mucus from the throat may be necessary. A darkened, quiet room with little disturbance may also help reduce the frequency and severity of the coughing or choking spells.

When to Call Your Doctor

Contact your doctor if your child comes into contact with another child who has had a recent diagnosis of whooping cough. For a child with pertussis, the caregiver should be prepared to closely monitor the child, as well as to follow respiratory isolation procedures. Pertussis is a serious illness and may be fatal, especially in young children.

For More Information
Contact your local health department for additional information about pertussis.

PHARYNGITIS

About Your Diagnosis

Pharyngitis is an inflammation of the throat that is most commonly caused by viral infections, but can also be caused by bacterial infections. The tonsils can also be involved. Diagnosis is usually done by obtaining a throat culture.

Living With Your Diagnosis

Signs and symptoms of the disease include fever, sore throat, difficulty swallowing, and general achiness.

Treatment

Antibiotics may be prescribed. Nonaspirin medications can be taken for the fever and pain. Gargle with a warm salt water solution to relieve the sore throat. A cool-mist vaporizer may help relieve the dry, tight feeling in the throat.

The DOs

- Take antibiotics, if prescribed, until finished.
- Take Tylenol or Advil for pain and fever.
- Gargle with a warm salt water solution to relieve sore throat (use 1/2 teaspoon of salt in 1 cup of warm water).
- Use a vaporizer to relieve the dry, tight feeling in the throat. Clean the vaporizer and change the water daily.
- Replace your toothbrush after treatment is started to prevent reinfection.
- Limit your activities until symptoms subside.
- Increase your fluid intake.
- Follow a liquid diet if swallowing is difficult (soups, jello, ice cream, and juices).

The DON'Ts

- Don't skip doses or stop antibiotics until finished.
- Don't give aspirin to a child younger than 16 years with a viral illness because of the risk of Reye's syndrome.
- Don't share food or drinking glasses.

When to Call Your Doctor

- If fever continues after treatment is started.
- If there is increased difficulty in breathing or swallowing.
- If a severe headache occurs.
- If a rash develops.
- If a cough develops that produces thick, yellow-green or bloody sputum.

For More Information

American Academy of Otolaryngology
One Prince Street
Alexandria, VA 22314
703-836-4444, Monday through Friday from 8:30 AM to 5 PM (EST).
American Lung Association
800-Lung-USA (800-586-4872)
National Jewish Center for Immunology and Respiratory Medicine
1400 Jackson Street
Denver, CO 80206
800-222-5864, Monday through Friday from 8:30 AM to 5 PM (MST), for a nurse to answer questions and send information, or 800-552-5864 for recorded information.

PHEOCHROMOCYTOMA

About Your Diagnosis

Pheochromocytoma is a tumor of the adrenal gland or the sympathetic nervous system chain that secretes adrenaline (epinephrine) or related compounds. This causes symptoms of high blood pressure, heart palpitations, headaches, and sweats that come and go over time.

Doctors do not know what causes pheochromocytomas to form. Most cases occur sporadically, but approximately 10% are part of familial endocrine tumor syndromes.

Pheochromocytomas are uncommon. They account for only 0.1% to 0.01% of all patients with hypertension.

Patients may complain of episodic spells of hypertension, headaches, sweats, or anxiety. Alternatively, a tumor may be noted on the adrenal glands while examining the abdomen for other reasons. Pheochromocytomas are diagnosed by measuring catecholamines in a 24-hour urine collection. It is important that the patient be in a nonstressful environment when this test is done, and that the patient not be consuming alcohol, caffeine, amphetamines, benzodiazepines, certain antidepressants, or lithium, which may falsely elevate urinary catecholamine levels. Once excess catecholamine secretion has been documented with the urine test, a magnetic resonance imaging (MRI) of the adrenal glands with T2-weighted images will localize the tumor. Ten percent of tumors lie outside the adrenals. These patients may require whole-body imaging with special nuclear medicine tests.

More than 90% of pheochromocytomas are curable by surgery because they are contained within the adrenal gland. Ten percent of these tumors, however, are malignant and are not curable with surgery. Such patients require a combination of treatments to control their disease.

Living With Your Diagnosis

Episodic headaches, anxiety, palpitations (strong heart beats), sweats, high blood pressure, heat intolerance, and dizziness when standing are common symptoms. Some individuals may have no symptoms.

Uncontrolled hypertension can cause loss of vision, heart disease, kidney disease, and strokes.

Treatment

More than 90% of pheochromocytomas are confined to the adrenal glands and are cured with surgery. The experience of the surgeon is critical for the success of the operation. Appropriate preoperative treatment must be instituted to ensure a safe operation. Complications from surgery include bleeding and infection, and transient low and high blood pressure reactions that can occur while the tumor is being removed. Rapid intraoperative response is required by the anesthesiologist. A catheter may be placed into a central vein to carefully monitor your cardiovascular status.

Patients should be started on a blood pressure medicine called phenoxybenzamine or another similar medicine preoperatively. Phenoxybenzamine may cause low blood pressure upon standing (orthostatic hypotension). Eat a high-salt diet and drink plenty of fluids to prevent this side effect. Phenoxybenzamine can also cause dry mouth, nasal congestion, and dizziness. The dose needs to be carefully adjusted preoperatively. A second medicine called a beta blocker may be added after the phenoxybenzamine has been started. Beta blockers help prevent racing heartbeats. Other blood pressure medicines may be used as well.

Malignant tumors should be surgically resected to remove as much tumor tissue as possible. Most patients will then be started on phenoxybenzamine postoperatively to control blood pressure. Usually, a combination of chemotherapy, radiation therapy, or other treatments are used to help control the spread of the disease.

The DOs

- Increase your fluid and salt intake preoperatively to prevent dizziness.
- Have your blood pressure checked both lying down and standing preoperatively.
- Rest as much as possible until your tumor has been removed to minimize extra stress to your heart.
- Inform your doctor if you have a history of pheochromocytomas, or other endocrine tumors in your family. Family members may need screening blood work or urine testing.

The DON'Ts

- Don't take a diuretic medicine (unless specifically ordered by your doctor) before your operation. This can lead to dehydration.
- Don't take the beta blocker medication if you are

not already on phenoxybenzamine or a similar compound. Beta blockers alone could lead to severely elevated blood pressures in patients with pheochromocytomas.

- Don't perform strenuous exercise until your pheochromocytoma has been removed.
- Don't expect that your high blood pressure will completely normalize after the operation. Some permanent changes may have already occurred in the kidneys and blood vessels.
- Don't forget to see your doctor on a regular basis to make sure that the tumor has not returned.

When to Call Your Doctor

- You have a change in your vision, a severe headache, weakness on one side of the body, chest pains, or increasing palpitations.
- You have ankle swelling or shortness of breath.
- You have weakness or dizziness when standing.
- Your symptoms return postoperatively.

For More Information

National Adrenal Diseases Foundation
505 Northern Boulevard, Suite 200
Great Neck, NY 11021
516-487-4992
The Endocrine Society
4350 East West Highway, Suite 500
Bethesda, MD 20814-4410
1-888-ENDOCRINE

PHOBIAS

About Your Diagnosis

In simple terms, a phobia is a fear of some behavior or some event. This fear is often accompanied by physical signs such as rapid heart rate, shortness of breath, feeling of a lump in the throat, tightness in the chest, and diarrhea. Individuals will often go to great lengths to avoid the stimulus that causes their fear or phobia, if that is possible. It is only when such fears become so intense that they interfere with social and occupational functioning that the attention of a psychiatrist is sought. In social phobia, there is a significant and long-lasting fear of one or more social situations in which individuals might be exposed to unfamiliar people or to possible scrutiny by others.

Living With Your Diagnosis

Individuals with a social phobia have a fear that they will act in a humiliating or embarrassing way. Such activities as writing a check in public, eating in a restaurant, and using a public restroom facility are examples of behavior that individuals with social phobia will try to avoid. If, however, these situations cannot be avoided, exposure to them almost always creates significant anxiety, which may even lead to a panic attack. Individuals with social phobia realize that the fear they are experiencing is unreasonable and excessive, but they are still unable to control it. Their only relief comes from avoiding the specific activity that they fear. An individuals' occupation may enhance exposure to the phobic event, such as individuals who work in a bank, or who are accountants or secretaries, where writing in full view of others may be part of the job. In that case, there can be a significant impairment in their occupational functioning.

The most common phobias are the specific phobias. Individuals with specific phobias have a marked, long-lasting fear which is excessive or unreasonable that is caused by the presence of a specific object or situation. The most common objects or situations that provoke specific phobias are fear of flying, fear of heights (acrophobia), fear of spiders (arachniphobia), fear of strangers (xenophobia), or fear of receiving an injection, fear of seeing blood, and fear of being in small spaces (claustrophobia). Exposure to one of these events or situations causes significant anxiety that can escalate into a full-blown panic attack. Therefore individuals try to avoid whatever might be causing the fear or phobia. In some situations, this is fairly easy. For those individuals who fear snakes, being a city dweller will greatly minimize their exposure to snakes. Therefore, avoidance of them will be easy. Other situations obviously are hard to avoid. Individuals who have a fear of closed in places often cannot ride an elevator, and cannot have certain procedures done that involve closed in areas, such as a magnetic resonance imaging (MRI) scan. These individuals will have more trouble avoiding phobic situations than those who have a specific fear of animals or blood.

Phobias are among the most common of all psychiatric disorders. The specific phobias are more common in women than in men, although there are some differences in terms of types of phobia in each group. The incidence of social phobias in males and females is about the same. Most phobias begin in the middle-to-late teenage years, but often phobias of animals, blood, storms, and water begin in early childhood. Phobias of height tend to begin in the teens, whereas situational phobias such as claustrophobia begin in the late teens to middle 20s.

If the occurrence rates of specific phobias in males and females are compared, we find that women are much more likely than men to have a fear of (1) spiders, bugs, mice, and snakes; (2) public transportation, such as buses and planes; (3) elevators; (4) water (being in a swimming pool or lake); (5) storms; and (6) closed places. Males and females are equally fearful of heights.

Men and women are equally affected by a fear of speaking to strangers or meeting new people, and by a fear of eating in front of others. Women are only slightly more likely to have a fear of public speaking.

There is no specific factor that may cause a phobia, although there probably is a genetic component because these disorders tend to run in families. Some phobias begin after a traumatic event, but many patients cannot recall the specific onset of their phobia. The onset of the phobia or fear can be sudden or gradual.

Treatment

In the treatment of phobia, the main goal is to decrease fear to a level that no longer causes significant distress, and to minimize the need to avoid the object or situation the patient fears, so that the ability to function is no longer impaired. Treatment also serves to improve some of the skills that phobic avoidance may have prevented the individual from obtaining or developing adequately, such as driving or social skills. Typically, an effective treatment for social phobia lasts several months, although the treatment of some specific social phobias, such as public speaking, may take less time. Specific phobias can be treated relatively quickly. In fact, the vast majority of individuals with phobias of animals, blood, or injections are able to overcome their phobias in one session of behavioral treatment.

Phobias can be effectively treated by using medications, behavioral techniques, or both. There is a marked difference in the response of social phobia and specific phobias to medication. Medication has generally been ineffective for the specific phobias. If medications are used, they are generally used to treat the consequences of the phobia, such as panic disorder, in which case the antidepressant imipramine and the serotonin drugs Paxil and Prozac are used. Therefore, medications that are effective for panic disorder may prove to be effective for situational phobias as well. In contrast to the specific phobias, the social phobias have been treated successfully with medication. The monoamine oxidase (MAO) inhibitor antidepressants, such as phenelzine (Nardil), are very effective for many patients with social phobias. The benzodiazepines such as clonazepam (Klonopin) and alprazolam (Xanax) have also shown some beneficial effects, as have the beta-blockers such as Atenolol and Inderal, which are used extensively for performance anxiety. Often, Inderal or Atenolol will be given to individuals who are stage performers just before their activity. These drugs decrease significantly some of the signs of anxiety, especially tachycardia or a sense of the heart pounding.

In contrast to drug therapy, numerous studies have shown that exposure-based treatments are effective for treating patients with specific phobias, including fear of blood, injections, dentists, animals, enclosed places, flying, heights, and choking. Also, the way in which individuals are exposed to these specific fears may make a difference in how well they respond to treatment. Exposure seems to work best when sessions are spaced close together, and prolonged exposure seems to be more effective than exposure for a short duration. During exposure to the object that is feared, patients should be discouraged from engaging in avoidance techniques such as distraction or thinking of something else, or overuse of different safety techniques such as being accompanied by someone during exposure. Gradual exposure to the feared object is the most common behavioral treatment for phobias and is very effective for the specific phobias. For instance, an individual with a fear of driving may initially spend some time washing a car, staying in the garage with a car, and then gradually advance to sitting in the car in the garage, sitting in the car in the driveway, backing the car out of the driveway, and so on. This gradual exposure to the feared event can offer the individual ways of dealing with the anxiety that comes from being near the feared object. Biofeedback often is helpful in helping the individual control his heart rate and breathing when exposed to the object.

In summary, there are three basic types of phobias: (1) agoraphobia, (2) social phobias, and (3) specific phobias. Agoraphobia is a fear of wide open spaces and the fear of being trapped without being able to return home. Social phobias are fears of performing certain activities in public or areas where the activity may be witnessed; for example, writing checks in public or eating in public. Specific phobias are fears of specific objects or situations, such as a fear of flying, fear of driving, fear of animals, fear of snakes, fear of strangers, fear of heights, and fear of closed places. It seems that the social phobias respond very well to medication, in particular to such drugs as the MAO inhibitor, Nardil. In contrast, the specific phobias respond much better to behavioral techniques, such as gradual exposure to the object and rating the anxiety produced by that, and then using biofeedback, hypnosis, or some other technique to diminish the anxiety.

There are side effects that can result from the medications used to treat phobias. In particular, patients who are taking the MAO inhibitor, Nardil, must follow certain dietary restrictions as well as avoid certain medications. Such patients cannot eat aged cheeses or fava beans and cannot drink red wine, especially Chianti wine. Also, patients should avoid the use of medications such as Demerol, any epinephrine-containing compounds, and cocaine while taking the MAO inhibitor. Patients must also avoid using any other antidepressants such as imipramine, Elavil, or Prozac within 2 weeks of being on the MAO inhibitor. If these dietary and medication restrictions are not followed, the MAO inhibitor may cause a severe hypertensive crisis. Therefore, patients who already have high blood pressure should not take this medication. Of course, the benzodiazepines such as Klonopin and Ativan can decrease respirations, so they should not be used in patients who have serious lung disease. They also tend to produce sedation, which may impair driving or activity that requires delicate machinery. The benzodiazepines have the additional problem of being potentially addictive. The tricyclic antidepressants such as imipramine can cause blurred vision, dry mouth, possible constipation, rapid heartbeat, and in some cases oversedation.

The DOs

If you do have a phobic disorder, it is very important to report this condition to your physician. Many individuals, especially some males, are embarrassed to admit their fear to certain objects. Specific phobias, however, can be successfully treated, often in a single session.

Because phobias are anxiety disorders, it is important to avoid undo stress. It is also important to minimize the use of stimulants, including caffeine and sugar in your diet. Getting plenty of exercise often provides an outlet for the anxiety associated with phobias, as well as relieving some of the consequences of phobias. If you do have a phobia of specific objects that can be successfully avoided without significant impairment of your functioning, such as snakes, then you should do so.

The DON'Ts

You should not take any medications without consulting with your physician. Many over-the-counter (OTC) medications have some stimulant properties and can increase the anxiety associated with phobias. Such OTC drugs as Valerian Root may interact with antidepressants.

When to Call Your Doctor

You should call your physician if you notice phobic attacks occurring more often, if you have physical complications from increased anxiety, or if you become depressed and suicidal because of a phobic condition.

For More Information

Most cities have phobic support groups, especially for specific phobias such as claustrophobia, and these can be contacted by calling your local crisis center line or talking to the psychiatry department at your local medical school.

For information online, try the Center for Anxiety and Stress Treatment @ http://www.cts.com/~health.

PHOTODERMATITIS

About Your Diagnosis

Photodermatitis is an itchy, scaly, blistery, reddening of the skin, caused by an increase of the skin's normal sensitivity to the effects of sunlight or ultraviolet rays A or B (UVA or UVB). This can be genetic (run in families), but most often the cause can be traced to chemicals found in medicines, cosmetics, and foods.

The tendency to photosensitization can be used therapeutically as well, as in the psoralen therapy used to treat psoriasis.

More than 10% of Americans have had some form of photodermatitis.

Living With Your Diagnosis

Signs of photodermatitis include redness, dryness, blistering, and bumpy rash. These may feel painful or itchy, and sometimes are hard to differentiate from the usual case of mild sunburn. There is always a pattern of exposure to the sun or ultraviolet radiation (e.g., from a tanning bed) preceding the onset of the skin problem, but often the time of exposure is minimal. Long-term effects of photodermatitis include chronic skin thickening and scarring, and increased risk of skin cancer in patients with a genetic source of their dermatitis.

Treatment

Prevention is the best treatment for this disease, when possible. Be sure to ask your doctor and pharmacist whether you should avoid sun exposure while taking medication. Check with your doctor before beginning any tanning ritual!

Once photodermatitis has occurred, the basis of therapy is to minimize the inflammation in the damaged skin while treating painful symptoms as well. Steroid creams or tablets may be prescribed. Antibacterial creams such as silvadene may be prescribed for burnlike reactions. Avoidance of the sun and elimination of the offending substance, if possible, is essential. Your doctor will review your medicines and inquire about new or different foods you may have eaten before the outbreak, and together you will agree on a plan to adjust your diet or medical regimen as necessary. Always use a sunblock for both UVA and UVB with an SPF of 15 or greater each morning.

The DOs

- Always take medications only as prescribed, and avoid ultraviolet light exposure as much as possible while using known photosensitizers .
- Do use PABA-free sunblocks, sunscreens, hats, and long sleeves to minimize the effects of unavoidable exposure.
- Do limit the amount of limes, celery, carrots, and figs in your diet, because these contain natural psoralens (sun sensitizers).
- Do avoid PABA- and musk-containing skin products.
- Do avoid "natural" fruit-based skin lotions and cosmetics, because they may contain sensitizers as well.
- Do check with your doctor before using any tanning device, no matter how "safe" the manufacturer says it is.

The DON'Ts

- Don't take sun exposure for granted. Once you have had photodermatitis, your skin will be sensitive to the combination of sun and the chemical you are sensitized to indefinitely.
- Don't rely on sun lotions and lightweight clothing to provide sun protection for prolonged periods.
- Don't rely on clouds for sunblock; they do not block ultraviolet rays.

When to Call Your Doctor

- If you have fever, chills, nausea or vomiting.
- If infection or pus is noted at the area of dermatitis.
- If dermatitis worsens despite treatment.
- If a stomachache or severe nausea occur while taking steroid medicines by mouth.
- If sudden bone pain develops while taking steroid medicines by mouth.

For More Information
American Academy of Dermatology
930 N. Meachum Road
Schaumburg, IL 60173
847-330-0230

PINWORMS

About Your Diagnosis

Pinworms are an intestinal infestation with a parasite. It is common worldwide. It is frequently found in children between the ages of 5 and 14 years. Crowded living conditions increase the chance of spread to several family members. It is generally more of a nuisance than a major health problem.

It is caused by a small worm that finds its way to the intestine to live. The female worm will travel to the anal area to lay eggs. The eggs are spread to others by contact on toilet seats, by hand-to-hand contact, or hand-to-mouth contact. Contact with contaminated clothing or bed linens could also spread them.

The infestation is detected by the description of symptoms, and a simple test using a special tape applied over the anal area that is then examined under the microscope for eggs. Pinworms are easily treated with medications.

Living With Your Diagnosis

Signs and symptoms include skin irritation and painful itching around the anal area, especially at night; interruption of sleep because of the itching; and, in females, a vaginal discharge with itching and discomfort if pinworms migrate to the vaginal opening. Complications are rare.

Treatment

Treatment is with an antiworm medication. All members of the family should be treated at the same time. Directions must be followed carefully. Notify your doctor if anyone is pregnant or has a seizure disorder. The medication must be taken on an empty stomach. Side effects of the medications include nausea, vomiting, and diarrhea. The bowel movements will be the color of the medication. Creams or lotions may be helpful to relieve itching and irritation.

The DOs

- Take the medication as directed by your doctor.
- Teach children good hand washing with soap after toileting and before eating.
- Notify the school nurse or day care if a child is affected.
- Keep fingernails clean and short.
- Shower daily and change underwear and bed linens daily.
- Use very hot water to wash dishes.
- Scrub all washable toys with a bleach solution.
- Scrub toilets thoroughly.
- Maintain a normal diet as tolerated.
- Follow-up with your doctor 2 weeks after treatment to make sure all parasites have been destroyed.

The DON'Ts

- Don't alter the medication schedule.
- Don't scratch the anal area.
- Don't allow other children to play or sleep over until treatment has been completed to prevent spread of the infestation.

When to Call Your Doctor

- If anyone has symptoms of pinworms again after treatment.
- If anyone has side effects from the medications that don't disappear quickly.

For More Information
National Institute of Allergy and Infectious Diseases
Office of Communications
Building 31 Rm 7A-50
9000 Rockville Pike
Bethesda, MD 20892
301-496-5717
Internet Site
www.healthfinder.gov (Choose SEARCH to search by topic.)

PITYRIASIS ROSEA

About Your Diagnosis

Pityriasis rosea is a common skin condition seen most frequently in children and young adults. The cause is unknown but may be from a virus; however, it is not considered to be contagious. The diagnosis is based on the history and physical examination. Pityriasis rosea usually resolves within 4–6 weeks and recurrences are rare.

Living With Your Diagnosis

Pityriasis rosea starts off with a small, round or oval patch with a red border and clearing in the center. (This may be confused with ringworm.) Within 2–10 days, a more general rash occurs in a Christmas tree pattern over the back, trunk, and chest. The neck, arms, legs, and face may also be involved. This rash is characterized by multiple small, oval spots. They may be pink, red, or tan but occasionally are a lighter color. New spots can appear for weeks. Itching can be very mild; rarely will itching be severe. Most cases resolve within 6 weeks but some can last for months. Some patients have mild fever and headaches and may feel tired. Pityriasis rosea heals without scarring. In dark-skinned individuals, there may be some long-lasting lighter brown spots.

Treatment

The aim of treatment is to decrease itching. Treatment does not shorten the course of pityriasis rosea. Over-the-counter medications such as calamine lotion, Benadryl, and Aveno Oatmeal baths can decrease the itching. Ultraviolet light treatments may also be prescribed. Exposure to sunlight may be helpful but sunburns should be avoided.

The DO's

- Apply calamine lotion two times per day to affected areas. Add one packet of Aveno Oatmeal to the tub and bathe for 10 minutes in lukewarm water.
- Try Benadryl for itching.
- Try over-the-counter hydrocortisone cream for itching if the above fails. Apply every 8–10 hours.

The DON'Ts

- Heat will worsen the itching, so don't take a hot bath or shower.
- If the skin becomes too dry, decrease the frequency of lotion use to once per day or every other day.
- Avoid strenuous activity if this aggravates the rash.

When to Call Your Doctor

- If the medications are not helping the itching after a few days of use.
- If not better in 6–8 weeks.
- If any signs of secondary infection occur, such as high fever, pus drainage, or swelling.

For More Information
American Academy of Dermatology
930 N. Meacham Road
Schaumburg, IL 60173
847-330-0230

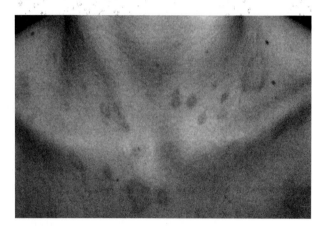

Pityriasis rosea. Note left supraclavicular herald patch and diffuse scaling papules and plaques in a Christmas tree distribution. (Courtesy of Department of Dermatology, University of North Carolina at Chapel Hill. From Goldstein BG, Goldstein AO: *Practical Dermatology*, vol 1. St. Louis, Mosby–Year Book, 1992. Used by permission.)

PNEUMONIA, BACTERIAL

About Your Diagnosis

Pneumonia is a term that refers to inflammation of the lung. Bacterial pneumonia means that inflammation is caused by a bacterial infection. Bacteria gain access to the lungs either through inhalation or via the bloodstream. Infections occur when the bacteria overwhelm the defense mechanisms. The following conditions may weaken your body's defense mechanisms and thus increase the risks for bacterial pneumonia:

- Old age.
- Smoking.
- Chronic alcohol use or misuse.
- Chronic lung disease.
- Congestive heart failure.
- Diabetes.
- Chronic kidney failure.
- Human immunodeficiency virus (HIV) infection.
- Use of drugs that are designed to lower your body's immune system, such as anticancer agents and prednisone.
- Recent viral respiratory tract infections.

Pneumonia can also occur in usually healthy individuals of all ages.

There are many different types of bacteria that can cause pneumonia. *Streptococcus* and *Mycoplasma* are common causes for pneumonia in otherwise healthy individuals. Those with chronic illnesses can be affected by *Staphylococcus, Haemophilus, Legionella*, and types of bacteria that are normally found in the intestinal tract. Bacteria normally found in the mouth can also cause pneumonia when they are accidentally inhaled into the lungs during seizures or coma.

Tests are performed to determine the cause and severity of pneumonia, including chest x-rays and analyses of sputum and blood. Despite these tests, the responsible bacteria is often not identified. Your doctor will then consider the circumstances in which the pneumonia began and the severity of the illness to help guide treatment. Other conditions may cause pneumonia-like symptoms, including heart failure, blood clot to the lungs, and cancer.

Living With Your Diagnosis

Pneumonia can range from a mild illness to a life-threatening condition. Common symptoms are fever, cough, chest pain, and shortness of breath. Phlegm may be yellow or green and contain blood. With some types of pneumonia, muscle aches, nausea/vomiting, fatigue, and weakness are prominent. Severe pneumonia is signaled by rapid breathing (greater than 30 breaths per minute), low blood pressure, temperature greater than 102°F, and confusion. Complications of pneumonia include inflammation and infection of the pleura (the layer of cells lining the outside of the lung), lung abscess, spread of infection outside the lung (to the brain, joints, etc.), and lung failure.

Treatment

Antibiotics are the mainstay of treatment and should be started as soon as pneumonia is suspected. For milder disease, oral antibiotics are used. Improvement is usually noted within 48–72 hours from starting therapy. More severely ill patients are hospitalized and receive several types of antibiotics administered intravenously. These patients are then switched to oral antibiotics when their condition stabilizes. Hospitalized patients may also receive supplemental oxygen and special respiratory care to help clear phlegm. If there is fluid buildup around the lung, this will be sampled to look for infection. Mechanical ventilation in an intensive care unit is used if the lungs are temporarily unable to take up oxygen and expel carbon dioxide.

Duration of antibiotic therapy ranges from 7 to 10 days in most cases. Therapy for 14–21 days or longer may be necessary for certain types of bacteria and in those individuals with other chronic medical conditions.

The DOs

- Take your antibiotics exactly as prescribed. If you miss a dose, simply resume with the next dose and continue to take the pills as scheduled until they are gone.
- Use acetaminophen and aspirin (except in children) to help decrease fever and to treat pain.
- Drink plenty of fluids (six to eight glasses per day) and/or breath moist air to help raise phlegm.
- Obtain a pneumococcal vaccine if you are older than 65 years or if you have a chronic illness. This vaccine is designed to improve your defense against *Streptococcus pneumoniae*, which is one of the most common causes of pneumonia.
- Let your doctor know about any allergic reactions to antibiotics that you have had.

The DON'Ts
- Home treatment of pneumonia with antibiotics should be avoided if the home environment is not stable and conducive to rest and recovery.

When to Call Your Doctor
- You suspect a pneumonia because of fever, green or yellow sputum production, increased shortness of breath, or chest pain.
- Symptoms continue or worsen after 48 hours of antibiotic therapy.
- If you note dusky-colored skin, lips, or fingernails.
- Nausea/vomiting prevent you from taking your antibiotics exactly as prescribed.
- Dehydration develops because of vomiting and/or diarrhea.

For More Information
American Lung Association
1118 Hampton Avenue
St. Louis, MO 63139
800-LUNG-USA
www.lungusa.org

PNEUMONIA, *MYCOPLASMA*

About Your Diagnosis

Mycoplasma pneumoniae is a bacteria that commonly causes pneumonia in individuals of all ages. *Mycoplasma* infections can occur throughout the year but are slightly more common during the winter months. Infection occurs after you inhale contaminated droplets coughed by someone who is also infected. Person-to-person transmission explains why *Mycoplasma* infections often spread quickly in close living situations, such as within families.

Living With Your Diagnosis

Symptoms usually begin 2–3 weeks after exposure to the *Mycoplasma* bacteria. Dry, persistent cough is the most common symptom. Fever and headaches also occur. Exposure to *Mycoplasma* may also cause ear and throat infections. *Mycoplasma* pneumonia usually completely resolves on its own, but this may take weeks. Only rarely are infections severe enough to warrant hospitalization.

Treatment

Oral antibiotics are often given to help speed healing. The duration of therapy is usually 5–14 days. Recommended antibiotics include erythromycin, clarithromycin, azithromycin, and tetracycline. Oral erythromycin may cause nausea. Tetracycline should be avoided in children and pregnant women. Nasal sprays and oral decongestants are often used to reduce nasal symptoms. Improvement usually begins within 1 or 2 days of starting antibiotics, although the cough may linger for weeks.

The DOs

- Take your antibiotics exactly as prescribed. If you miss a dose, simply resume at the next scheduled dose and continue to take the pills as scheduled until they are gone.
- Use acetaminophen or aspirin (except in children) for relief of fever and pain.
- Use a nonprescription cough suppressant as needed.
- Rest until you feel better.
- Drink plenty of fluids (six to eight glasses per day) and/or breath moist air to help raise phlegm.

The DON'Ts

- If you are ill, avoid contact with individuals who have chronic medical conditions because they may become very sick if they have *Mycoplasma* pneumonia.

When to Call Your Doctor

- If you suspect *Mycoplasma* pneumonia because of a generalized sense of illness, fever, shortness of breath, or phlegm production.
- If your symptoms fail to resolve or worsen after 48 hours of antibiotic therapy.
- If nausea prevents you from taking the prescribed antibiotics.
- If you note blood in the sputum.

For More Information
American Lung Association
1118 Hampton Avenue
St. Louis, MO 63139
800-LUNG-USA
www.lungusa.org

PNEUMONIA, *PNEUMOCYSTIS CARINII*

About Your Diagnosis

Pneumocystis carinii is a fungus that causes pneumonia only in individuals with impaired immune system function. It is a common cause of pneumonia in those with the human immunodeficiency virus (HIV), especially when the CD4 count (a type of immune system cell injured by HIV) drops below 200 mm^3. Others susceptible to *Pneumocystis carinii* pneumonia include those receiving cancer chemotherapy, long-term prednisone therapy, or immunosuppressant drugs to prevent transplant organ rejection, as well as those with rare inherited disorders of immunity. It remains unclear how *Pneumocystis carinii* pneumonia develops. Either the organism is spread person to person or lies dormant for years and then reactivates when the immune system is suppressed. There is no vaccine, but certain drugs can help prevent the development of *Pneumocysitis* pneumonia.

Living With Your Diagnosis

Symptoms usually develop slowly, and gradually become more severe over time. The most common symptoms are shortness of breath, dry cough, and fever. Chest x-rays and blood tests help to assess the severity of the illness. Specialized testing is required to diagnose *Pneumocystis* infection. The initial test is usually inspection of the sputum for *Pneumocystis*. If this test is inconclusive, then bronchoscopy is performed. During this procedure, your doctor inspects your lungs with a lighted tube guided through your nose or mouth. Lung fluids are collected and biopsy specimens may be taken. If *Pneumocystis* is present, it will be found by bronchoscopy in 90% of cases. Rarely, a surgical lung biopsy is required to confirm the diagnosis.

Pneumocystis is a serious, potentially life-threatening illness. More than 50% of patients will survive if treated with effective drugs, although the survival rate is lower in patients with more severe immune system dysfunction. *Pneumocystis* can recur after therapy if preventive drugs are not used.

Treatment

The combination of trimethoprim/sulfamethoxazole (TMP/SMX) is usually the drug of first choice. Other drugs are available, such as pentamidine, for those who are allergic to sulfa or who fail to improve with TMP/SMX. Symptoms may actually worsen during the first 2–4 days of treatment. Therapy is usually administered for up to 21 days. Steroids are used in severe cases to help reduce lung inflammation associated with infection.

Trimethoprim/sulfamethoxazole can be given either orally or intravenously. Milder cases can be treated on an outpatient basis. More severely ill patients are hospitalized for other supportive measures, such as supplemental oxygen. Mechanical ventilation in an intensive care unit may be used if the lungs temporarily are unable to adequately take up oxygen and expel carbon dioxide. The most common side effects of TMP/SMX include rash, nausea, fever, and low white blood cell counts.

Oral TMP/SMX is also very effective at preventing *Pneumocystis carinii* pneumonia. It is administered as infrequently as one tablet three times per week, but many individuals take it daily so as not to forget the medication. If you fit into any of the following groups, you should receive this preventive therapy.

- Patients who are HIV positive.
- Patients with CD4 counts less than 200 mm^3.
- Patients who have had a previous episode of *Pneumocystis carinii* pneumonia.
- Patients receiving long-term steroid therapy or other immunosuppressant drug therapy.

The DOs

- Take your prescription medications exactly as prescribed. Complete all courses of antibiotics.
- Use nonprescription cough suppressants as needed.
- Use acetaminophen or aspirin (except in children) to suppress fever and treat pain.
- If you are HIV positive, see your health care provider regularly for monitoring of immune function.

The DON'Ts

- Home treatment of *Pneumocystis carinii* pneumonia with antibiotics should be avoided if the home environment is not stable and conducive to rest and recovery.

When to Call Your Doctor

- If you suspect *Pneumocystis carinii* pneumonia because of a new fever, cough, or shortness of breath.

- If your symptoms worsen despite the prescribed therapy.
- If an unexplained rash develops (may signal a drug allergy).
- If nausea prevents you from taking the prescribed medications.

For More Information

American Lung Association
1118 Hampton Avenue
St. Louis, MO 63139
800-LUNG-USA
www.lungusa.org

PNEUMONIA, VIRAL

About Your Diagnosis

Viruses are frequent causes of many types of infections of the respiratory tract, such as the common cold, pharyngitis, laryngitis, and bronchitis. These illnesses are usually brief and resolve without specific therapy. It is thought that viral infections start after you inhale a contaminated droplet from an infectious individual, or that the virus is directly transferred to your nose, mouth, or eyes by your hands, which have previously touched a contaminated object. Viral pneumonia refers to an infection of the lung tissue that can be caused by many different types of viruses. Influenza virus, respiratory syncytial virus, adenovirus, parainfluenza virus, and varicella virus are some of the most common causes of viral pneumonia. Children and adults of all ages can be affected, sometimes as part of outbreaks. Smokers, the elderly, and those with chronic lung diseases may be most susceptible. Individuals with suppression of the immune system because of chemotherapy or because of drug therapy after organ transplantation are especially vulnerable to pneumonia caused by cytomegalovirus.

It is difficult to determine whether pneumonia is caused by a virus, as well as which specific virus is causing the pneumonia, because many viruses produce similar symptoms and there are few specific diagnostic tests. Viral pneumonias, especially those caused by influenza virus, can be followed quickly by the development of bacterial pneumonias because viruses can weaken the lung's defense mechanisms.

Living With Your Diagnosis

The most common symptoms of viral pneumonia include fever, chills, cough, shortness of breath, chest discomfort, muscle aches, fatigue, and poor appetite. Symptoms of runny nose, irritated eyes, and sore throat may also be present. Symptoms outside the respiratory tract may be present if the virus has infected other parts of the body. For instance, herpesvirus and measles virus may also cause rashes.

Some viruses can be found in respiratory secretions, whereas others can be detected by blood tests. However, in most cases, diagnostic tests are not performed to check for a specific viral cause. Instead, once your health care provider has established that pneumonia is present by examination of the chest and x-rays, analyses of the blood and sputum are usually performed to make sure a concomitant bacterial infection is not also present. Viral pneumonias in otherwise healthy individuals resolve within 1–2 weeks, but cough and fatigue may persist for many weeks. Viral pneumonias can be serious and potentially life threatening in those with other medical illnesses.

Treatment

Specific treatments are available for few viruses, so care measures are usually supportive. Options include:
- Bed rest.
- Acetaminophen or aspirin (not in children) for relief of fever and aches.
- Cough suppressants.
- Decongestant tablets or nasal sprays.

If a specific viral cause is found, antiviral drugs may be prescribed, such as amantadine or rimantadine for influenza A, acyclovir for herpesvirus, or ganciclovir for cytomegalovirus. Antibiotics are prescribed for concurrent bacterial infections. Seriously ill patients are hospitalized for treatment with intravenous fluids, supplemental oxygen, or breathing support by a mechanical ventilator.

The DOs

A vaccine is available to help decrease the risk of illness with influenza virus. Because influenza virus strains change yearly, this vaccine must be updated each fall. The vaccine is recommended for:
- Individuals older than 65 years.
- Adults or children with chronic lung, kidney, or heart disease; diabetes; or chronic anemia.
- Adults or children who live in chronic care facilities, such as nursing homes.
- Community workers such as police officers and firefighters.
- Health care workers.

The vaccine is given as a single injection into the shoulder region. Side effects are rare, but some individuals may experience slight fever and muscle aches shortly after the shot. The influenza vaccine can be given at the same time the pneumococcal vaccine is received. Individuals allergic to eggs and egg products should avoid the vaccine.

If viral pneumonia develops:
- Obtain plenty of bed rest.
- Drink at least six to eight glasses of liquid per day to avoid dehydration.
- Maintain proper nutrition.

The DON'Ts

- If you have viral respiratory tract infections, avoid contact with those who might be very vulnerable to illness such as infants, the elderly, and those with chronic diseases.
- Do not give aspirin to children younger than 16 years of age during viral infections because this may trigger Reye's syndrome (a rare, potentially life-threatening illness that affects the blood, brain, and liver).

When to Call Your Doctor

- If you have symptoms suggestive of viral pneumonia.
- If you have increasing shortness of breath.
- If your skin, lips, or fingertips are dusky.
- If there is blood in your sputum.
- If you have difficulty maintaining adequate liquid intake.
- If symptoms of fever and cough return after initially improving (this may signal the development of a new bacterial infection).

For More Information

American Lung Association
1118 Hampton Avenue
St. Louis, MO 63139
800-LUNG-USA

PNEUMOTHORAX

About Your Diagnosis

Pneumothorax occurs when air is present in the pleural space, which is the space between the lung and the inside of the chest wall. A small amount of fluid in the pleural space normally keeps the outside of the lung "stuck" against the inside of the chest cavity, keeping the lung expanded. This is similar to the effect that a small amount of water has in keeping two pieces of plastic stuck together when the water is between the two plastic sheets. When air enters the pleural space, the lung becomes unstuck and partially or completely collapses. Pneumothorax results when air leaks into the pleural space either from the outside through a puncture in the chest wall, or from an air leak in the lung that lets air escape.

Traumatic pneumothorax is the result of an injury that either causes a puncture wound through the chest wall, or a rib fracture that then allows a broken piece of rib to puncture the lung. A spontaneous pneumothorax can occur in individuals with emphysema, as well as in some tall, very thin individuals, when a hard cough causes a rupture of part of the lung and an air leak from the lung. Spontaneous pneumothorax may run in families. Around 9 of every 100,000 individuals in the United States will have a pneumothorax each year. A decrease in the loudness of breath sounds on one side of the chest detected with a stethoscope will raise suspicion of pneumothorax, and a chest x-ray will confirm it. Once found, it is fairly easy to treat.

Living With Your Diagnosis

The main symptoms of pneumothorax are increasing shortness of breath and chest pain. You may have a sense of tightness of the chest. You may become tired or fatigued more easily and may have a rapid heart beat. The lips or fingertips may appear blue with more severe cases. The result of pneumothorax is collapse of one lung, which makes that lung unable to take up oxygen when you breathe.

Treatment

A small pneumothorax can be treated by allowing the air to reabsorb on its own or inserting a needle into the air and drawing it out, which will re-expand the lung. A larger pneumothorax may need to have a tube (called a chest tube) inserted into the air. A suction machine is connected to the tube to draw out the air and re-expand the lung. If the leak is large, sometimes the tube may need to remain for a few days to keep the lung expanded till the leak has healed. The main side effect of the treatment is discomfort at the site that the needle or tube enters the chest wall. The main complications include a small risk of bleeding into the chest if insertion of the tube or needle injures a blood vessel. Infection at the puncture site is also a small risk.

The DOs

For a pneumothorax that requires a tube and suction, you will be admitted to the hospital. For a smaller pneumothorax that only requires drainage with a needle or that will reabsorb, you will probably go home. Your doctor will probably give you pain medicines, particularly if the pneumothorax is the result of an injury. If the pneumothorax is the result of a puncture wound or if pneumonia or bronchitis produced a severe cough that resulted in a spontaneous pneumothorax, you may receive an antibiotic. If you have a chest tube in, you need to keep your head elevated when you lie down. You should be at rest. More severe cases sometimes require oxygen. You should follow-up with your doctor as instructed because it is important to be sure that the pneumothorax is resolving.

The DON'Ts

You should avoid heavy exertion or coughing because both of these activities may increase air leaks. You should avoid smoking because this will interfere with your ability to draw oxygen from the air in the face of a partially or completely collapsed lung. In addition, smoking may cause coughing.

When to Call Your Doctor

You must call your doctor promptly if you are experiencing increasing shortness of breath. This could be a symptom of a collapsing lung. You should also call if you have a temperature of greater than 101.0°F. This may be a symptom of infection at the site of the needle or chest tube puncture, or at the wound site. It can also be a sign of developing pneumonia. As many as 50% of individuals who have had one spontaneous pneumothorax will have another. If you have a history of pneumothorax, you should call your doctor if symptoms reoccur.

For More Information
Description of the disease and pictures of x-rays
http://www.familyinternet.com/peds/top/000087.htm

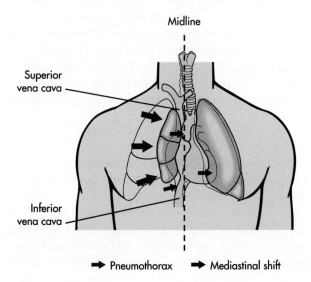

Midline

Superior
vena cava

Inferior
vena cava

➡ Pneumothorax   ➡ Mediastinal shift

Tension pneumothorax. As pleural pressure on the affected side
increases, mediastinal displacement ensures with resultant respiratory and cardiovascular compromise. (From Lewis SM, Collier
IC, Heitkemper MM: *Medical-Surgical Nursing: Assessment and Management of Clinical Problem,* vol. 4. St. Louis, Mosby–Year Book, 1995.
Used by permission.)

POLYCYTHEMIA VERA

About Your Diagnosis

Polycythemia vera is a malignant process that involves the stem cells (the cells that can produce white blood cells, red blood cells, or platelets) in the bone marrow (soft pink pulp in the long bones, ribs, and vertebrae where blood cells are formed). Polycythemia vera causes an increase in the number of red blood cells, white blood cells, and platelets and an enlarged spleen. The cause of this disease is unknown.

Polycythemia vera is an uncommon disease. Most patients are between 50 and 60 years of age. One of 100,000 persons has this disorder. There are families in which several family members have either polycythemia vera or another related problem, but these families are rare. This suggests that polycythemia vera can be transferred from parents to offspring genetically.

Polycythemia vera can be cured only by means of bone marrow transplantation. It is usually detected when an elevated red blood cell count, white blood cell count, and platelet count are found on a blood test.

Patients usually report fatigue, headache, drowsiness, forgetfulness, and vertigo. Itching after a bath is a common finding. Patients also may have nose bleeds or gastrointestinal bleeding. The eyes and face look red. There is an increased incidence of peptic ulcer disease among persons with polycythemia vera. An enlarged spleen is present in at least three fourths of patients with polycythemia vera. It gives a feeling of fullness in the abdomen. Enlargement of the liver is present among 40% of patients. Disturbances of vision, such as temporary blindness, double vision, specks, and bright points in front of the field of vision, are common.

Living With Your Diagnosis

Total blood volume is increased, which increases the thickness of the blood and gives rise to symptoms such as headaches, vertigo, dizziness, a sensation of fullness in the head, and tingling and numbness in the fingers and toes. Patients report shortness of breath on exertion. The skin of the face and neck redden. Blood clots can form in the veins, causing problems such as strokes and blood clots in the lungs and legs.

Treatment

Usually no treatment is needed by patients who feel well and have no symptoms. Phlebotomy (removal of blood by means of puncturing a vein) is the safest therapy for polycythemia vera. It can control the symptoms for most patients. One pint of blood is removed at periodic intervals to keep the hemoglobin and hematocrit within normal range. For older patients or patients with other medical problems, smaller volumes of blood are removed at one time, or other treatment possibilities are used.

Other options for symptomatic polycythemia vera are chemotherapy with agents such as hydroxyurea, chlorambucil, busulfan, and cyclophosphamide. Radiation therapy to the spleen and bones is another treatment option. Splenectomy (surgical removal of the spleen) can be considered in later stages of the disease if enlargement of the spleen causes fullness in the abdomen, discomfort, or worsening of anemia and thrombocytopenia.

Antihistamines such as diphenhydramine (eg, Benadryl) and hydroxyzine (eg, Atarax) are used for itching. H2 blockers such as cimetidine (eg, Tagamet) and famotidine (eg, Pepcid) are used for peptic ulcer disease.

Patients who are treated with phlebotomy are at increased risk for blood clot formation, because platelet production in the bone marrow increases when blood is removed. There are several other reasons for this problem, which should be discussed with a physician.

Chemotherapy destroys normal blood cells in addition to malignant cells and therefore can lower white blood cell count. This increases risk for infection and lowers red blood cell and platelet counts, causing anemia and risk for bleeding.

Chemotherapeutic agents can change the genetic structure of the cells, which can cause other cancers. Chemotherapy also causes thinning of the hair during therapy, but the hair grows back after treatment is stopped. Chemotherapy also causes nausea, vomiting, and diarrhea.

The DOs

- Undergo phlebotomy at periodic intervals to keep blood counts at the upper limits of normal.
- Participate in chemotherapy as recommended by your physician.
- Take antihistamines for itching as directed by your physician.

- Take H2 blockers for peptic ulcer disease as directed by your physician.
- Undergo routine clinical follow-up care with your physician.

The DON'Ts

- Do not use medications more frequently than recommended. Certain medications such as aspirin and dipyridamole increase risk for bleeding.
- Avoid uncooked vegetables, fresh fruits, and milk products. These products harbor bacteria, which do not cause problems for healthy persons but can cause severe infections if you have neutropenia.
- Avoid strenuous activity if your blood counts are low during chemotherapy or you have an enlarged spleen or anemia, because of risk for trauma to the spleen and decreased exercise tolerance.

When to Call Your Doctor

- If you have excessive fatigue, shortness of breath, severe headaches, bleeding from any orifice, severe abdominal pain, or sudden swelling of an arm or leg.

For More Information
American Cancer Society
URL: http://www.cancer
1599 Clifton Road, NE
Atlanta, GA 30329-4251
1-800-ACS-2345
Cancer Information Service (CIS)
1-800-4-CANCER
National Cancer Institute
Building 31, Room 10 A24
Bethesda MD 20892

POLYMYALGIA RHEUMATICA

About Your Diagnosis

Polymyalgia rheumatica (PMR) is a type of inflammation that produces pain and stiffness in the muscles around the neck, shoulders, buttocks, hips, and thighs. It seldom occurs in individuals younger than 50 years. No one knows what causes the inflammation in PMR, but it is not an infectious illness (like colds). Therefore you cannot "catch" it from another individual.

Polymyalgia rheumatica is diagnosed mostly by its symptoms. However, most individuals with PMR have evidence of inflammation as indicated by the results of two blood tests: the erythrocyte sedimentation rate (ESR) and the C-reactive protein (CRP). Because there are other diseases that can cause symptoms similar to those of PMR, your doctor will probably order other blood tests to be sure you do not have another problem.

Living With Your Diagnosis

Individuals with PMR commonly notice pain and stiffness (a feeling of restricted motion) in the muscles around the neck, shoulders, buttocks, hips, and thighs. The pain and stiffness are most noticeable in the morning and may improve with activity during the course of the day. Occasionally, PMR may also cause pain and swelling in the joints. In addition, PMR can also cause fatigue, poor appetite, fever, and sweats. Approximately 20% of individuals with PMR also have another condition called "temporal arteritis," which may cause headaches and sudden vision changes. Your doctor will determine whether you also have this condition. Fortunately, the treatment of PMR results in considerable improvement in nearly all of these symptoms within a few days. Although PMR responds to therapy, some patients may require treatment for more than 2 or 3 years.

Treatment

The most common treatment for PMR is corticosteroids (cortisone-like medicines such as prednisone). Nonsteroidal anti-inflammatory drugs (NSAIDs) such as ibuprofen are sometimes also used. Potential side effects of corticosteroids are increased appetite, weight gain, difficulty sleeping, easy bruising, and stomach upset. Longer term use of corticosteroids can lower your resistance to infection, and cause stomach ulcers and bone thinning (osteoporosis). Corticosteroids should always be taken with food to prevent stomach upset. In addition, patients should receive adequate amounts of calcium and vitamin D to help prevent osteoporosis.

The DOs

- Take your medicines as prescribed.
- Ask your doctor which over-the-counter medications you may take with your prescription medications.
- Inform your doctor and dentist that you are taking a corticosteroid (prednisone).
- Eat a well-balanced diet low in carbohydrates and fat to prevent excessive weight gain.
- Perform a physician-prescribed weight-bearing exercise program.

The DON'Ts

- Wait to see whether side effects from the medicines will go away.
- Stop taking the corticosteroid medicine unless your physician instructs you to do so.
- Overeat, because corticosteroids may increase your appetite.
- Continue an exercise program that causes pain.

When to Call Your Doctor

- You have any medication side effects.
- Your pain and/or stiffness return during treatment.
- You have new headaches, cramping in your tongue or jaw, or sudden changes in your vision.
- You run out of prednisone (cortisone).

For More Information

Contact the Arthritis Foundation in your area. If you do not know the location of the Arthritis Foundation, you may call the national office at 1-800-283-7800 or access the information on the Internet at www.arthritis.org.

POSTCONCUSSIONAL SYNDROME

About Your Diagnosis

Postconcussional syndrome is a syndrome (or collection of symptoms) that may follow a concussion. A jarring injury to the brain results in a concussion. This seems to cause a mild abnormality in normal function of the brain. It is diagnosed by noting the presence of the symptoms that make up the syndrome in an individual who has experienced a concussion. It does not produce any abnormalities on physical examination or on any tests such as computed tomography (CT) scan or magnetic resonance imaging (MRI) scan. It goes away on its own without treatment during a period ranging from weeks to months.

Living With Your Diagnosis

Postconcussional syndrome produces symptoms of headache, poor concentration, mild memory loss, irritability, trouble sleeping, bad dreams, and sometimes mild personality changes. These symptoms resolve completely during the course of weeks to months. Usually there is gradual improvement during this period. You should recover to your normal preinjury state. There are no permanent effects.

Treatment

Treatment consists of watchful waiting until the symptoms resolve. There is no known treatment that hastens the course of the syndrome.

The DOs

There are no medicines that will shorten the recovery time. Mild analgesics such as acetaminophen, aspirin, or ibuprofen are usually helpful for the headache. Strenuous exercise may aggravate the headache, but exercise in moderation may help with relaxation and help with sleep disturbances by inducing suitable fatigue. Some individuals find biofeedback and relaxation techniques helpful. Altering of work or school environments to minimize the effects of any memory loss or difficulties in concentration may be helpful. Support from friends and family to help the individual with the syndrome remember that this is a temporary condition may be helpful.

The DON'Ts

You should probably avoid medicines such as stimulants or decongestants because they may aggravate the irritability. Because this is a condition that will take some time to resolve, it would be well to avoid potentially habit-forming medications such as narcotics, sleeping pills, or tranquilizers. Strenuous activity may aggravate the headache. Although this condition may last for several months, it is important to remember that it will resolve. You should avoid making life-changing decisions such as quitting school or changing jobs because of the symptoms that you are experiencing. It is a very good idea to avoid activities that would result in another concussion while you are experiencing postconcussional syndrome. Evidence suggests that repeated concussions may result in permanent brain injury or even death.

When to Call Your Doctor

You should call your doctor if you are having increasing symptoms over time or if your symptoms have not improved over the course of several months. It would be especially worrisome if you start to have symptoms such as increasing dizziness, blurred or double vision, loss of strength or coordination, vomiting, or increasingly severe headaches.

For More Information

Brain Injury Association (formerly the National Head Injury Foundation)
1-800-444-6443
http://www.biausa.org

POSTTRAUMATIC STRESS DISORDER

About Your Diagnosis

Posttraumatic distress disorder (PTSD) applies to a situation in which a individual has been exposed to a traumatic event that involves actual or threatened death or serious injury, or a threat to the physical integrity of the patient or others. You may have experienced this event or merely witnessed it. In addition, if your response to this event involved fear, helplessness, or horror, you may later develop PTSD.

Living With Your Diagnosis

Frequently the traumatic event occurs again in your mind as flashbacks or memories, images, thoughts, or perceptions. These trauma flashbacks can occur at any time, and you are unable to voluntarily resist them. In addition, an individual with PTSD also generally has recurring distressing dreams of the event. During one of these flashbacks or dreams, you may feel you are actually reexperiencing the event again and may tell your physician, "It is like I'm back in the same situation." You will often have physical findings such as sweating, rapid heartbeat, and rapid respirations. As a result of fear of recurrence of these symptoms, you will often avoid stimuli that are associated with the trauma. For instance, if your PTSD is related to Vietnam era activities, you may avoid individuals of Asian descent, or may avoid airports where helicopters might be found. Occasionally, there is some amnesia or loss of memory about certain parts of the trauma. Other manifestations can include a decreased interest and participation in activities, a tendency to isolate yourself from previously established friends and family, an inability to trust or show loving feelings, trouble falling or staying asleep, extreme episodes of anger and rage, trouble concentrating, a feeling that someone is always watching you (hypervigilence), and a heightened sense of startle.

The event that triggers PTSD is most likely to be one that occurs outside the range of normal human experience. For instance, Vietnam War service is associated with PTSD, as are survival from natural disasters and from sexual assault (rape or incest). Posttraumatic stress disorder can occur in conjunction with other psychiatric disorders, such as phobias, anxiety disorders, and depression. Approximately 50% of individuals with PTSD will recover, and approximately 50% have a persistent, chronic form of the illness still present 1 year later.

Treatment

Treatment of PTSD is aimed at helping individuals gain some control over their impulses. This is often done by involvement in peer support groups composed of other disease sufferers, often those who experienced the same kind of traumatic event. There are also certain medications that are used to treat PTSD. At present, the most common drugs used are the tricyclic antidepressant drugs, such as imipramine. However, the monoamine oxidase (MAO) inhibitor drugs such as Nardil are also used, as well as the serotonin drugs such as Prozac, Zoloft, and Paxil. These medications do have side effects. The tricyclic antidepressants may cause blurred vision, dizziness, constipation, dry mouth, and lower blood pressure. The serotonin drugs may cause diarrhea, nausea and vomiting, and sexual dysfunction. Patients receiving the MAO inhibitor drugs require a special diet; they cannot drink Chianti wine or eat fava beans and aged cheeses. Also patients taking MAO inhibitors must avoid certain medications such as Demerol and epinephrine, and should not use stimulants such as cocaine or take OTC drugs like Valerian Root. Occasionally symptoms of PTSD will also respond to drugs such as the antihypertensive, propranolol (Inderal).

Cognitive therapy is also very important in the treatment of PTSD. Cognitive therapy involves trying to change the way you think so you will feel better. Usually, the more an individual tells someone about the event, the less tearful and anxious they will be. This is known as debriefing. Other traditional antianxiety techniques such as meditation, progressive muscle relaxation, imagery, and biofeedback are also helpful.

Some PTSD sufferers experience rage attacks, and anger control training may be helpful. There also is some evidence that chronic pain and PTSD are commonly associated, and there have been situations in which PTSD has occurred after serious physical injuries such as burns, head injury, or multiple fractures.

The lack of a supportive family or religious structure to allow for adaptation to trauma can also increase the likelihood of PTSD. The Vietnam era veterans who returned to the United States were not given the typical support that had been shown veterans of World War I and World War II; in fact, their behavior was criticized because it was an unpopular war. The lack of a supportive network for returning Vietnam veterans probably increased their likelihood of developing PTSD.

The DOs

It is very important to try to minimize stress. This can be done by the usual stress management techniques. Exercise is very important, and as with all anxiety conditions, you want to avoid drugs such as caffeine and other stimulants because they will increase anxiety symptoms. It is also important early on in PTSD for the individual to avoid situations that might produce flashbacks to a traumatic event. Although in some cases this may be impossible, often certain locations and certain events can be avoided without significant disruption of the patient's lifestyle.

The DON'Ts

Because PTSD is an anxiety syndrome, there is a high incidence of overuse of alcohol and other drugs, and a fairly high incidence of misuse of antianxiety drugs such as Valium, Librium, and Xanax. Thus, you should avoid becoming overly dependent on these medications. Because of the potential for episodes of uncontrolled rage and anger, family members of patients with PTSD need to consider whether it is wise to have weapons around the house.

When to Call Your Doctor

You should call your doctor if you notice an exacerbation of the anxiety symptoms associated with PTSD, if you notice feelings of homicide or suicide, or uncontrolled rage, and if you notice any psychotic features, especially paranoia. You should also contact your physician if you begin to develop any of the physical symptoms associated with PTSD such as asthma or ulcer disease (hypertension also associated with PTSD but usually has no symptoms).

For More Information
Contact your local mental health center, your local veteran's hospital, or sexual assault hot lines. Online, check out the following Web site:
Traumatic Stress Home page @:
http://www.long-beach.va.gov/ptsd/stress.htm/
There are links to the Vietnam Veterans home page and Gulf War Veterans home page at this site.

PREMATURE ATRIAL CONTRACTIONS

About Your Diagnosis

As the name suggests, premature atrial contractions (PACs) are contractions in the atria of the heart that occur too early in the rhythm sequence. Abnormal electrical impulses signal the atria to beat prematurely. PACs are very common and can happen in otherwise healthy persons. Most persons who have PACs never notice them. Because PACs occur out of the normal rhythm, this condition is an arrhythmia. The physician may notice an irregular pulse, or the PACs may be found on an electrocardiogram (ECG).

The most common cause of PACs among healthy persons is ingestion of caffeine, nicotine, or alcohol or exposure to stress. PACs are found more frequently among persons with heart disease such as ischemia (decreased blood flow to the heart muscle) or congestive heart failure (decreased pumping efficiency of the heart). Persons with heart disease are more likely to have PACs convert to atrial fibrillation or atrial flutter (two types of atrial arrhythmias). Chronic pulmonary disease may make PACs more frequent, as can electrolyte (salts in the blood) disturbances.

Treatment

Healthy persons with no symptoms of heart or lung disease need no specific treatment. The condition may resolve on its own or may be less frequent if one cuts down on caffeine, alcohol, nicotine, and stress. Persons with PACs can exercise safely and need no special dietary changes other than reductions in alcohol and caffeine. PACs may be controlled with anti-arrhythmic medications, but the main goal is to manage evident heart or lung disease.

The DOs

• Reduce your intake of caffeine, alcohol, and nicotine and your exposure to stress), especially if you have heart or lung disease.

The DON'Ts

• Do not neglect therapy for heart or lung disease.

When to Call Your Doctor

• If you have palpitations (rapid heartbeat), chest pain, shortness of breath, or fainting.

For More Information
Consult a textbook on cardiology at your local library or a medical school in your region. Call the American Heart Association at 1-800-242-8721 and ask for the literature department.

PREMATURE VENTRICULAR CONTRACTIONS

About Your Diagnosis

As the name suggests, premature ventricular contractions (PVCs) are contractions in the ventricles of the heart that occur too early in the rhythm sequence. Abnormal electrical impulses signal the ventricles to beat prematurely. PVCs are common and can happen in otherwise healthy persons. They occur more frequently among older persons. Most persons who have PVCs never notice them. Because PVCs occur out of the normal rhythm, this condition is an arrhythmia. A physician may notice an irregular pulse, or PVCs may be found on an electrocardiogram (ECG).

The most common cause of PVCs among healthy persons is intake of caffeine, nicotine, and alcohol and exposure to stress. PVCs occur more frequently among persons with heart disease such as ischemia (decreased blood flow to the heart muscle) or persons with congestive heart failure (decreased pumping efficiency of the heart). They also can occur because of toxicity from digitalis medications. Persons with PVCs may have the sensation of their heart missing a beat followed by a stronger beat.

Treatment

Healthy persons with no symptoms of heart or lung disease need no specific treatment. The condition may resolve on its own, or PVCs may become less frequent if caffeine, alcohol, nicotine, and stress are reduced. PVCs may be controlled with anti-arrhythmic medications if symptoms become disruptive.

The DOs

- Reduce caffeine, alcohol, nicotine, and stress.
- Exercise. Persons with PVCs usually can exercise safely; the PVCs may even stop during exercise. If the PVCs increase in frequency with exercise (evaluated with an exercise ECG), you may have heart disease.

The DON'Ts

- Do not forget to take your prescribed medications.
- Do not forget the main goal of treatment is to manage the underlying heart or lung disease. Persons with known heart disease and frequent PVCs are at risk for arrhythmias that cause sudden death.

When to Call Your Doctor

- If you have palpitations (rapid heartbeat), chest pain, shortness of breath, or fainting.

For More Information

Consult your local library for a textbook on cardiology. Contact the American Heart Association at 1-800-242-8721 and ask for the literature department.

PREMENSTRUAL SYNDROME

About Your Diagnosis

Premenstrual syndrome (PMS) is a group of symptoms that occur in some women during the second half of a menstruating women's cycle (after ovulation takes place). These symptoms include irritability, anxiety, depression, tension, emotional lability, and difficulty concentrating. Physical symptoms may also occur; the most common are feeling bloated (water retention), weight gain, breast tenderness or pain, lower abdominal swelling, headache, constipation, fatigue, and swollen hands and/or feet.

The exact cause of PMS is unknown. It is now felt that PMS is not caused by any excess or deficiency of hormones. However, the changing level of the hormones may trigger changes in chemicals made in the brain, causing some of the symptoms. Much research is being conducted to determine what causes PMS.

Premenstrual syndrome is very common. It is estimated that approximately 50% of women have some degree of PMS during their reproductive years (when they are having their periods).

Often PMS is diagnosed by keeping a calendar of periods and when the symptoms occur. If all the symptoms always occur within the 2 weeks before the period and the symptoms resolve during or after the period, then PMS is likely. There is no blood test or any other test that can confirm a diagnosis of PMS.

Living With Your Diagnosis

The symptoms of PMS are usually both behavioral and physical. The behavioral symptoms include irritability, depression, emotional lability (cries easily), tension, anxiety, difficulty concentrating on tasks, and possibly a change in sex drive. Physical symptoms include feeling bloated, breast tenderness, headache, lower abdominal swelling (many women complain of "feeling 5 months pregnant"), constipation, swelling of the hands and/or feet, and fatigue. The symptoms can vary from very mild to very severe. Most women are able to cope with mild symptoms. However, if the symptoms are very severe, then PMS can sometimes seriously affect family life, relationships with friends, and work.

You do not have to experience all the symptoms to have PMS. In addition, during some menstrual cycles the PMS may be mild and barely noticeable, whereas during other cycles the PMS may be more severe. Sometimes women will have PMS during their 20s and 30s; other women may not have PMS until they are in their 40s. It is very common for women who are perimenopausal to have an increase in their PMS symptoms. By definition, postmenopausal women do not have PMS.

Treatment

There are a variety of treatments for PMS. Sometimes one remedy will work for one individual but will not work as well for another. First, a healthy, well-balanced diet and plenty of exercise and adequate rest are recommended. It may be helpful to not schedule as many activities or commitments during the PMS period to minimize the stress and offset the fatigue. A diet especially high in complex carbohydrates (whole grain foods, i.e., pasta, breads, rice) may help alleviate some symptoms according to a recent study. An over-the-counter product called PMS Escape is available, which is simply a complex carbohydrate drink taken once or twice each day during the PMS period. There do not seem to be any side effects.

Another over-the-counter product which has been shown to be effective in a study is Evening Primrose Oil. This product can be found in health food stores. It usually comes as gelatin capsules. The recommended dose is 1.5–2.0 grams twice each day during the PMS period. There are no reported side effects. Evening Primrose Oil may also alleviate breast tenderness that may occur before periods.

Prescription antidepressants can also be used to treat PMS when symptoms are difficult to control with exercise, diet, and the over-the-counter remedies.

The DOs

- Eat a healthy, well-balanced diet. Especially take in a lot of foods high in complex carbohydrates (i.e., whole grain breads, pastas)
- Get lots of exercise regularly (even though this is the last thing you may feel like doing).
- Get plenty of rest and sleep during the PMS period.

The DON'Ts
- Avoid lots of sugar and caffeine.
- Don't stop your regular exercise routine.
- Don't schedule as many activities or commitments during the PMS period.

When to Call Your Doctor
- If your symptoms are interfering with your daily activities or ability to function at work or at home.
- If your symptoms are interfering with your relationships with your family or friends.

For More Information
Understanding Your Body: Every Woman's Guide to Gynecology and Health. Felicia Stewart, M.D., Felicia Guest, M.D., Gary Stewart, M.D., and Robert Hatcher, M.D., Bantam Books, 1987.

PRESSURE ULCERS (DECUBITUS ULCERS, BEDSORES)

About Your Diagnosis

A pressure ulcer is a sore that results from the death of the skin and its underlying tissue over areas of the body that receive pressure when the patient is sitting or lying still for long periods.

A pressure ulcer develops because the weight of the body or body part causes a slowing of the circulation in the skin over that pressure point. With decreased circulation and nutrition, the skin and eventually its underlying tissues such as fat and muscle will die, and an ulcer or sore will develop.

Other factors that contribute to the development of an ulcer are poor patient nutrition, wetness from urine and stool, and shear or friction from moving the patient over clothes and bedding.

Who gets pressure ulcers?
- Stroke patients.
- Patients with spinal cord injury.
- Anyone who spends long periods in bed or in a wheelchair.
- Individuals who cannot control their bowels or bladder.
- Individuals with illnesses that prevent them from changing position easily.
- Individuals who cannot tell a caregiver whether they are sore or need turning.
- Individuals with any of the above conditions and poor nutrition.

If a patient who has been immobile for some time is moved and turned, he may have an area of red skin (stage 1 ulcer) discovered. A deeper ulcer (stage 2 or 3) may be discovered if that part of the skin hasn't been inspected in a while, or if pressure continues on a stage 1 ulcer.

Living With Your Diagnosis

Pressure ulcers can be treated with a combination of good nursing care and the use of pressure-relieving devices. Special types of dressings that your physician may prescribe and sometimes surgery may be needed. Once the ulcer is resolved, it is imperative that prolonged pressure on that area be relieved.

Treatment

The treatment plan will depend on the stage of the ulcer.

Stage 1: redness with no break in the skin.
Stage 2: the outer layer of the skin is broken with blistering and drainage.
Stage 3: the sore extends into underlying tissue. It may have a white or black base. It can be painful around the edges and have foul-smelling drainage.
Stage 4: the sore reaches through to muscle or bone. It can be white or black at the base. It can have a bone infection and foul-smelling drainage.

All ulcers must be kept clean. This is best accomplished with sterile saline and an irrigation device such as a syringe or a "Water Pik" under the lowest pressure. The use of hydrogen peroxide, povodone-iodine solution (Betadine and others), liquid detergents, and bleach solutions all delay wound healing. Cleaning of hard scabs and dead tissue is done by several methods. Sharp debridement is done with a scapel or scissors by the doctor. Mechanical debridement is done by using wet-to-dry dressings, which pull off the scab when they are changed.

Enzymatic debridement is done with solutions that contain enzymes that digest dead tissue. Autolytic debridement is done by using moist wound dressings that are changed every several days.

Control of any infection is very important. The doctor may prescribe an antibiotic cream to be applied to the ulcer, an oral antibiotic to be taken by mouth, and in some cases, an injectable antibiotic is given.

The DOs
- PREVENTION IS BY FAR THE BEST TREATMENT!
- Know the pressure points that are likely to have areas of skin breakdown. These are areas that usually don't have much fat to pad them.
- Use pressure relief devices such as pillows, gel or foam cushions or mattresses, and foam or gel heel protectors.
- Move the patient or encourage the patient to move at least every 2 hours, and inspect the pressure points regularly. Write down a turning schedule.
- Keep the skin clean and lubricated but not moist.
- Manage stool and urine by a regular voiding or stooling schedule, or use incontinent devices.
- Use draw sheets or boards to keep down friction when the patient is moved.
- If the patient is bed bound, keep the head of the bed no higher that 30 degrees because this pre-

vents sliding and friction to the lower back and buttocks.

- Promote good nutrition. Liquid protein supplements and vitamin supplements may be necessary. Ask the patient's physician.

The DON'T'S

- Do not use donut-type cushions or devices.

When to Call Your Doctor

- The area of reddness around the ulcer increases.
- Drainage from the ulcer increases.
- Drainage from the ulcer is foul-smelling and looks like pus.
- Pain in the area of the ulcer increases.
- Fever and/or chills develop.
- Mental confusion, weakness, or rapid heartbeat develops.

For More Information

The wound care specialist with your local hospital or home health agency.
Preventing Pressure Ulcers: Patient Guide
Treating Pressure Sores: Consumer Guide
AHCPR Publications Clearing House
PO Box 8547
Silver Spring, MD 20907
800-358-9295
National Pressure Ulcer Advisory Panel
SUNY at Buffalo
3435 Main Street
Buffalo, NY 14214
716-881-3558
World Wide Web Sites
http://www.aafp.org/healthinfo
http://www.housecall.com/aafp (America's HouseCall Network)

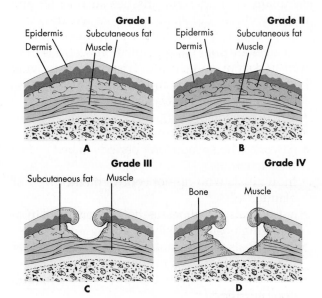

Staging of pressure sores. **A,** Stage I. Erythema not resolving within 30 minutes of pressure relief. Epidermis remains intact. Reversible with intervention. **B,** Stage II. Partial-thickness loss of skin layers involving epidermis and possibly penetrating into, but not through, dermis. May present as blistering with erythema and/or induration; wound base is moist and pink, painful, and free of necrotic tissue. **C,** Stage III. Full-thickness tissue loss extending through dermis to involve subcutaneous tissue. Presents as shallow crater unless covered by eschar. (If wound involves necrotic tissue, staging cannot be confirmed until wound base is visible.) May include necrotic tissue; undermining, sinus tract formation; exudate; and/or infection. Wound base is usually not painful. **D,** Stage IV. Deep tissue destruction extending through subcutaneous tissue to fascia and possibly involving muscle layers, joint, and/or bone. Manifests as a deep crater. May include necrotic tissue; undermining, sinus tract formation; exudate; and/or infection. Wound base is usually not painful. (From Lewis SM, Collier IC, Heitkemper MM: *Medical-Surgical Nursing: Assessment and Management of Clinical Problem,* vol. 4. St. Louis, Mosby–Year Book, 1995. Used by permission.)

PRIAPISM

About Your Diagnosis

Priapism is persistent erection of the penis. This disorder is most common among patients with sickle cell disease, infants or adults. The specific cause is unknown. There is speculation that once the erection is present, the abnormal red blood cells of sickle cell anemia perpetuate the episode. It is also known that once these cells are trapped inside the penis, the amount of oxygen on the blood also decreases. Acute attacks often begin during sleep, and a full bladder usually is an associated factor. Some episodes begin after sexual activity. However, there is frequently no identifiable event or cause.

Living With Your Diagnosis

There are three basic types of priapism, as follows:
1. Stuttering priapism is characterized by repeated erections that are usually reversible but painful. They come and go, do not last long, and cause no problem with sexual function once resolved. This is very common and occurs among 40% of patients.
2. Acute, prolonged priapism can last for several hours, but typically lasts for several days or weeks. The erection is painful, and induration may develop after the episode. This may cause impotence and necessitate a doctor's intervention.
3. Persistent priapism can last for weeks to years and usually develops after an acute attack as described in number 2. Persistent priapism is usually painless. It is characterized by enlargement or induration of the penis. It may also lead to partial or complete impotence.

Treatment

1. Stuttering priapism is often managed at home. The patient is encouraged to drink plenty of fluids and to empty his bladder frequently once the attack begins. Warm baths and exercise also are recommended. If the episode does not resolve in 3 hours, the patient should seek medical attention.
2. Acute, prolonged priapism necessitates hospitalization. Intravenous fluids and narcotics usually are prescribed to decrease the pain. The doctor may start blood transfusions immediately or opt to do a more complicated procedure called *exchange transfusion*. In this procedure a machine is connected to the patient that exchanges fresh blood with the patient's old blood. This may take one or two days to work; if it does not work, a surgical procedure may be indicated. The operation usually is performed with local anesthesia. The blood in the penis is drained through a small needle; the needle is removed, but the blood continues to drain until the patient experiences some relief. Transfusion and surgical treatment may decrease the incidence of loss of erection from 80% to 25% to 50%.
3. There is no standard treatment for persistent priapism. Patients usually are not in pain, but erection is impaired. Use of inflatable or fixed prostheses may have complications, but some patients have had good results. Some patients adjust to altered sexual function with the support of a partner, because ejaculation, orgasm, and fertility remain intact.

The DOs
• Empty your bladder as frequently as possible.

The DON'Ts
• Avoid prolonged dehydration and avoid extended sexual activity.

For More Information
MedWebHematology:http://www.gen.emory.edu/medweb.hematology.html
MedMark Hematology: http://medmark.bit.co.kr/hematol.html
National Heart, Lung, and Blood Institute Information Center
P.O. Box 30105
Bethesda, MD 20824-0105
301-251-1222
Sickle Cell Disease Association of America, Inc.
200 Corporate Point, #495
Culver City, CA 90230-7633
Operation Sickle Cell, Inc.
2409 Murchison Road
Fayetteville, NC 28301
910-488-6118
http://www.uncfsu.edu/osc/
Joint Center for Sickle Cell and Thalassemic Disorders
http://cancer.mgh.harvard.edu/medOnc/sickle.htm

PROLACTINOMA

About Your Diagnosis

A prolactinoma is a tumor of the prolactin-producing cells of the pituitary gland. The pituitary gland, or master gland, sits at the base of the brain and regulates normal growth, metabolism, and reproduction. One of the many hormones secreted by the pituitary is prolactin. Prolactin is the hormone that causes a woman's breasts to secrete milk after pregnancy. If a tumor develops in the prolactin-secreting cells of the pituitary, too much prolactin is secreted into the bloodstream.

One or two individuals in 10,000 will have a prolactinoma. There is no known genetic link for this disorder.

A prolactinoma is detected by measuring prolactin levels in the blood. It is important that patients are not taking certain medicines such as reserpine, alpha-methyldopa, metoclopramide, haloperidol, or trifluoperazine because prolactin levels could be falsely elevated. Prolactin levels may also be falsely elevated in patients with hypothyroidism or advanced kidney disease. The diagnosis is confirmed by obtaining a magnetic resonance imaging (MRI) scan of the pituitary gland.

Most prolactinomas are completely curable with medication or surgery.

Living With Your Diagnosis

Women may have changes in their menses, or have milk production when they are not pregnant. Elevated prolactin levels may decrease estrogen levels, leading to vaginal dryness and painful intercourse. Males may only notice impotence or decreased sex drive.

Untreated prolactinoma could lead to decreased bone mineral density or osteoporosis. It may also compress local nerves near the pituitary such as the optic nerves, which are important for vision. This causes a decrease in peripheral vision.

Treatment

The best treatment for a prolactinoma depends on the extent of the patient's symptoms as well as the extent of the tumor. The goal of treatment is to restore normal reproductive and pituitary function, as well as to minimize symptoms such as breast milky discharge and change in menstrual periods. Some patients with microadenomas of less than 10 mm who have no symptoms of their disease may be followed up clinically with annual MRI scans of the pituitary and annual prolactin levels. The vast majority of prolactinomas of this size do not progress to larger tumors.

Medication is required for symptomatic patients. Bromocriptine increases dopamine secretion from the hypothalamus, which leads to decreased prolactin levels and tumor shrinkage in most patients. Bromocriptine, 1.25 mg, is taken once at night with food for several days; the dose is then slowly increased until prolactin levels are normal or side effects, such as nausea or dizziness, become intolerable. Cabergoline is a newer longer-acting medication which may be better tolerated than bromocriptine.

If medical therapy is not tolerated or fails to control the growth of the prolactinoma, then surgery is required. This also has a very high success rate if the prolactinoma is identified early. Tumors may recur postoperatively. Complications of surgery include bleeding, infection, leaking cerebrospinal fluid (CSF), and hypopituitarism (an underactive pituitary) requiring hormone replacement.

The DOs

- Make sure your prolactin level was measured while you were fasting for at least 8 hours, and that there has not been recent breast stimulation.
- Obtain follow-up images of the pituitary to prove the prolactinoma is not growing.
- Start with a low dose of medication and increase the dose slowly.
- Find an experienced neurosurgeon if you require surgery for your prolactinoma. Success rates are highly dependent upon the experience and skill of the neurosurgeon.

The DON'Ts

- Don't give up on your medicine if you are having mild side effects. Instead, decrease your dose by one pill a day, and increase again 1 week later.
- Don't forget to use appropriate birth control if you are sexually active after beginning treatment for your prolactinoma. Women with irregular menstrual periods or men with low testosterone levels will have normalization of their reproductive status with treatment of their prolactinoma.

When to Call Your Doctor
- You experience any change in your vision.
- You have an unusual increase in headaches.
- You have nausea or dizziness as a result of the medicine.
- You are feeling excessively weak and tired or are urinating frequently after prolactinoma surgery.

For More Information
Pituitary Tumor Network Association
16350 Ventura Boulevard #231
Encino, CA 91436
805-499-9973
The National Institute of Diabetes and Digestive and Kidney Diseases
http://www.niddk.nih.gov/prolactinoma

PROSTATE CANCER

About Your Diagnosis

Prostate cancer is the most common cancer among men in the United States. Nearly 300,000 new cases are diagnosed each year. It is estimated that 1 in 5 men has a diagnosis of prostate cancer in his lifetime. The cause of prostate cancer is unknown. Abnormal findings during a digital rectal examination or an abnormal prostate-specific antigen (PSA) blood test usually leads the physician to ordering transrectal ultrasonography (TRUS). A biopsy of the prostate is performed to confirm the diagnosis of prostate cancer.

The PSA blood test can lead to early detection of prostate cancer even before there are any symptoms. This accounts for the high number of new cases diagnosed each year but also has led to controversy regarding therapy for early localized prostate cancer. The reason for the controversy is that prostate cancer generally is slow growing; some reports show that 80% of patients live 10 years without treatment. The decision is whether patients should undergo treatment, which places them at risk for complications, or undergo observation and be treated only when symptoms occur (watchful waiting), knowing that prostate cancer is curable if treated at an early stage.

Living With Your Diagnosis

Typical symptoms are difficulty starting the urine stream, waking up frequently at night to urinate, dribbling at the end of urination, blood in the urine, urinary urgency, and pain with urination. If the prostate cancer has spread (usually to bone), you may have back or hip pain.

Treatment

Once the diagnosis is made, staging is performed to determine whether the cancer is localized or has spread, or "metastasized" (Fig 1). Computed tomography (CT) of the abdomen and pelvis and a bone scan usually are ordered. If the tumor is confined to the prostate, the treatment options include the following:

1. Surgical removal of the prostate. The main complications are impotence (inability to have an erection) and urinary incontinence (leaking).
2. Radiation therapy. The main complications are diarrhea, blood-streaked stools and rectal and urinary urgency, frequency, and incontinence.
3. Radiation seed implants. Complications are similar to those of radiation therapy.

If the tumor has spread, treatment is focused on elimination of the male hormone testosterone, which increases prostate tissue growth. Removal of all testosterone stimulation has been shown to cause remission. The testes produce 95% of the testosterone in the body; the other 5% comes from the adrenal gland. Therefore, treatment of advanced prostate cancer includes the following:

1. Surgical removal of both testes (orchiectomy). Complications are impotence, hot flashes, and loss of libido (sexual drive).
2. Use of medicines, including hormones, that inhibit formation of testosterone, such as estrogens, leuprolide, and flutamide. Complications are similar to those of orchiectomy.

The DOs

- Be aware of the controversy about PSA screening. Some authorities recommend an annual PSA blood test with digital rectal examination for all men older than 50 years or sooner for men who have a family member in his 40s or 50s with prostate cancer. There is no answer to what age to stop checking PSA level. This becomes a judgment and discussion between you and your physician. Most prostate cancers are slow growing and produce no clinical symptoms for as long as 10 years.
- Ask yourself the following questions and have an active role in making decisions about your treatment: Do you believe your life expectancy is more than 10 years? A 50-year-old man would say yes, but an 80-year-old would think twice. What about a 70-year-old man? Do you want to find out if you have prostate cancer by undergoing a biopsy? Do you want to go through surgical treatment or radiation therapy and its complications?

The DON'Ts

- Do not forget your options if you have localized prostate cancer. They are watchful waiting, surgical treatment, or radiation therapy.
- Do not be afraid to ask for second opinions. You can ask opinions from an oncologist (cancer specialist), urologist (specialist who deals with diseases of the urinary and genital tract), and your primary care physician.

When to Call Your Doctor

- If you have blood in the urine.
- If you have difficulty initiating the urine stream or cannot urinate.
- If you have urinary frequency, urgency, or pain.
- If you have prostate cancer and new onset of back, hip, or bone pain.

For More Information
National Cancer Institute (NCI)
9000 Rockville Pike
Bethesda, MD 20892
Cancer Information Service
1-800-422-6237

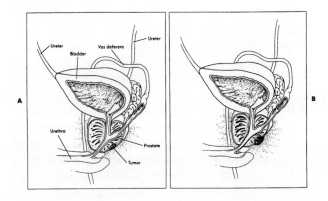

Four stages of prostatic cancer. (Illustrations by May S. Cheney. From LaFleur-Brooks ML: *Exploring Medical Language; A Student Directed Approach,* vol 3. St Louis, Mosby–Year Book, 1993. Used by permission.)

PRURITUS ANI

About Your Diagnosis

Pruritus ani is a burning or itching of the anus and genitals and the surrounding skin. Numerous conditions cause pruritis ani. Infections caused by yeast, herpes, genital warts, pinworms, scabies, and lice cause the condition. Skin conditions such as contact dermatitis, psoriasis, and seborrheic dermatitis may initially present as pruritis ani. Contact dermatitis may be caused by exposure to soaps, contraceptive jellies and foams, scented toilet paper, deodorant sprays, and douches. Individuals who have chronic diarrhea may have pruritis ani because of the difficulty keeping the area clean and dry. Diseases of the rectum such as hemorrhoids, fissures (tears), fistulas, or rectal prolapse may initially cause symptoms of pruritis ani. Women may have pruritis ani caused by a vaginal discharge or low estrogen levels if perimenopausal or postmenopausal. Excessive coffee drinking is also a known cause. However many times the cause cannot be identified.

Pruritis ani is common and affects both sexes and individuals of all ages. Individuals with diabetes may be at greater risk of developing this condition. It is most commonly detected by your observation of the symptoms. An examination by a doctor may be needed to confirm your suspicions. Occasionally laboratory studies are necessary to identify fungi, or microscopic examinations are necessary to look for pinworm eggs or scabies in skin burrows. With treatment, the symptoms can be controlled; however, the problem can reoccur.

Living With Your Diagnosis

The symptoms of pruritis ani include itching, redness of skin around the anus, and abrasions of the skin caused by scratching. The itching is often intense and worse at night. Complications such as skin thickening and chronic inflammation can occur. If the skin is damaged, a secondary bacterial infection can develop.

Treatment

The key to treatment is self care and the avoidance of predisposing factors. Keep the area clean, cool, and dry. You may use over-the-counter cortisone ointment or cream to control the itch. You should apply it three times a day and rub in gently until the medication disappears. You should stop using the cortisone when the itching stops. You should not use the cortisone for longer than 5 days because it may cause additional irritation and damage to the skin if used for longer periods. If you can not control the itch with the over-the-counter cortisone, you should see your doctor. Your doctor may prescribe a more potent topical cortisone drug or other agents to treat the cause of the pruritis.

Conditions such as yeast, herpes, genital warts, pinworms, scabies, and lice, must be specifically treated with the appropriate medications. Rectal diseases may require additional medical or surgical treatment.

The DOs

- Keep the area clean, cool, and dry.
- Use plain, unscented soaps if you must use soaps.
- Cleanse the area with moistened unscented tissue or tufts of cotton after bowel movements.
- Lose weight if overweight. Individuals who are overweight are at greater risk of developing pruritis ani.
- Wear loose clothing and cotton underclothing.
- Using tampons may be more comfortable than sanitary napkins for menstruating women.
- If scratching while asleep is an issue, wear soft mittens.

The DON'Ts

- Avoid contact with irritating substances that can cause pruritis ani.
- Avoid tight fitting underclothing.
- Avoid underclothing made from synthetic material.
- Avoid overdoing activities that could cause excess wetness or sweating in the area.
- Avoid spicy or highly seasoned foods that may irritate the area.
- Avoid excess coffee consumption.
- Avoid laxatives

When to Call Your Doctor

- If the area seems to be infected.
- If fever occurs.
- If symptoms persist, despite self-care.

For More Information
Contact your primary care physician

PSEUDOGOUT

About Your Diagnosis

Pseudogout is an abrupt and often very painful form of arthritis generally affecting individuals older than 60 years. It usually affects only one joint at a time such as a knee, ankle, wrist, elbow, or shoulder. Because it resembles gout but has a different cause, it is called pseudogout, meaning "false gout."

Pseudogout "attacks" are caused by the release of "crystals," made of calcium and phosphorus, into a joint. These crystals cause inflammation in the joint, leading to pain and swelling. No one knows why some individuals get pseudogout and others do not. It is not caused by an infection. In other words you cannot "catch" it. The only way to be certain of the diagnosis of pseudogout is to place a needle into the affected joint, remove joint fluid, and look for the pseudogout crystals under a microscope.

Living With Your Diagnosis

Individuals with pseudogout frequently have pain, swelling, warmth, and redness develop rapidly in the affected joint. The pain is often constant and it gets worse if the joint is moved a lot. Everyday activities such as walking, dressing, and lifting may be difficult. In some cases more than one joint may be affected. Some individuals experience fever and fatigue with the arthritis.

There is no way to know when or how many attacks an individual will have once they have had their first attack. Attacks may occur at any time; however, certain events such as surgery or an acute illness can trigger attacks. Once the attacks are treated, the symptoms generally resolve within days; untreated they may last for several weeks or more. Between attacks the symptoms resolve completely for most individuals.

Treatment

Nonsteroidal anti-inflammatory drugs (NSAIDs) such as ibuprofen, naproxen, or indomethacin are commonly used to treat pseudogout. Potential side effects of NSAIDs include stomach upset, ulcers, constipation, diarrhea, headaches, dizziness, difficulty hearing, and skin rash. Occasionally, a more potent anti-inflammatory medicine such as prednisone, a cortisone-like medicine, is necessary. Potential side effects of cortisone-like medicines are increased appetite, weight gain, difficulty sleeping, easy bruising, and stomach upset. Colchicine is another type of anti-inflammatory medication used to treat pseudogout. Colchicine's potential side effects include stomach cramps, nausea, vomiting, and diarrhea. Removal of the joint fluid from the affected joint followed by a cortisone injection into the joint is another common treatment for pseudogout. Cortisone injections usually provide the most rapid and complete relief of pain and swelling. Aside from the discomfort of the injection, there are very few side effects with cortisone injections. Regardless of the specific treatment used, it is important to rest the affected joint until the symptoms begin to subside.

The DOs

- Rest the affected joint until the symptoms begin to improve.
- Take your medicines as prescribed.
- Ask your doctor which over-the-counter medications you may take with your prescription medications.

The DON'Ts

- Wait to see whether side effects from medications will go away.
- Give up; ask your doctor about other treatment options if your symptoms are not going away on their own.

When to Call Your Doctor

- You experience any medication side effects.
- The treatment is not decreasing your symptoms in a reasonable amount of time.
- You begin to lose full motion in the affected joint.
- You experience worsening warmth, redness, or pain after a cortisone injection.

For More Information

Contact the Arthritis Foundation in your area. If you do not know the location of the Arthritis Foundation, you may call the national office at 1-800-283-7800 or access the information on the Internet at www.arthritis.org.

PSEUDOMEMBRANOUS COLITIS

About Your Diagnosis

Pseudomembranous colitis is an inflammatory disorder of the small and large bowel. It is associated with antibiotic use. The most commonly associated antibiotics are the penicillins, cephalosporins, clindamycin and sulfa drugs. However any antibiotic may be associated with the disease. When an individual is given an antibiotic to treat an infection, the bacteria in the bowel can be affected. Certain bacteria such as *Clostridium difficile* and *Staphylococcus* can flourish and cause the disease. Pseudomembranous colitis affects 6 per 100,000 individuals treated with antibiotics. It occurs more commonly in hospitalized and nursing home patients. Patients who have had recent surgery or are undergoing cancer treatments are at greater risk.

The condition is detected by stool cultures that grow the bacteria. A sigmoidoscopy or colonoscopy, a procedure where a lighted flexible instrument is inserted into the rectum to view the colon, is done to look for the abnormal findings of this disease. Tissue samples are taken from the colon and sent for microscopic examination. Most individuals will respond to treatment within a couple of days and have no long-term effects. If untreated, the condition can be fatal.

Living With Your Diagnosis

Pseudomembranous colitis presents with diarrhea that is classically watery, green, foul smelling, and bloody. Abdominal cramps and pain occur commonly. Fever also occurs. The symptoms usually start 4–10 days after beginning antibiotics; however, a significant portion of individuals do not have symptoms until after the antibiotics are stopped. There will be an elevated white blood cell count because of the infection. If severe, symptoms of shock, low blood pressure, weak pulse, and increased heart rate may be present.

Treatment

The key to treatment is stopping the antibiotics and bed rest. If symptoms are severe, hospitalization with intravenous fluid and nutrition may be necessary. The diet is then gradually returned to normal. In severe cases, antibiotics such as metronidazole and vancomycin are given to help treat the condition.

The DOs

- Stop all antibiotics.
- Bed rest is important.
- Avoid Dairy Products (may worsen diarrhea).

The DON'Ts

- Do not use antidiarrheal agents unless prescribed by your doctor.
- Do not have a barium enema x-ray done. It can cause complications.
- Avoid inappropriate use of antibiotics.

When to Call Your Doctor

- If you have symptoms of pseudomembranous colitis, particularly when taking or just finishing a course of antibiotics.
- If symptoms do not resolve after 4 days of treatment.
- If new symptoms appear during treatment.

For More Information
National Digestive Diseases Information Clearinghouse
2 Information Way
Bethesda, MD 20892-3570
www.niddk.nih.gov
nddic@aerie.com

PSORIASIS

About Your Diagnosis

Psoriasis is a chronic skin disorder with frequent recurrences and remissions characterized by silvery white, scaly plaques. Your psoriasis can vary from mild to severe, depending upon the type of psoriasis and the extent of involvement.

The exact cause is unknown. Psoriasis is likely autoimmune (i.e., a condition in which your immune system mistakenly attacks normal parts of the body, resulting in tissue injury or disease).

This condition is common, affecting about 2% of individuals in the United States. It is less common in individuals of African, Asian, and Native American descent. It affects men and women equally. It typically begins in adolescence or early adulthood and persists throughout life.

This condition is hereditary but is not infectious or cancerous. Other members of your family may have psoriasis. Minor injury, including scratching or rubbing, can provoke an outbreak of the lesions. Other factors that can increase your risk for an episode of psoriasis include stress, infections, cold and dry climates, obesity, and other autoimmune conditions.

Diagnosis is usually based upon the appearance of the skin lesions. Your doctor may perform a skin biopsy (i.e., removal of a small piece of skin or other tissue) for laboratory evaluation to assist in diagnosis.

Psoriasis is not curable. Psoriasis is a chronic condition in which episodes may persist for days to months. Periods of remission occur between episodes. The severity may decrease during pregnancy. Treatment aims to control symptoms and lessen the severity and duration of skin lesions, but does not cure psoriasis.

Living With Your Diagnosis

Skin lesions are slightly raised, silvery white scales with red or pink margins. The lesions can develop painful fissures (cracks). Lesions may be single, localized to certain areas of the body, or generalized. They are typically bilateral (i.e., involve both sides of the body). Psoriasis can affect any part of the body. It most commonly involves the skin of the scalp, face, elbows, hands, knees, feet, chest, lower back, and the folds between the buttocks. Fingernails and toenails are frequently involved. Nails often show discoloration and pitting.

Itching is common, particularly in the scalp. Joint pain occasionally occurs, especially if psoriasis involves the fingernails and toenails. Rarely, you may have fever, chills, arthritis, and a generalized pustular psoriasis.

Secondary bacterial infections can occur, especially if you scratch the lesions. These infections often require antibiotic therapy. You may also experience social embarrassment because of your skin's appearance: "the heartbreak of psoriasis." Other complications include arthritis and pustular psoriasis.

Treatment

Specific treatment depends upon the type, location, and severity of your psoriasis, its impact on the quality of your life, and your response to therapy. Treatment does not cure psoriasis, but it lessens the severity of your condition and prevents complications. Treatment includes the avoidance of precipitating factors, general measures, and medications.

Treatment of mild-to-moderate psoriasis includes topical creams, lotions, and ointments to reduce inflammation, scaling, and itching. Shampoos and lotions are frequently used to treat psoriasis of the scalp. Be cautious when using topical medications because they may be absorbed through your skin into your bloodstream, thereby causing toxic effects. Do not exceed prescribed doses of your medicine.

General measures include:
1. Maintaining good skin hygiene.
2. Avoiding skin injury.
3. Avoiding excessive skin dryness.
4. Exposing your skin to moderate amounts of sunlight.
5. Considering moving to areas with a warmer climate.
6. Oatmeal baths to loosen scales, which can improve the appearance of your skin and enhance the effects of topical medications.

Your doctor may prescribe a variety of medications to reduce inflammation, scaling, and itching and to lessen the severity and duration of outbreaks of psoriasis. These medications include:
1. Ointments and shampoos containing coal tar. These medications are effective for psoriasis of the scalp and for mild-to-moderate cases.
2. Topical steroids and other topical anti-inflammatory agents. These agents are effective in mild-to-moderate cases and as combination therapy for more severe cases. Before using these agents,

soak the affected areas in water to loosen and to remove scales, which increases the effectiveness of the topical medications. Your doctor may recommend placing occlusive dressings over the topical medications to increase their effects. Side effects include skin atrophy, formation of abnormal, small blood vessels, and absorption of medication through the skin into the bloodstream, which can cause toxic effects. To decrease the risk of side effects, do not exceed the recommended dose prescribed by your doctor.

3. Salicylic acid in mineral oil. This helps to remove plaques, thereby maximizing the effects of topical medications.

4. PUVA (combination of the medicine psoralen and exposure to ultraviolet light wavelength A [UVA]).

5. Combination of emollients or tar baths with ultraviolet light wavelength B (UVB).

6. In severe cases, immunosuppressive agents (i.e., medications that lessen the effects of your immune system) such as methotrexate, isotretinoin, and etretinate. These medications are effective but do carry the risk of toxic effects to the liver and kidney. Therefore, your doctor will closely follow laboratory tests to monitor your response to these medications and to check for side effects. Isotretinoin can be toxic to a developing fetus and should not be used in women who are pregnant or who may become pregnant.

7. Antihistamines to relieve itching. They may cause drowsiness, so use these agents cautiously when driving or performing other activities in which you must be awake and alert. 8. Antibiotics to treat secondary bacterial infections. A rare form of psoriasis, known as guttate psoriasis, is caused by a strep infection. Prompt antibiotic therapy is indicated for individuals with this type of psoriasis.

The DOs

- Take medications as prescribed by your doctor.
- Inform your doctor of all other medications, including over-the-counter medicines, that you are taking. Continue these medications unless your doctor instructs you to stop them.
- Read the labels of medicines and follow all instructions. Consult your doctor if you have any concerns or if you have possible side effects caused by the medication.
- Frequently expose your skin to *moderate* amounts of sunlight.
- Maintain good skin hygiene to reduce outbreaks of psoriasis and to decrease the risk of secondary bacterial infection.
- Oatmeal baths (one cup of oatmeal in a bathtub of warm water) loosens scales, which can improve the appearance of your skin and enhance the effects of topical medications.
- Consider moving to a warmer climate.
- Keep scheduled follow-up appointments with your doctor; they are essential to monitor your condition, your response to therapy, and to screen for possible side effects of treatment.
- Monitor your skin for healing and for evidence of secondary bacterial infection. Signs and symptoms of infection include redness around the skin lesions, purulent discharge (pus), increased pain or swelling of lesions or lymph nodes, and fever.
- Individuals with psoriasis frequently become depressed or experience other psychological conditions. If you feel depressed or are having difficulty adjusting to your psoriasis, talk to your doctor about the best treatment options, including psychological counseling.

The DON'Ts

- Do not stop your medicine or change the prescribed dose without consulting your doctor.
- Do not exceed recommended doses of medicines, because higher doses can increase the risk of toxic effects.
- Do not use potent topical steroids on the skin of the face or genitals, because these areas are most prone to skin atrophy.
- Do not abruptly stop steroids or immunosuppressive therapy because you may have a rebound worsening of your condition. In particular, do not suddenly stop steroids because this action can have serious effects to your health. Consult your doctor before stopping these medications.
- Do not drive or perform other potentially hazardous activities when taking medications that cause drowsiness or sedation (e.g., antihistamines and pain medications).
- Avoid skin injuries, including scratching, rubbing, or scrubbing, which can trigger outbreaks.
- Avoid skin dryness to reduce the frequency of outbreaks.
- Avoid activities that can cause infection of skin lesions.

When To Call Your Doctor

- If you have any signs or symptoms of infection (see above).
- If you notice that lesions are becoming worse or if new lesions appear despite appropriate therapy.
- If you notice pustules on the skin, especially if accompanied by fever, fatigue, muscle aches, or joint pain/swelling.
- If you have new or unexplained symptoms.

For More Information

Contact the National Psoriasis Foundation
6415 Southwest Canyon Court
Suite 200
Portland, OR 97221
503-244-7404

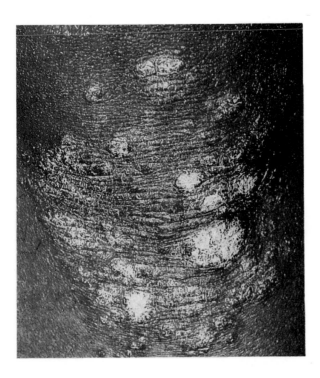

Psoriasis. Note scaly plaques characteristic of this condition. (From Thibodeau GA, Patton KT: *The Human Body in Health & Disease*, vol 2. St. Louis, Mosby–Year Book, 1996.Used by permission.)

PYELONEPHRITIS

About Your Diagnosis

Pyelonephritis means infection of the kidney. This usually starts as a urinary tract infection (UTI). A UTI is an inflammation that occur when germs get into the urinary tract. These germs usually enter the the urinary tract through the urethra (tube that carries urine out of the body). These germs may then go up to the urinary bladder (the organ where urine is stored before it is passed out of the body) and sometimes to the kidney. When they go to the kidney, it is called pyelonephritis. Sometimes germs may reach the kidneys from the bloodstream. Infections of the kidney are less common; however, they are more serious. Repeated kidney infections may hurt the kidney and lead to scarring. Very rarely, when an individual has a block or other problem in the urinary tract, then infection may continue to damage the kidneys and cause what is called chronic pyelonephritis. This can cause kidney failure. Certain individuals have a greater risk of getting UTIs. These include:

- Women.
- Older individuals.
- Individuals with a tube called a catheter placed in the bladder to help drain urine.
- Individuals with diabetes.
- Individuals with blockage of their urinary tract with stones or an enlarged prostate gland.

Living With Your Diagnosis

You may have fever, feel sick to your stomach, and have pain in your back or side below the ribs. You will be treated with antibiotics. Your doctor will follow-up closely to ensure the infection has been cleared. In more complicated cases, the underlying cause such as obstruction or infection needs to be treated. Your doctor will see you periodically once you get better to ensure that the infection does not come back.

Treatment

You are usually admitted to the hospital and treated with antibiotics given into your vein. The antibiotics are administered through your vein until you improve. They may then be switched to antibiotics in tablet form, which may need to be continued for 3–4 weeks. You will be given pain relief and fluids through your vein if you are dehydrated.

If you have repeated UTIs, you may be treated with low doses of antibiotic daily for a period of 6 months or more to prevent infections.

The DOs

- Do tell your doctor if there is a history of kidney infections in your family. Certain tests can be done in infants to detect conditions that may result in future infections and kidney damage.
- Do drink plenty of water.
- Drinking large amounts of cranberry juice is sometimes advised because it makes the urine more acidic and slows the growth of germs.
- Do not put off going to the bathroom when you feel the need.
- Do go to the bathroom after having sex and observe clean hygiene.
- Do ask your doctor about any questions you may have regarding this condition.

The DON'Ts

- Don't stop taking your medication before checking with your doctor.
- Don't take over-the-counter medication unless you have checked with your doctor. Some of these medicines may not be safe with your kidney condition.
- Don't take any herbal preparations that you may find at health food stores. Some of these preparations have been known to cause kidney disease.
- Don't hesitate to ask your doctor any questions about your disease or its treatment that may concern you.

When to Call Your Doctor

Always call your doctor if you feel unwell. He may be able to assess whether you need to be seen right away or whether a change in medication is necessary.

For More Information

Your doctor can help answer specific questions you or your family may have about UTIs, pyelonephritis, symptoms, and medicines. He can order the tests needed to find out whether you have an infection and why you have an infection. Your national Kidney Foundation affiliate can give you further information about types of treatment available; their address can be obtained from your doctor or The National Kidney Foundation, Inc., 30 East 33rd Street, New York, NY 10016.

RAYNAUD'S PHENOMENON

About Your Diagnosis

Raynaud's phenomenon causes temporary decreased blood flow to the fingers, toes, and ears, and less often the tip of the nose. Raynaud's phenomenon usually occurs with exposure to cold temperatures when blood flow decreases in the fingers and toes. The skin in the area involved will first turn white because there is no blood in that area. Next, the skin may turn blue, and once the blood flows back the skin becomes purple or red. If Raynaud's is not treated, sores or ulcers may develop in the areas with the decreased blood flow. If the blood flow is decreased for a long time, the skin in the affected areas could turn black and die. Rarely, Raynaud's phenomenon affects organs inside the body.

Raynaud's phenomenon may occur at any age but usually occurs between the ages of 20 and 40 years. It occurs more frequently in women than in men. Although we do not know the cause of Raynaud's, it is not an infectious illness. To diagnose Raynaud's, a physician obtains a medical history and performs a physical examination. There are no specific blood tests to diagnose Raynaud's, but a physician may perform certain blood tests to determine whether Raynaud's phenomenon is associated with other conditions.

Living With Your Diagnosis

Raynaud's phenomenon may cause pain and numbness when the affected areas turn white. Some individuals have swelling, warmth, or a throbbing pain when the affected areas turn purple or red. To prevent these problems, you should keep the body warm and avoid any unnecessary exposure to cold. If you have a job that involves working outside or that exposes your body to cold temperatures indoors, you should see whether your job can be modified or explore other employment options.

Treatment

The best way to manage Raynaud's phenomenon is through a combination of therapies and preventive measures. To keep the body warm you should dress in layers, wear lined mittens rather than gloves, wear a hat and scarf, and always carry a sweater with you to adjust to the room temperature. To avoid exposure to cold, have someone warm up your car in the winter, use an oven mitt to get items out of the refrigerator/freezer, and warm up the bathroom by letting the warm water run for a while before you take a shower or bath. Smoking also causes the blood vessels to close down, leading to less blood flow in the affected areas and a greater chance of sores or an infection developing in those areas. Therefore, individuals with Raynaud's must stop smoking. If emotional stress seems to cause a Raynaud's attack, relaxation and biofeedback may be helpful to increase the circulation in certain areas of the body. If the Raynaud's is severe, a physician may prescribe a medication such as nifedipine that can improve the blood flow. The most common side effects of this medication may include swelling in the hands and feet, lightheadedness or dizziness, and a rash. If these medications do not help and your symptoms are severe, your physician may suggest a type of surgery called a sympathectomy. This surgery involves cutting the nerves that cause the blood vessels to close down, thereby increasing blood flow.

The DOs

- Call your doctor if you are experiencing side effects from medications.
- Ask your doctor what over-the-counter medication you may take or should avoid.
- Stop smoking.
- Examine your fingers, toes, nose, and ears daily for any new sores or infections.
- Moisturize your affected areas at least daily with lots of ointments.

The DON'Ts

- Wait to see whether a possible medication side effect will go away on its own.
- Continue smoking.
- Expose yourself unnecessarily to cold.

When to Call Your Doctor

- You experience side effects that you believe may be caused by your medications.
- The medication and other treatments are not helping to improve your symptoms.
- You are concerned about a sore in an affected area.
- You need a referral to a stop smoking program.
- You believe you need a referral to a vocational rehabilitation specialist to explore other job options.

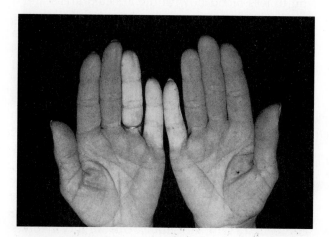

Whiteness from blood vessel constriction in primary Raynaud's phenomenon. **B** and **C**, Puffy, swollen fingers and sores on the fingertips. (From Noble J: *Textbook Primary Care Medicine*, vol 2. St. Louis, Mosby–Year Book, Inc., 1995. Used by permission.)

REITER'S SYNDROME

About Your Diagnosis

Reiter's syndrome is a form of arthritis that typically affects younger adults. This condition not only affects the joints but can also affect other areas including the spine, eyes, urinary tract, skin, and tendons.

Although the cause of Reiter's syndrome is not always known, a number of infections may trigger the condition. The infections may not be apparent to the individual who has them. Other times, a diarrheal illness or a sexually transmitted disease might be the cause.

Reiter's syndrome is diagnosed by a medical history and physical examination. There are no specific tests to diagnose this condition; however, certain blood tests and x-rays can assist in making the diagnosis.

Living With Your Diagnosis

Reiter's syndrome may cause low-grade fevers, fatigue, joint pain with swelling, muscle aches, and low back pain. Stiffness in the joints and back are very noticeable, especially early in the morning and after prolonged periods of rest. Usually only a few joints are affected at any given time. The knees, ankles, feet, wrists, toes, and fingers are most commonly affected and may make work and daily activities harder to perform. Heel pain is caused by tendinitis of the Achilles tendon. Low back pain and stiffness make walking, bending, and lifting difficult.

Other symptoms may include eye inflammation causing "pink eye" or blurry vision. Rashes can occur on the tip of the penis and soles of the feet. Discharge from the penis and pain with urination may occur with the other symptoms. This may or may not be caused by an infection. Although uncommon, leaky heart valves develop in some individuals with Reiter's syndrome.

Treatment

The treatment of Reiter's syndrome is individualized but involves medicines, exercises, and physical therapy. If an infection can be identified or suspected, it is treated with antibiotics. Nonsteroidal anti-inflammatory drugs (NSAIDs) such as indomethacin improve pain, stiffness, and swelling caused by inflammation. Individuals with persistent arthritis may need other medicines such as sulfasalazine or methotrexate. Sometimes cortisone injections into joints are helpful.

Potential side effects of NSAIDs include stomach upset, ulcers, constipation, diarrhea, headaches, dizziness, difficulty hearing, and rash. The most common side effects of sulfasalazine are rash, stomach pain, and nausea. Methotrexate can cause poor appetite, nausea, headaches, mouth sores, and diarrhea. Routine blood counts and liver function tests are necessary to monitor for side effects with both methotrexate and sulfasalazine.

A very important part of treating Reiter's syndrome is physical therapy and exercises. Swollen joints should be rested for a short period until the inflammation begins to improve. Simple stretching and strengthening exercises may be taught by a physical therapist. It is also important to learn and maintain good posture to lessen pain and maintain normal motion in joints and the spine.

Some individuals completely recover from Reiter's syndrome; the symptoms improve and never return. However, even with treatment, many individuals have recurrent episodes of arthritis, back pain, rashes, and urinary symptoms.

The DOs
- Take your medicines as prescribed.
- Ask your doctor which over-the-counter medications you may take with your prescription medications.
- Perform stretching exercises everyday.
- Perform exercises to maintain joint motion and preserve strength.
- Learn and maintain good sitting, standing, and sleeping posture. Be aware of and check your posture throughout the day.

The DON'Ts
- Wait to see whether side effects from medications will go away.
- Sleep with pillows under your legs or neck if you are having difficulty maintaining posture through the day.
- Continue an exercise program that causes pain. If pain after exercise continues, it usually means the exercise program needs to be modified specifically for you.

When to Call Your Doctor

- You experience any medication side effects.
- The medication and treatments are not decreasing the pain.
- You believe you need a referral to a physical or occupational therapist.

For More Information

Contact the Arthritis Foundation in your area. If you do not know the location of the Arthritis Foundation, you may call the national office at 1-800-283-7800 or access the information on the Internet at www.arthritis.org.

RENAL ARTERY STENOSIS

About Your Diagnosis

Obstruction of the main artery that brings clean blood to your kidney is called renal artery stenosis. The artery to one or both kidneys may be blocked. This usually, but not always results in high blood pressure. In individuals older than 50 years, buildup of atherosclerotic material inside the blood vessels, which occurs with age, can gradually block the artery. In young women, a condition called "fibromuscular hyperplasia" can cause blockage of the artery and high blood pressure. This is also a form of renal artery stenosis. If this condition is not diagnosed and treated in a timely manner, it may result in a progressive decrease in kidney function and complete kidney failure.

Living With Your Diagnosis

You may not have any symptoms from your condition. Your doctor may suspect that you have this condition if you have high blood pressure. Special tests are necessary to diagnose this condition. The test that is most helpful is putting some dye in an artery in your groin and then taking pictures of your kidney blood vessels. You have to take your blood pressure medicine regularly.

Treatment

Some artery blocks can be dilated with a balloon, whereas others may require surgery. Occasionally blood pressure will be controlled with drug therapy. Your doctor will examine you often to ensure that your blood pressure is well controlled. He will also follow your kidney blood tests closely. If your blood pressure is poorly controlled with medicines or your kidney function starts to worsen, you may need the balloon treatment or surgery. Sometimes you may also receive blood-thinning medicines.

The DOs

- Do not smoke. Smoking makes cells called platelets in your blood sticky. This worsens blood pressure control and may increase your chances of getting heart disease.
- Do take your medicine regularly. It is the most important thing you can do to delay or prevent worsening of your kidney function.
- Do keep your appointments with your doctor.
- Do exercise regularly. This will decrease the risk of complications, such as heart disease, that result from high blood pressure.
- Do eat healthy food. Follow your dietitian's advice because it is possible that your blood cholesterol level is high. A high cholesterol level increases your risk of heart disease, especially with high blood pressure.
- Do ask your doctor about any questions you may have regarding this condition.

The DON'Ts

- Don't stop taking your medication before checking with your doctor.
- Don't take over-the-counter medication, especially drugs similar to ibuprofen, unless you have checked with your doctor. Some of these medicines may not be safe with your kidney condition and may actually make it worse.
- Don't take any herbal preparations that you may find at health food stores. Some of these preparations have been known to cause kidney disease.
- Don't hesitate to ask your doctor any questions that may concern you about your disease or its treatment.

When to Call Your Doctor

Always call your doctor if you feel unwell. He may be able to assess whether you need to be seen right away or whether a change in medication is necessary.

For More Information

Your national Kidney Foundation affiliate can give you further information about types of treatment available; their address can be obtained from your doctor or The National Kidney Foundation, Inc., 30 East 33rd Street, New York, NY 10016.

RENAL CALCULI

About Your Diagnosis

Kidney stones are a very common problem. About 12% of men and 5% of women will have at least one kidney stone in their lifetime. Most kidney stones contain calcium. Other substances such as oxalate are necessary to remain in solution in the urine. Stones are typically caused by an imbalance in the urinary system: too little water, too much oxalate, or too much calcium. Rarely are stones related to too much calcium in the blood. There are also other types of stones that can develop, such as uric acid, magnesium ammonium phosphate, or cystine stones.

There are some rare stone types that are inherited in families, although these usually are seen in children. Your physician can determine that you have a stone by a variety of means. It might show on an x-ray of the abdomen, an ultrasound examination, or by intravenous pyelography (IVP, a procedure where dye administered into a vein highlights the "road map" of the kidneys and ureters).

Living With Your Diagnosis

For most patients a stone is an isolated event. The small piece of calcium or uric acid travels down the ureter (the tube connecting kidney and bladder) and causes crampy pain, typically in the flank, that may be severe. Some patients vomit with the discomfort, whereas others are simply aware of an ache in the groin. In some cases there is a history of a previous stone; in others, the stone does not cause many symptoms until it is complicated by infection. In this case, the patient will be quite ill with high fever, chills, pain in the side, and burning on urinating.

Treatment

The treatment depends on the location and size of the stone. Small stones may pass spontaneously over 24–48 hours; larger stones might require shockwave therapy or rarely surgery to retrieve them. Once the problem has been treated, the main role is in preventing recurrence. About 50% of patients will have another stone within 5 years of the first episode.

The essentials are to maintain a high-volume, dilute urine output to discourage "stagnation" of urine. Keeping the urine as clear as water is a good clue that your fluid intake is sufficient.

As so many stones are formed because of an imbalance of calcium and oxalate, your doctor may treat you with high doses of calcium supplements (e.g., calcium carbonate) or dairy products. This therapy is effective and goes against the common belief that patients with a history of stones should avoid calcium in their diet. Depending on the type of stone you have, your physician may have to use other medications such as hydrochlorothiazide (HCTZ, a diuretic) or allopurinol (a drug that reduces the formation of uric acid, which accounts for about 5% to 15% of stones), depending on the type of stone that is identified by the laboratory.

There are a few side effects of the treatment. Calcium pills can be chalky and hard to swallow, but otherwise are well tolerated. Hydrochlorothiazide is a mild diuretic that can result in impotence (less than 20% of users), high cholesterol levels, high blood calcium levels, low potassium or magnesium, or worsening diabetes. Allopurinol may rarely cause a rash or a lowering of blood cell counts.

If you undergo shockwave treatment, the stone will break up in the ureter and may cause some discomfort as it travels out. Rarely, some patients have had hypertension after this therapy.

The DOs
- Do drink lots of water every day; 1–2 pints a day is recommended. If you have recurring stones, it's advisable to drink more than this: enough so your urine looks as dilute as water all the time.
- Do take calcium supplements as recommended, to avoid the "imbalance" that might exist.
- Do take the preventive therapy your doctor may prescribe, such as allopurinol or HCTZ.
- Always ask questions regarding your treatment or any side effects you are experiencing.
- Do remember to bring water with you, especially if exercising or working in hot weather.

The DONTs
- Don't get dehydrated.
- Don't forget to choose your food with care. Your physician may suggest a diet rich in calcium and water. Some patients will have an animal protein restriction to avoid making too much uric acid (which can go on to form stones).

- Don't forget the medications prescribed to reduce the risk of further stones forming, such as calcium supplements, HCTZ, or allopurinol.
- Don't use painkillers in excess of the amount prescribed by your health care provider because they can accumulate and make you ill.
- Don't drink too much coffee or tea because they can lead to further dehydration, especially in warm weather.

When to Call Your Doctor

Call your doctor if you have fevers or chills, if you are not able to control the pain on the standard treatment, or if you are vomiting and unable to keep food down. You should also call if you are unable to void urine, or if doing so is painful or causes burning. There may be some bleeding with a kidney stone; call the doctor if there is persistent or more blood noticed in the urine.

For More Information

You can read the pamphlet on kidney stones available from the National Kidney Foundation. Your local office of the National Kidney Foundation may be reached at 1-800-622-9010 or by writing the Head Office at 30 East 33rd Street, New York, NY 10016.

RENAL FAILURE, ACUTE

About your diagnosis

Acute renal failure is an abrupt decline in kidney function resulting in retention of nitrogenous end products of metabolism in the body. There are many causes of acute renal failure, including conditions that have a secondary effect on the kidneys (e.g., a drop in blood pressure that could occur from many causes), as well as an obstruction of the kidneys at any level. Direct injury to the kidney by certain drugs and radiographic dyes, for example, is the third major cause of acute renal failure. Conditions such as acute glomerulonephritis (inflammation of the kidney) can also cause acute renal failure. It is a serious illness.

Living With Your Diagnosis

You will most likely be admitted to the hospital with this diagnosis, or you may have acute renal failure develop as a complication of the original condition for which you were hospitalized. You may require treatment in an intensive care unit. You may find that your urine output is very low, although this is not always the case. You may be short of breath and cough because of extra fluid in your lungs. Your blood pressure may be high. You may even require supportive treatment with breathing machines and artificial kidney machines (Fig 1). Complete recovery of kidney function is possible and may sometimes take as long as 6 weeks.

Treatment

Because the causes of acute renal failure are diverse, management depends on the underlying condition. The common thread of treatment involves giving medicines that may help increase the amount of urine you make, and putting you on the artificial kidney machine. You will have blood tests done very frequently (daily) to assess your response to treatment. Your doctor may ask you to reduce your intake of protein, salt, and potassium, and to take blood pressure pills and calcium supplements. You may be discharged home once you are stable on medicines and dialysis. This treatment would need to be continued until your kidneys improve or recover completely.

The DOs

- Do tell your doctor of any exposure you may have had to toxins such as chemicals or drugs.
- Do follow dietary advice because it is very important in preventing complications from your disease. You may have to eliminate fruit, chocolate, and nuts from your diet because these foods have high amounts of potassium in them. When your kidneys are not working, high potassium levels have to be prevented because they are dangerous for your heart.
- Do keep to the fluid restriction you have been advised because otherwise you could have fluid buildup in your lungs. This could be dangerous to your immediate health.
- Do let your doctor know of all the medication you are taking, such as over-the-counter medicines and herbal preparations.
- Do exercise within your capacity to do so.

The DON'Ts

- Don't stop taking your medication before checking with your doctor.
- Don't take over-the-counter medication unless you have checked with your doctor. Some of these medicines may not be safe with your kidney condition.
- Don't take any herbal preparations that you may find at health food stores. Some of these preparations have been known to cause kidney disease.
- Don't hesitate to ask your doctor any questions that may concern you about your disease or its treatment.

When to Call Your Doctor

Always call your doctor if you feel unwell. He may be able to assess whether you need to be seen right away or whether a change in medication is necessary.

For More Information

Many patients with kidney failure are able to go back to a normal lifestyle after getting used to their treatment. Your national Kidney Foundation affiliate can give you further information about types of treatment available; their address can be obtained from your doctor or The National Kidney Foundation, Inc., 30 East 33rd Street, New York, NY 10016.

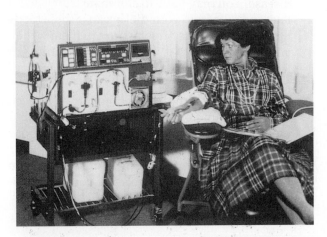

A, Hemodialysis (artificial kidney machine). **B,** Peritoneal dialysis (removal of nitrogenous end products through the abdomen). (From Thibodeau GA, Patton KT: *The Human Body in Health & Disease,* vol. 2. St. Louis, Mosby–Year Book, 1996. Used by permission.)

RENAL FAILURE, CHRONIC

About Your Diagnosis

Your doctor is treating you for chronic renal failure (CRF). This means there is an abnormality in your kidney function. The kidneys are important in many ways: they regulate the amount of water and byproducts of the body's metabolism; they excrete certain waste products, whose accumulation would be detrimental; they maintain your body water, blood salt, and calcium levels; and they help the bone marrow to make blood.

Chronic kidney failure may be caused by a variety of diseases: long-standing diabetes; hypertension; certain drugs you may have taken; and chronic inflammation of the kidneys. It is a very common problem. Many Americans live with this diagnosis, the only inconvenience being regular trips to the doctor, close attention to your blood pressure control, and being careful of the foods you eat. Rarely, you may have an inheritable form of kidney disease passed on from parent to child (polycystic kidney disease); your doctor will be able to tell you whether your disease fits this type.

Often kidney disease is diagnosed incidentally, or by a routine urine or blood test. Some patients are seen by their physician because their blood pressure is very high, needing urgent treatment. Kidney physicians and other researchers are working to find means to cure CRF. At this time the best treatment is to take care of the kidney function you have left, by avoiding certain medicines, treating your blood pressure, and avoiding certain foods.

Living With Your Diagnosis

Although often without symptoms, as kidney failure progresses it can lead to fatigue, lack of energy, anemia, shortness of breath, and nausea. Keeping regular appointments with your doctor for blood tests and treatment changes are vital to avoid these distressing problems. You may feel tired and depressed with kidney disease. Occasionally, patients are seen at the hospital because of complications arising from noncompliance: getting too much water, potassium, or phosphorous into the body that cannot be eliminated.

Treatment

Your doctor will advise you of the optimum treatment to help treat your failing kidneys. He will use blood and urine tests to follow your progress.

Generally, patients with CRF do well to avoid foods containing potassium, phosphorous, or too much salt or protein. Your dietitian can help you plan your diet.

It's very important to keep your blood pressure under good control; your physician will help choose a therapy that suits you. You might also need iron pills or calcium pills to boost your body stores; CRF plays a role in depleting our body stores of nutrients.

Sometimes your physician might want to refer you to a kidney specialist for further advice. The treatments for CRF are the same as for those of the underlying cause. Often, patients need diuretics ("water pills") to keep from gaining excess fluid, in addition to caring for the stores of iron, calcium, and vitamins in the body.

We know that patients who don't take care of themselves do worse than those who do; some patients need to receive dialysis treatments if the conservative measures fail. Dialysis is essentially a treatment where the patient is placed on an artificial kidney two or three times per week (Fig 1). There are other excellent alternatives available. Your physician can describe these in detail.

The DOs

- Do keep taking your blood pressure medicines. If you find a medication disagrees with you, consult your doctor for an alternative.
- Do keep to your diet. Your dietitian will show you how to restrict items like bananas, fruits, dairy products, or excess meat protein.
- Do exercise as much as you can within your tolerance.
- If your doctor has advised restricting fluid intake, be careful to follow that advice. He may be prescribing calcium supplements to boost your stores and reduce the amount of phosphorous in your blood. These are important too.
- Do give up smoking, and prolong your life. Patients with kidney failure are more prone to abnormal cholesterol, hypertension, angina, and heart attacks.

The DON'Ts

- Don't forget to ask questions about drug side effects.
- Don't eat foods you should avoid; a potassium buildup in the blood can make you very ill.
- Don't take over-the-counter drugs without checking first that they are safe.
- Don't overdo exercise to exhaustion. Call if you are feeling unwell, nauseous, chest pains, or shortness of breath.
- Don't drink too much water or liquids if you have been placed on a restriction, because you may gain too much fluid in the tissues, leading to worsening edema and hypertension.

When to Call Your Doctor

You should call your doctor if you develop shortness of breath, nausea, vomiting, or chest pains. Chronic kidney failure is an often silent disease; you should be sure and keep appointments so your blood tests can be done.

For More Information

You can read the pamphlet on chronic renal failure available from the National Kidney Foundation. Your local office of the National Kidney Foundation may be reached at 1-800-622-9010 or by writing the Head Office at 30 East 33rd Street, New York, NY 10016.

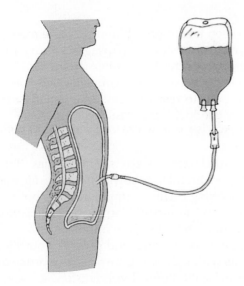

A, Hemodialysis (artificial kidney machine). **B,** Peritoneal dialysis (removal of nitrogenous end products through the abdomen). (From Thibodeau GA, Patton KT: *The Human Body in Health & Disease,* vol. 2. St. Louis, Mosby–Year Book, 1996. Used by permission.)

RHABDOMYOLYSIS

About Your Diagnosis

Rhabdomyolysis is a condition that happens when muscle is damaged. This releases pigments from the muscle and blood into the bloodstream. The kidney filters the pigments out of the blood. The pigments accumulate in the kidney, blocking up the filtering portion of the kidney. The kidney then fails. Conditions that cause rhabdomyolysis include crushing injuries to muscle, seizures, and exercise-related heat stroke. Other causes include severe frostbite, alcoholism, drug overdose, cocaine use, and as a side effect of some medicines. Occasionally, excessive high-endurance exercise by someone who is not trained adequately can also result in rhabdomyolysis.

A history of one of the above causes followed by red or brown urine is diagnostic. Some blood work and a urinalysis will confirm the diagnosis. If rhabdomyolysis is diagnosed before the kidneys fail, it can usually be treated effectively in the hospital.

Living With Your Diagnosis

The main symptom of rhabdomyolysis is red or brown urine following one of the above causes. It may then proceed to decreased or absent urine production. This is a serious sign that should cause you to seek immediate medical care because this is a symptom of developing kidney failure.

Treatment

Treatment takes place in the hospital. Initially, high volumes of intravenous fluids are administered to try to keep urine flow greater than 6 ounces an hour to flush the pigments through the kidney. Medicines are then given to make the urine alkaline and to increase urination, again with the goal of flushing the pigments out of the kidney. The main adverse effect of this treatment is fluid overload if the kidneys have already started to fail before starting treatment. If this is the case, dialysis (a kidney machine) may be necessary to remove fluid and wastes and to rest the kidney until it has time to recover. This may take weeks to months depending on the severity.

The DOs

If you have had one of the causes of rhabdomyolysis, particularly a crushing muscle injury or exercise-related heat stroke, you should seek medical care immediately if you notice red or brown urine. If you notice a recurrence of colored urine or a decrease in urine output after treatment for rhabdomyolysis, you should also seek immediate medical care. In any case, you need to stay well hydrated and drink plenty of fluids.

The DON'Ts

If you are at risk of rhabdomyolysis, you should not let yourself become dehydrated. This will increase the risk of pigments building up in the kidney. This is especially important if you have experienced exercise-induced heat stroke, because you are already dehydrated.

Do not participate in high-endurance sporting events without adequate training.

When to Call Your Doctor

You should call your doctor for any onset or recurrence of red or brown urine. You should also seek immediate medical care if urination decreases or is absent.

For More Information

Information on exercise-related rhabdomyolysis
http://www.gssiweb.com/library/sse/sse42S1.html

RHEUMATIC FEVER

About Your Diagnosis

Rheumatic fever is an inflammatory response to a previous streptococcal infection, which may have been mild or untreated. It affects the heart, nervous system, skin, and joints. It usually occurs in children younger than 18 years. Rheumatic fever is not contagious, but the strep infections that caused it is. The strep infection is curable with antibiotic treatment. Blood tests may be helpful in diagnosing the disease.

Living With Your Diagnosis

Signs and symptoms include fever, loss of appetite, mild rash, fatigue, paleness, small bumps under the skin over bony areas (such as the hands, wrists, elbows, and knuckles), and joint inflammation that is characterized by pain, swelling, and warmth. If the heart is involved, there may be shortness of breath, swelling of the ankles and around the eyes, and a rapid heartbeat. There may be uncontrolled jerky movements.

The most common complication of this disease is damage to the heart valves, resulting in a heart murmur. In some cases the damaged valves may need surgical replacement.

Treatment

Bed rest is required until the disease has subsided. This could take 2–5 weeks. Antibiotic treatment over a long period is needed. Let your doctor know if you are allergic to penicillin. In the early stages, a liquid or soft diet may be better tolerated, with progression to a normal diet high in calories, protein, and vitamins. Aspirin or other anti-inflammatory drugs are given for the muscle and joint pain. Common side effects of these drugs are ringing in the ears and stomach upset. After the initial infection is over, a daily dose of penicillin is necessary.

The DOs

- Take antibiotics as prescribed until finished.
- Take the daily dose of penicillin as instructed.
- Rest. Use a bedside commode so trips to the bathroom will be minimal.
- Encourage fluid intake while the fever is present.
- Resume activity gradually. It will be necessary to schedule rest periods and naps.
- Seek treatment for any sore throats in the future.

- Inform doctors or dentists of your history of the disease because you will need antibiotics before any surgical procedures.

The DON'Ts

- Don't skip or stop antibiotics until finished.
- Don't have any dental surgery or other surgeries until antibiotics are taken first.
- Don't resume activity until fever and other symptoms subside.

When to Call Your Doctor

If during treatment you have:
- Swelling of the legs or ankles.
- Shortness of breath.
- Vomiting or diarrhea.
- A dry hacking cough.
- Severe abdominal pain.
- A temperature of 101°F or higher.

For More Information
National Heart, Lung, and Blood Institute
Information Center
P.O. Box 30105
Bethesda, MD 20824-0105
Information Line 800-575-WELL
Internet Sites
www.healthanswers.com
www.healthfinder.gov

RHINITIS, ALLERGIC

About Your Diagnosis

In individuals with allergic rhinitis, the nasal passages are much more sensitive to environmental irritants or allergic triggers. Symptoms may be seasonal (especially in the spring and/or fall) or continuous (perennial). Allergic rhinitis is also known as "hay fever." The diagnosis of allergic rhinitis is based on the clinical presentation and positive allergy skin tests (especially to house dust, animal danders, or pollen). In patients with more constant or long-term problems, sinus changes, nasal polyps, loss of sense of smell, and itchy red eyes may also be present.

Although there are many irritants that produce nasal symptoms in individuals without allergies, irritants such as smoke and smog may cause more problems in individuals with allergic rhinitis. Other common triggers, especially in individuals with seasonal symptoms, may result from exposure to certain pollens, molds, or dust. This condition is not contagious or curable but may require medication and other forms of allergy treatment for control.

Living With Your Diagnosis

Symptoms may be seasonal (especially in the spring and/or fall) or continuous (perennial), and can range from being mild to interfering with daily activities. Sneezing, runny nose, nasal congestion, and an itchy nose, often with itchy eyes and a scratchy throat, are the most common symptoms. In severe cases, frontal headaches, sinus involvement, and sleep deprivation caused by nighttime symptoms are seen.

Treatment

The best treatment usually involves reducing or avoiding exposures to the potential allergens, in combination with the use of antihistamines and topical intranasal steroids. In more severe cases, a short course of oral corticosteroids and nasal decongestants may be required. Preventive therapy with agents such as cromolyn, as well as the use of a mask, may also be helpful. Finally, allergy injections (desensitization) for specific types of allergic rhinitis may be considered for individuals who have a poor response to drug therapy. Possible side effects may include excessive sleepiness (especially with oral antihistamines), palpitations or changes in blood pressure control (oral decongestants), and occasional thinning of the nasal mucosa (intranasal steroids).

Surgery by an ear, nose, and throat specialist may be necessary if problems persist despite trying the previous measures.

The DOs

It is important to work with your care provider in trying to identify possible triggers of your nasal symptoms. Keeping a diary of indoor and outdoor activities in relation to any nasal symptoms may provide clues for avoidance in the future. For individuals with seasonal symptoms, starting your preventive medications at least 2–3 weeks before the season that gives you problems may reduce the potential for a severe flare. For patients who have asthma and nasal polyps, additional precautions may be required, because some of these individuals are also sensitive to aspirin and aspirin-type products; for example, ibuprofen.

The DON'Ts

Overuse of nasal decongestant preparations may lead to reactive "after congestion," excessive heart rate or high blood pressure, and nosebleeds. It is important to review your medication use and options with your doctor and pharmacist, especially if you are taking other medications. Avoiding the possible allergic triggers is very helpful but not always practical.

When to Call Your Doctor

Call your doctor if your symptoms become constant and keep you awake, your nasal discharge becomes thickened and colored (especially if associated with fever and sinus headaches), or you think you are having a problem with your medications. Your doctor may refer you to an allergist for possible immunotherapy (allergy shots), or to an ear, nose, and throat specialist for advice on long-term management.

For More Information
American Academy of Allergy, Asthma, and Immunology
64 East Wells Street
Milwaukee, WI 53202-2887
800-822-2762
Asthma and Allergy Foundation of America (AAFA)
1125 15th Street NW
Suite 502
Washington, DC 20005
800-727-8462
American Lung Association
1118 Hampton Avenue
St. Louis, MO 63139
800-LUNG-USA
www.lungusa.org

RINGWORM

About Your Diagnosis

Ringworm is a general term used to describe a very common type of skin infection. It is not caused by a worm at all but is actually caused by a fungus. Fungi are extremely small and can only be seen under a microscope. Fungi are found everywhere and they are contagious. They are transmitted from other individuals or animals. They can also be found in towels, carpet, bedding, showers, and baths. Ringworm is much more common in hot, humid weather. The diagnosis of ringworm can usually be made by its typical appearance on the skin. In unusual cases, a small scraping of an affected area can be examined under a microscope to confirm the diagnosis. Ringworm is curable but takes 2–4 weeks of treatment, sometimes longer.

Living With Your Diagnosis

Ringworm can occur anywhere on the body. On the skin, ringworm starts as slightly raised, red-to-brown round patches that itch. Ringworm is categorized by where it occurs.

- Tinea corporis: ringworm of the body.
- Tinea pedis: ringworm of the feet (athlete's foot).
- Tinea capitis: ringworm of the scalp. This type of ringworm requires treatment with prescription medications; over-the-counter antifungal medications will usually not cure tinea capitis.

As the patch enlarges a central clearing develops. Small blisters can occur with ringworm of the groin or feet. Itching is common and can be severe. Scratching can cause secondary infection.

Treatment

Mild cases of ringworm can be treated with over-the-counter medications. Apply a small amount of antifungal cream, ointment, or powder to affected areas two times a day. Continue for 7 days after the areas have healed. If itching is severe, use calamine lotion twice a day. Aveeno Oatmeal bath can also help relieve itching. Benadryl taken by mouth every 4–6 hours is also helpful. If ringworm is not responsive to over-the-counter medicines, your doctor can prescribe a more potent cream to apply to the skin. Continue to use this for 7 days after the infection appears to be resolved to prevent recurrences. In severe cases that do not respond to medicine applied to the skin, a medicine taken by mouth once or twice a day can be used. Take this according to your doctor's instructions. Ringworm of the scalp usually requires weeks to months of treatment with a medication taken by mouth.

The DOs

- Bathe or shower daily. Gently wash affected areas with a cloth, dry off, then apply cream or ointment.
- Always wear clean, dry clothing. Cotton or other absorbent clothing is best. Avoid man-made fabrics such as nylon.
- Keep moisture away from skin. It is very important to keep areas infected with ringworm clean and dry.

The DON'Ts

- Don't share towels, clothing, or bedding.
- Avoid scratching because this can spread the infection or cause secondary infection.
- Avoid wearing clothing that chafes the skin.

When to Call Your Doctor

- If the rash has not improved after 2 weeks of treatment.
- If signs of a secondary infection develops such as fever, pus drainage, oozing, crusting, or swelling.
- If skin changes occur such as scarring or bleeding.

For More Information
American Academy of Dermatology
930 N. Meacham Road
Schaumburg, IL 60173
847-330-0230

ROCKY MOUNTAIN SPOTTED FEVER

About Your Diagnosis

Rocky Mountain spotted fever is an acute illness caused by a microorganism called rickettsia that is transmitted to humans by an infected tick. It is common during the spring and summer months. It is not spread from person to person. Dogs and rodents can carry the tick that carries the organism, so it can be found in urban areas as well as rural areas.

Living With Your Diagnosis

Signs and symptoms usually occur within 2–5 days after being bitten by an infected tick. They include a high fever with chills; a red rash that first appears on the hands and feet, then spreads to the wrists and ankles, and finally spreads to the legs and trunk of the body; weakness with muscle aches and headaches; nausea and vomiting; shortness of breath with a cough; and mental confusion.

Treatment

Hospitalization may be necessary during the acute phase of the illness. Antibiotics such as tetracycline or chloramphenicol may be prescribed. Aspirin products should be avoided to prevent possible bleeding complications. Patients should rest in bed until the fever is gone. A regular diet can be followed as tolerated. Extra fluid intake should be encouraged. Milk and antacids should not be given with the antibiotics.

The DOs

- Continue the antibiotics until finished. Usually they are needed for a week after the fever is gone.
- Increase your fluid intake, especially while you have a fever.
- Rest in bed as much as possible while you have a fever.
- Try a heating pad to relieve the muscle aches.
- Use only nonaspirin products to reduce fever and for minor pain.
  In the future:
- Try to avoid exposure to ticks. Wear light-colored clothing with long sleeves and legs, and use insect repellant that is effective against ticks.
- Inspect your body frequently during outdoor activities.
- Remove a tick by using tweezers to gently grasp and pull it off; don't crush the tick during removal. You can also apply oil to the tick body before pulling with a tweezer.
- Immediately report a rash or fever that occurs after a tick bite.

The DON'Ts

- Don't skip doses or stop taking the antibiotics until finished.
- Don't use aspirin or aspirin-containing medications. They may cause bleeding complications.
- Don't drink milk or take antacids within 2 hours of taking the antibiotics.

When to Call Your Doctor

- If chest pain or increased shortness of breath occurs.
- If it is difficult to tolerate fluids, and there are signs of dehydration—dry skin, coated tongue, and decreased urge to urinate.
- If any area of the rash appears infected.
- If nonaspirin medications don't decrease the fever.
- If a severe headache or seizures occur.
- If severe abdominal pain is present.
- If any bleeding occurs.

For More Information
National Heart, Lung, and Blood Institute Information Line
800-575-WELL
National Institute of Allergy and Infectious Disease
301-496-5717

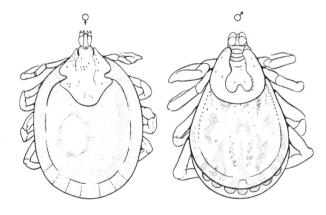

Dermacentor andersoni, the tick that causes Rocky Mountain spotted fever, demonstrating the difference in appearance between males and females. (From Auerbach PS: *Wilderness Medicine-Management of Wilderness and Environmental Emergencies,* vol 1. St. Louis, Mosby–Year Book, 1992. Used by permission.)

ROSACEA

About Your Diagnosis

Rosacea is a skin disease that affects patients between 30 and 60 years of age. The cause is unknown, but it is in part hereditary. Alcohol, hot beverages, and certain foods can worsen the disease. The diagnosis is made by a doctor based on the characteristic appearance. Rosacea is treatable, and the symptoms can be controlled with medications in most cases. It is usually not curable.

Living With Your Diagnosis

Rosacea affects the skin of the nose, cheeks, and forehead. It can cause redness, swelling, and pimples or pustules. The skin can become oily. In more severe cases it causes larger bumps on the nose. Rarely it can affect the eyes and eyelids, causing swelling, redness, dry eyes, and burning. Small blood vessels under the skin can become enlarged and be very noticeable. These are seen as thin red lines on the face or nose.

Treatment

Mild cases can sometimes be treated with an antibiotic cream applied to the affected areas. Antibiotics taken by mouth such as tetracycline or erythromycin are used to treat rosacea. Some patients will clear up in less than 1 month, whereas others take longer. Recurrences are common and may require a smaller dose of medication taken regularly to keep symptoms under control. Early treatment may slow down the progression of rosacea. Pustules can be treated with special sulfur preparations.

Sometimes a combination of medications is used to control symptoms. Severe nose enlargement is occasionally treated with corrective surgery.

The DOs

- Wash your face two times a day with a washcloth and mild soap such as Dove.
- Follow your doctor's recommendations for soaps, sunscreens, and medications. Early treatment may prevent some of the long-term effects of rosacea.

The DON'Ts

- Avoid foods that aggravate your condition. These may include hot liquids and spicy foods, chocolates, cheeses, nuts, iodized salt, and seafood.
- Avoid alcohol.
- Avoid exposure to sun and extreme heat and cold.

When to Call Your Doctor

- If you have any symptoms involving your eyes or eyelids.
- If treatment is not helping after 3 or 4 weeks.

For More Information
American Academy of Dermatology
930 N. Meacham Road
Schaumburg, IL 60173
847-330-0230

ROSEOLA (EXANTHEMA SUBITUM)

About Your Diagnosis

Roseola has been diagnosed in your child by your doctor. Another name for this common illness of small children is exanthem subitum. It is important that you know that this illness is not "measles" or "German measles." Both of these illnesses are more serious for either the child or a pregnant woman. Roseola is generally not a serious illness.

Roseola is thought to be infectious, possibly caused by a type of herpes virus. Your child, however, may not have a history of exposure to others with the illness, which is usually the case. Roseola does not pose any special risk to pregnant women.

Living With Your Diagnosis

The illness is most prevalent in the child from 6 months to 3 years old. It is never seen after the age of 5 years. The illness begins with the sudden onset of fever. The child may have a temperature up to 105°F. In spite of the high temperature, the child usually does not look or act very ill. The fever will last from 2 to 5 days but most frequently for 3 or 4 days. Suddenly the child will break out in a rash, and the fever will go away. The rash is rose-pink and blotchy. It appears first on the chest and upper back, then spreads to the arms and neck. At this point, the fever has disappeared and the child acts totally well.

Treatment

Because this common childhood illness is caused by a virus, there is no specific treatment. You can make your child more comfortable by treating the fever with acetaminophen or children's ibuprofen in the doses listed in Table 1 and 2.

Other things you can do for the fever are to give your child lukewarm baths, have your child wear lightweight clothing, keep your child quiet, and give your child cool drinks.

Because of the rapid onset of the fever, an occasional child may have what is referred to as a febrile convulsion or seizure. If this should occur, contact your physician immediately.

The DOs

Because this is such a mild illness, you should treat your child as normally as possible. There is nothing that can be done to make the illness go away any quicker. There is no special diet that the child should eat.

The DON'Ts

Because roseola is a viral infection, there is nothing that you can do to make the rash go away any faster. Therefore, do not put any cortisone creams, calamine lotion, or Vaseline on the rash. Acetaminophen or children's ibuprofen, as discussed above, can be used to help make your child more comfortable.

When to Call Your Doctor

- If the illness does not follow the course as outlined.
- If your child becomes more ill, acts as if he is in pain, or does not eat or drink fairly normally. This may indicate that the child has another virus or a very rare complication.

For More Information
The American Medical Association Family Medical Guide, 3rd edition. Also available on a CD-ROM.
American Academy of Family Physician's Family Health and Medical Guide, Word Publishing Co., 1997.

Table 1.

Age	Weight (lb)	Dose of Acetaminophen
4-7 months	13-17	80 mg every 4 hours
8-18 months	18-23	120 mg every 4 hours
1.5-3 years	24-32	160 mg every 4 hours

Table 2.

Age	Weight (lb)	Dose of Ibuprofen
4-7 months	13-17	Not recommended
8-18 months	18-23	50-100 mg every 6-8 hours
1.5-3 years	24-32	100 mg every 6-8 hours

ROTATOR CUFF TENDINITIS/TEAR

About Your Diagnosis

Rotator cuff diseases include inflammation (tendinitis) and possibly a partial- or full-thickness tear of the tendon (Fig 1). This causes marked pain in the shoulder region, which may worsen at night or with activities in which the arms are held over the head. Rotator cuff problems are caused by cumulative trauma throughout one's lifetime. It is believed to be partially caused by impingement of the tendon on a bone spur within the shoulder. Rotator cuff tendinitis or tear is fairly common. It is usually detected by means of placing the shoulder through ranges of motion that reproduce the pain. The diagnosis is generally made by means of history and physical examination. Magnetic resonance imaging (MRI) is helpful when a tear is suspected. Rotator cuff tendinitis or tear can be managed to the point that pain can usually be completely alleviated.

Living With Your Diagnosis

Signs and symptoms of rotator cuff tendinitis and possible tear include pain in the shoulder that worsens with activities such as lying down to sleep at night or working with one's arms over one's head. The tendinitis not only causes pain in the shoulder region but also can eventually lead to a tear in the rotator cuff tendon itself. When that happens, the shoulder becomes much weaker, and it becomes quite difficult to perform any activities above your head.

Treatment

Rotator cuff tendinitis generally can be managed successfully with nonsurgical methods. Nonsteroidal anti-inflammatory drugs (NSAIDs) can help not only to control inflammation but also to relieve pain. Exercise, specifically physical therapy focused on rotator cuff rehabilitation to strengthen the internal and external rotator tendons of the shoulder can make a difference in the overall pain (Fig 2). Surgical decompression or possible repair of the torn tendon is considered when physical therapy does not make a difference or should the tendon actually sustain a tear. Surgical treatment may have complications, and you should discuss them thoroughly with your physician before you undergo this form of treatment.

The DOs

- Take your medications as prescribed.
- Perform your exercises as directed.

The DON'Ts

- Avoid addictive pain medications as long-term therapy for rotator cuff tendinitis or tear.
- Avoid activities that necessitate using your hands above your head.
- Do not attempt to strengthen the shoulder with push-ups. This has not been found to make a difference and may worsen the pain.

When to Call Your Doctor

- If pain is severe enough to prevent you from sleeping satisfactorily at night and is not controlled with over-the-counter medications.

For More Information
http://www.sechrest.com/mmg/shoulder/cufftear.html

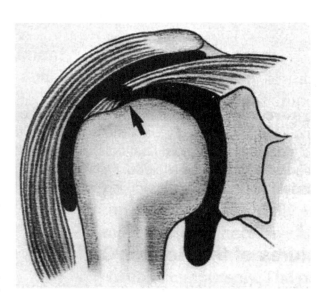

Rupture of the rotator cuff *(arrow)*. (From Mercier LR: *Practical Orthopedics*, vol 4. St. Louis, Mosby–Year Book, 1995. Used by permission.)

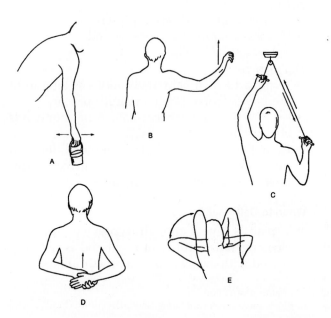

Shoulder exercises. **A,** pendulum exercises. **B,** wall-climbing exercise. **C,** pulley exercises. The normal arm assists in the elevation of the stiffened arm. **D,** exercise for restoring internal rotation. **E,** exercise for restoring external rotation. Each exercise should be performed hourly or at least four times a day. Applying moist heat before the exercise may be helpful. In addition, activities that aggravate the pain, such as overhead work, should be avoided. For sitting work, a chair that supports the arms and shoulders should be used, and the patient should sit as close to the working surface as possible. (From Mercier LR: *Practical Orthopedics,* vol 4. St. Louis, Mosby–Year Book, 1995. Used by permission.)

RUBELLA (GERMAN MEASLES)

About Your Diagnosis

Rubella, or German measles, is a mildly contagious disease caused by a virus. It affects the lymph glands and skin. It occurs most commonly in children aged 5–9 years and young adults. The number of cases have decreased because of the use of vaccines. The most common complication of rubella is serious birth defects if a pregnant woman has the disease in the first 3–4 months of pregnancy. It is spread by direct contact with an infected individual. Patients with rubella are usually contagious for 1 week before the rash develops until 1 week after it fades.

Living With Your Diagnosis

Signs and symptoms of rubella are a mild fever, headache, fatigue, a red rash on the body that lasts for 2–3 days, and swollen lymph glands in the neck. Adults may have joint pain also.

Treatment

Recovery occurs in 1 week. No specific treatment is necessary. An increase in fluid intake and extra rest may be all that is needed. If anyone who is pregnant is exposed, notify them immediately so they can contact their doctor. Nonaspirin products such as Tylenol can be used for fever and aches.

The DOs
- Rest until the fever is gone.
- Limit activities for 1–2 days after the rash disappears.
- Avoid contact with others for 1 week after the rash is gone.
- Notify any pregnant woman who may have been exposed.
- Increase fluid intake.
- Use nonaspirin products such as Tylenol to reduce fever and aches.

The DON'Ts
- Don't Give aspirin to a child younger than 16 years. Aspirin given during a viral infection has been shown to increase the risk of Reye's syndrome occurring.
- Don't send a child to school until the rash has been gone for 1 week.
- Avoid exposing a pregnant woman to the disease.

When to Call Your Doctor
- A high fever develops.
- A cough or shortness of breath develops.
- Increased drowsiness, weakness, or headache develops.
- Any unusual bleeding occurs 1–4 weeks after recovery.

For More Information
Center for Disease Control and Prevention
Voice Information System (24-hour automated)
404-332-4555
National Institute of Allergy and Infectious Diseases
9000 Rockville Pike
Bethesda, MD 20892
301-496-5717
Internet Sites
www.healthfinder.gov (Choose SEARCH to search by topic.)
www.healthanswers.com

SALIVARY GLAND TUMORS

About Your Diagnosis

Salivary glands produce saliva to keep the mouth moist and to lubricate the food as it is chewed. Salivary gland tumors may be benign or malignant (cancerous). The salivary glands are classified into major and minor glands.

The major salivary glands are the parotid gland in front of your ear and under the skin of your cheek; the submandibular glands under your jaw bone; and the sublingual salivary glands under you tongue. There are more than 500 minor salivary glands, and most are in the roof of the mouth.

Salivary gland tumors are rare. They are not contagious, and the cause is not. The only sure way to diagnose salivary gland tumors is to remove the tumor completely with a surgical procedure and examine the tissue with a microscope. Salivary gland tumors can be cured if detected and removed before the cancer has spread.

Living With Your Diagnosis

A lump or mass is the usual first sign that a tumor is present. Salivary gland cancers tend to spread locally by invading surrounding tissue. For parotid tumors, local spread may involve the facial nerve, which crosses through the parotid gland. This can lead to facial paralysis with facial droop and inability to close the eye on the affected side. Other salivary cancers spread into the muscles at the floor of the mouth, base of the skull, and to local lymph glands. This causes facial pain, ear pain, headache, and swollen lymph glands. In advanced cases, the cancer can spread to the blood stream and metastasize to the lungs and bones.

Treatment

Computed tomography (CT) or magnetic resonance imaging (MRI) and a physical examination give a good idea whether the cancer is malignant. Nevertheless, the treatment of all major and minor salivary gland tumors is removal of the entire gland and surrounding involved structures. In the case of the parotid gland, the involved lobe is removed, but care is taken not to cut the facial nerve. If the cancer has spread to the local lymph nodes, these nodes are removed. Complications of surgical treatment include cutting important nerves, such as the facial nerve and the nerve that goes to the tongue.

Radiation therapy can be used to manage advanced inoperable tumors or tumors that return. Complications are dry, red, itchy skin; loss of ability to produce saliva, which causes dry mouth, sore throat, and difficulty swallowing; loss of facial hair growth; and loss of the sense of taste.

The DOs

- Seek an experienced surgeon who specializes in tumors of the head and neck.
- Understand the importance of nutrition after treatment. Because of pain, loss of saliva, and loss of taste, you can lose a substantial amount of weight. It is important to take nutritional supplements and to drink lots of fluids to stay hydrated.
- Remember to keep all appointments during and after treatment to monitor any side effects or recurrence of the cancer.
- Remember the earlier the cancer is detected, the better is the prognosis. The 10-year survival rate is 90% for salivary gland tumors less than 2 centimeters (0.8 inches) in diameter and localized to the gland without any spread. It is 25% when the tumor is larger than 2 centimeters (0.8 inches) and has spread to a lymph node.

The DON'Ts

- Do not ignore any lumps in your mouth, cheek or neck.
- Do not ignore any swollen lymph glands.
- Do not forget that 80% of tumors of the parotid gland are benign, whereas 80% of tumors of the minor salivary glands are malignant.

When to Call Your Doctor

- If you notice a lump anywhere in your head or neck.
- If you suddenly notice facial droop with the inability to close your eye on the same side. This can be paralysis of the facial nerve.
- If you have facial or ear pain.
- If you need emotional support.

For More Information
Cancer Information Service
1-800-422-6237 (1-800-4-CANCER)

SALMONELLOSIS

About Your Diagnosis

Salmonellosis is a gastrointestinal infection caused by the *Salmonella* bacteria. It is one of the most common infections in the United States. The infection is transmitted by eating contaminated or inadequately processed foods, especially eggs, chicken, turkey, or duck, or by drinking contaminated water. The bacteria can survive freezing. Thorough cooking helps to decrease the risk but doesn't completely eliminate it. It can be spread from person to person. Pet turtles can also carry the bacteria. The disease is detected by a culture done on a stool specimen. Most infections are curable with treatment in 24–48 hours.

Living With Your Diagnosis

An epidemic can occur when many individuals eat the same contaminated foods, such as at a restaurant or a social function. The signs and symptoms appear within 6–48 hours after eating the contaminated food. They include nausea, vomiting, fever, and diarrhea accompanied by abdominal cramping.

Treatment

If possible, infected individuals should be isolated, or at least have them use a separate bathroom. Good hand washing is essential to prevent the spread of the disease. Antibiotic treatment may be needed for patients who have a prolonged fever. If the fever is high, use tepid sponge baths to reduce it. Don't give Tylenol or other such medications because they may mask the symptoms. Bed rest should be maintained until the symptoms subside. Increased fluid intake is needed to prevent dehydration. A liquid diet including Gatorade or Pedialyte should be followed until the diarrhea stops; then regular foods should be resumed, gradually increasing caloric intake until recovery is complete.

The DOs

- Have the infected individual use a separate bathroom or clean the bathroom after each use (use gloves).
- Rest in bed until the symptoms subside.
- Use tepid sponge baths to reduce fever. Don't use Tylenol.
- Maintain fluid balance. Drink Gatorade or Pedialyte to replace lost fluids because of the diarrhea.
- Use a heating pad or hot water bottle wrapped in a towel to help ease abdominal pain.
- Resume a regular high-calorie diet after the diarrhea stops.
- Wash hands before eating, and before and after preparing raw poultry.

The DON'Ts

- Don't use Tylenol or other such medications because it may mask symptoms.
- Don't let others use the same bathroom unless it has been thoroughly cleaned.
- Don't eat raw or undercooked poultry or eggs, or drink unpasteurized milk.
- Don't forget to wash your hands thoroughly before eating and after handling poultry.

When to Call Your Doctor

- If signs of dehydration are present, such as dry, wrinkled skin and dark or decreased urine.
- If symptoms last longer than 48 hours.
- If the temperature goes higher than 102°F.
- If diarrhea worsens.
- If the skin or eyes turn yellow.

For More Information
Intestinal Disease Foundation
412-261-5888, Monday through Friday from 9:30 AM to 3:30 PM (EST).
National Institute of Allergy and Infectious Diseases
301-496-5717
Internet Sites
www.healthanswers.com
www.healthfinder. gov (Choose SEARCH to search by topic.)

SARCOIDOSIS

About Your Diagnosis

Sarcoidosis is a disease caused by inflammation. It can appear in almost any body organ but most often starts in the lungs or lymph nodes. It is associated with granulomatous lesions of unknown cause. The term granuloma refers to a special type of tissue inflammation seen under the microscope by a pathologist. Many conditions are associated with granulomas, including sarcoidosis. Sarcoidosis may affect any organ or organ systems, but is not contagious and is usually easily treatable.

The diagnosis of sarcoidosis is tricky to make because patients may not have any symptoms, and other causes of granulomas need to be excluded. The chest x-ray is often abnormal because the lung is one of the most common sites of involvement. The physical examination is often normal, but it depends on which organs are involved and how extensive or active the sarcoidosis is. Your doctor may order blood tests including a serum angiotensin converting enzyme level (ACE), breathing tests, a computed tomography (CT) scan of the chest, a tissue biopsy, and tests for tuberculosis (TB). If tissue sampling of the lung is necessary, bronchoscopy or mediastinoscopy is often performed.

Living With Your Diagnosis

Most patients with sarcoidosis do not have any symptoms, but some may have shortness of breath, dry cough, generalized aching of the joints, or tender red areas over the legs. Virtually any organ can be involved with sarcoidosis. In complicated cases, inflammation of the eye, high serum calcium levels, liver and kidney problems, heart rhythm problems, or various skin lesions may be found.

Treatment

Sarcoidosis usually responds to oral steroids (prednisone) within 1–3 months, but close follow-up and dose adjustments are necessary. In "earlier" stages and asymptomatic patients, there is a 50% to 80% chance of spontaneous recovery within 2 years. Side effects from prednisone include rapid mood swings, weight gain, facial puffiness, easy skin bruising, high blood pressure, increased blood sugar, cataracts, osteoporosis, and increased susceptibility to infections.

Prednisone is usually given for at least 6–12 months in symptomatic patients. It is generally tapered to the lowest dose necessary for control of the sarcoidosis. Response to therapy is judged by any changes in symptoms, chest x-ray findings, breathing test measurements, and any additional parameters that were abnormal at the time of diagnosis. Unfortunately, there is no one single measure for determining the activity level of sarcoidosis, and relapses may occur.

The DOs
- Obtain an influenza vaccination each fall.
- Obtain/update the pneumococcal vaccination.
- Maintain close contact with your health care provider.
- Monitor your blood sugar carefully, especially if diabetic and taking prednisone.

The DON'Ts
- Avoid vitamin D or calcium supplements.
- Avoid excessive direct sun exposure.
- Stop smoking.

When to Call Your Doctor
- If you have excessive thirst, urination, or weight change.
- If coughing produces discolored sputum or blood.
- If fever or chills are present.
- If you have any concerns about the effects of the medications you are taking.

For More Information
American Lung Association
1118 Hampton Avenue
St. Louis, MO 63139
800-LUNG-USA
www.lungusa.org
Facts About Sarcoidosis, 1985

SCABIES

About Your Diagnosis

Scabies is an extremely itchy rash caused by a tiny mite that burrows into the skin. Although the mite is only slightly larger than the head of a pin and only burrows a short distance into the skin, it causes an intense itching. The condition is very widespread and although anyone can catch scabies, it is much more common in young children. Often children will bring the mite infection home and spread it to family members. It is also common in individuals who live close together, such as those in nursing homes and extended care facilities. The infection is transferred from person to person.

Fortunately scabies is easy and quick to treat. It is not a dangerous infection and does not usually lead to permanent damage. Excessive scratching, however, can cause the scabies rash to become infected with bacteria. This bacterial infection may lead to serious cellulitis and scars. Therefore prompt and correct treatment is necessary.

Physicians are able to make the diagnosis by close skin examination. Occasionally the tiny mite can be seen, but in most cases it is necessary to painlessly scrape the skin. This will bring the mite onto a slide for microscopic examination.

Living With Your Diagnosis

The itchy rash of scabies can occur almost anywhere on the body. Because it is an allergic reaction, there may or may not be mites in the rash site. The rash is often identified by its linear nature, following the burrow of the mite. It consists of little red bumps, bites, or pimples often in a row. The most common areas of the body for infection by the mite are in the body creases or where straps and bands constrict the skin. These areas are primarily the hands, wrists, ankles, groin, waist, and arm pits. Nonetheless, because the rash is allergic, it can appear anywhere. The earliest and most common symptom of scabies is nighttime itching, even before the rash appears.

Treatment

The standard treatment of scabies consists of applying an insecticide lotion on the skin, such as permethin, lindane, crotamiton, or sulfur. These lotions require total body application and must be left on for a specific length of time (varies depending on lotion). The lotion is then washed off. The lotion must cover the entire body below the face including the genital area, hands, breasts, and feet.

These medications are usually safe, but caution is especially important with infants younger than 2 years and with pregnant women. All such medicine should be used under a physician's supervision.

All close family contacts should be treated at the same time.

Careful washing of all clothes, bedding, and toys with hot, soapy water is required. You do not have to boil clothes or bedding.

The itching usually disappears rapidly within a week or two of treatment. If symptoms do not go away, retreatment may be needed. The severe itching may be treated with antihistamines or topical emollients and/or steroids.

If it is determined that a secondary bacterial infection has occurred, you will need to be treated with antibiotics.

The DOs

- See a physician immediately. Anyone can get scabies. It is not a reflection on your personal cleanliness.
- Wash clothing, bed linens, towels, and toys in hot, soapy water and machine dry.
- Vacuum entire house and dispose of bag.
- Follow precisely your physicians directions for use of lotions and medications; wash off thoroughly when time is up.
- Wash hands frequently to avoid spreading the mites.

The DON'Ts

- Don't treat with home remedies such as detergents, scrubbing, or kerosene; these often make it worse.
- Don't use steroid creams unless prescribed by your doctor.
- Try to avoid scratching heavily or picking at the rash.

When to Call Your Doctor

- The rash shows signs of infection (redness, pus, swelling, or pain) after treatment.
- Persistent itching or pain 1–2 weeks after treatment.
- New unexplained symptoms.

For More Information

American Academy of Dermatology
930 N. Meachum Road
Schaumburg, IL 60173
847-330-0230

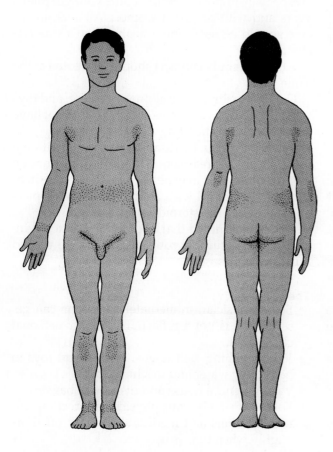

Characteristic distribution of scabies lesions. (From Goldstein BG, Goldstein AO: *Practical Dermatology*, vol 1. St. Louis, Mosby–Year Book, 1992. Used by permission.)

SCARLET FEVER

About Your Diagnosis

Scarlet fever occurs mainly in children and is characterized by a bright red rash. It is caused by a reaction to a toxin produced by a specific type of strep infection. Not everyone that has a strep infection will have scarlet fever develop. It is contagious and is spread by direct contact. It can be detected by a throat culture.

Living With Your Diagnosis

Signs and symptoms usually occur during a 3– to 6-day period. First a high fever, sore throat, enlarged lymph glands, cough, and vomiting develop. Next, a bright red rash is seen on the face, and the tongue becomes red. The rash then spreads to the body. Finally, by the sixth day, the rash begins to fade and the skin begins to peel. This continues for 10–14 days. If untreated complications can occur.

Treatment

Treatment include antibiotics such as penicillin or erythromycin. Bed rest is needed. The child should be kept away from others to prevent the spread of the disease. No special diet is needed, but fluid intake should be increased. Using a cool-mist vaporizer as well as gargling with warm salt water can help ease the sore throat.

The DOs

- Keep the child away from others. Generally he can return to school in 2 weeks.
- Take the antibiotics until finished.
- Rest in bed until symptoms subside.
- Use a cool-mist vaporizer and a warm salt-water gargle to ease the sore throat.
- Use Tylenol or tepid sponge baths to reduce fever.
- Increase fluid intake. Offer liquid or soft foods until the sore throat subsides.

The DON'Ts

- Don't skip doses or stop antibiotics until finished.
- Don't send a child to school until the infection is cleared.
- Don't expose others to the disease.

When to Call Your Doctor

- If the fever returns (temperature greater than 101°F) after it has been gone for a few days.
- If nausea or vomiting develops.
- If a severe headache or earache develops.
- If chest pain and a cough that produces thick sputum develop.
- If the areas of peeling skin show signs of infection.

For More Information

National Institute of Allergy and Infectious Diseases
9000 Rockville Pike
Bethesda, MD 20892
301-496-5717
Request information from:
The American Academy of Pediatrics
141 NW Point Blvd.
Elk Grove Village, IL 60007-1098
National Institute of Child Health and Human Development
31 Center Dive
MSC 2725 Building 31/2A32
Bethesda, MD 20892
301-496-5133
Internet Sites
www.healthfinder.gov (Choose SEARCH to search by topic.)
www.healthanswers.com

SCHIZOPHRENIA

About Your Diagnosis

Schizophrenia is a condition that affects about 1% of the population. It usually begins in the late teenage years to early adulthood, and it seems to occur as frequently among males as among females. Schizophrenia is a chronic condition that leads to progressive loss of intellectual function and social isolation.

Living With Your Diagnosis

The main features of schizophrenia include ambivalence (i.e., difficulty making decisions), problems displaying and expressing emotions, marked impairment of ability to function in social situations, and abnormal thinking. The abnormal thinking can occur in many different forms. It may include hallucinations—that is, touching, seeing, hearing, feeling, and smelling things that are not there. The most common form of hallucinations in schizophrenia involves hearing voices of individuals not actually present, so-called auditory hallucinations. The voices may actually tell the patient to do some act that the patient may feel uncomfortable about, such as killing oneself or others. In addition to hallucinations, schizophrenic patients may believe that someone is following them, controlling their thoughts, or making fun of them, and therefore, they may be paranoid. Less commonly, patients may believe that they have special powers, or that there is some physical condition affecting them, although there is no evidence of a medical problem. Cancer and AIDS are the most common imagined condition for these individuals.

The cause of schizophrenia is unknown, but it probably occurs more commonly in cases where someone else in the family, particularly parents, has had schizophrenia diagnosed. There is, however, no blood test to confirm the diagnosis, and no genetic tests that can determine who will likely become schizophrenic. Schizophrenia is not curable; however, many of the symptoms of this disease can be successfully treated by the use of medications in conjunction with counseling.

Treatment

The treatment of schizophrenia usually involves the use of drugs designed to stop psychotic features such as hallucinations and paranoia. These drugs are called antipsychotics, and they include such drugs as Thorazine, Mellaril, and Haldol. The medication must be taken every day; if the patient does so, the hallucinations and other abnormal thinking will improve significantly. The antipsychotic medications do have some side effects, including blurred vision, drowsiness, restlessness, occasional constipation, dry mouth, and sexual dysfunction. More serious, but less common complications include effects on the heart, liver, and blood pressure, and the production of seizures. Many of the side effects of the antipsychotics can be treated by lowering the dose of the drug, changing to a different drug, or adding a drug to treat side effects, such as Cogentin, Artane, or Benadryl. Occasional schizophrenic patients get their medications (Haldol, Prolixin) by injection once or twice a month. The psychosocial treatment of schizophrenia often involves having a counselor to help with different aspects of daily living, including getting the patient to their appointments and helping the patient with medication. Frequently, it is helpful for the patient to be involved in a support group with other schizophrenic patients. Support groups can be helpful as far as teaching the patient social skills.

The DOs

It is important that schizophrenic patients avoid the use of alcohol because it may intensify the effects of their medication. Drugs such as cocaine, amphetamines, and PCP may produce psychotic features and lead to hospitalization, so these drugs should also be avoided. It is important for schizophrenic patients to avoid stress because stressful situations, lack of sleep, poor diet, and use of caffeine may make them more likely to have psychotic features. Above all, schizophrenic patients should always take their medication as prescribed.

The DON'Ts

Schizophrenic patients should avoid the use of any medications, including over-the-counter medications, without first checking with their physician.

When to Call Your Doctor

You should contact your doctor if you have any side effects from the medication (especially fever or muscle stiffness), if you begin to hear voices, feel paranoid, or have other unusual thoughts, if you notice that your sleep has decreased, or if depression/suicidal thoughts occur.

For More Information

Contact your local mental health association or crisis center line, or the About Schizophrenia Web site at: WWWGopher://Nightingale.con.utk.edu:70/11/ Communications/Discussion - groups/Mental/Schizoph

SCLERODERMA (PROGRESSIVE SYSTEMIC SCLEROSIS)

About Your Diagnosis

Scleroderma is a multisystem connective tissue disease in which the skin and a variety of internal organs progressively degenerate, thicken, and lose flexibility. It is characterized by widespread inflammation, stiffness, and loss of function of the connective tissue (the framework for all body tissues). It affects multiple organs and tissues, including the skin, blood vessels, joints, heart, kidneys, lungs, esophagus (the food tube connecting the throat to the stomach), fingers, and toes.

The exact cause is unknown. Scleroderma is an autoimmune disorder (i.e., a condition in which your immune system mistakenly attacks normal parts of the body, resulting in tissue injury and disease).

Scleroderma is uncommon. It affects women four times more frequently than men. It typically begins in adults aged 30–50 years. The transmission of this condition is unknown, although it may be genetic. Individuals with scleroderma tend to have poor circulation. As a result, exposure to extremely cold weather and air conditioning may aggravate your scleroderma.

Diagnosis is usually based upon the inflammation, degeneration, thickening and stiffness of your skin and other internal organs. Your doctor may order blood tests and perform a skin biopsy (removal of a small piece of skin or other tissue) for laboratory evaluation to assist in diagnosis.

No cure is known. Scleroderma is a chronic condition in which the skin and multiple internal organs slowly and progressively degenerate, lose function, and become thick and stiff. Treatment aims to control symptoms and to lessen the severity of inflammation, but does not cure scleroderma.

Living With Your Diagnosis

Individuals with scleroderma frequently have multiple symptoms because of the widespread nature of the disease. The skin typically loses flexibility and becomes coarse and thickened. These changes produce a masklike appearance of the face, thinning of the lips, and furrowing around the mouth. The fingers become thickened and stiff, resulting in pain as well as loss of mobility. Many individuals have pain, swelling, and stiffness of the joints, muscle aches, weakness, and fatigue. Other symptoms include heartburn, difficulty swallowing (especially with solid foods), constipation or diarrhea, abdominal bloating, and weight loss. With lung involvement, symptoms include shortness of breath with mild activity, and a dry cough.

Some individuals with scleroderma have the CREST syndrome:

- *Calcinosis*: calcification of the skin, especially the fingers and hands, associated with drainage of white paste from ulcerations.
- *Raynaud's phenomenon*: a disorder of the blood vessels resulting from inflammation, thickening, and loss of flexibility. It typically affects the small arteries of the hands and feet. Symptoms include discoloration of the fingertips and toes (pale, blue/purple, or red) with exposure to cold temperatures. Other symptoms include pain, tingling, and coldness of the fingers and toes.
- *Esophageal dysfunction*: heartburn, difficulty swallowing (especially solid foods), and gastroesophageal reflux (acid from the stomach irritates the lining of the esophagus).
- *Sclerodactyly*: thickening and stiffness of the skin of the fingers and toes, associated with a waxy and shiny appearance.
- *Telangiectasia*: a cluster of dilated, small blood vessels of the skin.

Because scleroderma is so widespread, it can cause multiple complications. The most common cause of death is kidney failure. Other complications include heart failure, abnormal heart rhythms, high blood pressure, poor lung function, poor wound healing, gangrene, bleeding, and bruising.

Treatment

Scleroderma is incurable, and its course is characterized by a gradual and relentless progression of skin and internal organ damage. Treatment aims to control symptoms, lessen the severity of your illness, and to treat/prevent complications. Your treatment will depend on the type and severity of your symptoms. Treatment consists of general measures and medications.

General measures to follow include:

1. Stop smoking, because smoking can worsen the function of your heart, lungs, and blood vessels, as well as irritate the lining of your digestive system.
2. If you have heartburn or gastroesophageal reflux, several measures may reduce the severity of your symptoms. Eliminating or reducing ciga-

rette smoking, as well as the intake of alcohol and caffeine, can decrease reflux and heartburn. Also, avoid eating within 2 hours of bedtime or lying down. When lying down, raise the head of your bed by 6–8 inches and sleep on two or three pillows.

3. Avoid exposure to extremely cold temperatures, and be careful of air conditioning, which may worsen poor circulation. Wear warm, protective clothing, especially gloves and socks.

4. Avoid skin injuries and burns. Adjusting the hot water heater in your home to limit the water temperature to a maximum of 120°F reduces your risk of sustaining burns. Also, check the water temperature with a body part that has good circulation before exposing fingers and toes with poor circulation.

5. Apply heat to improve joint pain and stiffness.

6. Individuals with scleroderma frequently become depressed or experience other psychological conditions. If you feel depressed or are having difficulty coping with your illness, talk to your doctor about the best treatment options, including psychological counseling. Biofeedback techniques are also effective in increasing circulation in some individuals.

The following medications are helpful in treating scleroderma:

1. Corticosteroids can relieve inflammatory symptoms. Side effects are more likely with higher doses and include increased susceptibility to infection, swelling, diabetes mellitus, osteoporosis (thinning of your bones), and injury to the lining of the digestive system. Do not stop steroid medication without first consulting your doctor because abrupt cessation can result in severe weakness, fatigue, and low blood pressure.

2. Skin lotions, moisturizers, and bath oils are useful in softening the skin.

3. Over-the-counter antacids or prescription medications are useful in treating gastroesophageal reflux.

4. Your doctor may prescribe other medications to treat complications of other organ systems. Examples are blood pressure medicines, antibiotics for infections, and aspirin or anti-inflammatory medications for arthritis.

The DOs
- Take medications as prescribed by your doctor.
- Inform your doctor of all other medications, including over-the-counter medications, that you are taking. Continue these medications unless your doctor instructs you to stop them.
- Read the labels of medicines and follow all instructions. Consult your doctor if you have any concerns or if you have possible side effects caused by the medications.
- When lying down, raise the head of your bed by 6–8 inches and sleep on two or three pillows.
- Regular exercise improves blood pressure and circulation and maintains heart and lung function. Exercise also helps keep the skin and joints flexible and maintains good muscle tone. Exercise regularly as your strength permits.
- Stop smoking, because smoking can worsen the function of your heart, lungs, and blood vessels, as well as irritate the lining of your digestive system.

The DON'Ts
- Do not stop your medicine or change the prescribed dose without consulting your doctor.
- Do not exceed recommended doses of medicines, because higher doses can increase your risk of toxic effects.
- Do not abruptly stop corticosteroids because you may experience a rebound worsening of your condition. Abrupt cessation of these medicines can result in severe weakness, fatigue, and low blood pressure. Consult your doctor before stopping these medicines.
- Avoid skin injury, burns, and cuts to reduce your risk of skin ulceration, infections, and gangrene.
- If you have gastroesophageal reflux symptoms or heartburn, eliminate cigarette smoking, as well as your intake of alcohol and caffeine, to reduce the irritation of the lining of the esophagus and to decrease your symptoms. Avoid eating within 2 hours of bedtime to reduce symptoms. Avoiding spicy foods can also improve symptoms.

When To Call Your Doctor
- If you have any signs or symptoms of infection, including redness around a wound or skin lesion, purulent discharge (pus) from a wound, increased pain or swelling of wounds or lymph nodes, and fever.
- If you notice that signs or symptoms of your condition are becoming worse, or if new signs or symptoms develop.

- If you have signs or symptoms of systemic illness, including fever, lethargy, confusion, or respiratory distress.
- If you have new or unexplained symptoms, which may indicate a complication of your condition or side effects from medications.

For More Information

The Scleroderma Association
P.O. Box 910
Lynnfield, MA 01940
508-535-6600
The Scleroderma Federation
1182 Teaneck Road
Teaneck, NJ 07666
201-837-9826

SCOLIOSIS

About Your Diagnosis

Scoliosis is defined as a lateral, or sideways, curvature of the spine that measures more than 10 degrees (Fig 1). It usually begins during childhood or adolescence and may continue to slowly worsen into adulthood. Typically, the greater the angle of the curvature, the greater is the risk that it will progress. Curves less than 30 degrees at the end of growth rarely progress and do not usually necessitate close observation. Curves greater than 50 to 75 degrees are at a high risk for progression and may necessitate aggressive therapy.

Pain is the most common reason that adults seek treatment of scoliosis. Although the pain is believed to be caused by muscle fatigue along the outside of the curve, the true source of the pain remains unclear. Some patients may notice a loss of height, an increase in the prominence of a rib, or changes in their waistline, which can signal a progression of the curve.

A series of radiographs (x-rays) taken over several years is the most accurate method for monitoring the curve. A slowly progressive curve may remain nonpainful and as a result not necessitate formal treatment. However, a rapidly progressive curve that produces pain and deformity may necessitate more aggressive management.

Living With Your Diagnosis

The diagnosis of scoliosis includes a wide range of deformities from mild to painful and severe. Although the deformity may not be noticeable until late in the course of the progression of the curve, the emotional aspects of this disease may be quite severe, particularly for adolescents. Breathing difficulties may develop with large curves but are usually preceded by pain and fatigue.

Treatment

Analgesics and anti-inflammatory drugs may reduce the pain of scoliosis. There are no medications, injections, diets, or exercises that affect the curve itself. The nonoperative management of scoliosis includes routine radiographs taken at regular intervals to monitor for progression. Bracing can be effective in preventing progression but does not correct a curve that has already developed. Exercises have not proved to be of benefit in this diagnosis, nor has electrical stimulation of muscles. An operation is indicated when the curve progresses or results in severe pain. When the curve is not progressive, you have to decide whether the pain warrants a complex surgical procedure. The surgeon must be sure that there is not some other cause for the back pain that may be unrelated to the scoliosis.

The DOs

- Take your medications as prescribed.
- Wear your brace as directed, but be aware that many curves can progress despite bracing.

The DON'Ts

- Do not stop wearing your brace without your doctor's recommendation.

When to Call Your Doctor

- If you notice a change in the deformity, such as an increased rib prominence, change in leg length, or new onset of pain.

For More Information
http://www.yahoo.com/Health/Diseases_and_Conditions/ Scoliosis<L#>Fig 1
Scoliosis. (Courtesy of the American Orthopaedics Association. From LaFleur-Brooks ML: *Exploring Medical Language—A Student Directed Approach.* vol 3. St. Louis, Mosby–Year Book, 1993. Used by permission.)

SEIZURE DISORDER, GRAND MAL

About Your Diagnosis

A seizure is caused by abnormal signals in the brain. This may be brought on by a head injury, stroke, brain infection, or tumor, but more than half the time the cause is unknown. During a grand mal seizure, patients may lose consciousness as well as bowel and bladder control. They may stop breathing or may become injured during the severe muscle contractions.

Living With Your Diagnosis

Grand mal or tonic-clonic seizures are characterized by four phases. Recognizing these may be important. Grand mal seizures are often preceded by an odd feeling, strange taste or odor, or headache. These warning signs are known as auras (phase 1). Not all grand mal seizures are preceded by an aura. This type of seizure generally begins with a rigid stiffening of the body, lasting a minute or less, and loss of consciousness. This is known as the tonic phase (phase 2). This is followed by the tonic-clonic phase that appears as strong muscle contractions and convulsions (phase 3). The tonic-clonic phase may last several minutes. A tonic-clonic seizure generally causes a loss of consciousness, vigorous muscle contractions, and loss of control of your bladder and/or bladder. Persistence of tonic-clonic seizure activity is a medical emergency called status epilepticus. Immediately after the seizure is the postictal phase where the patient gradually returns to consciousness from a level of stupor and confusion (phase 4).

When epilepsy is newly diagnosed, you must take several precautions until you have confidence that your seizure disorder is well controlled. If you live alone, you should make arrangements for someone to stay with you until your physician believes it is safe for you to resume living alone.

Treatment

Initially, your physician may want to get a computed tomography (CT) scan of your brain and a brain wave study (electroencephalogram, [EEG]) to determine whether there is a known cause for your seizures. The primary treatment for seizures is medication. Sometimes more than one antiseizure (anticonvulsant) medication may be used.

Your physician may have to obtain blood samples at times to ensure that you are receiving the correct dose of medication. Your dose schedule may be adjusted to achieve a protective blood level of medication. There are several different medications that may be used, and your physician will give you information about the side effects associated with each medication prescribed. Often, the medication will decrease the frequency and severity of the seizure but some individuals, despite medication, continue to have seizures.

The DOs

- Take your medication as prescribed to prevent seizures.
- Wear an ID bracelet indicating that you have a seizure disorder and listing the medications you are taking.
- Teach your family and friends about your disorder and what to do if you have a seizure.
- If you feel a seizure coming on, tell someone near you and lie down.

The DON'Ts

- Don't operate dangerous machinery or drive unless your physician has approved.
- Don't swim alone.
- Don't climb on ladders or roofs or anything that may be dangerous should you have a seizure.

When to Call Your Doctor

- If the patient is injured during a seizure, has difficulty breathing, or does not regain consciousness shortly after the seizure.
- If the patient has continuous tonic-clonic seizures. This is a medical emergency called status epilepticus. Call "911" for an ambulance.
- If you have any problems associated with your medications.
- If your seizures become more frequent or severe.

For More Information
Epilepsy Foundation of America (EFA)
4351 Garden City Drive
Landover, MD 20785-4951
800-EFA-1000
301-459-3700
e-mail: postmaster@efa.org
World Wide Web
http://www.efa.org

SEIZURE DISORDER, JACKSONIAN

About Your Diagnosis

A seizure is caused by abnormal signals in the brain. This may be brought on by a head injury, stroke, brain infection, or tumor, but more than half the time the cause is unknown. Jacksonian, or simple partial, seizures are usually limited to one area of the body. This form of seizure generally starts in your arm or leg and progressively moves upward to other areas on that side of the body.

Living With Your Diagnosis

A Jacksonian seizure generally does not impair consciousness or awareness. You will probably remain aware of the seizure as it occurs. However, a Jacksonian seizure may lead to a full-body (tonic-clonic or grand mal) seizure. A tonic-clonic seizure generally causes a loss of consciousness, vigorous muscle contractions, and loss of control of your bladder and/or bowel.

When epilepsy is newly diagnosed, you must take several precautions until you have confidence that your seizure disorder is well controlled. If you live alone, you should make arrangements for someone to stay with you until your physician believes it is safe for you to resume living alone.

Treatment

Initially, your physician may want to get a computed tomography (CT) scan of your brain and a brain wave study (electroencephalogram, [EEG]) to determine whether there is a known cause for your seizures. The primary treatment for seizures is medication. Sometimes more than one antiseizure or anticonvulsant medication may be used. Your physician may have to obtain blood samples at times to ensure that you are receiving the correct dose of medication. Your dose schedule may be adjusted to achieve a protective blood level of medication. There are several different medications that may be used, and your physician will give you information about the side effects associated with each medication prescribed. Often, the medication will decrease the frequency and severity of the seizure, but some individuals, despite medication, continue to have seizures.

The DOs

- Take your medication as prescribed to prevent seizures.
- Wear an ID bracelet indicating that you have a seizure disorder and listing the medications you are taking.
- Teach your family and friends about your disorder and what to do if you have a seizure.
- If you feel a seizure coming on, tell someone near you and lie down.

The DON'Ts

- Don't operate dangerous machinery or drive unless your physician has approved.
- Don't swim alone.
- Don't climb on ladders or roofs or anything that may be dangerous should you have a seizure.

When to Call Your Doctor

- If the patient is injured during a seizure, has difficulty breathing, or does not regain consciousness shortly after the seizure.
- If the patient has continuous tonic-clonic seizures. This is a medical emergency called status epilepticus. Call "911" for an ambulance.
- If you have any problems associated with your medications.
- If your seizures become more frequent or severe.

For More Information...

Epilepsy Foundation of America (EFA)
4351 Garden City Drive
Landover, MD 20785-4951
800-EFA-1000
301-459-3700
e-mail: postmaster@efa.org
World Wide Web
http://www.swlink.net/ mayhall/les2.html
http://www.uic.edu/depts/cnr/ref g.html:
http://www.efa.org

SEIZURE DISORDER, PETIT MAL

About Your Diagnosis

A seizure is caused by abnormal signals in the brain. This may be brought on by a head injury, stroke, brain infection, or tumor, but more than half the time the cause is unknown. Petit mal seizures generally respond well to antiseizure medication.

Living With Your Diagnosis

Petit mal or absence seizures are characterized by a period of altered consciousness, which may only appear as a blank stare. They may occur in adults but are more common in children. Petit mal seizures may be mistaken for a lack of attention or daydreaming. Seizures may be preceded by a warning sign such as a strange feeling, an unusual taste or odor, or a headache. Rarely, a petit mal seizure may lead to a full-body (tonic-clonic or grand mal) seizure. A tonic-clonic seizure generally causes a loss of consciousness, vigorous muscle contractions, and loss of control of your bladder and/or bowel.

When epilepsy is newly diagnosed, you must take several precautions until you have confidence that your seizure disorder is well controlled. If you live alone, you should make arrangements for someone to stay with you until your physician believes it is safe for you to resume living alone.

Treatment

Initially, your physician may want to get a computed tomography (CT) scan of your brain and a brain wave study (electroencephalogram, [EEG]) to determine whether there is a known cause for your seizures. The primary treatment for seizures is medication. Sometimes more than one antiseizure or anticonvulsant medication may be used. Your physician may have to obtain blood samples at times to ensure that you are receiving the correct dose of medication. Your dose schedule may be adjusted to achieve a protective blood level of medication. There are several different medications that may be used, and your physician will give you information about the side effects associated with each medication prescribed. Often, the medication will decrease the frequency and severity of the seizures, but some individuals, despite medication, continue to have seizures.

The DOs

- Take your medication as prescribed to prevent seizures.
- Wear an ID bracelet indicating that you have a seizure disorder and listing the medications you are taking.
- Teach your family and friends about your disorder and what to do if you have a seizure.
- If you feel a seizure coming on, tell someone near you and lie down.

The DON'Ts

- Don't operate dangerous machinery or drive unless your physician has approved.
- Don't swim alone.
- Don't climb on ladders or roofs or anything that may be dangerous should you have a seizure.

When to Call Your Doctor

- If the patient is injured during a seizure, has difficulty breathing, or does not regain consciousness shortly after the seizure.
- If the patient has continuous tonic-clonic seizures. This is a medical emergency called status epilepticus. Call "911" for an ambulance.
- If you have any problems associated with your medications.
- If your seizures become more frequent or severe.

For More Information
Epilepsy Foundation of America (EFA)
4351 Garden City Drive
Landover, MD 20785-4951
800-EFA-1000
301-459-3700
e-mail: postmaster@efa.org
World Wide Web
http://www.swlink.net/ mayhall/les2.html#abscense
http://www.efa.org

SEIZURES, FEBRILE

About Your Diagnosis

Febrile seizures occur in about 2% to 4% of children, and represent one of the most common neurologic disorders of childhood. The usual age of occurrence is between 6 months and 3 years, and this condition is somewhat more common in boys. There is a genetic tendency toward febrile seizures in some families. In most cases, this type of seizure occurs during a fever associated with a normal childhood illness and, by definition, a minimum body temperature of 37.8°C or 100.1°F is required for a seizure to be considered a febrile seizure.

It is important to remember that febrile seizures are not the same as epilepsy. The occurrence of a febrile seizure does slightly increase the risk for having an epileptic seizure disorder. In infants or children whose neurologic status is not normal, the risk for having epilepsy is much greater. Recurrent febrile seizures occur in approximately 30% of infants and children who have had one febrile seizure. The risk of recurrence is greatest in the first 6–12 months after a febrile seizure.

Living With Your Diagnosis

Febrile seizures almost always involve the entire body, causing rigid muscles followed by generalized shaking or tremors of the arms and legs. Carefully protect the child from injury during the seizure. Most seizures stop spontaneously shortly after they begin. After a febrile seizure, a child may appear listless or very sleepy.

Treatment

If a febrile seizure lasts more than a couple of minutes, treatment should be directed at controlling the convulsion with anticonvulsant medications similar to those used for initially stopping other types of seizure activity. Once a febrile seizure has occurred, the best treatment is to reduce the fever by sponging with tepid water to prevent another seizure.

The DOs

- Monitor your child's temperature closely during an illness. Rectal temperatures are the most accurate measure of body temperature.
- Treat fevers promptly with over-the-counter infant or child fever medications (acetaminophen or ibuprofen every 4 hours).
- Be sure that your child drinks plenty of water or juice during an illness with fever because fever increases the body's needs for fluids.
- Carefully protect your child from injury during a seizure.

The DON'Ts

- Don't use ice baths to cool your child if the fever is high. It is better to completely undress your child and continuously sponge him with tepid water.

When to Call Your Doctor

- If your child has a temperature of greater than 102°F that does not decrease with fever medications.
- If a febrile seizure does not stop within a few minutes.
- If your child is too ill to keep fluids down.
- If you notice signs of dehydration such as a dry mouth or a decrease in the number of wet diapers.

For More Information
National Institute of Neurological Disorders and Stroke
9000 Rockville Pike
Building 31, Room 8A16
Bethesda, MD 20892
301-496-5751
World Wide Web
http://www.ninds.nih.gov

SHIGELLOSIS

About Your Diagnosis

Shigellosis is an infection of the intestinal tract caused by a bacteria. It can be spread from individual to individual with close contact. It is transmitted through contaminated food or water. Shigellosis commonly affects children and can rapidly spread through day-care centers. There are more than 20,000 cases per year in the United States. Diagnosis is made by obtaining a stool culture.

Living With Your Diagnosis

Signs and symptoms include fever, which can be high in children; abdominal cramps; watery diarrhea; nausea or vomiting; muscle aches and pains; and mucus or blood in the stools.

Treatment

If possible, infected individuals should use a separate bathroom. If not possible, use gloves and scrub the toilet with a bleach solution after each use. Good hand washing is necessary to avoid the spread of the disease. Make sure children wash their hands with soap and water after using the bathroom and before eating. Fluid intake should be increased. Initially, a liquid diet (jello, ice cream, soups) is appropriate; subsequently, the diet should be increased gradually, avoiding raw fruits and vegetables. Antibiotics may be given, such as ampicillin, ciprofloxacin, or tetracycline. Don't give antidiarrheal medicines because they can prevent the bacteria from being eliminated and prolong the diarrhea and fever. Bed rest is needed, except for trips to the bathroom, until the fever and diarrhea are gone. Wash soiled bed linens and clothes in soap and the hottest water possible.

The DOs

- Take antibiotics if prescribed until finished.
- Wash hands well after using the bathroom and before eating.
- Encourage fluid intake to prevent dehydration. Use preparations such as Gatorade or Pedialyte.

The DON'Ts

- Don't use over-the-counter medications to stop the diarrhea. They will prolong the disease.
- Don't give solid foods until the diarrhea slows.
- Don't eat raw fruits and vegetables until the infection is completely cleared.
- Don't forget to wash hands frequently.

When to Call Your Doctor

- If abdominal pain becomes severe and the abdomen swells.
- If the temperature is more than 102°F during treatment.
- If there is blood in the stools.
- If signs of dehydration are present, such as weight loss, dry skin, sunken eyes, or a decreased need to urinate.
- If other symptoms develop, such as sore throat, earache, shortness of breath, or swollen joints.

For More Information

National Institute of Allergy and Infectious Disease
9000 Rockville Pike
Bethesda, MD 20892
301-496-5717
Internet Sites
www.healthfinder.gov (Choose SEARCH to search by topic.)
www.healthanswers.com

SHORT BOWEL SYNDROME

About Your Diagnosis

Short bowel syndrome is a malabsorption disorder that is a complication of extensive surgical resection of the small bowel. After surgery there is not enough bowel to absorb nutrients. If more than half of the bowel is removed during surgery, the risk of small bowel syndrome is great. Small bowel diseases that may require surgical intervention include Crohn's disease and necrotizing enterocolitis in infants.

The condition is detected by the patient's history and an upper gastrointestinal (GI) barium x-ray study. On this study, the barium moves rapidly through the small bowel. The symptoms of short bowel syndrome may improve over time but will always require close attention to diet.

Living With Your Diagnosis

The key symptoms of short bowel syndrome are large amounts of foul-smelling diarrhea and weight loss. Crampy abdominal pains and weakness accompany the diarrhea and weight loss. The symptoms usually begin 3–10 days after abdominal surgery.

Treatment

The treatment for small bowel syndrome is nutritional support. Hospitalization may be required. The initial treatment commonly is intravenous hyperalimentation (TPN). This will allow the bowel to rest and recover somewhat. A histamine-2 (H_2) blocker medication is given to help prevent the secretion of acid from the stomach. Usually after 1–4 weeks, the diarrhea will resolve and the appetite will return. At this time enteral feedings (mixtures put through a tube into the stomach) can resume. This is a slow process as the gut learns to work again. After weeks to months of this, you are able to slowly advance to oral feedings. Close monitoring of the diet will be key. A high-calorie, low-fat, low-residue diet is necessary. In some cases lifelong TPN is required. Supplementation of fat-soluble vitamins and minerals is also necessary.

The DOs

- If you have the condition, be patient. This condition takes months to slowly resolve.
- Be prepared for a long hospital stay. Many patients' stays exceed 8 weeks.
- Once able to eat, watch the diet closely.
- Take vitamin and mineral supplements as prescribed.

The DON'Ts

- Avoid high-fat diets

When to Call Your Doctor

- If after bowel surgery you have diarrhea.
- If being treated for short bowel syndrome and the symptoms worsen or return.

For More Information
PedBase–Short Bowel Syndrome
www.icondata.com/health/pedbase/files/SHORTBOW.HTM

SIALADENITIS

About Your Diagnosis

Sialadenitis is an acute bacterial infection of the salivary glands. Often the duct leading from the gland under the tongue becomes obstructed with mucus or a stone and then becomes infected. It is generally associated with a chronic illness or dehydration. It can be detected by using ultrasound or computed tomography (CT) scan.

Living With Your Diagnosis

Signs and symptoms include acute swelling of the salivary gland, with pain and swelling increasing with meals. There may be tenderness and redness of the duct opening.

Treatment

Treatment with antibiotics is necessary, as well as measures to increase the flow of saliva to clear the duct. These measures include increasing fluid intake to correct and prevent dehydration, applying warm compresses to the gland, massaging the gland, and sucking on hard candies and lemon drops to stimulate saliva production. A liquid or soft diet may help to decrease pain when eating. Dilation of the duct may be needed if other measures fail.

The DOs

- Take antibiotics as prescribed until finished.
- Take Tylenol or Advil for minor pain.
- Try a liquid or soft diet until the duct is clear.
- Increase your fluid intake to 8–10 glasses of water per day.
- Apply warm compresses to the swollen gland.
- Suck on hard candies or lemon drops to help stimulate saliva and clear the duct.

The DON'Ts

- Don't skip doses or stop taking the antibiotics until finished.
- Don't avoid liquids. If you can't tolerate eating, then try a liquid diet of soups, juices, and ice cream, and continue to drink water to avoid further dehydration.

When to Call Your Doctor

- If a fever develops.
- If pain becomes severe and is not relieved by medication.
- If the symptoms don't improve after 3 days of starting the antibiotics.

For More Information

National Oral Health Information Clearinghouse
301-402-7364, Monday through Friday from 9:30 AM to 5:30 PM (EST).
National Institute of Dental Research
301-496-4261
American Dental Association
Department of Public Education and Information
211 E. Chicago Avenue
Chicago, IL 60611
www.ada.org/

SILICOSIS

About Your Diagnosis

The inhalation of silica dust may cause lung disease called silicosis. Silica exposures usually occur in the workplace. Industries where workers are potentially at risk include foundries, mining, excavation, quarrying, sandblasting, stoneworking, and ceramics manufacturing. Initially, small rounded nodules develop when the silica deposits in the lung. Later, the number and size of the nodules may increase. The nodules eventually can join together to form large masses and lung scarring, which can interfere with lung function. This condition is called progressive, massive fibrosis.

Diagnosis is usually established by occupational history and chest x-ray. Occasionally a lung biopsy is necessary to make the diagnosis or to exclude such complications as tuberculosis or lung cancer. Breathing tests may be obtained to help assess the impact of silicosis on lung function.

Living With Your Diagnosis

The risk of developing silicosis is determined primarily by the intensity and duration of silica exposure. Years of exposure are usually necessary for development of illness, yet symptoms may occur in months with shorter but more intense inhalations.

The symptoms may vary. Early in the disease, silicosis does not cause symptoms or impair lung function. The disease may stay at this point and never threaten life span. In some individuals, the disease may progress, even after silica exposures have stopped. Shortness of breath and dry cough are the most common symptoms associated with progressive, massive fibrosis. Severe respiratory disability may lead to premature death.

Treatment

There are no treatments known to decrease the number of silica nodules in the lung, or to reliably prevent the development of progressive, massive fibrosis. Lung transplantation is considered in certain individuals. Those workers whose chest x-rays reveal silicosis changes should take the necessary steps to avoid further silica exposures.

Silicosis is known to increase the risk of tuberculosis. If silicosis is diagnosed, a tuberculin skin test should be performed. If the test is positive (meaning there has been a prior exposure to the organism that causes tuberculosis), a course of medications is required to help prevent the development of tuberculosis.

The DOs

- Obtain an influenza vaccination each fall.
- Obtain/update the pneumococcal vaccination.
- Maintain good cardiovascular fitness by participating in an exercise program.
- Maintain close contact with your health care provider.
- No special diet requirements.

The DON'Ts

- Avoid all further exposures to inhaled silica by following special industrial protection measures, such as wearing dust masks.
- Avoid individuals with acute respiratory tract infections.
- Avoid other conditions known to irritate the lungs, such as exposures to smoke, fumes, and very cold or very humid air.
- Stop smoking.

When to Call Your Doctor

- If you suspect that you have a lung infection as suggested by an abrupt worsening of cough, yellow or green sputum production, increased shortness of breath, and fever or chills.
- If you have weight loss, chest pain, or blood in the sputum (tests may be necessary to make sure tuberculosis or cancer is not present).
- If you have dusky-colored skin, fingertips, or lips.
- If you have new ankle swelling.

For More Information
American Lung Association
1118 Hampton Avenue
St. Louis, MO 63139
800-LUNG-USA
www.lungusa.org
Centers for Disease Control
National Institute for Occupational Safety and Health
800-35-NIOSH

SINUSITIS

About Your Diagnosis

Sinusitis is an inflammation of the sinuses (the air pockets in the facial bones that are connected to the nose). It can be an acute or chronic infection often caused by bacteria, allergies, pollution, or nasal polyps. The sinuses usually affected are located between the eyes and the cheekbones. Sinusitis sometimes occurs after a viral infection such as a cold.

Living With Your Diagnosis

Signs and symptoms include pain over the sinuses affected, such as the cheek, upper teeth, behind the eyes, or over the eyebrows; a nonproductive cough; low-grade fever; nasal congestion with a thick green-yellow discharge; a severe headache that is worse in the morning; and fatigue.

Treatment

Your doctor may prescribe antihistamines if the sinusitis is caused by allergies, or antibiotics if the sinusitis is caused by a bacterial infection. Nasal sprays and decongestants will help to decrease the congestion. Increasing your fluid intake will help to thin the secretions. Resting with your head elevated slightly will help promote drainage. For minor pain use medications such as Tylenol or Advil. An acute bout of sinusitis will usually clear completely in 2–3 weeks with treatment.

The DOs

- Take all of your antibiotics; stopping them can result in a recurrence of the infection.
- Rest with your head slightly elevated (no more than 30 degrees).
- Increase your fluid intake to help thin secretions. Drink at least 8 glasses of water a day.
- Use a vaporizer or inhale steam from a shower to help relieve congestion.
- Use warm compresses over the sinus area four times a day for one- or two-hour intervals.
- Use nonprecription medications such as Tylenol or Advil for minor pain.

The DON'Ts

- Don't use nonprescription nose sprays because they can make symptoms worse.
- Don't allow anyone else to use your nasal sprays or drops.
- Don't rest sitting up. Elevate your head only slightly to help the sinuses to drain.
- Don't travel in an airplane during an acute attack because the pressure changes can make symptoms much worse. Check with your doctor first if you must fly.

When to Call Your Doctor

- If you have fever and chills during treatment.
- If you have swelling of the face over the sinuses.
- If you have blurred vision or a severe headache that is not relieved with nonprescription medications.

For More Information
American Academy of Otolaryngology
One Prince Street
Alexandria, VA 22314
703-836-4444, Monday through Friday from 8:30 AM to 5 PM (EST), or send self-addressed stamped envelope with request for pamphlet "Sinus Pain, Pressure and Drainage."
Internet Sites
www.healthfinder.gov (Choose SEARCH to search by topic.)
www.healthanswers.com

SJOGREN'S SYNDROME

About Your Diagnosis

Sjogren's syndrome refers to inflammation that can lead to dry eyes, dry mouth, and dry skin. It can also lead to inflammation of the joints, lungs, kidneys, blood vessels, nerves, and muscles. Very rarely it may lead to lymphoma (a type of lymph node cancer).

Although certain hereditary and environmental factors may increase an individual's risk of developing Sjogren's, the exact cause of this disease is unknown. Sjogren's syndrome is not an infectious illness. In other words, one cannot "catch" it from another individual.

Sjogren's syndrome affects more than 1 million adults in the United States. It occurs nine times more frequently in women than in men, and rarely develops before 20 years of age. To diagnose Sjogren's syndrome, a physician obtains a medical history, performs a physical examination, and orders laboratory tests. Laboratory tests may include an erythrocyte sedimentation rate (ESR), which measures inflammation in the body, a complete blood cell count (CBC), and Sjogren's syndrome antibodies called SS-A and SS-B. The SS-A and SS-B tests are positive in only 50% of individuals with Sjogren's. A doctor may perform a "Schirmer's test" to determine the amount of tears in the eyes and/or a lip biopsy to confirm the diagnosis of Sjogren's.

Living With Your Diagnosis

One of the first signs of Sjogren's syndrome is dry eyes and dry mouth. The amount of dryness varies by individual. Dry eyes may cause a sandy feeling under your eyelids, burning of the eyes, increased sensitivity to light, decreased tearing, and in severe cases, ulcers of the eye. A dry mouth may cause difficulty chewing and swallowing dry foods, and an increased susceptibility to tooth decay, gingivitis (gum disease), and infections of the mouth. Women may have vaginal dryness that can cause pain with intercourse and can increase susceptibility to vaginal yeast infections. The nose may also become dry and lead to inflammation of the sinuses. If there is joint pain, it may be difficult to do some daily activities. There is no cure for Sjogren's. However, with improved medications and comprehensive treatment, individuals with Sjogren's can lead a full life.

Treatment

The best way to manage Sjogren's syndrome is through a combination of medications and therapies. Over-the-counter moisturizing products for dry eyes, dry mouth, and dry vagina may be very helpful. Nonsteroidal anti-inflammatory drugs (NSAIDs) may help decrease joint pain and swelling. Potential side effects of NSAIDs include stomach upset, ulcers, diarrhea, constipation, headache, dizziness, difficulty hearing, and a rash. Sometimes an ophthalmologist will suggest "plugging" the tear ducts to increase the amount of tears in the eyes. If the joint pain becomes severe, a physician may prescribe hydroxychloroquine. Potential side effects of this drug include nausea, diarrhea, and rash, and rarely it may affect the eyes. Prednisone or methotrexate may be used if the lungs, kidneys, and blood vessels are affected. Prednisone may cause skin bruising, high blood sugar, increased blood pressure, difficulty sleeping, weight gain, and thinning of the bones. Methotrexate may affect the blood and liver and may cause a rash.

The DOs

- Take your medication as prescribed.
- Call your doctor if you are experiencing side effects from medications.
- Ask your doctor what over-the-counter products are available to decrease dryness. If an artificial tear preparation burns the eyes, switch to another product or to one without a preservative. If the eyes dry out at night, an eye ointment may be more beneficial. Vaginal lubricants used throughout the day or before intercourse can be helpful.
- Use a cream or ointment for dry skin because these help "seal in" moisture.
- See a dentist regularly and brush and floss the teeth at least twice a day.
- Use a humidifier at night to prevent dryness of the eyes, mouth, and nose.

The DON'Ts

- Wait to see whether a medication side effect will go away. Always call your doctor if you have any questions.
- Give up. If a medication or product doesn't help, discuss this with your physician until you find a medicine or product that does.
- Eat a diet of sugary, sticky foods. This may accelerate dental cavities and gingivitis.

When to Call Your Doctor

- You have any side effects listed above from any of the medications or products.
- The medications or products are not helping.
- You need a referral to an opthamologist and/or dentist.

For More Information

Contact the Arthritis Foundation in your area. If you do not know the location of the Arthritis Foundation, you may call the national office at 1-800-283-7800 or access the information on the Internet at www.arthritis.org. The Sjogren's Syndrome Foundation may be reached at 1-800-475-6436.

SLEEP APNEA, OBSTRUCTIVE

About Your Diagnosis

Obstructive sleep apnea refers to a condition of repetitive episodes of stoppage of breathing during sleep because of blockage of the throat area. Whether through the nose or mouth, all air we breathe must pass through the throat region (pharynx) on its way to and from the lungs. The muscles of the pharynx naturally relax during sleep, causing some narrowing of the throat. Snoring occurs when the structures of the throat vibrate as the air moves through the narrowed throat region. Apnea occurs when the pharyngeal muscles cannot keep the throat open and the structures collapse on themselves, preventing the flow of air. After about 15–30 seconds of trying unsuccessfully to breathe against a blocked upper airway, a brief arousal from sleep will occur. The muscles of the throat will reestablish an open passage, and breathing will resume. Unfortunately, the cycle will begin as soon as the individual falls back to sleep. These recurring episodes of arousal are usually not remembered, but they prevent sustained, restorative sleep from occurring, so affected individuals wake up unrefreshed and feel sleepy during the day. An estimated 4% of middle-aged men and 2% of women have sleep apnea.

Factors that increase the likelihood of airway obstruction during sleep include:
- Obesity (for men a collar size greater than 17 inches is associated with an increased risk for obstructive sleep apnea).
- Use of alcohol.
- Use of sleeping pills.
- Nasal congestion.
- Sleeping on the back.
- Sleep deprivation.

Living With Your Diagnosis

The clinical features of obstructive sleep apnea include:
- Loud snoring.
- Breathing pauses during sleep with loud snorts/gasps as breathing resumes.
- Daytime sleepiness, especially in such permissive situations as reading, watching television, highway driving, and after meals.
- Headache, dry mouth, or sore throat upon awakening from sleep.
- Shortness of breath during the night.
- Irritability or difficulty concentrating during the day.

Diagnosis is made by a sleep study conducted overnight in a sleep disorders clinic. In some areas, these sleep studies are conducted in the patient's home. During the test, brain activity, breathing patterns, oxygen level, and heart rate are recorded. The technician conducting the study may ask the patient to turn during sleep to see whether position affects the frequency of snoring and stopped breathing episodes. Despite all the recording equipment, most individuals sleep well during the study.

Detecting sleep apnea is very important. Untreated sleep apnea increases the risk for high blood pressure, stroke, heart disease, and premature death. Patients with sleep apnea are also at higher risk for involvement in car accidents because of sleepiness behind the wheel.

Treatment

Treatment varies depending on the severity of the situation. Weight loss, avoidance of alcohol and sleeping pills, use of nasal decongestants, and not sleeping on the back are usually recommended for those who stop breathing infrequently during sleep. A 10% reduction in body weight is a reasonable initial weight loss goal. Sleeping on the back can be prevented by wearing a T-shirt during sleep that has a pouch in the back filled with tennis balls. An inexpensive way to make a T-shirt with tennis balls is to fill a large sock with three or four tennis balls and then safety pin the sock to the back of a T-shirt.

For many patients, continuous positive airway pressure (CPAP) is prescribed. This system consists of a mask for the nose connected to a bedside fan via a flexible hose. Air from the fan travels under pressure through the hose and mask and into the throat, keeping the passages open. Continuous positive airway pressure is usually first tried during the sleep study. The pressure is adjusted by the technician to find the optimal level. Continuous positive airway pressure is very effective when used on a nightly basis and is the most widely prescribed form of therapy.

There are several alternatives to CPAP. Oral appliances can be made by a dentist that advance the jaw during sleep (the effect can be simulated by jutting your jaw forward). This forward movement of the jaw helps keep the throat open. Various surgeries to keep the airway open during sleep are possible, ranging from partial removal of some of the structures of the throat area to full facial reconstruction. These surgeries are not consistently effective, and it is difficult to predict beforehand who will benefit.

The DOs

If CPAP is prescribed:
- The goal should be all night, every night use.
- Wash the mask and tubing in warm, soapy water daily, then let thoroughly air dry.
- If your nose becomes too dry with CPAP, try a room humidifier or get a humidifier that plugs directly into the CPAP unit. Coating your nostrils liberally with a water-soluble jelly (such as K-Y jelly) before putting the CPAP mask on at night will also help reduce dryness.
- If you experience nasal congestion, runny nose, or sneezing with CPAP, a nasal steroid spray prescribed by your doctor will help.
- If the bridge of your nose gets too sore with the prescribed CPAP mask, you may be clamping the mask down too tightly. Try a Band-Aid or piece of cotton over the tender area of your nose. Eventually, you may need to change mask styles.

The DON'Ts

- Avoid further weight gain and alcohol use when using CPAP because they may render the prescribed CPAP pressure inadequate.
- Avoid sleep deprivation. The goal should be 7–8 hours in bed per night.

When to Call Your Doctor

- If you have signs or symptoms of obstructive sleep apnea syndrome.
- If your bed partner still hears you snore while using CPAP (this means that the prescribed pressure is not adequate).
- If you continue to feel sleepy despite regular use of CPAP and adequate time in bed; persistent sleepiness may signal the presence of another sleep disorder.

For More Information
American Lung Association
1118 Hampton Avenue
St. Louis, MO 63139
800-LUNG-USA
www.lungusa.org
American Sleep Disorders Association
1610 14th Street NW
Suite 300
Rochester, MN 55901
507-287-6006
www.asda.org.

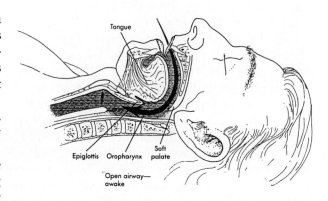

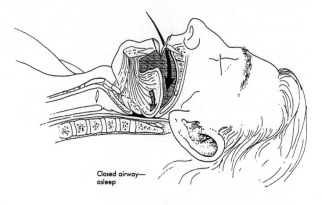

Obstructive sleep apnea. During sleep the absence of activity of the pharyngeal muscle structure allows the airway to close. (From LaFleur-Brooks ML: *Exploring Medical Language—A Student Directed Approach.* vol 3. St. Louis, Mosby–Year Book, 1993. Used by permission.)

STEVENS-JOHNSON SYNDROME

About Your Diagnosis

Stevens-Johnson syndrome is an acute inflammatory skin disease. Most cases have a strong association with exposure to specific medications. It occurs 1–3 weeks after the first drug exposure. It is fairly uncommon and is not infectious. The disease can be severe and may require treatment in the intensive care unit of a hospital.

Living With Your Diagnosis

Stevens-Johnson syndrome begins with a fever and flulike symptoms. After 1–3 days, skin lesions appear. Mild-to-moderate skin tenderness and burning or itching of the eyes are present. There may be painful mouth lesions that impair swallowing. Sensitivity to light and anxiety may be present. There may be painful urination. The rash consists of raised target-type lesions, which will look like blisters. These lesions will peel off, exposing red, oozing skin. Fingernails may also shed.

Treatment

If the blistering and peeling is extensive, hospitalization may be needed. Topical ointments to the areas will be needed. Prevention of infection is the primary concern. Mouth lesions can be treated with a rinse consisting of a mixture of Benadryl liquid and Kaopectate.

The DOs

- Prevent infection by careful hand washing by anyone caring for the lesions.
- Maintain adequate nutrition. A liquid diet may be needed if swallowing and pain are a problem.
- Maintain adequate fluid intake to prevent dehydration.
- Avoid the medication suspected of causing the episode.
- Wear a Medic Alert bracelet stating the medication suspected of causing the episode.

The DON'Ts

- Don't scratch the lesions or "peel" the loose skin.
- Don't use the medication suspected of causing the episode.

When to Call Your Doctor

- If high fever occurs.
- If adequate fluids and nutrition cannot be maintained because of the mouth lesions.
- If any of the symptoms worsen.

For More Information
National Institute of Arthritis, Musculoskeletal and Skin Diseases of the NIH
301-495-4484
American Academy of Allergy and Immunology
800-822-2762
National Health Information Center
800-336-4797, Monday through Friday from 9 AM to 5 PM (EST).
Internet Site
www.healthfinder.gov (Choose SEARCH to search by topic.)

STOKES-ADAMS ATTACKS (ADAMS-STOKES-MORGAGNI SYNDROME; CARDIAC FAINTS)

About Your Diagnosis

Stokes-Adams attacks are a type of syncope (fainting) of cardiac origin resulting from a sudden reduction in blood flow from the heart to the brain. Syncope may result when a patient's pulse suddenly becomes exceptionally slow or fast because the brain does not receive adequate blood flow. Stokes-Adams attacks occur most frequently in patients with complete atrioventricular heart block and a pulse of 40 or less per minute.

Living With Your Diagnosis

Cardiac faints of the Stokes-Adams variety may recur several times a day, at any time of the day or night regardless of the position of the body. They may last for a few seconds or in some instances longer, in which case the patient may require resuscitation.

Treatment

Treatment must be undertaken by a qualified cardiologist. Medication and/or a cardiac pacemaker may be required to prevent the sudden heart rate changes that prevent adequate flow of blood to the brain.

The DOs

- Keep a record of the cardiac faints to share with your doctor.
- Take your medications as prescribed.
- Eat a well-balanced diet.

The DON'Ts

- Don't engage in any type of work or activity that may put you or someone else at risk of injury
- Don't drive until you get your doctor's approval.
- Don't ignore these cardiac faints. Seek assistance from your doctor immediately.

When to Call Your Doctor

- If you continue to have Stokes-Adams attacks.
- If you awaken from an attack feeling confused, especially weak or ill.
- If you have any difficulty related to your medication.

STOMATITIS

About Your Diagnosis

Stomatitis is a generalized inflammation of the mouth. It involves the oral mucosa, lips, tongue, and palate. There are many causes of stomatitis. Acute herpetic stomatitis and aphthous stomatitis are the two most common causes. Other causes include allergic reactions, smoking, dental disease, vitamin deficiencies, systemic diseases, medications, and other viral and bacterial infections. Stomatitis is a common condition found in all age groups.

An examination is the best way to detect stomatitis. Occasionally if the cause is not clear or there is no improvement with treatment, a biopsy is done. In most cases, stomatitis will resolve with outpatient treatment.

Living With Your Diagnosis

There are variable signs and symptoms associated with stomatitis. There is inflammation of the mouth that may be associated with varying amounts of pain. Sores (ulcers) in the mouth are associated with some causes. You may also have bad breath (halitosis). There may also be symptoms of fever, malaise, headache, and loss of appetite.

Treatment

The treatment will vary depending on the cause. The key, no matter the cause, is providing symptomatic relief. Analgesics such as acetaminophen and topical anesthetic agents should be used. Mouth rinses with a half teaspoon of baking soda and 8 oz of warm water can provide relief. If symptoms are so severe that you are not able to drink fluids, intravenous fluids may be given. The other treatment options are dependent on the cause. If the cause is bacterial infection, antibiotics are necessary. If the cause is nutritional deficiencies, vitamin supplementation is the treatment. If the symptoms are severe, corticosteriods taken by mouth may be necessary.

The DOs

- A bland or liquid diet may be needed.
- Good oral hygiene is necessary. Brush and floss teeth and clean the tongue after each meal. See a dentist regularly.
- If you wear dentures, they should be fitted properly.

The DON'Ts

- Avoid foods that are spicy, hard, sharp, or dry.
- Avoid foods or other agents that can cause allergic reactions in the mouth.
- Avoid smoking.

When to Call Your Doctor

- If you have symptoms of stomatitis.
- If symptoms worsen after treatment begins.
- If symptoms do not resolve after 7–14 days of treatment.

For More Information
American Dental Association
211 E. Chicago Avenue
Chicago, Illinois 60611
312-440-2500
Fax: 312-440-2800

SYNCOPE

About Your Diagnosis

Syncope (pronounced sink-o-pee) means fainting. The term is often used for near fainting or lightheadedness. Syncope can have many causes but is generally related to insufficient blood flow (and therefore decreased oxygen delivery) to the brain. Damaged or stiffened blood vessels may reduce blood flow. Reduced blood flow also can be caused by an arrhythmia (abnormal heart rhythm) that disrupts the normal beating of the heart.

Low blood pressure, inefficient pumping by the heart because of heart disease (heart failure), or heart valve abnormalities may cause syncope. Dehydration, anemia (low red blood cell count in the blood), low blood oxygen from lung disease, and some medications (especially medications for lowering blood pressure) can cause syncope. Hyperventilation, low blood sugar, and some neurologic conditions are noncardiac causes that must be addressed.

Venous pooling (blood collecting in the veins in the lower body from the effects of gravity) or straining maneuvers (Valsalva) may prevent blood from moving up to the brain when needed. *Vasovagal syncope* refers to overstimulation of the vagus nerve. This causes reflex lowering of blood pressure through opening of more blood vessels. This may occur with anxiety, pain, urination, or coughing.

Living With Your Diagnosis

For a healthy person a single episode of syncope that resolves by itself usually requires no attention. Multiple episodes or episodes among persons with cardiovascular disease require further evaluation. The physician performs a physical examination and electrocardiogram (ECG) and takes the blood pressure in different positions (lying, sitting, standing, after exercise). Tilt-table testing sometimes is ordered to check for symptoms of syncope in different positions. Blood glucose and hematocrit (blood count) may be checked. A Holter monitor is a device that is worn for continuous monitoring of heart rhythm and may be used to help make the diagnosis.

Treatment

Management of syncope depends on the cause. If cardiac output (blood being pumped out) is low, the cardiac condition must be evaluated. The most common cause of a single event is a lightheaded sensation from hyperventilating or standing up too fast. The most common causes of frequent episodes of syncope are related to hypotension (low blood pressure) or cardiac disease. Lowering of blood pressure with changes in position is called *orthostatic hypotension*. Any medications believed to be causing the condition are discontinued on a trial basis. All illnesses and medical conditions should be managed. Blood pressure monitoring is recommended.

The DOs

- Record the setting of episodes of syncope; for example, it happens when you suddenly stand from a seated position.
- Ensure a proper, regular diet and adequate fluid intake, because these are essential to avoiding syncope caused by low blood sugar and dehydration.
- Sit or lie down if you feel faint, because this helps improve blood flow to the brain. Drink cool water once you are able to drink. Eat something to help replenish glucose if you have a history of low blood sugar.

The DON'Ts

- Avoid situations known to aggravate your symptoms.

When to Call Your Doctor

- If episodes of syncope become more frequent or do not respond to home treatment.
- If you have syncope and chest pain, shortness of breath, or a history of heart disease.

For More Information

Consult your local library or medical school for more information regrading the specific cause of your syncope. Call the American Heart Association at 1-800-242-8721 and ask for the literature department.

SYNDROME OF INAPPROPRIATE ANTIDIURETIC HORMONE SECRETION (SIADH)

About Your Diagnosis

Antidiuretic hormone (ADH) is an important hormone in maintaining normal water balance. Too little ADH results in diabetes insipidus, which is manifested by large volumes of water in the urine. Too much ADH results in the syndrome of inappropriate antidiuretic hormone secretion (SIADH), with water retention and decreased blood sodium levels.

Many different conditions and drugs may cause SIADH. Antidiuretic hormone may be produced by certain tumors such as a lung cancer, or may result from chronic lung diseases. A long list of medicines has been associated with SIADH including such common medicines as antidepressants, antianxiety agents, antipsychotic agents, seizure medicines, and desmopressin (DDAVP).

Many individuals have a mild form of SIADH that causes no symptoms. More advanced cases with markedly decreased serum sodium levels usually occur in hospitalized patients who are undergoing surgical procedures or being treated for brain tumors, seizure disorders, lung cancers, or other chronic conditions.

The diagnosis is established through a combination of blood and urine tests performed under certain specified conditions. The patient must not be dehydrated or volume overloaded. The patient must have a low serum sodium and plasma osmolality level, and an inappropriately concentrated urine (increased urine osmolality level) to have SIADH diagnosed. These tests indicate an excess of body water relative to the amount of body sodium. In other words, ADH is inappropriately holding onto too much water. It is important to eliminate other causes of a low sodium level, such as hypothyroidism or adrenal insufficiency, before settling on a diagnosis of SIADH.

Curing SIADH is possible by removing the offending drug or tumor, and by treating the underlying condition.

Living With Your Diagnosis

Early SIADH has no symptoms; however, if left untreated, SIADH may cause lethargy, weakness, seizures, and coma. Symptoms are worse in those patients whose serum sodium levels fall rapidly.

Most individuals tolerate SIADH well with no effects. However, it may progress to coma and death if untreated.

Treatment

Water restriction is the cornerstone of treatment. Decreased water intake allows the serum sodium level to rise normally. The maximum amount of water that patients with SIADH are allowed to drink is just slightly more than the amount of urine they produce. Patients must have regular serum sodium measurements to ensure that the water restriction has been effective. Some patients may require a diuretic such as furosemide if further treatment is needed. Another medicine called demeclocycline is also effective for SIADH.

The most concerning potential side effect from treatment is dehydration. This occurs when water restriction is maintained in a patient with increased fluid requirements because of fever, exercise, or other reasons. Therapy with furosemide may lead to a low blood potassium level, which, if not corrected, can cause cardiac arrhythmias. Demeclocycline causes a nephrogenic diabetes insipidus (kidney resistance to ADH). Kidney function must be carefully monitored in patients receiving this medicine.

The DOs

- Restrict the amount of water you drink if you have SIADH. This may be the only treatment necessary.
- Understand the reason for your SIADH. If you treat the underlying cause, the SIADH will go away.
- Ask your doctor to eliminate any medicines that may be causing SIADH, whenever possible.
- Follow-up regularly for serum sodium measurements.

The DON'Ts

- Don't assume you have SIADH just because you have a low blood sodium level. Other disorders must be excluded first.
- Don't take medication for SIADH unless absolutely necessary. Careful water restriction is a better treatment.

When to Call Your Doctor
- You feel weak or lethargic.
- You have an illness with a fever.
- You are scheduled for elective surgery or a radiologic procedure.

For More Information

The Endocrine Society
4350 East West Highway, Suite 500
Bethesda, MD 20814-4410
1-888-ENDOCRINE
Pituitary Tumor Network
16350 Ventura Boulevard, Suite 231
Encino, CA 91436
1-800-642-9211

SYPHILIS

About Your Diagnosis

Syphilis is a chronic sexually transmitted disease that causes tissue destruction. It is caused by a bacteria called *Treponema pallidum*. Syphilis affects the genitals, skin, and central nervous system. It can be transmitted from an infected mother to her newborn. There are five stages of the disease: incubation, primary, secondary, latency, and late stages. Syphilis is spread to another individual during sexual intercourse with someone who has primary- or secondary-stage syphilis. It can be detected with a blood test.

Living With Your Diagnosis

Signs and symptoms in the first stage include a painless, chancre sore that appears on the genitals, rectum, or mouth. This usually heals on its own in 1–5 weeks. The secondary stage lasts 2–6 weeks and can include headache; enlarged lymph glands in the armpit, groin, or neck; fever; nausea; and rash with small, red scaly bumps that appear on the penis, vagina, or mouth. The latent stage may last 1–40 years with no symptoms. The late stage includes destructive lesions and may affect the nervous system.

Treatment

With treatment, syphilis is usually curable in about 3 months. Without treatment, widespread tissue destruction and death can occur. Penicillin is the drug of choice, and usually only 1 injection is required if syphilis is in the early stage. If syphilis has been present for more than a year, an injection every week for 3 weeks may be needed. If you are allergic to penicillin, you may be given tetracycline or erythromycin orally for 15–38 days. After the injection, some individuals may experience a reaction to the toxin released from the dying organisms, which includes fever, headache, and nausea.

The DOs

- Finish taking all the prescribed oral antibiotic.
- Make sure all sexual partners are notified.
- Return to your doctor for follow-up testing in 1 month and then every 3 months for 1 year.
- If you have a reaction after the injection, notify your doctor, rest, increase your fluid intake, and take Tylenol for the fever.

- Avoid sexual intercourse for at least 2 weeks after treatment or until cleared by your doctor.
- Use latex condoms during intercourse.
- Get tested for other sexually transmitted diseases.

The DON'Ts

- Don't have unprotected sex with a new partner.
- Don't hesitate to see your doctor if new symptoms appear after treatment.

When to See Your Doctor

- If after treatment you have a rash, a fever, a sore throat, or swelling in any joint.
- If you have had syphilis in the past and have not had a checkup in the past year.

For More Information
The CDC National STD Hotline
800-227-8922, Monday through Friday from 8 AM to 11 PM (EST).
American Social Health Association
800-972-8500, to request pamphlets about sexual health or information about support groups
Internet Sites
www.healthfinder.gov (Choose SEARCH to search by topic.)
http://sunsite.unc.edu/ASHA/

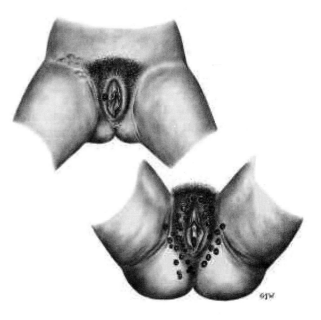

Syphilis. **A,** primary stage: chancre with inguinal adenopathy. **B,** secondary stage: condylomata lata. (From Lowdermilk DL, Perry SE, Bobak IM: *Maternity & Women's Health Care*, vol 6. St. Louis, Mosby–Year Book, 1996. Used by permission.)

SYSTEMIC LUPUS ERYTHEMATOSUS

About Your Diagnosis

Systemic lupus erythematosus (SLE) is a disease that causes inflammation in various parts of the body. The first signs of SLE may be joint pain or stiffness and/or fatigue. The joints most frequently affected are the hands, wrists, and knees. The fatigue can be severe. In other individuals a rash may occur on sun-exposed areas of the body, frequently on the face. This rash on the cheeks and nose is sometimes called a "butterfly rash (fig 1)." Some individuals with lupus have "Raynaud's phenomenon," which can cause pain and discoloration in the fingers. Systemic lupus erythematosus may also cause inflammation in other parts of the body including the heart, lungs, blood vessels, kidneys, nervous system, and blood cells.

Although certain hereditary and environmental factors may increase an individual's risk of developing lupus, the exact cause of SLE is unknown. Research indicates that SLE occurs more frequently in close relatives. Systemic lupus erythematosus is not an infectious illness. In other words, you cannot "catch" it from another individual.

Systemic lupus erythematosus affects about 1 in 2,000 individuals and occurs 5 times more frequently in women than in men. The disease usually occurs in individuals between the ages of 15 and 40 years. African Americans and individuals of Asian and Hispanic ancestry develop SLE more frequently than Caucasians.

To diagnose SLE, a physician obtains a medical history, performs a physical examination, and orders laboratory tests and possibly x-rays. Laboratory tests may include an erythrocyte sedimentation rate (ESR), which measures inflammation in the body; a complete blood cell count (CBC), which measures the white and red blood cell counts and the platelet count (platelets are cells that help control bleeding); and an antinuclear antibody (ANA). The ANA is usually positive in individuals with SLE, but sometimes is positive in individuals without SLE. Therefore, this test is not 100% accurate in confirming a diagnosis of SLE. If the ANA is positive, the doctor may order an anti-DNA test, which is more specific for SLE. Urine tests are done to identify kidney problems.

Living With Your Diagnosis

Systemic lupus erythematosus affects each individual differently. Systemic lupus erythematosus of the joints may decrease your ability to write, open jars, and dress. If you have Raynaud's phenomenon, your fingers may turn white and blue and become painful when exposed to cold. Some individuals have pleurisy (inflammation of the lining of the lungs), which can make breathing painful. If SLE affects the skin, you will need to avoid exposure to the sun. The fatigue of SLE may interfere with your activities at home and at work. If the kidneys are affected, you may have high blood pressure. Systemic lupus erythematosus may affect your memory and mood. This may cause stress or confusion in the family and at work. There is no cure for SLE. However, with earlier detection, improved medications, and comprehensive treatment, individuals with SLE can lead a full life.

Treatment

Medications help decrease the inflammation that causes pain. Nonsteroidal anti-inflammatory drugs (NSAIDs) are often the first line of therapy. If these medications do not adequately control the disease, a physician may prescribe "disease-modifying" medications that can slow down the disease process. These medicines include hydroxychloroquine, methotrexate, azathioprine, and cyclophosphamide. Because these medications may take up to a few months to be effective, the doctor may prescribe prednisone. Prednisone is a strong anti-inflammatory medication that works quickly.

All medications can cause side effects. The NSAIDs may cause stomach upset, ulcers, diarrhea, constipation, headache, dizziness, difficulty hearing, or a rash. Hydroxychloroquine may cause nausea, diarrhea, and a rash, and rarely may affect the eyes. Methotrexate and azathioprine may affect your blood, liver, and kidneys and may cause a rash. Cyclophosphamide may be given by mouth or through a vein and may affect your blood, kidneys, and bladder. Prednisone may cause skin bruising, high blood sugar, increased blood pressure, difficulty sleeping, cataracts, weight gain, and thinning bones.

Learning about SLE is essential because you may have it for a long time, maybe for the rest of your life. Exercise is important to maintain joint movement and muscle strength. Alternating periods of rest and activity helps to manage fatigue.

The DOs
- Take your medication as prescribed.
- Call your doctor if you are experiencing side effects from medications.
- Ask your doctor which over-the-counter medications you may take with your prescription medications.
- Exercise to maintain range of motion of your joints and muscle strength.
- Alternate periods of rest and activity to manage fatigue.
- Take your blood pressure regularly.

The DON'Ts
- Wait to see whether a possible medication side effect will go away on its own.
- Give up. If one medication doesn't work for you, discuss with your physician other medicines that might help decrease your pain, stiffness, and fatigue.
- Continue an exercise program that causes pain and fatigue. Increased pain and fatigue after exercise usually indicate that the exercise program needs to be modified.

When to Call Your Doctor
- You experience side effects that you believe may be caused by your medications.
- The medication and other treatments are not helping the pain, stiffness, or fatigue.
- You believe you may need a referral to a physical or occupational therapist for exercise or joint protection, or a referral to a counselor to discuss family and social problems that have occurred because of this diagnosis.
- You are interested in vocational rehabilitation for job retraining.

For More Information
Contact the Arthritis Foundation in your area. If you do not know the location of the Arthritis Foundation, you may call the national office at 1-800-283-7800 or access information on the Internet at www.arthritis.org. The Lupus Foundation of America may be reached at 1-301-670-9292 or www.lupus.org/lupus.

TAPEWORM INFESTATION

About Your Diagnosis

Tapeworms are a parasite usually obtained by eating undercooked meat or fish. It cannot be spread from individual to individual. Usually it is acquired when traveling to a foreign country; it is uncommon in the United States. It can be detected through a stool sample examined in a laboratory.

Living With Your Diagnosis

Many times individuals don't have any symptoms. However, they should be checked for tapeworms if they have recently traveled outside the United States and then have the following symptoms and signs: diarrhea, pain in the upper abdomen, unexplained weight loss, or anemia.

Treatment

Your doctor will prescribe a drug to kill the parasite. One dose is usually all that is required. A repeat stool specimen should be examined in 3–6 weeks to make sure you are cured. There are no restrictions in activity or your diet. You may have side effects from the medication such as headache, drowsiness, nausea, vomiting, and loss of appetite. Stomach upset can be lessened by taking the medication with food.

The DOs

- Take the medication as directed.
- Have a follow-up examination in 3–6 weeks.
- Have all family members checked for the infection.
- Avoid undercooked meat and fish.
- Buy only meats that have been inspected.

The DON'Ts

- Don't skip your follow-up examination.
- Don't eat undercooked meats or fish while traveling in a foreign country.

When to Call Your Doctor

- If you have any symptoms after treatment.

For More Information
Further information regarding the proper cooking of meats is available form the following organizations:
The National Center for Nutrition
800-366-1655
The Department of Agriculture, Meat and Poultry Hotline
800-535-4555

TARSAL TUNNEL SYNDROME

About Your Diagnosis

Tarsal tunnel syndrome is a relatively rare condition that produces burning pain along the medial (inside) aspect of the ankle and down into the bottom of the foot. It is generally caused by compression on a nerve that travels in this area (Fig 1). Although the name is similar to carpal tunnel syndrome, it is much less common, and the physician considers this diagnosis only after other potential causes of pain in these areas are excluded. A physical examination is all that is usually needed to confirm or exclude the diagnosis. However, electrical testing, such as electromyography (EMG) can sometimes be helpful. You can be treated for tarsal tunnel syndrome after it has been appropriately diagnosed. Surgical decompression may be necessary.

Living With Your Diagnosis

Signs and symptoms of tarsal tunnel syndrome include pain along the inside of the ankle that extends down into the bottom of the foot. Numbness or tingling also may occur in this distribution. Compression on the nerve can sometimes lead to decreased function of the nerve but does not usually cause any permanent paralysis of the foot. This is usually a painful condition and eventually begins to limit your ability to walk or stand for prolonged periods. The symptoms usually come and go and are usually related to activity level.

Treatment

When the diagnosis of tarsal tunnel syndrome has been confirmed, treatment can include rest, elevating the extremity, and, sometimes, injections in an effort to decrease the inflammation that can occur around the nerve. Anti-inflammatory medications can sometimes be helpful. No vitamins, diets, or exercises have been proved to decrease the pressure on the nerve once it occurs. An attempt to determine the cause of the symptoms, including critical evaluation of shoes and activities, may be of benefit. Surgical release of the nerve can be considered when the other forms of treatment fail. There can be risks with surgical treatment, including failure to relieve the pain. Pain sometimes can be relieved initially with surgical treatment, but the symptoms quickly recur. Scarring around the nerve after an operation is common and can lead to long-term difficulties.

The DOs
- Take your medications as prescribed.
- Rest and elevate the leg.

The DON'Ts
- Do not perform aggressive exercise usually worsens the condition.

When to Call Your Doctor
- Should your symptoms change from intermittent to constant, then a physician should be sought out who has a fair amount of experience dealing with this relatively rare diagnosis.

For More Information
http://www.sechrest.com/mmg/foot/tarstun/tarstun.html

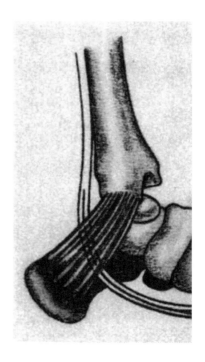

The tarsal tunnel. The posterior tibial nerve runs beneath the flexor retinaculum. (From Mercier LR: *Practical Orthopedics,* vol 4. St. Louis, Mosby–Year Book, 1995. Used by permission.)

TEMPOROMANDIBULAR JOINT DISORDER

About Your Diagnosis

The temporomandibular joints (TMJs) are the two joints near the ears that allow the jaw to open and close. Individuals with TMJ disorder (TMD) may have pain, noises, and clicking around the jaw, and they often have abnormal movement of the mouth or jaw. TMD usually occurs as a result of strain and spasm of the muscles that open and close the mouth but can also result from changes in the joints themselves. TMD occurs for different reasons, but usually stress and jaw clenching are involved. Other reasons for strain and fatigue are changes in the alignment of the jaw from already diagnosed forms of arthritis.

TMD is a common problem that affects women more often than men. It is diagnosed by obtaining a medical history and performing a physical examination. Occasionally, x-rays or other types of scans such as a magnetic resonance imaging (MRI) scan are needed.

Living With Your Diagnosis

Individuals with TMD often have symptoms in one or more locations including pain in the face or jaw, difficulty opening or closing the mouth, problems aligning the jaw, and clicking or popping noises in the TMJ near the ear. The pain is worse with movement of the jaw, chewing, yawning, and clenching the teeth. TMD can be associated with headaches, ear pain, neck pain, and ringing in the ears.

Treatment

Anti-inflammatory medication and heat or ice will decrease the pain. A soft diet that requires less vigorous chewing will reduce the strain and fatigue in the jaw muscles. Your dentist might fit you with a mouth piece to modify jaw clenching, especially at night. Some individuals require a dental evaluation to determine whether there are any abnormalities in the alignment of the teeth or jaw. Jaw exercises can help to relax the jaw. A roll-shaped pillow can help with neck pain. If these treatments are not effective, different pain medications such as amitriptyline, physical therapy, relaxation training, or biofeedback might be recommended.

The DOs

- Take your medicines as prescribed.
- Use your mouth piece if it is prescribed.
- Follow other treatment instructions.
- Ask your doctor which over-the-counter medications you may take with your prescription medications.

The DON'Ts

- Wait to see whether side effects from medications will go away.

When to Call Your Doctor

- You have any medication side effects.
- The treatment is not decreasing your symptoms in a reasonable amount of time.
- Your jaw "locks" open or closed.

For More Information

Access the American Dental Association on the Internet at www.ada.org.

TENDINITIS

About Your Diagnosis

Tendinitis is inflammation or irritation in a tendon. Tendons connect muscles to bones (Fig 1). Tendinitis is a common cause of shoulder, elbow, wrist, and ankle pain. It usually results from overuse or abnormal use of a tendon or muscle. It is diagnosed by obtaining a medical history and performing a physical examination of the painful area. X-rays and blood tests are seldom helpful in making the diagnosis.

Living With Your Diagnosis

Tendinitis causes pain and occasionally swelling around the painful area. In more severe cases it may restrict movement of the joint. The pain is worse with activities and improves with resting the painful area. Tendinitis, depending on its location, may make it difficult to perform everyday activities such as dressing, grooming, reaching, lifting, writing, or walking. Most often, tendinitis is easily treated and gets better with time.

Treatment

Treatment of tendinitis includes rest, ice, heat, strengthening and stretching exercises, splints, acetaminophen or nonsteroidal anti-inflammatory medications (NSAIDs), ultrasound treatment, or "cortisone" injections. Occasionally, a therapist will provide exercises and/or splints to strengthen muscles and reduce strain on certain tendons.

Potential side effects of NSAIDs include stomach upset, ulcers, constipation, diarrhea, headaches, dizziness, difficulty hearing, and rash. Cortisone injections usually work quickly but require injecting a needle through the skin. Rarely, they can cause irritation under the skin or infection. The other treatments uncommonly cause side effects.

The DOs
- Follow your doctors treatment instructions.
- Rest the painful area as recommended by your doctor.
- Ask your doctor which over-the-counter medications you may take with your prescription medications.

The DON'Ts
- Wait to see whether a side effect from your medication or injection goes away.

- Continue an exercise program that causes excessive or prolonged pain. If this occurs, the program needs to be modified specifically for you.

When to Call Your Doctor
- You experience any medication side effects.
- The medication or treatments are not decreasing the pain.
- You believe you may need a referral to an occupational therapist or a physical therapist.
- You have worsening warmth or redness of the skin after a cortisone injection.

For More Information
Contact the Arthritis Foundation in your area. If you do not know the location of the Arthritis Foundation, you may call the national office at 1-800-283-7800 or access the information on the Internet at www.arthritis.org.

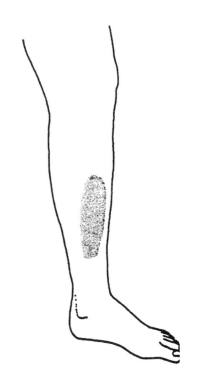

Fig 1. The area of tenderness and pain with posterior tibial tendinitis. (From Mercier LR: *Practical Orthopedics,* vol 4. St. Louis, Mosby–Year Book, 1995. Used by permission.)

TESTICULAR CANCER

About Your Diagnosis

Testicular cancer or germ cell tumors are cancers that begin in the testes (testicles). The testes are the male sex glands that produce and store sperm and the male hormone testosterone. Approximately 7500 new cases of testicular cancer are diagnosed each year in the United States. Most patients are men between the ages of 20 and 40 years. The cause is not known. Some patients, however, are at higher risk for testicular cancer than are others. Men who were born with an undescended testicle (cryptorchidism; the testicle remains in the abdomen instead of descending into the scrotum) are more likely to have testicular cancer than are other men. Testicular cancer is not contagious.

The best way to detect testicular cancer is by performing a self-examination of the testicles (Fig 1).

This is important because the first sign of testicular cancer usually is a lump in the testicle. If you feel a lump in your testicle, you should notify your primary care physician, who proceeds with further evaluation. The next step usually is testicular ultrasonography. If this examination shows a solid testicular mass (lump), the primary care physician refers you to a urologist, who removes the testicle (orchiectomy) and makes a definitive diagnosis. Nearly 90% of newly diagnosed testicular cancers are curable. Even cancers that have spread have a very good cure rate of 70% to 80%.

Living With Your Diagnosis

The first sign of testicular cancer usually is a lump in the testicle. Other signs and symptoms are pain, swelling, and enlargement of the testis. Cancer that spreads to the back and lungs produces low back pain and shortness of breath.

Treatment

Testicular cancers are divided into two types, seminomatous and nonseminomatous. This is important to know because the tumors spread differently and are managed differently. Once the diagnosis is made during an operation, staging is performed to find out the extent of spread of the disease. Staging is commonly performed with special blood tests, computed tomography (CT) of the abdomen and pelvis to look for spread to lymph nodes, and possibly an operation to remove lymph nodes (retroperitoneal lymph node dissection; RPLND).

Stage I disease is confined to the testis. Stage II is disease that has spread to local lymph nodes. Stage III disease has distant spread. Depending on the type of tumor (seminomatous or nonseminomatous) and the stage of disease (I, II, III), specific treatment with surgical, radiation, or chemotherapy is recommended.

Seminomatous tumors are sensitive to radiation. If there is no distant spread, irradiation is the recommended treatment. If there is distant spread, chemotherapy is advised. Typical side effects of radiation are dry, red, itchy skin in the area of radiation. Because radiation is in the abdominal area, diarrhea, bloody stools, urinary frequency and discomfort, and nausea may occur. Chemotherapy can cause easy bruising and bleeding, hair loss, nausea, vomiting, and fevers.

Nonseminomatous tumors in the early stage are managed with a surgical procedure (RPLND) and observation. For more advanced disease, chemotherapy is added to surgical treatment.

The DOs

- Learn and perform testicular self examinations.
- Ask for second opinions. You must feel comfortable with the decisions about treatment, and learning about the disease helps relieve anxiety.
- Understand the importance of nutrition after surgical treatment and chemotherapy.
- Ask about emotional support groups.

The DON'Ts

- Do not miss follow-up appointments with your physicians. Special blood tests usually are ordered to help detect whether the cancer has recurred. Radiographs (x-rays) and scans are obtained regularly to make sure there is no recurrence.
- Do not forget to perform testicular self-examinations on the remaining testicle; there is a 1% chance that cancer will develop in that testis.
- Do not be afraid to ask about sex. An operation to remove one testicle does not make you infertile, sterile, or impotent (inability to have an erection). An operation to remove the lymph nodes has no affect on your ability to have an erection but can cause sterility.
- Do not wait if you feel a lump on your testicle.

When to Call Your Doctor
- If you feel a lump on your testicle.
- If you have swelling or pain in your testicle.
- If you have a fever after chemotherapy.
- If you have back pain or shortness of breath.
- If you have excess drainage from the surgical site.

For More Information

National Cancer Institute (NCI)
9000 Rockville Pike
Bethesda, MD 20893
Cancer Information Service
1-800-422-6237 (1-800-4-CANCER)
American Cancer Society
1599 Clifton Road, N.E.
Atlanta, GA 30329
1-800-ACS-2345

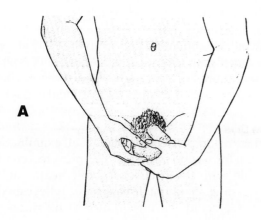

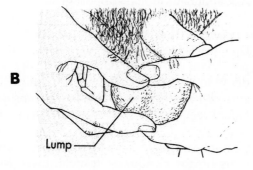

Testicular self-examination. **A,** Grasp testis with both hands; palpate gently between thumb and fingers. **B,** Abnormal lumps or irregularities are reported to physician. (From Phipps WJ, Long BC, Woods NF: *Medical-Surgical Nursing, Concepts and Clinical Practice,* ed 1. St. Louis, Mosby–Year Book, 1987. Used by permission.)

THALASSEMIA MINOR

About Your Diagnosis

Thalassemic anemia is a term that defines a genetically transmitted anemia common to certain populations worldwide. Thalassemia minor is a hereditary disease. That means one or both of your parents must have the abnormal gene for the offspring to have the disease. The more severe types are called *thalassemia intermedia* and *thalassemia major*. These conditions are easily recognized, usually occur among infants and children, necessitate many blood transfusions, and have other findings such as skeletal changes or an enlarged liver and spleen. *Thalassemia minor* usually is asymptomatic. Patients have mild anemia that usually is found during a routine blood analysis. A blood smear also shows characteristic changes consistent with the diagnosis.

Anemia happens when one of the necessary tools for the production of red blood cells is either deficient or decreased in number. Thalassemia belongs to the first category. Because of an alteration on the gene responsible for production of a main component of the red blood cells, these cells are destroyed, and anemia occurs.

Thalassemia is subdivided into alpha and beta types. Alpha-thalassemia is transmitted by four different genes, two inherited from the father and two from the mother. When two of the four are absent, thalassemia minor occurs. Beta-thalassemia is transmitted by two genes, one from the father and one from the mother. When one is absent thalassemia minor occurs.

It is speculated that red blood cells that have the thalassemia characteristics are less susceptible to infestation by certain parasites, specifically the malaria parasite. This confers an advantage in some areas of the world, and it is there that thalassemia is most common. These areas are Africa, the Mediterranean, and Southeast Asia. Patients whose ancestors came from these areas also are at increased risk.

The most important aspect of thalassemia minor is prevention of the more severe types. Being aware of carrying the genetic alteration always raises the question of transmitting it to one's offspring. It is recommended that persons with thalassemia minor ask their partners to undergo medical evaluation, especially if they belong to any of the risk groups. If both partners have thalassemia minor, there is risk for transmitting thalassemia intermedia or thalassemia major to their offspring. The percentage varies according to the number of genes missing. There are centers that can study the blood in detail to give accurate numbers, and many of these specialized centers even offer fetal testing.

Living With Your Diagnosis

Thalassemia minor is usually asymptomatic. It is diagnosed either when a routine blood test shows mild anemia or microcytosis (small red blood cells) or through examinations of family members of patients with more severe forms of thalassemia. Rare patients with thalassemia minor may have mild symptoms of anemia, such as fatigue or shortness of breath with exercise.

Because thalassemia minor is a genetic disorder, persons who have it may transmit it to their children. This is usually not a problem for the child, unless both parents have a genetic red blood cell abnormality, in which case, the child may be affected by a severe form of thalassemia (thalassemia major, thalassemia intermedia, or sickle thalassemia, to name a few). Therefore persons with thalassemia minor and their partners may want to consider genetic counseling when they decide to have a baby.

Treatment

Patients with thalassemia minor usually do not need treatment.

The DOs

- Take folic acid supplements as prescribed by your physician if you are pregnant.
- Stop exercising if you become fatigued.
- Seek genetic counseling if you are planning to start a family to determine your risk for having a baby with this condition.

The DON'Ts

- Do not take a vitamin supplement that contains iron without consulting your physician. Some types of thalassemia are associated with increased absorption of iron, and taking iron supplements for a prolonged period of time may lead to iron overload.
- Avoid overexertion.

When to Call Your Doctor

- If you experience severe fatigue, chest pain, or shortness of breath. Because the anemia of thalassemia minor is mild, most persons with this disorder do not have medical emergencies due to the thalassemia.

For More Information
MedWeb Hematology: http://www.gen.emory.edu/medweb.hematology.html
MedMark Hematology: http://medmark.bit.co.kr/hematol.html
National Heart, Lung, and Blood Institute Information Center
P.O. Box 30105
Bethesda, MD 20824-0105
301-251-1222
Joint Center for Sickle Cell and Thalassemic Disorders
http://cancer.mgh.harvard.edu/medOnc/sickle.htm

THYROID NEOPLASMS

About Your Diagnosis

The thyroid is a gland in the neck that lies in front of and to the sides of the Adam's apple. The thyroid produces hormones that regulate your metabolism. The cells that make up the thyroid gland are called *follicular* and *parafollicular cells*. Thyroid cancers (neoplasms) are generally divided into those originating from the follicular cells (papillary, follicular and anaplastic) and those originating from the parafollicular cells (medullary carcinoma of the thyroid). Approximately 10,000 new cases of thyroid cancer are diagnosed each year in the United States.

Thyroid cancer is not contagious. Radiation exposure poses a risk for this cancer, especially among children who undergo radiation therapy to the head, neck, or upper chest during infancy or childhood.

In most instances, a thyroid nodule or lump is the first sign of the cancer. For a definite diagnosis, cells are removed from the lump (fine needle aspiration) and examined with a microscope. Thyroid cancers if detected and diagnosed early, before they spread beyond the thyroid gland, can be cured. The anaplastic type of thyroid cancer, however, is aggressive and resistant to treatment.

Living With Your Diagnosis

A lump in the neck is the first sign. As thyroid cancers grow, they usually spread to nearby structures, causing hoarseness, difficulty swallowing, swollen lymph glands, and neck pain.

Treatment

Sometimes the cells removed by fine needle aspiration can suggest cancer but the findings are not conclusive. In this case the physician orders a thyroid scan and an ultrasound scan of the thyroid. These two studies give clues about whether the lump is cancerous. Once the diagnosis of thyroid cancer is confirmed, treatment can be a surgical procedure, radiation therapy, or chemotherapy, depending on whether the cancer has spread beyond the thyroid gland.

Removal of the thyroid gland is called *thyroidectomy*. Surgical treatment is important because it helps determine the extent of the disease, whether the cancer has spread to nearby lymph nodes, and the type of thyroid cancer found. Complications of surgical treatment are injury to the vocal cords and removal of the small glands behind the thyroid gland called the parathyroid glands.

The nuclear material called *radioactive iodine* can be used after surgical treatment or to treat patients with known spread of the cancer to kill the cancer cells. A side effect of use of radioactive iodine is that it kills normal thyroid cells in addition to cancer cells.

Chemotherapy is used to treat patients who do not respond to surgical treatment or therapy with radioactive iodine. The side effects of chemotherapy are easy bruising, bleeding, infection, nausea, vomiting, and hair loss.

The DOs

- Take the prescribed medication after surgical treatment. Because your thyroid gland is removed, you no longer produce thyroid hormones and must take thyroid supplements.
- Find a surgeon who is experienced in thyroid operations. Surgical treatment is important, and the procedure may vary depending on the size of the tumor.
- Understand the importance of nutrition and exercise after surgical treatment.
- Remember the earlier thyroid cancer is detected, the higher are the chances of cure with treatment. It is important to evaluate any lump in the neck to look for thyroid cancer.

The DON'Ts

- Do not miss follow-up appointments with your physicians. Careful neck examinations are performed to look for lumps that may have recurred. Blood tests and thyroid scans are performed to look for evidence that the cancer has returned.
- Do not forget there are different types of thyroid cancers. The papillary type is the most common and occurs among young persons. The follicular type occurs among an older group of patients. The medullary type can occur sporadically or in a hereditary form. The hereditary form tends to be associated with other diseases that produce excess hormones (adrenaline, parathyroid hormone) called pheochromocytoma and hyperparathyroidism. A blood test (calcitonin level) helps determine whether the medullary type of thyroid cancer has returned after surgical treatment.

When to Call Your Doctor
- If you notice a lump in your neck.
- If you have hoarseness.
- If you have hand tremors (hands shaking), diarrhea, sweats, and palpitations. This may mean you are taking too much thyroid medication after surgical treatment.
- If you have an intolerance to cold, a raspy voice, constipation, loss of hair over the eyebrows along with weight gain. This may mean you are taking too little thyroid medication.
- If after an operation you notice numbness around your mouth, the tips of your fingers, and feet along with muscle spasms of your hands, legs, or face. This can indicate a low calcium level. This can happen when the parathyroid glands are removed with the thyroid gland.

For More Information
National Cancer Institute (NCI)
9000 Rockville Pike
Bethesda, MD 20892
Cancer Information Service
1-800-422-6237 (1-800-4-CANCER)
American Cancer Society
1599 Clifton Road, N.E.
Atlanta, GA 30329
1-800-ACS-2345

THYROID NODULE

About Your Diagnosis

A thyroid nodule is any discrete lump on the thyroid gland.

Thyroid nodules may be caused by a localized infection, a cyst, a benign tumor, or a malignant tumor of the thyroid. The vast majority of nodules are benign tumors or fluid-filled cysts; however, some are a thyroid cancer. For this reason, all thyroid nodules should be investigated.

Thyroid nodules are extremely common, occurring in up to 5% of the population. Many individuals do not realize they have a nodule.

Thyroid nodules may be noticed by patients when they look in the mirror, or by a physician at a routine office visit. Nodules may be noted by radiologists when images are taken of the chest or neck. Once detected, two important questions must be answered:
- Is the thyroid functioning normally?
- Is the nodule benign or malignant?

Thyroid function blood tests will determine whether the thyroid is functioning normally. If it is overactive, a special test called a radioactive iodine scan is performed to see whether this is a solitary, hyperfunctioning nodule that requires medical treatment.

Most patients have normal thyroid function and require a fine- needle aspiration biopsy (FNAB) to ensure that the nodule is not a cancer. This may be performed directly or under ultrasound guidance, depending on the location of the nodule.

The majority of nodules are benign and easily treated with medications that help prevent nodule growth. Some patients may require surgery to remove benign thyroid nodules if they cause local compressive symptoms in the neck. Thyroid cancer is cured by surgery when detected before spread outside of the thyroid gland. Long-term survival is the rule, even in patients in whom the entire cancer cannot be removed at surgery. Certain types of thyroid cancers are more aggressive, however.

Living With Your Diagnosis

Some patients may have no symptoms of their disease. Others may notice a soft, painless swelling in the area of the thyroid gland. Hot nodules cause symptoms of anxiety, sweating, weight loss, hunger, and tremor. A rock-hard nodule that rapidly grows and is associated with hoarseness or difficulty swallowing is suggestive of cancer, especially if other lumps are noted elsewhere in the neck.

Most nodules are benign cold nodules, having no effect on an individual's health. Hot nodules may cause hyperthyroidism. Cancerous nodules may spread beyond the thyroid.

Treatment

Large nodules that compress the windpipe, or nodules found to be suspicious of cancer at FNAB, are surgically removed. If tumor was left behind in the neck, radioactive iodine is given as a single tablet by mouth to destroy the remaining cancer cells. This treatment will make the patient hypothyroid, and replacement thyroid hormone therapy is given with levothyroxine. Cystic nodules that contain fluid are drained at the time of FNAB. Benign, solid nodules are diagnosed by FNAB and treated with levothyroxine to help prevent further nodule growth.

Possible complications of surgery include local bleeding, infection, a low calcium level caused by parathyroid gland damage, or vocal damage caused by cutting a nerve that runs through the neck to the vocal cords. In experienced hands, complications occur in less than 2% of operations. Excess hormone replacement for benign nodules can lead to mild hyperthyroidism. Radioactive iodine therapy may cause swelling and drying of the parotid or salivary glands. Very high doses have been associated with chronic lung disease.

The DOs
- Obtain a FNAB of any prominent nodule in the thyroid.
- Find an experienced surgeon if necessary.
- Examine your neck regularly.
- Tell your doctor if you have had a history of radiation therapy to the neck, or a family history of thyroid cancer.

The DON'Ts
- Don't speak or swallow while the doctor performs the FNAB.
- Don't obtain a radioactive iodine scan to evaluate the nodule unless blood tests confirm that you are hyperthyroid. You will still need a FNAB unless you are hyperthyroid as a result of a hot nodule.

When to Call Your Doctor

- You notice any new nodule in the thyroid or any rapid growth of an old nodule, even if a biopsy specimen of this nodule had been obtained in the past and found to be benign.
- You have hoarseness, difficulty swallowing, or difficulty breathing.
- You have bleeding, fever, or infection after FNAB or surgery.
- You feel weak or notice facial twitching, or numbness around the lips after thyroid surgery. These are signs of a low blood calcium level and require immediate attention.

For More Information

Thyroid Foundation of America, Inc.
Ruth Sleeper Hall, RSL 350
40 Parkman Street
Boston, MA 02114-2698
1-800-832-8321
Thyroid Society for Education and Research
7515 South Main Street, Suite 545
Houston, TX 77030
1-800-THYROID
The American Thyroid Association
http://www.thyroid.org/patient
American Association of Clinical Endocrinologists
701 Fisk Street, Suite 100
Jacksonville, FL 32204
904-353-7878
http:\\www.aace.com

THYROIDITIS

About Your Diagnosis

The thyroid is a small gland located in the center of the neck and is important for regulating metabolism. Thyroiditis literally means inflammation of the thyroid. The inflammatory reaction may result in either an overactive or an underactive thyroid gland.

The most common type of thyroiditis is called Hashimoto's thyroiditis. This occurs when the body's own immune system attacks the thyroid cells, leading to decreased hormone production (hypothyroidism). Subacute and silent thyroiditis result in an overactive thyroid (hyperthyroidism), which resolves spontaneously over several weeks. Finally, postpartum thyroiditis occurs in women who were recently pregnant. Patients may go through both a hyperthyroid and hypothyroid phase of several weeks' duration before returning to normal thyroid function. Some patients, however, may remain permanently hypothyroid.

Hashimoto's thyroiditis is a common disorder, occurring approximately 10 times more commonly in women than men. Up to 2% of women in the United States may be affected. Silent and subacute thyroiditis are much less common than Hashimoto's disease, but recent evidence suggests that postpartum thyroiditis may occur in up to 5% to 7% of normal pregnancies, especially affecting those women who have a history of thyroid abnormalities before they were pregnant.

Thyroiditis is detected through a careful medical history, physical examination, and measurement of blood tests, including thyroid hormone (T4 and T3), thyroid-stimulating hormone (TSH), and antithyroid antibodies. A radioactive iodine uptake (RAIU) may be measured in certain circumstances to help establish the diagnosis. In Hashimoto's disease, the thyroid gland is mildly enlarged and has a lumpy texture. The T4 and T3 levels are low, and TSH levels are high, indicating hypothyroidism. The majority of patients have antibodies detected in the blood that react against the thyroid. Subacute thyroiditis occurs after a viral infection; the thyroid gland is enlarged and painful. An elevated erythrocyte sedimentation rate (ESR) is noted. The T4 and T3 levels are elevated and the TSH is suppressed. The RAIU is low. Silent thyroiditis has a presentation that is similar to subacute thyroiditis, except that the physical examination is normal. Postpartum thyroiditis is diagnosed in women 3–8 months after pregnancy. Depending on the timing of the blood work, the patient may be either hyperthyroid or hypothyroid. The RAIU is low.

Thyroiditis is curable with appropriate medical treatment.

Living With Your Diagnosis

Signs and symptoms of thyroiditis vary depending on the type of thyroiditis and gland activity. Symptoms of hyperthyroidism, seen in silent, subacute, or early postpartum thyroiditis include weight loss, increased appetite, diarrhea, irregular menses, racing heart beat, anxiety, heat intolerance, and tremulousness. Patients who are hypothyroid, such as those with Hashimoto's or late postpartum thyroiditis, may have weight gain, decreased appetite, constipation, fatigue, depression, cold intolerance, and weakness.

If not treated, Hashimoto's can progress to severe hypothyroidism with a decreased blood pressure and coma (myxedema). Silent thyroiditis usually resolves spontaneously after several weeks. Subacute thyroiditis may cause neck pain and swelling. Postpartum thyroiditis may have no effects, or may cause anxiety in the hyperthyroid phase, and depression and fatigue in the hypothyroid phase.

Treatment

Hashimoto's disease is treated by replacing the missing thyroid hormone. Most patients require between 75 and 150 micrograms of levothyroxine daily. Geriatric patients may require significantly less medicine. Levothyroxine is safe and well tolerated. Rapid replacement may exacerbate underlying coronary artery disease. Silent and subacute thyroiditis may resolve spontaneously without treatment or may require anti-inflammatory medicines, such as a nonsteroidal anti-inflammatory drug (NSAID) or prednisone for pain. A beta-adrenergic blocking drug such as Inderal or atenolol may be required for rapid heartbeats. This medication should be slowly tapered once symptoms abate.

The DOs

- Learn about the type of thyroiditis you have and whether your thyroid is overactive or underactive.
- Take your medication treatment as prescribed.
- Tell your doctor if you are pregnant or breastfeeding or wish to become pregnant soon.

The DON'Ts

- Don't wait to seek treatment if you feel poorly.
- Don't expect overnight response to treatment. Treatment requires 4–6 weeks before patients begin to feel better.
- Don't have an RAIU if you are pregnant or breast-feeding.
- Don't exercise vigorously if you are symptomatically hyperthyroid or hypothyroid.
- Don't overeat.

When to Call Your Doctor

- You have chest pain, chest pressure, or palpitations after starting thyroid hormone replacement.
- You are pregnant, breast-feeding, or planning to become pregnant.
- You have a high fever or other severe illness.
- You have a rash or other reaction to your medications.
- You continue to feel poorly despite treatment for several weeks.

For More Information

American Thyroid Association
Montefiore Medical Center
111 East 210 Street, Room 311
Bronx, NY 10467
718-882-6047
http:\\www.thyroid.org\patient\.
Thyroid Foundation of America, Inc.
Ruth Sleeper Hall, Room 350
40 Parkman Street, Boston, MA 02114-2698
1-800-832-8321 or 617-726-8500
Thyroid Society for Education and Research
7515 South Main Street, Suite 545
Houston, TX 77030
1-800-THYROID or 717-799-9909
The Thyroid Foundation of Canada http://home.ican.net/~thyroid/guides.

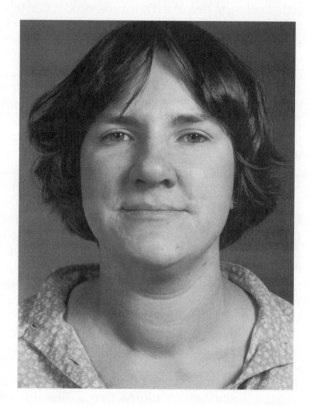

Thirty-year-old patient with Hashimoto's thyroiditis and hypothyroidism. Presenting complaint was thyroid enlargement. T4=4.5 µg/dl, TSH=84 µU/ml. Note puffiness of face and visible goiter. (From Noble J: *Textbook Primary Care Medicine*, vol 2. St. Louis, Mosby–Year Book, Inc., 1995. Used by permission.)

TINEA CAPITIS

About Your Diagnosis

Tinea capitis of the scalp is a common childhood disease that is often confused with other conditions of the scalp. It frequently results in patchy hair loss. Although usually called ringworm because of its round appearance, tinea capitis is actually caused by a very common fungus. It rarely affects infants and adults. The most common age for infection is 2–10 years. It is transmitted by contact with other infected humans or from infected animals. Because symptoms are frequently minimal, it can go untreated for long periods. Tinea capitis is readily cured but usually requires weeks to months of treatment with medication taken by mouth. It is usually diagnosed by a doctor with a skin examination and cultures of a small sample of hair or infected skin. These are examined under a microscope. Culture results are usually available in 3 or 4 weeks.

Living With Your Diagnosis

Symptoms may be mild and initially include redness and swelling of the scalp, followed by hair loss. Pustules may be present. In some cases, a tender, swollen area with drainage may be present. When severe, tinea capitis can also cause fever and enlarged lymph nodes.

Treatment

Tinea capitis of the scalp should always be treated under the direction of your doctor. Medications by mouth can cure tinea capitis, but treatment usually takes weeks to months. It is very important to continue the entire course of treatment and follow your doctor's instructions until your doctor tells you to stop treatment; otherwise you will be prone to have recurrences. Medications by mouth are taken once or twice a day. Rarely these medications cause changes in liver function tests, and your doctor may periodically examine your stomach or order laboratory tests if necessary. Your doctor may also prescribe special creams or shampoos if necessary.

The DOs
- Avoid contact with infected individuals.
- Wash hair after every haircut.
- Continue treatment until your doctor tells you to stop.

- Check pets for skin infection or irritation, and consult your veterinarian if present.
- Check brothers and sisters for ringworm of the scalp.

The DON'Ts
- Don't share combs, brushes, or hats.
- Close haircuts, shaving the head, or wearing caps are not necessary as long as you are taking your medication.

When to Call Your Doctor

- If fever, pus drainage, or swelling occurs.
- If other areas of the scalp or body become involved, despite treatment.
- If tinea capitis recurs after you have completed the course of treatment.

For More Information
American Academy of Dermatology
930 N. Meacham Road
Schaumburg, IL 60173
847-330-0230

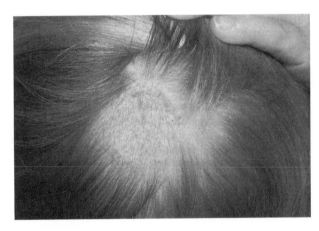

Tinea capitis. Note scaling and alopecia. (Courtesy of Department of Dermatology, University of North Carolina at Chapel Hill. From Goldstein BG, Goldstein AO: *Practical Dermatology*, vol 1. St. Louis, Mosby–Year Book, 1992. Used by permission.)

TINEA CORPORIS

About Your Diagnosis

Tinea corporis is a common superficial skin infection caused by a fungus. Although frequently called ringworm, it is actually caused by a very common fungus. This minor skin infection occurs worldwide and is usually transmitted by contact from infected humans and animals, as well as from clothing, towels, or anywhere the fungus may come to rest, such as showers. Tinea corporis is usually diagnosed on visual inspection, but occasionally a microscopic analysis or culture may be helpful. It is usually cured with 2–4 weeks of treatment.

Living With Your Diagnosis

Involved areas on the skin are well-defined, slightly raised, somewhat circular patches. They are usually red or discolored and have a central clearing. There can be scaling or small blisters present. Itching is common. Scratching can cause swelling, weeping, and secondary infection. Scratching can also cause the infection to spread to other parts of the body.

Treatment

Apply a topical antifungal cream or ointment available without a prescription from any pharmacy, or use the medication prescribed by your doctor. Creams should be continued for 7 days after the area has cleared to prevent recurrence. Treat all affected areas no matter how small, even those that may have just started. If you have been prescribed medication to take orally, be certain to complete the entire course of therapy.

The DOs

- Keep all affected areas clean and dry.
- Wash and dry off, then apply cream.
- Wash towels and bedding more frequently while infected with tinea corporis.
- Check pets for infection. If frequent scratching or abnormal-appearing skin or hair loss exists, consult your veterinarian.
- Wear cotton clothing. Change clothing frequently to prevent skin from becoming damp or moist skin.
- Periodically inspect skin for early recurrences and treat promptly.

The DON'Ts

- Don't share bath towels.
- Don't wear nylon or synthetic clothing over affected areas because this keeps moisture in contact with the skin.
- Avoid wearing clothing that chafes the skin.
- Avoid direct contact with individuals with tinea corporis.

When to Call Your Doctor

- If the rash is not improved after 1–2 weeks of treatment.
- If any signs of a secondary infection exist, such as fever, pus drainage, oozing, crusting, or swelling.
- If any scarring or bleeding occur.

For More Information
American Academy of Dermatology
930 N. Meacham Road
Schaumburg, IL 60173
847-330-0230

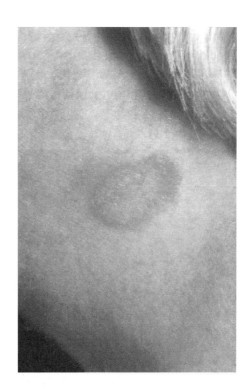

Tinea corporis. Note well-demarcated erythematous plaques with central clearing and peripheral scale. (Courtesy of Department of Dermatology, University of North Carolina at Chapel Hill. From Goldstein BG, Goldstein AO: *Practical Dermatology*, vol 1. St. Louis, Mosby–Year Book, 1992. Used by permission.)

TINEA CRURIS

About Your Diagnosis

Tinea cruris is a very common superficial fungal infection of the skin in the area of the groin and upper thighs. It occurs most often in men and adolescent boys. Factors that increase risk for infection include tinea pedis (athlete's foot), obesity, hot humid weather, and use of public baths or showers. Tinea cruris is caused by a very common fungus. The diagnosis is usually made by examination of the skin, but cultures or inspection under a microscope may occasionally be helpful. Tinea cruris can be cured in 2–3 weeks with appropriate treatment.

Living With Your Diagnosis

Involved skin is usually slightly raised, red to brown, and itches. There may be patches, scaling, or small blisters. Both sides of the groin are usually affected. Itching is a common symptom. As long as redness and scaling are present, you are contagious. Scratching can cause oozing, swelling, and secondary infection.

Treatment

Apply a topical antifungal cream or ointment available without a prescription from any pharmacy, or use the medication prescribed by your doctor. Continue the cream for 7 days after the area has cleared. If you have been prescribed medication to be taken orally, be certain to complete the course of therapy as prescribed.

The DOs

- During and after treatment to help healing and prevent recurrence, always dry the groin first and the feet last after bathing or showering.
- Wear loose-fitting, washed cotton underwear. Change underwear daily or more often to keep the groin dry.

The DON'Ts

- Don't share towels.
- Don't touch or scratch feet and then touch the groin area.
- Don't wear nylon or other synthetic underwear that keep moisture in the groin area.
- Avoid wearing garments that chafe the skin.

When to Call Your Doctor

- If the rash is not improved after 1–2 weeks of treatment.
- If signs of a secondary infection occur, such as fever, pus drainage, oozing, crusting, or swelling.
- If any scarring or bleeding is present.

For More Information

American Academy of Dermatology
930 N. Meacham Road
Schaumburg, IL 60173
847-330-0230

TINEA PEDIS

About Your Diagnosis

Tinea pedis is an infection of the foot caused by a fungus. It is one of the most common infections in humans. Tinea pedis is most frequently seen in adolescents and adults during the warm months, but can occur at any time. Certain factors increase risk for this infection including moist, sweaty feet and socks, hot humid weather, and use of public showers. The diagnosis is usually made based on the clinical examination, although occasionally fungal cultures may be obtained if necessary. Tinea pedis can be cured in 2–3 weeks, but recurrence is frequent without strict preventive measures.

Living With Your Diagnosis

The most common symptoms are cracked and boggy skin between the toes, associated with itching. Scaling, dead skin, and small blisters are sometimes present, as well as musty or unpleasant odor. Scratching can cause an inflamed or weeping rash to occur.

Treatment

It is important to keep the feet dry. Wear sandals or go barefoot if possible. Wash feet and then remove scales and dead skin. Apply an antifungal powder, cream, or ointment, available without a prescription from any pharmacy, or use a topical antifungal medication prescribed by your doctor. To prevent recurrence, continue the medication for 1 week after the symptoms and rash disappear.

The DOs

- During treatment and to prevent recurrence, wash and dry feet at least once per day.
- Always wear clean, dry socks made of cotton or wool.
- Change socks daily or more often if necessary to keep feet dry.
- Wear sandals instead of going barefoot when in public places such as locker rooms or showers.
- Wash and dry your feet immediately after exercising.

The DON'Ts

- Don't scratch your feet.
- Don't wear synthetic socks. These keep moisture around the feet.

When to Call Your Doctor

- If rash does not improve after treating for 1 week.
- If signs of a secondary infection occur, such as fever, pus drainage, or red streaks on the foot.

For More Information

American Academy of Dermatology
930 N. Meacham Road
Schaumburg, IL 60173
847-330-0230

Tinea pedis. Note erythematous, scaling plaques. (Courtesy of Department of Dermatology, University of North Carolina at Chapel Hill. From Goldstein BG, Goldstein AO: *Practical Dermatology*, vol 1. St. Louis, Mosby–Year Book, 1992. Used by permission.)

TINEA UNGUIUM

About Your Diagnosis

Tinea unguium is a fungal infection of the nails. It most commonly affects the toenails, rarely the fingernails. Tinea of the toenail occurs most often in patients with recurrent attacks of tinea of the feet (athlete's foot). It is seen most often in the elderly but can be seen in young adults. The diagnosis is usually made by inspection, but may be confirmed by obtaining a culture of the infected toenail or by examining it under a microscope. Tinea unguium is not life threatening unless a serious secondary infection occurs in patients such as diabetics. Tinea unguium is difficult to eliminate even with prescription medication, and many patients learn to "live" with this disease.

Living With Your Diagnosis

Patients with tinea unguium have thickened and deformed or distorted toenails. The nail frequently begins to detach at the end or side. Secondary infection can occur, especially with poorly fitting shoes. Secondary infection requires treatment with prescription antibiotics.

Treatment

Tinea of the fingernails can frequently be cured with an extended course of medications taken by mouth. Take these for as long as you doctor has prescribed. Occasionally these medications cause changes in the liver; therefore your doctor may request periodic laboratory tests and close follow-up. Tinea of the toenails is usually not curable, and therefore medications by mouth are usually not used. Trimming of thick nails can provide relief of discomfort. This should be done under the direction of your physician. If you are diabetic or have other medical diseases associated with poor circulation, consult your doctor before trimming your toenails.

The DOs

- Inspect your feet daily. Report any signs of infection such as swelling or drainage to your doctor.
- Wash your feet daily and keep them clean and dry.
- Wear cotton socks that absorb sweat.

The DON'Ts

- Don't share nail-trimming instruments.
- Don't wear tight-fitting shoes.

When to Call Your Doctor

- If pus drainage, swelling, or redness occurs in the area of the nail.
- If the nail becomes painful to touch.

For More Information
American Academy of Dermatology
930 N. Meacham Road
Schaumburg, IL 60173
847-330-0230

TINEA VERSICOLOR

About Your Diagnosis

Tinea versicolor is a common skin disorder caused by a type of yeast. This yeast is normally found on the skin of most individuals. During hot, humid weather the yeast can overgrow and cause changes in the skin. Tinea versicolor is not considered to be contagious. It is usually diagnosed on visual inspection, but examination of a small sample of infected skin under a microscope can be helpful. Tinea versicolor is treatable but cure usually takes weeks to months.

Living With Your Diagnosis

Tinea versicolor starts as small, tan, scaly patches on the skin, most commonly on the back and upper chest. The neck and arms can also be affected. These can grow and come together to form large patches. When exposed to the sun, the patches do not tan, so they appear lighter than surrounding skin.

Treatment

Lotions such as selenium suspension 2<cf1/2>% are usually prescribed to treat tinea versicolor. First bathe and dry off. Apply the lotion to all the involved areas. Wash the medicine off after 24 hours, and repeat once a week for 4 weeks. Retreatment every 3 months may be necessary in some cases.

If selenium suspension irritates sensitive skin, then apply for 10 minutes only. Repeat this every day for 3 days, then once a week for 1 month. Your doctor may prescribe other topical lotions or creams if selenium does not work. In cases that do not respond to topical medications, your doctor may prescribe an antifungal medication to be taken orally. Antifungal pills taken by mouth rarely cause changes in liver function tests, and your doctor may periodically check your stomach.

The DOs

- Take all medications as prescribed, and follow your doctor's recommendations for follow-up.
- Keep skin clean and dry; dampness causes tinea versicolor to grow faster.
- Bathe and dry off every day, and wear clean cotton clothing.
- When your skin is improved, inspect it weekly for recurrences and begin treatment early. It is easier to treat smaller areas.
- Be patient. Even after treatment it can take months for pigment to return to the affected areas.
- Use sunscreen during treatment, and wear a hat and long- sleeve shirt when in the sun.

The DON'Ts

- Don't apply lotions or creams to red, inflamed, or swollen areas on the skin, or to any break in the skin.
- Avoid the sun especially from 11 AM to 3 PM. Sun tanning will cause tinea versicolor to look worse.

When to Call Your Doctor

- If not improved after 3 or 4 months.
- If any other symptoms occur such as skin redness or swelling.

For More Information
American Academy of Dermatology
930 N. Meacham Road
Schaumburg, IL 60173
847-330-0230

TONSILLITIS

About Your Diagnosis

Tonsillitis is an inflammation of the tonsils (the cluster of soft tissue at the back of the throat), caused by a viral or bacterial infection. It generally occurs in children 5–10 years of age. The duration of the disease is usually 4–6 days. Tonsillitis is contagious and is spread by direct contact with infected respiratory secretions.

Living With Your Diagnosis

Signs and symptoms include throat pain (may be mild or severe), chills and fever, swollen lymph glands, difficulty swallowing, headache, and earache.

A throat culture is needed to determine the cause and proper treatment of tonsillitis. Possible complications of tonsillitis are abscess of the tonsils; chronic tonsillitis; and rheumatic fever, if the cause is a strep infection and it is not treated.

Treatment

The best treatment includes rest and adequate fluids. If the cause is bacterial (strep), antibiotics will be prescribed for 10 days. Tylenol or Advil can be used for the pain and fever. Gargling with a salt water solution or other soothing liquid may help with the pain and irritation. A cool-mist vaporizer may also help relieve the cough and irritation. Side effects of the antibiotics include stomach upset, nausea, vomiting, or diarrhea.

The DOs

- Take antibiotics until finished.
- Increase fluid intake.
- Follow a liquid diet with soups and milkshakes if swallowing is difficult. Gradually progress to solid foods as tolerated.
- Rest in bed until the fever subsides.
- Avoid contact with others until symptoms are gone.
- Practice good hand washing to avoid spreading the infection to other family members.
- Avoid eating or drinking from the same utensils.
- Increase activity gradually after the fever has been gone for 2–3 days.

The DON'Ts

- Don't stop antibiotics until finished. Symptoms may disappear before the bacterial infection is completely cleared.
- Don't share drinking glasses or food.
- Don't give aspirin to a child because it has been shown to be associated with the development of Reye's syndrome.
- Don't eat spicy or irritating foods.

When to Call Your Doctor

- If severe swelling of the tonsils occurs and breathing becomes difficult.
- If your fever has gone away for a few days and suddenly returns (temperature greater than 101°F).
- If new symptoms appear, such as a rash, nausea, vomiting, chest pain, shortness of breath, or a cough that produces thick or discolored sputum.

For More Information
The American Academy of Pediatrics
141 NW Point Blvd.
Elk Grove Village, IL 60007-1098
Send a self-addressed, stamped, business-sized envelope to request a copy of "Tonsils and Adenoids."
Internet Site
www.healthanswers.com

TOURETTE'S SYNDROME

About Your Diagnosis

Tourette's syndrome is a type of nervous tic (habit spasm) that results in brief, purposeless, semivoluntary or involuntary movement or vocalizations that occur repeatedly in the same way. Little is known about the cause of this syndrome.

Initially the tics may be controlled, but persistent tics become automatic. The face, shoulders, or arms are most often affected. Common nervous tics of Tourette's syndrome include twitching of the corner of the mouth or eye, blinking, grimacing, shoulder shrugging, or arm movements. The most severe form of the syndrome includes bizarre noise-making, uncontrollable swearing, and troublesome sexual and aggressive impulses.

Living With Your Diagnosis:

There seems to be family clustering of this syndrome because it has been observed in other family members in one third of patients with the syndrome.

Tourette's syndrome usually begins in childhood and gradually worsens in extent and severity. During the teenage years, uncontrollable grunting, barking, sniffing, and shouting may develop. The course of this disorder is unpredictable, but in many cases it stabilizes by adulthood. In some patients the syndrome subsides and long remissions occur.

Treatment

Neuroleptic medications are most commonly used to treat this disorder. These may be prescribed independently or in combination with other medications to prevent side effects of the neuroleptic medications. New medications are currently being investigated.

The DOs

- Take your medications as prescribed.
- Monitor and record your symptoms and side effects as your medications are adjusted to assist your doctor in determining their effectiveness.
- Get an adequate amount of sleep and rest regularly.
- Become informed about support groups and other resources for patients with Tourette's syndrome.

The DON'Ts

- Don't adjust your medications without your doctor's approval.
- Don't ignore side effects of your medications.
- Don't ignore worsening of your symptoms.

When to Call Your Doctor

- If you have any difficulty associated with your medications.
- If your symptoms worsen significantly.
- If you need assistance or resources to educate others (teachers, friends, fellow employees) about the syndrome.

For More Information

World Wide Web
http://neuro-www2.mgh.harvard.edu/tsa/tsamain.nclk
Tourette Syndrome Association, Inc.
42-40 Bell Blvd., Ste. 205
Bayside, NY 11361-2820
Phone: 718-224-2999
800-237-0717
Fax: 718-279-9596
Tourette Syndrome Foundation of Canada
3675 Keele Street, Suite 203
Toronto, Ontario, CANADA, M3J 1M6
Phone: 416-636-2800
800-361-3120
Fax: 416-636-1688

TOXIC SHOCK SYNDROME

About Your Diagnosis

Toxic shock syndrome is a severe form of blood poisoning caused by toxins released by staphylococcal bacteria. It can affect both sexes, resulting from wounds or infections of the skin, lungs, throat, or bones. However, the most well-known type is associated with females using tampons during their menstrual periods.

Living With Your Diagnosis

Signs and symptoms include sudden shaking and a high fever (temperature greater than 104°F); intense muscle pain; vomiting and diarrhea; thirst; rapid pulse; a deep red rash; severe weakness; headache; sore throat; or confusion.

Treatment

Early diagnosis and hospital treatment is essential for a full recovery. Complications of the disease often include peeling of the skin of the hands and feet, loss of hair and nails, kidney failure, congestive heart failure, and respiratory distress.

Hospital treatment will include administration of intravenous fluids as well as antibiotics; management of the respiratory problems with oxygen and mechanical ventilation if needed; and dialysis if there is kidney failure.

Once the symptoms are under control and the initial dangers are over, home care can begin. Antibiotics may still be needed. Rest is important. Activities should be increased gradually. Fluid intake should be increased, and a well-balanced diet followed to regain strength. The antibiotics may have side effects such as stomach upset and diarrhea.

The DOs

- Seek treatment immediately if you have symptoms of toxic shock.
- Change tampons frequently.
- Seek medical treatment for any wounds that appear infected.
- Rest and increase activity gradually.
- Continue antibiotics until finished.
- Increase fluid intake and eat a well-balanced diet.
- Wash hands thoroughly before inserting tampons, because staph bacteria are found on the skin, especially on the hands.

The DON'Ts

- Don't skip doses or stop antibiotics unless ordered by your doctor.
- Don't ignore a wound if it looks red, swollen, or has pus.
- Don't use superabsorbant tampons, especially overnight; alternate them with sanitary napkins.
- Don't use tampons if you have a skin infection, especially near the genital area.

When to Call Your Doctor

- If you have any symptoms of toxic shock syndrome. It progresses rapidly and may be fatal if not treated.

For More Information
National Womens Health Network
202-628-7814, Monday through Friday from 9 AM to 5 PM (EST).
• Centers for Disease Control
404-639-2215
National Institute of Allergy and Infectious Disease
9000 Rockville Pike
Bethesda, MD 20892
301-496-5717

TOXOPLASMOSIS

About Your Diagnosis

Toxoplasmosis is an infection caused by a protozoa (a microscopic organism) that is found in birds, animals, and humans. The disease is most dangerous for an individual with a suppressed immune system (someone receiving chemotherapy, a patient with AIDS, or a transplant recipient) or a pregnant woman. It affects the gastrointestinal tract, heart, nerves, and skin. The disease can be transmitted by eating undercooked meat from an infected animal, especially lamb and pork, or by handling cat litter if the cat harbors the organism.

Living With Your Diagnosis

Most healthy individuals do not have any symptoms and do not require treatment. Others may have fever, fatigue, muscle aches, headache, and swollen lymph glands. Treatment is necessary for children younger than 5 years to prevent eye complications. Other complications that can occur include inflammation of the brain, heart and lung damage. Complications are more frequent in patients with a suppressed immune system. If a pregnant woman has the infection in the early stages of her pregnancy, she may miscarry, have a stillbirth, or the infant may be born with birth defects.

Treatment

Most individuals don't require treatment. Others may need prescription drugs such as sulfadiazine, trisulfapyrimidines, or pyrimethamine for 4–6 weeks. These drugs can cause side effects such as an upset stomach, sun sensitivity, bleeding, or bruising. Your doctor will do blood tests frequently to monitor the side effects. Activity levels will depend on the type of symptoms experienced. Tylenol or tepid sponge baths can be used to reduce the fever. No special diet is needed, but fluid intake should be increased.

The DOs

- Use Tylenol for aches and fever.
- Use tepid sponge baths to help reduce fever.
- Rest until symptoms subside, and gradually increase your activity.
- Continue your medication until finished or stopped by your doctor.
- Take the medication with food to decrease stomach upset.
- Keep appointments for follow-up blood work.
- Use sunscreen when outdoors because the medication may make you more sensitive to the sun.
- Have someone else change the litter box if you suspect you are pregnant, or you have a suppressed immune system.
- Properly cook meats.
- Wash your hands frequently.
- Keep a child's sandbox covered to keep cats out.
- Keep flies away from food.

The DON'Ts

- Don't eat undercooked meats, especially lamb and pork, uncooked eggs, or unpasteurized milk.
- Don't change the cat litter box if you are pregnant, have had an organ transplant, are receiving chemotherapy, or have AIDS.
- Don't stop taking your medication before it is finished unless ordered by your doctor.
- Don't stay in the sun for long periods or forget your sunscreen.

When to Call Your Doctor

- If the symptoms don't improve after you start treatment.
- If you experience any bleeding or bruising.
- If you start to have visual changes or increased weakness.

For More Information
National Heart, Lung and Blood Institute
800-575-WELL
National Institute of Allergy and Infectious Diseases
9000 Rockville Pike
Bethesda, MD 20892
301-496-5717
Internet Sites
www.healthfinder.gov (Choose SEARCH to search by topic.)

TRACHEITIS

About Your Diagnosis

Tracheitis is an inflammation of the trachea, or wind pipe. It is usually caused by a viral infection such as influenza. It may resemble croup but occurs in adults. The inflammation is treatable and resolves within a few days.

Living With Your Diagnosis

Signs and symptoms of tracheitis include a nonproductive cough that becomes worse at night; pain while inhaling, especially cold air; fever, headache, and body aches; and loss of appetite. The throat may be reddened, and there may be tenderness of the trachea.

Treatment

Rest until the symptoms subside. Nonaspirin medications such as Tylenol or Advil can be taken for the fever and body aches. A cool-mist vaporizer will help to soothe the irritated air passages. Cough syrups and lozenges may also ease the soreness. Fluid intake should be increased. If solid foods are not tolerated, a liquid or soft diet should be taken until symptoms improve. Antibiotics are not necessary unless a secondary infection occurs.

The DOs
- Rest.
- Use nonaspirin products to reduce the fever and aches.
- Use a cool-mist vaporizer at the bedside, but remember to change the water and clean the unit daily.
- Increase your fluid intake.

The DON'Ts
- Don't eat spicy foods or drink acidic juices or alcohol that may irritate the throat.

When to Call Your Doctor
- If you have a high fever.
- If you experience difficulty breathing.
- If you have difficulty swallowing liquids.

For More Information

American Lung Association
800-LUNG-USA (800-586-4872)
National Jewish Center for Immunology and Respiratory Medicine
1400 Jackson Street
Denver, CO 80206
800-333-5864, Monday through Friday from 8AM to 5 PM (MST), for a nurse to answer questions and send information; or 800-552-5864, for recorded information.
Internet Sites
www.healthfinder.gov (Choose SEARCH to search by topic.)
www.healthanswers.com

TRANSIENT ISCHEMIC ATTACK

About Your Diagnosis

Transient ischemic attacks, by definition, are focal neurologic abnormalies of sudden onset and brief duration (less than 24 hours). Most TIAs last less than 10 minutes and may be caused by a temporary interruption or reduction of blood flow to a specific part of the brain. The symptoms depend upon the part of the arterial blood system to the brain that is affected. Consciousness remains intact throughout the episode.

Transient ischemic attacks are often caused by a plaque or blood clot in the artery that blocks blood flow. The body naturally breaks down these plaques, restoring blood flow and allowing the symptoms to resolve. Transient ischemic attacks are most common in the middle-aged and elderly but, although rare, may occur in young individuals with heart disease.

The attacks are usually recurrent and may forecast an impending stroke.

Living With Your Diagnosis

The following are some of the more common symptoms of a TIA:
- Weakness or numbness on one side of the face or body (face, arm, leg).
- Changes in vision.
- Confusion.
- Dizziness.
- Binocular blindness.
- Double vision.
- Slurred speech, inability to talk, or difficulty swallowing.
- Loss of coordination or balance.

In 70% of cases, the symptoms of a TIA will resolve in less than 10 minutes, and in 90% they will resolve in less than 4 hours. A TIA is a warning sign that you are at risk for a stroke.

Treatment

In addition to treating the underlying conditions (high blood pressure, diabetes, tobacco abuse, sedentary lifestyle, and high cholesterol level), the treatment of TIAs is aimed at preventing strokes. For most patients this will involve medications to prevent blood clot formation in the heart or arteries supplying the brain. Often this is as simple as taking a small amount of aspirin each day. However, if the symptoms are severe or frequent, a more potent "blood thinner" may be needed. Some TIAs are caused by plaques or clots in the large arteries of the neck. An ultrasound study of the arteries in your neck may be necessary to determine the probable cause of your symptoms, and whether surgery is necessary.

The DOs

- Take note of the conditions and symptoms when you have a TIA.
  - What kind of activity were you doing when it occurred?
  - Exactly what symptoms did you have?
  - How long did your symptoms last?
  - When did they occur?
- Take only the medications prescribed by your doctor. Some of these medications may require you to get blood tests on a regular basis.
- If you have other medical problems, such as diabetes, a high cholesterol level, or high blood pressure, be sure that your physician is aware of those problems and that they are being managed as well.
- Keep your follow-up appointments with your doctor.

The DON'Ts

- Don't use tobacco products because they promote and accelerate the development of vascular disease and will increase your risk of stroke.
- Don't eat a high-fat diet.
- Avoid driving or doing any activity in which a sudden onset of the symptoms described above could put you or others in danger.
- Don't delay in reporting recurrent symptoms to your doctor.
- Avoid strenuous activities and exertion.

When to Call Your Doctor

- If you have another TIA after beginning medication.
- If you have an unusually severe headache.
- If you have any problems associated with your medication.

For More Information

National Stroke Association
96 Inverness Drive East, Suite I
Englewood, CO 80112-5112
303-649-9299
World Wide Web
http://neuro-www.mgh.harvard.edu/
Robert's Neurology Listings on the Web http://
mediswww.meds.cwru.edu/dept/neurology/robslist.html

TRICHINOSIS

About Your Diagnosis

Trichinosis is an infection caused by the larvae of a parasitic roundworm that lives in the intestines of pigs. It is transmitted to individuals when they eat the meat of an infected animal and the meat has not been cooked well enough to kill the parasite. Within 2 days of eating infected meat, the parasite matures and the female burrows into the intestinal wall to produce living larvae. By the seventh day, they are carried into the bloodstream and live in the muscles. Trichinosis is curable with treatment. Complications can include congestive heart failure, respiratory failure, or kidney damage.

Living With Your Diagnosis

In the early stage of the infection, diarrhea, a low-grade fever, nausea, and vomiting occur. Seven to 10 days later, the eyelids and face may become puffy. Muscle pain, headache, weakness, shortness of breath, high fever, and itching and burning of the skin also occur.

Treatment

Medications to kill the parasite should be taken as prescribed by your doctor. Tylenol or tepid sponge baths can be used to reduce fever. You should rest in bed until the symptoms subside, and gradually resume normal activities. Maintaining proper nutrition is important. Your appetite will be decreased, so it may be helpful to eat small frequent meals.

The DOs

- Take the medication as directed.
- Bed rest is most important until symptoms are gone.
- Resume normal activities gradually after symptoms are gone.
- Use Tylenol for fever and pain.
- Maintain proper nutrition by eating small, frequent meals.
- Increase fluid intake to prevent dehydration.

The DON'Ts

- Don't drive or operate heavy machinery while taking antiparasitic medications. Most of these can cause drowsiness, dizziness, nausea, or diarrhea.
- Don't skip doses of the medication. Usually the course of medication is short, but if you cannot tolerate it notify your doctor.
- Don't eat undercooked meat to prevent infections in the future.

When to Call Your Doctor

- If you are having side effects from the medication and cannot tolerate them.
- If you have a temperature of more than 104°F, shortness of breath, or an irregular heartbeat.

For More Information

National Institute of Allergy and Infectious Diseases of the NIH
Office of Communications
9000 Rockville Pike
Bethesda, MD 20892
301-496-5717
Internet Sites
www.healthfinder.gov (Choose SEARCH to search by topic.)
www.healthanswers.com
For information regarding the proper cooking of meats:
The National Center for Nutrition
800-366-1655
The Department of Agriculture, Meat and Poultry Hotline
800-535-4555

TRICUSPID REGURGITATION

About Your Diagnosis

The tricuspid valve is between the right atrium and right ventricle in the heart. The valve opens when the atrium contracts to allow blood to flow into the ventricle. It closes when the ventricle contracts to prevent back flow (regurgitation) of blood into the atrium. If there is regurgitation, blood does not flow through easily, which makes the ventricle work too hard. Abnormalities in the tricuspid valve are unusual. When present, they often exist with abnormalities of other valves, such as mitral stenosis. The damage may be congenital (present at birth) or caused by enlargement of the right ventricle. It may be from infections in the heart such as rheumatic fever (from a previous streptococcal infection) or bacterial endocarditis.

Living With Your Diagnosis

There may be no symptoms of tricuspid regurgitation. However, because tricuspid regurgitation often exists with mitral stenosis, symptoms may develop. Symptoms that do occur usually begin many years after the bout with rheumatic fever and are associated with symptoms of heart failure. Swelling in the legs or abdomen (causing tenderness in the liver) or difficulty with breathing, especially when you are lying down, may occur. Other symptoms include irregular heartbeat, coughing up blood, or chest pain. Atrial fibrillation may develop, and the atrium does not contract normally. Because blood pools in the atrium if the atrium is not contracting normally, clots may form. These blood clots may travel out of the heart when normal contractions resume. Because of this possibility, some patients undergo an operation to have their valve widened or replaced.

Heart valve disease is diagnosed on the basis of symptoms and findings at a physical examination. Blood moving abnormally through the valve makes an abnormal sound called a *murmur*. The timing of the murmur in the cardiac cycle and the location of the murmur help determine which valve is affected. An echocardiogram (ultrasound examination of the heart) shows the abnormal valve and is used to assess blood flow through the valve. Chest radiographs (x-rays) often show the right atrium and ventricle enlarged from overfilling and leakage of fluid into the lungs. An ECG may show arrhythmias such as atrial fibrillation, which occur if the changes in the atrium affect the electrical system of the heart. This may cause palpitations or a rapid heartbeat.

Treatment

Treatment varies depending on severity. If the condition is mild, attempts are made to prevent possible complications. An abnormally functioning valve may be a target for an infection in the heart called *endocarditis*. Antibiotics are routinely given to patients with known mitral regurgitation for dental or surgical procedures and for bacterial infections. Digitalis (digoxin) may be given for atrial fibrillation and heart failure. Some patients with atrial fibrillation also are given anticoagulant medications to try to prevent a blood clot from forming in the atrium. If there is evidence of heart failure, diuretics reduce fluid volume in the blood so the heart does not have to work as hard. Vasodilators such as nitrates, hydralazine, captopril, or enalapril may be used when heart failure becomes more prominent. If the heart failure becomes unmanageable with medication or the ability of the heart to keep working is threatened, heart valve replacement may be needed.

Side effects of the medications include allergies to antibiotics or the other drugs listed. Digoxin levels in the blood have to be checked periodically. Diuretics cause frequent urination and can cause dehydration and electrolyte (salt) abnormalities in the blood. Extra potassium pills may be needed with the diuretics, and these can cause nausea, vomiting, or diarrhea. Nitrate medications may cause headaches or dizziness. The other vasodilators may cause lightheadedness, fatigue, and intestinal problems.

The DOs

- Take your medications as prescribed.
- Restrict the fluid and salt in your diet if symptoms of heart failure are present.
- Remember to take antibiotics as prescribed before and after dental or surgical treatments, including tooth cleanings.
- Exercise as tolerated.

The DON'Ts

- Do not overexert yourself. If easy exercise is becoming difficult, rest until examined by your doctor.

When to Call Your Doctor

•If you have side effects to your medications or have new or worsening symptoms such as chest pain, shortness of breath, palpitations or rapid heartbeat, or swelling in the legs or abdomen.
•If you are taking anticoagulants and have a cut that does not stop bleeding or sustain a head injury.

For More Information
Contact the American Heart Association at 1-800-242-8721 and ask for the literature department.

TRICUSPID STENOSIS

About Your Diagnosis

The tricuspid valve is between the right atrium and right ventricle in the heart. Stenosis is a narrowing in the opening of the valve. The valve opens when the atrium contracts to allow blood to flow into the ventricle. It closes to prevent back flow of blood into the atrium when the ventricle contracts. If the opening is narrow, blood does not flow easily. This makes the atrium work too hard. An abnormality in this valve is unusual; when present, it often exists with abnormalities of other valves, such as mitral stenosis. The damage may be congenital (present at birth) or from infections in the heart such as rheumatic fever (from previous streptococcal infection) or bacterial endocarditis.

Living With Your Diagnosis

There may be no symptoms of tricuspid stenosis. However, because the condition often exists with mitral stenosis, symptoms may develop. Symptoms that do occur usually begin many years after the bout with rheumatic fever and are associated with symptoms of right heart failure. Difficulty with breathing, especially when lying down, commonly occurs. Other, more severe symptoms include irregular heartbeat, coughing up blood, or swelling in the legs and abdomen. Atrial fibrillation may develop, and the atrium does not contract normally. Because blood pools in the atrium if the atrium is not contracting normally, clots may form. This may cause blood clots to travel out of the heart when normal contractions resume. Because of this possibility, some patients undergo an operation to have the valve widened or replaced.

Heart valve disease is diagnosed on the basis of symptoms and findings at a physical examination. Blood moving abnormally through the valve makes an abnormal sound called a *murmur*. The timing of the murmur in the cardiac cycle and the location of the murmur help determine which valve is affected. An echocardiogram (ultrasound examination of the heart) shows the abnormal valve and is used to assess blood flow through the valve. Chest radiographs (x-rays) often show the right atrium and ventricle enlarged from overfilling and leakage of fluid into the lungs. An electrocardiogram (ECG) may show arrhythmias such as atrial fibrillation. These occur if the changes in the atrium affect the electrical system of the heart.

Treatment

Treatment varies depending on the severity of the stenosis. If the condition is mild, attempts are made to prevent possible complications. Abnormally functioning valves may be a target for an infection in the heart called *endocarditis*. Antibiotics are routinely given to patients with known mitral regurgitation for dental or surgical procedures and for bacterial infections. Digitalis (digoxin) may be given for atrial fibrillation and heart failure. Some patients with atrial fibrillation take anticoagulant medications to try to prevent a blood clot from forming in the atrium. If there is evidence of heart failure, diuretics reduce the fluid volume in the blood so the heart does not have to work as hard. Vasodilators such as nitrates, hydralazine, captopril, or enalapril may be used when heart failure becomes more prominent. If the heart failure becomes unmanageable with medication or the ability of the heart to keep working is threatened, heart valve replacement may be needed.

Side effects of the medications include allergies to antibiotics or the other drugs listed. Digoxin levels in the blood have to be checked periodically. Diuretics cause frequent urination and can cause dehydration and electrolyte (salt) abnormalities in the blood. Extra potassium pills may have to be taken with the diuretics, and these can cause nausea, vomiting, or diarrhea. Nitrate medications may cause headaches or dizziness, and the other vasodilators may cause lightheadedness, fatigue, and intestinal problems.

The DOs
- Take your medications as prescribed.
- Restrict fluid and salt in your diet if you have symptoms of heart failure.
- Remember to take antibiotics as prescribed before and after dental or surgical treatments, including tooth cleanings.
- Exercise as tolerated.

The DON'Ts
- Do not overexert yourself. If easy exercise is becoming difficult, rest until examined by your doctor.

When to Call Your Doctor
- If you have side effects to your medications or have new or worsening symptoms such as chest pain, shortness of breath, palpitations or rapid

heartbeat, or swelling in the legs or abdomen.
• If you are taking anticoagulants and have a cut that does not stop bleeding or sustain a head injury.

For More Information
Contact the American Heart Association at 1-800-242-8721 and ask for the literature department.

TRIGEMINAL NEURALGIA

About Your Diagnosis

Trigeminal neuralgia is a disorder that causes intense, stabbing, "electric shock–like" pain in the areas of the face where the nerve is distributed—jaw, lips, eyes, nose, scalp, forehead, and face. It rarely occurs in patients younger than 50 years, and it is nearly twice as common in women. In most cases the cause is unknown, although some patients have had this disorder after tooth extraction, facial nerve injury, herpes virus infection, or compression from a blood vessel or tumor.

Living With Your Diagnosis

Trigeminal neuralgia can often be relieved with medication. For those patients who do not get adequate relief or who have unacceptable side effects from their medication, there are several surgical options available that may provide partial or complete relief of pain. Many patients learn what the "trigger points" are that cause their pain and learn ways to avoid stimulating these areas that set off the pain.

Treatment

There are several medications that may be tried independently or in combination to achieve relief of pain. Surgical treatment options are reserved for tumors or blood vessels that press on the trigeminal nerve, or for patients that do not respond to medical treatment. These procedures include noninvasive radiosurgery (focused radiation therapy), treatment of the nerve by injection or electrical stimulation, and open operation for removing pressure on the nerve.

The DOs

- Take your medication as prescribed.
- Keep all scheduled follow-up appointments so that you can be checked for side effects of your medication.
- Report the improvement or worsening of symptoms to your doctor.

The DON'Ts

- Don't despair. There are many new treatments and support groups available.
- Don't adjust your medication without your physician's approval.

When to Call Your Doctor

- If your symptoms do not improve with the medication that you were prescribed.
- If you have any side effects associated with your medication.
- If you have any new symptoms such as double vision, facial weakness, or changes in hearing or balance.

For More Information

Trigeminal Neuralgia Association
P.O. Box 340
Barnegut Light, NJ 08006
609-361-1014
World Wide Web
http://www.mco.edu/neuro/tripage.html Medical College of Ohio
http://www.neurosurgery-neff.com/Trigeminal Neuralgia.html
Samuel Neff MD, Neurosurgery.

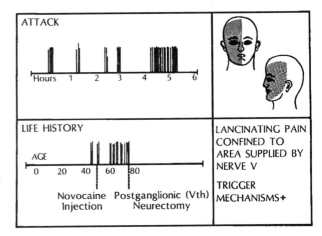

Profile of trigeminal neuralgia. (From Noble J: *Textbook Primary Care Medicine,* vol 2. St. Louis, Mosby–Year Book, Inc., 1995. Used by permission.)

TUBERCULOSIS, PULMONARY

About Your Diagnosis

Pulmonary tuberculosis is a lung infection that is produced by an acid-fast bacillus (AFB) called *Mycobacterium tuberculosis*. Tuberculosis continues to be one of the most common infectious diseases around the world, especially in low-income countries and areas of AIDS. The tuberculosis organism is most often transmitted through the air by coughing. Patients with live organisms detected in their sputum or in any skin lesions are considered potentially contagious, and special precautions are necessary.

The diagnosis of tuberculosis is suspected in patients who have unexplained cough, lung infiltrates, weight loss, or fever. Your doctor will inquire about places you have been or individuals you have spent a lot of time with, usually within 3 months of developing symptoms; any prior tuberculosis history or skin test results; coexisting risk factors (especially human immunodeficiency virus [HIV] risks); foreign travel; use of medications that suppress the immune system; and job situation. Tuberculosis can involve any organ or organ systems, but most often the upper lung areas. Your doctor may order a chest x-ray, sputum sampling, bronchoscopy, and a tuberculosis skin test. Testing for HIV may also be advised. Although preliminary sputum (AFB stain) results may be obtained within a few hours, routine tuberculosis culture and drug susceptibility results take several weeks. Rapid diagnostic testing for tuberculosis is now available in some countries and will greatly help detection and isolation/control efforts. Most patients with tuberculosis can be cured with earlier detection, improved control, and compliance with effective drug treatment.

Living With Your Diagnosis

The importance of early diagnosis and effective long-term treatment of this very serious public health problem (tuberculosis) is critical, especially in individuals with HIV. The emergence of multiply drug-resistant tuberculosis is a real challenge for patients, their families, and the public. In most individuals with active tuberculosis, symptoms and infectivity rapidly dropped with the taking of antituberculous medication. It is extremely important to work with your health care provider and maintain close follow-up to ensure complete response to treatment. In a small proportion of cases, surgical removal of the infected area is required. Family members and other close contacts, as well as caregivers, may also require screening for tuberculosis after an exposure.

Treatment

The treatment of tuberculosis involves notifying public health officials, starting a minimum of three antituberculosis drugs, and monitoring for any drug effects.

Your doctor will likely request additional tests including blood work, sputum samples, chest x-rays, and an eye examination as part of the monitoring while you are taking tuberculous medications. Treatment often is prolonged, with a minimum of 6 months.

The DOs

Anyone concerned about being exposed to tuberculosis should seek medical attention as soon as possible. If you have received a diagnosis of tuberculosis, it is very important to follow the isolation and treatment program outlined by your health provider. Taking the right amount of medication for the right time is very important while maintaining close contact with your health care provider. Do try to understand your tuberculosis problem and how it may impact others as well as yourself.

The DON'Ts

- Do not forget to take your tuberculous medications as prescribed.
- Do not forget to notify your health care provider if you have any concerns about possible medication side effects or if you miss more than one or two doses of medication.
- Do not assume you are not infective unless informed by your doctor.
- Do not drink any alcohol or take other medication unless previously discussed with your physician.
- Do not forget that tuberculosis can involve areas other than the lung.

When to Call Your Doctor

- If you have excessive thirst, urination, or weight change.
- If coughing brings up discolored sputum or blood.
- If you have fever or chills.

- If you have any concerns about the effects of medications.
- If persistent or worsening symptoms are present despite starting antituberculous medication.
- To clarify when to return to work, school, or a health care facility.

For More Information
American Lung Association
1118 Hampton Avenue
St. Louis, MO 63139
800-LUNG-USA
www.lungusa.org
Tuberculosis: What You Should Know, 1994.
Understanding Tuberculosis, Krames, 1994.

TYPHOID FEVER

About Your Diagnosis

Typhoid fever is an infection of the intestinal tract caused by a bacteria. It can also affect the nervous system. Typhoid is transmitted to humans when they eat contaminated food, water, ice, eggs, or undercooked meat. Also, individuals who have or carry the bacteria can transmit the bacteria to others when they handle food without properly washing their hands after using the bathroom.

Typhoid fever is more common in countries that don't have adequately purified water systems. The infection is usually curable in 2–3 weeks with treatment. Typhoid can be fatal if not treated, especially in children.

Living With Your Diagnosis

Signs and symptoms include diarrhea that is often severe, muscle aches, headache, fever, and a rash. Sometimes a child will have abdominal cramps and bloody diarrhea.

Treatment

Antibiotics such as sulfa drugs or ampicillin may be prescribed. Bed rest should be maintained until after symptoms subside; activity can then be gradually increased. During the diarrhea phase, increase fluid intake as tolerated and stay on a liquid diet. As the symptoms subside, gradually change your diet to a well-balanced, high-calorie diet. Isolation may not be possible, but if available use a separate bathroom. If another bathroom is not available, someone will need to scrub the toilet with a bleach solution after each use, using gloves. Hand washing is essential to prevent spreading the disease. Don't give aspirin or aspirin derivatives for the fever because they can irritate the intestinal tract even more. Instead, use tepid sponge baths.

The DOs

- Take the antibiotics as ordered and until finished.
- Increase fluid intake and stay on a liquid diet until the diarrhea stops.
- Advance to a high-calorie diet after the diarrhea stops.
- Isolate the patient or have him use a separate bathroom.
- Scrub the bathroom with a bleach solution after use.

- Wash hands thoroughly and frequently.
- Use tepid sponge baths to reduce fever.
- Rest in bed until symptoms subside.

The DON'Ts

- Don't skip doses or stop antibiotics until finished.
- Don't use aspirin or aspirin derivatives for fever because these medications irritate the intestinal tract.
- If the water supply is of questionable safety, don't eat raw fruits or vegetables unless you peel them yourself.

When to Call Your Doctor

If during treatment, any of the following occurs:
- Sore throat.
- Severe cough.
- Shortness of breath.
- High fever (temperature greater than 102°F).
- Severe abdominal pain.
- Severe headache or earache.

For More Information
National Institute of Allergy and Infectious Diseases
9000 Rockville Pike
Bethesda, MD 20892
301-496-5717
Internet Site
www.healthfinder. gov (Choose SEARCH to search by topic.)

ULCERATIVE COLITIS

About Your Diagnosis

Ulcerative colitis (UC) is a chronic inflammatory disease of the colon. Granulomatous colitis is another name for this disease. It is one of two disorders listed under the category of inflammatory bowel disease. The other disorder is Crohn's disease. Ulcerative colitis causes tiny ulcers and small abscesses to form in the inner lining of the colon. The cause of UC is not known. It affects men and women equally and appears to run in some families. About 250,000 Americans have UC. The most commonly affected individuals are between the ages of 15 and 35 years.

Detection of UC is by a flexible sigmoidoscopy, a procedure where a lighted flexible instrument is inserted into the rectum to view the rectum and the lower portion of colon. Tissue samples are taken from the colon and sent for microscopic examination. Alternative detection methods are colonoscopy, a procedure similar to a flexible sigmoidoscopy but with a longer instrument, or barium enema x-ray. Ulcerative colitis is a lifelong condition in most individuals. About half of the patients will have only mild symptoms. Others experience more frequent and severe attacks. Medications can control the symptoms. This condition is sometimes curable with surgery.

Living With Your Diagnosis

Abdominal pain and bloody diarrhea with mucus are the most common symptoms of UC. The abdominal pain is usually on the left side. A bowel movement may help relieve the pain. As the condition worsens, the diarrhea increases in frequency, Up to 20 stools a day is common. Symptoms of UC may alternate with periods of remission. Over 75% of patients will have relapses.

Other symptoms include fatigue, weight loss, loss of appetite, and fever. Symptoms are not limited to the colon. About 15% to 20% of individuals will have joint pains. The most commonly affected joints are the knees, ankles, and wrists. Eye problems occur in up to 10% of individuals. Complications of UC include severe hemorrhage (blood loss), perforation of the bowel, megacolon (dilatation of the colon), and peritonitis (infection of the abdomen). Individuals with UC are at greater risk for having colon cancer.

Treatment

The goal of treatment is to relieve the symptoms, control the inflammation, and prevent complications. Anti-inflammatory drugs are the main medications used; these include sulfasalazine, mesalamine, olzalazine, and corticosteroids. Sulfasalazine is used to maintain remissions and control minor-to-moderate symptom flares. Corticosteroids are used for major flares and to maintain remissions. This drug can be given as an enema if needed. If symptoms are severe, hospitalization is necessary. The bowel is put at rest (no food orally) and intravenous nutrition given.

About 20% to 25% of UC patients require surgery at some time. Patients who do not respond to medications or have severe disease are good candidates for surgery. The surgery involves removing the affected portion of the colon and joining the two ends of bowel.

The DOs

- Maintain normal physical activity except when symptoms require bed rest.
- Take medications as prescribed.
- A heating pad or hot water bottle placed on the abdomen may help with pain and cramping.
- See your physician regularly. Evaluation of the bowel by colonoscopy to monitor for cancerous changes is important.

The DON'Ts

- Avoid aspirin. This medication can cause bleeding.
- Avoid antidiarrheal medications except for minimal symptoms. These medications can cause megacolon.
- Avoid raw fruits and vegetables. They can cause the symptoms to worsen.
- Avoid spicy foods, coffee, and alcohol. They can cause diarrhea symptoms to worsen.

When to Call Your Doctor

- If you have symptoms of UC.
- If fever or chills develop.
- If the number of bowel movements increase or if bleeding increased.
- If the abdomen becomes distended, the pain increases, or vomiting starts.

For More Information

National Foundation for Ileitis and Colitis
444 Park Avenue S, 11th Floor
New York, NY 10016-7374
800-343-3637
Crohn's and Colitis Foundation of America
386 Park Avenue South, 17th Floor
New York, NY 10016-7374
800-923-2423
National Digestive Diseases Information Clearinghouse
2 Information Way
Bethesda, MD 20892-3570
www.niddk.nih.gov
nddic@aerie.com

URETHRITIS

About Your Diagnosis

Urethritis is an inflammation of the urethra (the tube that carries urine from the bladder) caused by an infection. It may also be present during a bladder infection. Urethritis is caused by bacteria, trauma, or as a reaction to bath oils and bubble baths. It can be detected by testing the urine or by examining a discharge, if there is any.

Living With Your Diagnosis

Signs and symptoms include urinating more frequently and in smaller amounts; pain or burning upon urination; a discharge of cloudy mucus (can also be yellow-green); painful intercourse; and in older men, dribbling of urine.

Treatment

Antibiotics are needed to clear the infection. Sitz baths several times a day will help ease the pain. Nonprescription medications such as Tylenol or Advil can be taken for the pain.

No special diet is needed, but fluid intake should be increased to eight glasses of water a day. Acidify the urine by drinking cranberry juice. Avoid alcohol and caffeine because they irritate the urethra. Avoid sexual intercourse until the infection is cleared. You will need a follow-up urine culture to verify this.

The DOs

- Take antibiotics as ordered until finished.
- Increase your fluid intake to include eight glasses of water per day.
- Avoid sexual intercourse until the infection is cleared.
- Avoid bubble baths and bath oils that may irritate the urethra.
- Keep the genital area clean, but use nonscented plain soaps.

The DON'Ts

- Don't stop taking the antibiotics until finished. If the infection is not cleared, it could become a chronic problem.
- Don't have sexual intercourse until the infection is cleared.
- Don't use bubble baths, bath oils, or scented soaps.
- Don't drink beverages containing alcohol or caffeine.

When to Call Your Doctor

- If a high fever develops.
- If blood is seen in the urine.
- If symptoms don't improve in 1 week.

For More Information
Bladder Health Counsil
300 W. Pratt St., Suite 401
Baltimore, MD 21201
National Kidney and Urologic Disease Information Clearinghouse
301-654-4415
Internet Site
www.healtfinder.gov (Choose SEARCH to search by topic.)

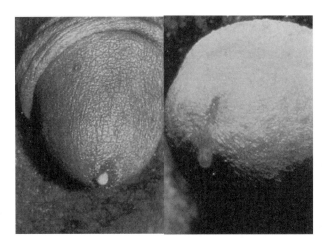

Urethritis in men. Gonococcal urethritis classically produces a profuse and purulent discharge **(A)**, whereas nongonococcal urethritis more often results in a scant mucoid discharge **(B)**. (From Noble J: *Textbook Primary Care Medicine*, vol 2. St. Louis, Mosby–Year Book, Inc., 1995. Used by permission.)

URINARY INCONTINENCE

About Your Diagnosis

Urinary incontinence is the uncontrollable loss of urine. The two most common types of incontinence are "stress incontinence" and "urge incontinence." If you lose urine in a spurt or gush with a cough or sneeze, you probably have stress incontinence. If you lose urine on the way to the toilet because you waited too long or run to the toilet frequently (every 1–2 hours), you probably have urge incontinence.

Stress incontinence can be caused by childbirth or growing older. Urge incontinence can be caused by medication, too much caffeine or alcohol, or growing older. Many women notice bladder problems worsen at the time of menopause.

Urinary incontinence is very common. It is estimated that up to 60% of women have incontinence. The type of urinary incontinence can be diagnosed with "urodynamic testing." Fortunately, most cases of urinary incontinence can be cured or at least improved significantly.

Living With Your Diagnosis

If you occasionally leak a very small amount of urine with a cough or sneeze, or on the way to the toilet, you have very mild incontinence and you may not be interested in treating it. Usually, treatment requires some time and effort. If you leak daily and/or wear a pad for protection, you have mild-to-moderate incontinence and may definitely be interested in treatment options. If you can soak a pad when you lose urine and do it frequently (several times each day), you have severe incontinence. If you have moderate or severe incontinence, you may have found yourself restricting your activities or not going out as much as previously.

Treatment

Fortunately, there are many treatment options available for urinary incontinence. Strengthening the pelvic floor muscles is usually the first step to cure stress incontinence. Contracting the pelvic floor muscles is called "Kegel" exercise. A Kegel is done by pulling in the pelvic floor muscles; it should feel like you are pulling in your rectum or "sucking up water with you pelvic floor." Make sure you are performing the Kegel exercises correctly by having someone observe you who knows what a correct Kegel is. Usually, 40–50 Kegels are recommended each day, i.e., 10 Kegels in a row, 4 or 5 sets each day. Also, it is very important that you try to Kegel (tighten your pelvic floor muscles) when you cough, sneeze, or lift something.

If Kegel exercises do not seem to help, you may be referred for physical therapy to help improve bladder control. Specialized physical therapy for the pelvic floor muscle includes biofeedback and/or functional electrical stimulation. This type of physical therapy is usually done in special centers.

More recently, special types of pessaries have been designed to treat stress incontinence. Sometimes pessaries are very useful for women who only lose urine during certain activities such as jogging, aerobics, and horseback riding, but are otherwise fine. These incontinence pessaries can be placed before the activity and then removed after the activity or left in all day.

Usually, the first step in treating urge incontinence is bladder training. Bladder training is done by voiding (emptying your bladder) at certain intervals. The intervals are gradually lengthened. The goal is to be able to go 3 hours before voiding during the daytime without any episodes of leaking. Sometimes medication is prescribed to help with the bladder training. Medications used to treat urge incontinence may cause some dryness of the mouth or eyes. This side effect is expected and as long as the dryness is tolerable, the medication can be continued.

Surgery can also be used to resolve stress incontinence. There are a variety of different types of surgical procedures. The type of surgical procedure that is best for you should be discussed by you and your specialist. The specialist may be a gynecologist or a urologist.

The DOs

- Do your Kegel exercises as directed. Sometimes a good place to remember to do them is in the car every time you come to a red light or stop sign.
- Take your medication (if one is prescribed) as directed.

The DON'Ts

- Avoid drinking lots of liquids with caffeine in it such as coffee, black tea, and sodas with caffeine (Coca Cola, Pepsi). Caffeine is a diuretic; it makes the kidneys produce more urine at a faster-than-normal rate. This will make both stress and urge incontinence worse, and can cause frequent urination as well.

- Avoid drinking excessive amounts of alcoholic beverages such as beer and wine. Alcohol is a diuretic as well, so it will also make stress and urge incontinence worse. Alcohol can also cause increased urinary frequency.
- Avoid drinking excessive amounts of liquid during the day; most individuals do not need more than 64 ounces (eight 8-ounce glasses) of liquid each day. Also, avoid drinking a lot of fluid at one time. It is better to space out fluid intake evenly during the day.
- If you get up more than twice during the night to urinate, avoid drinking liquids after 7–8 PM.

When to Call Your Doctor
- If your symptoms are not improving.
- If you cannot tolerate the side effects of any prescribed medication.

For More Information:
Alliance for Aging Research
2021 K Street, N.W., Suite 305
Washington, DC 20006
202-293-2856
Help For Incontinent People
PO Box 544
Union, SC 29379
803-579-7900
Simon Foundation for Continence
Box 835
Wilmette, IL 60091
800-23-SIMON or 708-864-3913

URINARY TRACT INFECTION

About Your Diagnosis

Urinary tract infection is a bacterial infection that can affect the bladder or kidneys or both. The most common cause is a bacteria called *Escherichia coli*, which is found in the gastrointestinal tract.

Urinary tract infection is not contagious. The bacteria can find their way into the urinary tract by way of catheters or tubes used during medical treatment, when there is blockage of the urinary tract by stones or congenital abnormalities, or when women have vigorous sexual activity, which allows the bacteria to enter the urethra and bladder. Urinary tract infection can also occur when an infection elsewhere in the body travels through the bloodstream to the kidneys. Urinary tract infection can be detected by culturing a urine specimen.

Living With Your Diagnosis

Signs and symptoms of an infection include burning upon urination, frequency and urgency to urinate, fever and chills, cloudy or bloody urine, lower back pain and lower abdominal pain, and fatigue.

Treatment

Antibiotics will be needed for 7–10 days. The drugs commonly used are ampicillin, ciprofloxacin, Bactrim or Septra, and Macrodantin. Fluid intake should be increased to help flush the urinary system. Caffeine and alcohol should be avoided because they will irritate the urinary system. Analgesics for the urinary system such as pyridium may be prescribed. This drug will turn your urine orange. Sitz baths may also ease the discomfort. Bed rest should be encouraged until fever and pain are gone. No special diet is needed, but drinking juices to acidify the urine can help, such as cranberry or prune juice. Taking Vitamin C can also help.

The DOs

- Take the antibiotics until finished. A repeat urine culture may be needed after the antibiotics are completed to make sure the urine is free of bacteria.
- Take the antibiotics with food to help relieve any stomach upset they may cause.
- Increase your fluid intake. Include cranberry or prune juice.
- Urinate frequently during the day and after intercourse to help avoid infections.
- Use sitz baths to help ease discomfort.
- Rest in bed until fever and pain subside.
- Wipe from the vaginal area toward the rectum after bowel movements to avoid introducing bacteria to the urethral area.

The DON'Ts

- Don't skip doses or stop taking antibiotics before they are finished.
- Don't resume sexual relations until the fever and symptoms have cleared.
- Don't hold your urine for long periods.
- Don't drink caffeinated beverages or alcohol.

When to Call Your Doctor

- If your fever continues after 48 hours of antibiotic therapy.
- If your symptoms return after you complete your antibiotics.

For More Information
National Kidney and Urologic Disease Information Clearinghouse
301-654-4415
Bladder Health Council
388 W. Pratt St., Suite 401
Baltimore, MD 21201
Internet Sites
www.healthfinder.gov (Choose SEARCH to search by topic.)
www.healthanswers.com

UTERINE MALIGNANCY

About Your Diagnosis

The uterus (womb) is located between the bladder and rectum. It is made up of the cervix, which connects the uterus to the vagina, and the body (corpus), from which the fallopian tubes extend. Cancer of the uterus can start from the cervix or from the inner layer of the uterus (the endometrium).

Malignant tumors of the uterus also can start from the muscular body of the uterus or from its connecting tissue and are called uterine sarcoma. Uterine sarcoma is rare, occurring among 1 in 100,000 women. The cause of uterine sarcoma is unknown. Uterine sarcoma can be divided into one of three types, which can be diagnosed only by means of a biopsy and tissue examination. Uterine sarcoma is difficult to cure, but if detected early, the chance for cure is better than if the cancer has spread.

Living With Your Diagnosis

Uterine sarcoma usually becomes apparent with abnormal vaginal bleeding among women who have gone through menopause. Other symptoms include abdominal fullness, bloating, and pain. Urinary symptoms of frequency, urgency, and discomfort can occur. Uterine sarcoma usually spreads local and invades nearby organs, such as the vagina, ovaries, rectum, and bladder.

Treatment

To confirm the diagnosis a D & C is performed to remove tissue for examination with a microscope. D & C means to dilation (widening) of the cervix for insertion of a curette (a spoon-shaped instrument with sharp edges) to remove tissue. Once the diagnosis is made, the physician determines the extent of disease by staging the cancer. Staging tells whether the disease has spread. Blood tests, radiographs (x-rays) of the chest, and computed tomography (CT) of the abdomen and pelvis are performed to look for disease outside the uterus. Stage I means the sarcoma is confined to the uterus. Stage II means the sarcoma extends to the cervix. Stage III means the sarcoma extends to structures in the pelvis. Stage IV means the sarcoma extends beyond the pelvic structures.

Treatment depends on the stage of the disease and can be surgical, radiation, hormonal, or chemotherapy. A surgical procedure is the main treatment. It consists of removing the uterus, fallopian tubes, and ovaries (hysterectomy with bilateral salpingo-oophorectomy). A surgical procedure is generally performed for early-stage disease. The decision to use radiation or chemotherapy depends on the type of uterine sarcoma and the stage of disease. The type of radiation or combination of chemotherapy should be discussed with an oncologist (physician specializing in cancer).

Side effects of surgical treatment are pain and soreness in the pelvic area and problems emptying the bladder or moving the bowels. Side effects of radiation therapy are dry, red, itchy skin, nausea, vomiting, diarrhea, vaginal dryness, pain with intercourse, and frequency, urgency and discomfort with urination. Side effects from chemotherapy are nausea, vomiting, easy bruising and bleeding, infections, fever, and hair loss.

The DOs

- Find a surgeon and oncologist who have experience in the treatment of uterine sarcoma. This cancer is so rare you should seek a cancer center with a team of physicians and healthcare personnel who deal with all aspects of treatment.
- Keep your appointments during and after treatment to monitor for side effects and determine whether the cancer has returned.
- Remember that you will no longer have periods (menstrual cycles) after your operation. If your ovaries are removed or if damage is caused by irradiation, menopause occurs, and you may experience symptoms of menopause such as hot flashes.

The DON'Ts

- Do not ignore any vaginal bleeding after menopause.
- Do not ignore abnormal vaginal bleeding (excess bleeding or bleeding between periods) if you have not gone through menopause.
- Do not believe you will have no sexual desire or not be able to have sexual intercourse after surgical treatment. Sexual intercourse and normal activity can be resumed 4 to 8 weeks after the operation.

When to Call Your Doctor

- If you have any vaginal bleeding or abnormal vaginal bleeding.

- If you have any abnormal vaginal discharge (smell, quantity, color).
- If you need emotional support.
- If you have any side effects of treatment (surgical, radiation, or chemotherapy).

For More Information

Cancer Information Service
1-800-4-CANCER
American Cancer Society
1599 Clifton Road, N.E.
Atlanta, GA 30329
1-800-ACS-2345

UTERINE MYOMAS

About Your Diagnosis

Uterine myomas also called "fibroids" are tumors that grow from the wall of the uterus. The wall of the uterus is made of muscle tissue, so a fibroid is a tumor made of muscle tissue. The fibroids start off very small, actually from one cell, and generally grow slowly over years before they cause any problems. Most fibroids are benign; malignant fibroids are rare. The cause of fibroids is unknown, although it is known that fibroids have a tendency to run in families. Fibroids are very common, with an estimated 50% of women having them. Fibroids can be diagnosed by pelvic examination or by ultrasound.

Fibroids do not have to be removed unless they are causing symptoms such as heavy periods, irregular bleeding, or severe cramps with periods. Also, sometimes the size alone causes enough discomfort so that removal is necessary. Once women go through menopause, fibroids do not usually cause any further problems.

Living With Your Diagnosis

The most common symptoms are:
- Cramping with periods.
- Heavy flow or clots with periods.
- Discomfort, such as pressure, as well as being unable to lie on your stomach and being unable to button your clothing easily, caused by the mass of the fibroids.

Other, less common symptoms include irregular bleeding and urinary frequency caused by the pressure on the bladder from the fibroids.

If your periods are very heavy, you may become anemic and an iron supplement may be recommended.

Treatment

If fibroids become symptomatic enough, they can be removed surgically. The most common surgical approach is to perform an "abdominal myomectomy. An incision is made in the lower abdomen into the abdominal cavity, and the fibroids are removed from the uterus and the uterus stitched closed. If the uterus is no longer necessary (the woman is finished having her family) and the woman desires her uterus removed, a hysterectomy (removal of the uterus) can be performed. (A "hysterectomy" is removal of the uterus and cervix, not removal of the ovaries. Therefore, a woman who has a hysterectomy does not necessarily go through menopause.) If a "submucous" fibroid is diagnosed, then the removal of the fibroid can be performed through the cervix. This is called a "hysteroscopic myomectomy." Because the instrument goes through the cervix, there is no cutting. It is usually a same-day procedure, which means you come in on the day of the procedure and go home the same day, with a minimal recovery period.

If you are very anemic or the fibroids are very large, you may be treated before surgery with a medication called Depot Lupron. This medication puts you into a temporary menopause, thus decreasing your estrogen levels and causing the fibroids to shrink. Unfortunately, this medication does not shrink the fibroids permanently, so it can not be used as a permanent solution.

The DOs

- Keep your follow-up appointments so that your doctor can check your fibroids regularly.
- Take your iron supplement if one has been recommended. This will prevent anemia. It is also helpful to eat a diet rich in iron in addition to the iron supplement.
- If your period cramps are uncomfortable, over-the-counter ibuprofen can be very effective in relieving the cramps. Over-the-counter ibuprofen comes in 200-milligram tablets. You can start with 2 tablets every 4 hours. However, if this does not relieve the cramps enough, you can take 3 tablets (600 milligrams) every 6 hours or 4 tablets (800 milligrams) every 8 hours. You should always take ibuprofen with some food on your stomach to avoid stomach irritation. (Obviously, you should not take ibuprofen if you have an allergy to it, have been told you should not take it or any aspirin-like products, or have a history of ulcer or gastritis.)

The DON'Ts

- If you take birth control pills, you and your doctor may want to consider another birth control method because the estrogen in the birth control pills sometimes stimulate the fibroids to grow more quickly.

When to Call Your Doctor

- If your periods become heavier, either heavier flow or more or larger clots.

- If you have irregular periods/bleeding.
- If the ibuprofen does not relieve enough of the cramps.
- If you feel that the fibroids are suddenly larger, or the mass causes discomfort.

For More Information

Understanding Your Body: Every Woman's Guide to Gynecology and Health. Felicia Stewart, M.D., Felicia Guest, M.D., Gary Stewart, M.D., and Robert Hatcher, M.D., Bantam Books, 1987.

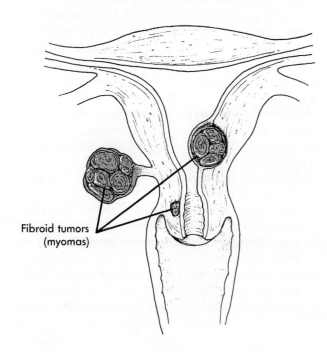

Fibroid tumors (myomas). (From LaFleur-Brooks ML: *Exploring Medical Language—A Student Directed Approach.* vol 3. St. Louis, Mosby–Year Book, 1993. Used by permission.)

VAGINITIS, *CANDIDA*

About Your Diagnosis

Candida vaginitis or "yeast infection" is caused by the fungus *Candida*. It is very common and can occur in women of all ages. Taking antibiotics can make it more likely to develop a yeast infection because antibiotics "kill" the "healthy, protective" bacteria. Lack of the healthy bacteria allows the yeast to grow. When yeast organisms are present in large amounts, they cause symptoms. Women who are diabetic or who are receiving chronic steroid treatment may be more susceptible to yeast infections. Any medical condition in which the immune system is suppressed will increase the risk of developing a yeast infection.

Controversy exists as to whether yeast infections can be sexually transmitted. Recent studies indicate that they are not sexually transmitted in most cases.

Candida vaginitis is diagnosed by examining the vaginal discharge under a microscope or sending a specimen for culture. In most cases, it is easily treated with vaginal creams, suppositories, or oral medication. A few women have recurrent yeast infections.

Living With Your Diagnosis

The most common symptoms are:

- Vulvar and/or vaginal itching.
- White, often clumpy discharge, sometimes described as "cottage cheese–like." (However, yeast infections can be present with minimal discharge as well.)
- Vulvar and/or vaginal burning.

Treatment

Yeast infections can be treated by using a vaginal cream, suppository, or an oral medication. The vaginal creams and suppositories are available without a prescription, whereas the oral medication is only available by prescription. The over-the-counter medications are just as effective, in most cases, as the prescription medication. Some women find the oral medication more convenient to use than vaginal medications. Side effects from any of the medications are uncommon. Occasionally, some women may experience vaginal or vulvar "burning" with the medication.

The DOs

- Take or use all the medication as directed. If you do not finish a complete course, the yeast infection may not be completely treated and may recur.
- If you have a lot of vulvar itching and discomfort, doing "sitz baths" (soaking the vulvar area for 10–15 minutes in plain water that is at a comfortable temperature), then patting the area dry and gently blow-drying the vulvar area can sometimes help relieve the symptoms more quickly.
- Eating 8 ounces of yogurt with live acidophilus bacteria daily may help prevent recurrent yeast infections. (And yogurt is a good source of calcium anyway!)

The DON'Ts

- Don't have intercourse while being treated.
- Avoid wearing tight, "nonbreathing" clothing; for example, panty hose and tight pants.

When to Call Your Doctor

- If symptoms persist after you have finished the complete course of medication.
- If you experience any adverse reaction to the medication, such as vaginal/vulvar burning.

For More Information
Understanding Your Body: Every Woman's Guide to Gynecology and Health. Felicia Stewart, M.D., Felicia Guest, M.D., Gary Stewart, M.D., and Robert Hatcher, M.D., Bantam Books, 1987.

VAGINITIS, *TRICHOMONAS*

About Your Diagnosis

Trichomonas vaginitis is a sexually transmitted vaginal infection. However, it does not cause the serious health problems often associated with other sexually transmitted diseases (such as chlamydia or gonorrhea). It is caused by a "protozoan" (a microscopic living organism). It is a very common infection. It is diagnosed by examining the vaginal discharge under a microscope or by sending a culture specimen to the laboratory. It is usually completely curable by taking the appropriate medication.

Living With Your Diagnosis

The most common symptoms are:
- Intense vaginal/vulvar itching.
- Increased vaginal discharge that may be yellow-greenish or gray.

Treatment

The treatment is metronidazole (Flagyl). Metronidazole can be either taken in a dose of 2 grams all at once, "stat," or in a dosage of 250 milligrams three times each day for 7 days. Both regimens are equally effective. The 2-gram stat dose is easier to take, but the 7-day treatment may be better tolerated by some. Occasionally, metronidazole can cause mild nausea. *Trichomonas* vaginitis has to be treated with oral metronidazole because vaginal metronidazole is not effective.

Your partner (if you have a partner) should be treated at the same time. This is very important. If your partner is not treated, you will get *Trichomonas* again.

Anytime an antibiotic is used, a vaginal yeast infection may follow. (The antibiotic "kills" the "healthy, protective" bacteria as well as the "unhealthy" bacteria, allowing the yeast to grow.) If you experience vulvar or vaginal itching after treatment, you can purchase an over-the-counter antiyeast medication, such as Monistat, Femstat, or Gynelotrimin, or purchase the generic equivalent (just as effective as brand names) and use it as directed. If the itching does not resolve, call your doctor.

The DOs
- Take all your medication as prescribed.
- If you have a partner, make sure your partner is treated.

The DON'Ts
- Refrain from sexual activity (intercourse) while being treated.
- Do not drink any alcoholic beverages while taking the medication. You can become very nauseated!
- Do not take metronidazole if you think you may be pregnant.

When to Call Your Doctor
- If you become very nauseated and cannot take the medication.
- If you have persistent symptoms after you finish the medication.

For More Information
Understanding Your Body: Every Woman's Guide to Gynecology and Health. Felicia Stewart, M.D., Felicia Guest, M.D., Gary Stewart, M.D., and Robert Hatcher, M.D., Bantam Books, 1987.

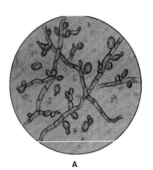 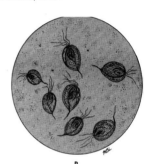

A   B

Microscopic views. **A,** *Candida (Monilia) albicans,* a fungus. **B,** *Trichomonus,* a protozoan or microscopic animal. (From Ingalls AJ, Salerno MC: *Maternal and Child Health Nursing,* vol 7. St. Louis, Mosby–Year Book, 1990. Used by permission.)

VAGINOSIS, BACTERIAL

About Your Diagnosis

Bacterial vaginosis is a vaginal disorder in which women experience infection-like symptoms, although technically it is not an infection. It occurs when the "unhealthy" bacteria in the vagina multiply and outnumber the "healthy" bacteria that normally grow there. Currently, it is the most common vaginal disorder in the United States. It is diagnosed by examining the vaginal discharge under a microscope and checking the pH in the office. It can also be diagnosed by sending a sample of the discharge to a laboratory to be tested. Bacterial vaginosis is completely curable with appropriate treatment; however, it can recur.

Bacterial vaginosis may occur spontaneously, sometimes after resuming sexual activity or after changing partners. Controversy exists as to whether it is actually sexually transmitted. If it recurs after treatment, it may be helpful if your partner is treated.

Living With Your Diagnosis

Symptoms of bacterial vaginosis include:
- Increased vaginal discharge that may be gray.
- Vulvar and/or vaginal irritation.
- A "fishy" odor.

Treatment

Bacterial vaginosis can be treated by using a vaginal antibiotic cream or by taking an oral antibiotic. Both ways are equally effective. You and your doctor can discuss the pros and cons of oral versus vaginal treatment. Taking the antibiotic orally can occasionally cause mild nausea. Some women dislike the cream because it is "messy." Whichever treatment you select, do take or use all the medication as directed. If you stop before you complete treatment, even if the symptoms have resolved, bacterial vaginosis may recur.

Anytime an antibiotic is used, orally or vaginally, a yeast infection may follow. (This is because the antibiotic "kills" the "healthy, protective" bacteria as well as the "unhealthy" bacteria, allowing the yeast to grow.) If you experience vulvar or vaginal itching after treatment, you can purchase an over-the-counter antiyeast medication, such as Monistat, Femstat, or Gynelotrimin, or purchase the generic equivalent (just as effective as brand names) and use it as directed. If the itching does not resolve, call your doctor.

The DOs

- Take or use all your medication as prescribed. If you do not finish the medication, the bacterial vaginosis may be incompletely treated, so it may recur.
- There is some evidence that eating yogurt with live acidophilus bacteria may help keep the vagina healthier and help prevent infection. So you may want to eat 8 ounces of yogurt daily, especially if you are having problems with recurrent vaginal infections. (Yogurt is a great source of calcium anyway! And all women should take in 800 mg of calcium daily. Eight ounces of yogurt has 300 mg of calcium.)

The DON'Ts

- Refrain from intercourse while you are being treated.
- Do not drink any alcoholic beverages if metronidazole (Flagyl) is prescribed; you could become very nauseated.

When to Call Your Doctor

- If you become nauseated and cannot take the medication.
- You continue to have symptoms after you have completed the course of treatment.
- If you treated yourself for a presumed yeast infection and the itching has not resolved.

For More Information
Understanding Your Body: Every Woman's Guide to Gynecology and Health. Felicia Stewart, M.D., Felicia Guest, M.D., Gary Stewart, M.D., and Robert Hatcher, M.D., Bantam Books, 1987.

VENTRICULAR SEPTAL DEFECT

About Your Diagnosis

The ventricles are the lower chambers of the heart. The septum is the heart muscle wall that divides the left and right sides. A defect in the septum produces a hole in the heart. These defects develop before birth (congenital) and may persist as a hole into adulthood. The defect usually closes or is surgically closed in childhood. If the defect is near the aortic valve, damage to the valve may occur as one grows.

The left side of the heart normally pumps under higher pressure than the right side. The ventricular septal defect produces a left-to-right shunt that allows blood from the two sides of the heart to mix. This causes blood with less oxygen to be pumped to the body and oxygenated to travel back to the lungs. This can overload the circulation on the right side of the system (pulmonary hypertension). If the defect is small, it may not cause a problem. Large defects eventually overload the right heart system. This results in heart failure (inefficient pumping of the heart) and causes fatigue, difficulty breathing, especially with exertion, or chest pain. Cyanosis, a bluish tone to the skin, sometimes occurs when the poorly oxygenated blood reaches the skin. Abnormal heart rhythms (arrhythmias) may develop.

Living With Your Diagnosis

Ventricular septal defects are the most common type of congenital heart abnormality and are more common among girls than boys. The defect may close as you grow, but it may persist into adulthood. If you have a small defect or the defect closes, you may never have symptoms and usually need no treatment. If the defect persists, you may have symptoms that necessitate treatment to correct the defect.

Ventricular septal defect is diagnosed on the basis of symptoms and findings at a physical examination. An electrocardiogram (ECG) may show some abnormalities. A chest radiograph (x-ray) may be abnormal, showing enlargement of the lung vessels and an enlarged heart. An echocardiogram (ultrasound examination of the heart) is used to assess the structure and pumping function of the heart and to measure ventricular function and relative pulmonary (lungs) to systemic (body) blood flow.

Treatment

Persons with ventricular septal defects are usually referred to a cardiologist. Treatment of patients with excessive pulmonary flow involves an operation to correct the defect. Heart failure if it develops may be managed with diuretics to reduce excess blood volume or with digitalis medicines to help the contracting efficiency of the heart. Vasodilator medications may be used to reduce the pressure against which the ventricle pumps. Arrhythmias may be managed with antiarrhythmic drugs.

Sometimes replacement of the aortic valve is needed. If there is no other heart disease, correcting the defect usually allows a normal life span and lifestyle.

If you have an open ventricular septal defect or have undergone surgical closure of the defect, antibiotics are required before and after dental or surgical procedures. This helps prevent bacterial endocarditis, an infection of the lining of the heart muscle.

The DOs
- Take your regularly prescribed medications.
- Take antibiotics as prescribed before and after dental and surgical procedures.

The DON'Ts
- Do not neglect worsening symptoms. Seek medical attention for evaluation.

When to Call Your Doctor
- If you have symptoms of ventricular septal defect.

For More Information
The American Heart Association has more information on heart valve disease. Call 1-800-242-8721 and ask for the literature department.

VITILIGO

About Your Diagnosis

Vitiligo is a disorder that causes loss of skin pigment. It is a relatively common problem, affecting 1% of the population. Half of all cases begin before 20 years of age. The cause is not known. In one fourth of cases, there is a family history of vitiligo. Some cases are related to sunburns, trauma, or physical illness. Vitiligo is not contagious. Vitiligo can cause serious cosmetic changes in the skin. It is not life threatening but is sometimes associated with other illnesses such as thyroid diseases, which if present should be treated. Vitiligo is not curable, but some skin pigment may return on the face and neck.

Living With Your Diagnosis

Vitiligo can occur anywhere on the body, but most commonly occurs on the face, hands, and feet. This disorder slowly worsens over time, but remissions (temporary improvements) are common. Vitiligo does not cause any other problems, but it can be associated with disorders such as thyroid disease and diabetes. Vitiligo starts as small, white spots on the skin with no pigment they grow to larger spots and the spots sometimes come together to form larger areas without pigmentation. It occurs on both sides of the body. Common areas of involvement are the nostrils, mouth, eyes, nipples, belly button, and anus. Vitiligo can also affect the hair.

Treatment

Treatment is not always necessary for patients who have mild involvement.

Treatment involves a combination of cosmetics, prescription creams, and specialized light therapy.

Patients with limited areas of involvement can do well with cosmetic stains and makeup. Fair-skinned individuals may benefit from avoidance of tanning. This can be achieved by using sunscreens with an SPF of 15 or greater and avoiding direct sunlight.

For limited areas of involvement, a steroid cream applied once per day can be helpful. Best results may take 3 or 4 months. Steroid creams should not be applied to eyelids, armpits, or groin areas.

Specialized light therapy, or PUVA therapy, consists of application of a solution of medication called psoralens, followed by ultraviolet light therapy. Psoralens can also be taken in pill form. This treatment is most helpful for vitiligo of the face, neck, trunk, upper arms, and upper legs. This is a slow process; results begin after 25–50 treatments depending on the areas of involvement. The major side effect is severe sunburning and blistering.

The DOs

- Mild cases may not require treatment, but if your disorder worsens, seek the advise of your doctor.
- If you will be in the sun, use a sunscreen with an SPF of 15 or higher, and wear a hat, a long-sleeve shirt, and pants.

The DON'Ts

- Avoid direct sunlight especially between 11 AM and 3 PM during summer months.
- Avoid sunburns or tanning. The skin that is not affected by vitiligo will darken with sun tanning, and the affected areas will become more obvious.

When to Call Your Doctor

- If severe reddening or blistering occurs during treatment.
- If any new symptoms occur.

For More Information
American Academy of Dermatology
930 N. Meacham Road
Schaumburg, IL 60173
847-330-0230

VON WILLEBRAND'S DISEASE

About Your Diagnosis

Von Willebrand's disease is an inherited bleeding disorder of variable severity that may manifest itself only with trauma or a surgical procedure. The cause of bleeding is deficiency or abnormality in the von Willebrand factor. This complex factor provides the important interaction between platelets that stops bleeding.

An estimated 1% to 3% of the population carries the gene for von Willebrand's disease. The disease affects men and women equally and affects different ethnic groups. A subtype that constitutes a severe deficiency is rare and affects one in a million persons.

Von Willebrand's disease is inherited from one's parents. It can manifest in all generations (autosomal dominant type) or skip generations (autosomal recessive).

Persons who report easy bruising, bleeding from the mouth or nose, or excessive bleeding after a surgical or dental procedure need to be tested for von Willebrand's disease. Special tests can be performed that measure bleeding time and the amount and quality of von Willebrand factor in the blood. First-degree relatives of patients with the disease benefit from the same tests.

Von Willebrand's disease cannot be cured, but it can be effectively managed to prevent bleeding. Most persons with this disease need treatment only if they need an operation or experience serious trauma. A very small percentage of patients need constant treatment.

Living With Your Diagnosis

There are three subtypes of von Willebrand's disease. Patients with Type I have a mild deficiency and may have excessive bleeding during operations, dental extractions, or trauma. Type II is characterized by production of von Willebrand factor with abnormal function. Most of those patients have mild manifestations. Only patients with Type III, which is very rare, have virtually no von Willebrand factor. They may have spontaneous bleeding from the gums, mouth, nose, and even into muscles or joints.

Once the diagnosis of von Willebrand's disease is made, appropriate treatment and precautions usually prevent excessive bleeding. For patients with mild or moderate disease, there is no limitation on regular exercise.

Treatment

Most patients with Type I and Type II disease do not need treatment. However, in the setting of an elective surgical procedure or serious trauma, treatment is indicated. Patients with Type III von Willebrand's disease need routine supplementation. Desmopressin (DDAVP) is a synthetic hormone that stimulates release of von Willebrand factor from the "storage cells" into the blood stream. It is essential to repeat special blood tests after DDAVP therapy to demonstrate efficacy for every patient. Response to DDAVP can vary.

DDAVP most frequently is administered through intravenous infusion in a hospital or surgical center. It is also available as a nasal spray (Stimate). Stimate can be used at home for on-demand control of minor bleeding and prophylactically before activities that are likely to produce bleeding or minor surgical procedures. DDAVP cannot be used more frequently than once every 48 hours.

For patients who do not respond well to DDAVP, replacement with von Willebrand factor from human plasma is indicated. Cryoprecipitate or special factor concentrates (intermediate purity virus inactivated factor VIII) are used for this purpose.

Other medications used to stop bleeding, such as aminocaproic acid (e.g., Amicar) and tranexamic acid (Cyklokapron), are important during surgical procedures on the oral cavity or gastrointestinal tract.

Patients receiving DDAVP need to be monitored for blood pressure elevations. Some patients experience headaches, nasal congestion, and nausea. Transfusion of cryoprecipitate or factor VIII concentrates carries the risks of use of any blood product. The risks are infection, especially viral infections, and allergic reactions. Virus inactivated products are protected from most viral agents.

The DOs

- Have DDAVP treatment prescribed and monitored by a physician.
- Use Stimate nasal spray according to the instructions. Keep Stimate away from children. A physician monitors the infusion of plasma concentrates in the hospital.
- Be vaccinated for hepatitis A and B virus before transfusions.
- Use medical alert identification.

The DONT's
- Do not use Stimate more frequently than indicated.
- Avoid using anti-inflammatory medications, such as aspirin or ibuprofen (eg, Motrin), without consulting a physician. They can worsen bleeding.
- Avoid interactive sports and games, which can lead to trauma.

When to Call Your Doctor
- If you are going to undergo any operation or dental procedure or participate in a sporting event that can lead to bleeding. Report immediately any bleeding that cannot be controlled with your regular medication.

For More Information
National Heart, Lung, and Blood Institute Information Center
P.O. Box 30105
Bethesda, MD 20824-0105
301-251-1222
National Organization for Rare Disorders
P.O. Box 8923
New Fairfield, CT 06812
203-746-6518
MedWeb Hematology: http://www.gen.emory.edu/medweb.hematology.html
MedMark Hematology: http://medmark.bit.co.kr/hematol.html
World Federation of Hemophilia: http://www.wfh.org/

WARTS

About Your Diagnosis

All warts, no matter where they grow on the body or what they look like, are caused by the same family of viruses called the human papillomavirus (HPV) group. Although in the same family, different types of these viruses tend to infect different areas of the body.

Warts are classified by their characteristic appearance as well as where they appear on the body.

- Common warts: warts that frequently occur on the hands, arms, and legs. The warts often look like little rough cauliflowers.
- Periungual warts: warts around the fingernails.
- Flat warts: warts are flat, slightly elevated, and flesh colored, and occur on the face, knees, and elbows of children and young women.
- Genital warts: warts on the genital and rectal area, often transmitted sexually.
- Plantar warts: warts on the bottom of the feet, often transmitted by bare feet.
- Filiform warts: warts that are small with hairlike projections.

Warts may look different and occur in different places on the body, but they are all caused by the HPV family.

Warts are extremely common, especially in individuals 10–20 years of age. The majority of these warts (up to 65%) will disappear on their own without treatment within 2 years. Unfortunately warts often come back even when treated.

Because warts are an infection, you can catch warts from another individual and you can give warts to someone. You can also infect other parts of your body by scratching and picking warts. Skin that is moist from prolonged soaking, or skin that has been open by cuts or scratches is more likely to become infected by virus and form warts.

Treatment of warts is usually but not always successful. The treatment itself can often cause problems such as pain, infection, and scarring. With the high number of warts that go away on their own (65% in 2 years), not all warts need treatment. However, depending on where the wart is, how big it is, how many there are, and your degree of concern about it (physical and emotional), as well as to prevent spread of the wart, treatment may be needed. Your doctor should be consulted if you have any questions.

Living With Your Diagnosis

Most warts are little more than unsightly tumors on the skin. At times they are in places where they can catch and bleed, such as on the face and head. The long-term effects of most warts are usually not serious or dangerous, but warts are not pretty and can spread. If you decide to get rid of your warts, you must treat carefully. The treatment often takes several weeks, and in some cases can cause pain, blistering, and infection. Self-treatment for some warts can be done by yourself using over-the-counter medications. Other warts, especially genital warts that may lead to cancer, need to be treated by your doctor.

Treatment

Treatment depends to some extent on where the warts are located.

Warts of the common variety on the arms, hands, and legs can initially be treated by salicylic acid and lactic acid in solution (Duofilm, Dalactic Film, Viranol Solution, Wart Solution). You should apply the solution each night directly on the wart. Peel off any dead skin from the previous night's treatment. If redness or pain occurs, the treatment needs to be stopped for a few days. Usual treatment is from 2 to 3 weeks. If satisfactory results are not obtained, stronger medication may be needed from your doctor.

Plantar warts can be treated with application of 40% salicylic acid plasters. Cut the plaster to the size of the wart and place on the wart; remove weekly, cleaning all dead skin. The wart should begin to go away in 2–3 weeks; if not, you may need to see your doctor to obtain stronger medication.

Flat warts are often treated with skin peeling using acne medications. This will require seeing your doctor.

Genital warts almost always require the evaluation of your doctor to ensure the warts have not spread. Treatment is usually with a blistering agent that will require your doctor's application and follow-up. Your sexual partner will need to be examined also.

Other treatments include freezing the warts, injecting them with drugs that stimulate the immune system, surgically cutting the warts, and burning the warts with a laser or electricity. Your doctor will know which method is best for your particular warts.

The DOs
- Do treat warts early to improve response to treatment.
- Do wash hands after touching your warts if you must touch them at all.
- Do use salicylic acid solution on common warts as directed.
- Do use salicylic acid plasters on plantar warts.

The DON'Ts
- Don't bite fingernails, pick cuticles, or soak hands for long periods.
- Don't pick at, dig at, or pull warts.
- Don't cut or scrape warts.
- Don't let your skin come in contact with warts.
- Don't shave or cut hair over warts.

When to Call Your Doctor
- If you have warts that cannot be treated by over-the-counter preparations of salicylic acid.
- If after several weeks of treatment your warts are no better.

For More Information
American Academy of Dermatology
930 N. Meachum Road
Schaumburg, IL 60173
847-330-0230

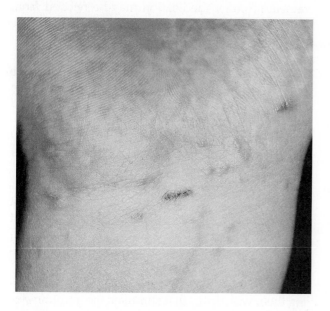

Common warts. (Courtesy of Thomas Habif, M.D. From Thibodeau GA, Patton KT: *The Human Body in Health & Disease,* vol 2. St. Louis, Mosby–Year Book, 1996. Used by permission.)

WARTS, PLANTAR

About Your Diagnosis

All warts including plantar warts are caused by the family of viruses called the human papillomavirus (HPV) group. Certain HPV viruses are more likely to infect one area of the body than the other. In the case of plantar warts, the HPV virus infects the bottom of the foot.

Anyone can get warts; they are very common in the United States. The most likely group of individuals to get warts are those between the ages of 10 and 20 years. Plantar warts are often obtained by walking barefoot in public locker rooms, showers, and pool areas. Individuals with plantar warts leave the virus behind on the moist floor, which is then picked up by bare feet.

Plantar warts can be a big problem because they are on the bottom of the foot. When we stand on them, the warts are like a big lump in our shoe and it hurts. The pain can become so severe that simply standing becomes difficult.

Living With Your Diagnosis

A plantar wart begin as a thickening of the skin on the bottom of the foot. At first this may seem like a small callous or bunion, but over time the plantar wart becomes larger, hurts, and takes on a very sharp border. It is flat, usually flesh colored, but can bleed and become brown or blackish.

The plantar wart will often grow and make walking, running, and even standing very painful. A large number of plantar warts will go away on their own; more than 65% of all warts will go away in 2 years with no treatment.

Treatment

Because the plantar wart forms on the sole of the foot, it is often covered by thick skin. After soaking in a shower or bath, gentle abrasion with a coarse cloth or pumice rock will remove some of this thick skin. This will help the medication to get to the wart but not go too deeply and cause soreness or bleeding.

The usual medication placed on a plantar wart is 40% salicylic acid in plaster form (Duoplast). Salicylic acid ointment can also be applied and covered with an occlusive tape. The premade plaster (Duoplast) is easier to use. The plaster is cut to the size of the plantar wart and applied once a week. The acid will kill the wart and the skin around it.

Each time the plaster is taken off, the underlying whitish dead skin must be removed. Sometimes the plaster will cause inflammation and tenderness. If this occurs you should stop the treatment for 2 or 3 days. Treatment should be continued until the wart is gone. This may take several weeks.

If the plantar wart does not go away, or if it becomes very sore with treatment, you need to call your doctor. Your doctor has other treatments that may be more successful. Warts can come back even after a cure. You must remember to avoid reinfection if at all possible.

The DOs
- Do treat plantar warts early; waiting makes treatment more difficult.
- Do wear protective footwear (flip flops, sandals) in public showers, locker rooms, and pool areas.
- Do gently remove dead skin overlying the wart.
- Do use salicylic acid plasters or ointment on plantar warts.
- Do wash hands after touching your plantar warts.

The DON'Ts
- Don't cut, dig, or pick at your plantar warts.
- Don't put your feet in contact with warts on other parts of the body.
- Don't cause your warts to bleed.
- Don't continue treatment of your plantar warts if they become painful or sore.

When to Call Your Doctor
- If your wart does not go away with salicylic acid treatment, or if it becomes worse.

For More Information
American Academy of Dermatology
930 N. Meachum Road
Schaumburg, IL 60173
847-330-0230

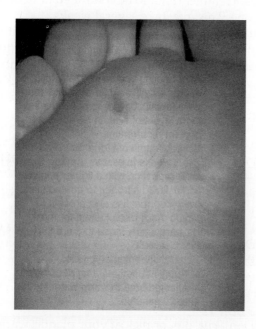

Plantar warts. Note disruption of skin lines. (Courtesy of Beverly Sanders, M.D. From Goldstein BG, Goldstein AO: *Practical Dermatology*, vol 1. St. Louis, Mosby–Year Book, 1992. Used by permission.)

WEGENER'S GRANULOMATOSIS

About Your Diagnosis

Wegener's granulomatosis is an inflammatory condition that affects many tissues in the body. It was originally described as a "flu-like" illness in the first patients in whom this condition was diagnosed, because its principal symptoms are similar to those of a viral illness. The dominant organs involved in the inflammatory process are the lungs, kidneys, eyes, and muscles. The disease ranges in severity from mild pain and weight loss to sudden kidney failure, shortness of breath with pneumonia, or severe eye pain (because of inflammation of those tissues).

There is no known substance or agent that gives rise to this condition. It is classified as an autoimmune disease, which means that the body develops immune proteins (called antibodies) that attack various cells and cause damage. Wegener's granulomatosis is a rare disease, although the exact incidence is unknown. Typically, the patient is older than 40 years at the time of presentation, and women are affected more often than men, although it is not clear why.

There is no tendency for the condition to be passed on to children. It does not have a vector for transmission. Often patients have Wegener's granulomatosis diagnosed because of the "constellation" of symptoms present that raises the doctor's concern: some patients initially have mild kidney failure, fatigue, fevers, and a pneumonia on chest X-ray. In others, Wegener's granulomatosis is more dramatic in its presentation, and affected patients require hospitalization for close care. There is an antibody that can be detected in the blood of most affected patients (called the ANCA antibody). The presence of this antibody has been closely linked to the presence of Wegener's granulomatosis.

With modern treatments, patients do extremely well in disease remission.

Living With Your Diagnosis

Patients with Wegener's granulomatosis may have kidney failure, shortness of breath, or fevers and weight loss. The treatment offered today seems to alleviate most of the symptoms. As with most chronic inflammatory diseases, patients can become debilitated over time, especially if they don't respond to or comply with medical therapy. Depression may occur, and patients who don't take care of themselves can become malnourished.

Treatment

Your physician will be offering you two principal treatments. All patients require steroid medication in the form of prednisone. In addition, studies have shown a better cure rate with potent medicine called cyclophosphamide(Cytoxan) or azathioprine (Imuran). Trimethoprim-sulfamethoxazole (Bactrim, Septra) may reduce the incidence of relapses of Wegener's granulomatosis.

If you have severe Wegener's granulomatosis, your doctor may admit you to a hospital to treat you with intravenous medications and a special form of blood treatment, called plasmapheresis. This is where the antibodies in the blood are removed quickly, and fresh proteins are administered.

All treatments carry risk of side effects.

Steroids may raise blood pressure; raise blood sugar (induce diabetes in some patients); cause stomach ulcers; cause bruising; increase susceptibility to infection; cause flushing; and with long-term therapy, may cause cataracts or worsen osteoporosis. There are more potential side effects your physician can describe for you.

Cytoxan may cause nausea, hair loss, a lowering of blood cell counts (with more chance of infection), and rarely infertility in women.

The DOs

- Medications: prednisone is best taken with milk to avoid irritating the stomach. It is very important to take the prescribed steroid course becaues abrupt cessation can be harmful. Do wear a Medic-Alert bracelet, or some alternative, to let others know you are receiving this important treatment.
- Diet: do eat well and take supplementary calories as necessary, to avoid getting debilitated. Your dietitian can help. • If your blood sugar goes up with prednisone, your doctor may place you on a type of diet used in diabetic patients. Do stick to the diet to avoid serious complications of high blood sugars.
- Exercise: do stay as active as possible to minimize the time spent recuperating. Patients who are bed bound are slower to recover from the illness.
- Your doctor will need to keep a close eye on you and your blood counts during treatment: it's very

important to keep the appointments you set. Patients on these drugs need close supervision.

The DON'Ts

- Don't take over-the-counter medications unless you receive the doctor's advice to do so. Some medications should be avoided until your body is healed.
- Don't skip doses of prednisone. To do so can be harmful to you.
- Don't cheat on any dietary advice you might receive. Patients with high blood glucose levels (mild diabetes) and kidney problems need to restrict their food intake to avoid serious illness. The provider and his team will let you know of any restrictions you should observe.
- Don't overdo work/exercise to exhaustion. That will drain your reserves further.

When to Call your Doctor

Should you experience any symptoms associated with treatment, or if you cannot tolerate or forget to take the treatment, you should call. Also, you should call if you experience new symptoms that you are concerned about, such as cough, shortness of breath, pain (especially ulcer pains), difficulty swallowing, and sore throat. Finally, if you get a fever or chills during your treatment, call if you have any concerns.

For More Information

You can read the pamphlet on Wegener's granulomatosis available from the National Kidney Foundation. Your local office of the National Kidney Foundation may be reached at 1-800-622-9010 or by writing the Head Office at 30 East 33rd Street, New York, NY 10016. They will enable you to reach a support group.

WHIPPLE'S DISEASE

About Your Diagnosis

Whipple's disease is a rare condition. It is also known by the names lipophagic intestinal granulomatosis, intestinal lipodystrophy, and secondary nontropical sprue. It is a systemic disease that affects many organ systems (heart, lung, brain, joints, gastrointestinal, and eye). It almost always involves the small intestine causing malabsorption. Malabsorption is the inadequate absorption of nutrients. The cause is not fully understood but is probably caused by a bacterial infection. Despite being a bacterial infection, the disease does not appear to be contagious. It appears that the patient's own immune system plays a role in the cause of the disease. The disease affects primarily middle-aged men. Whipple's disease occurs in about 1 in 100,000 individuals. It is more common in blacks.

To detect this condition, lymph node or small intestine biopsies are done. A special stain technique (periodic acid–Schiff) is used before the microscopic examination is done. The biopsy specimens show macrophages containing bacteria. Without treatment, the condition is progressive and usually fatal. Treatment improves the chances of a good outcome.

Living With Your Diagnosis

The onset of symptoms is usually slow. The four most common symptoms are weight loss, diarrhea, joint pain, and abdominal pain. The joints most commonly affected are the ankles, knees, shoulders, and wrist. The joint pain tends to be migratory (move from joint to joint). The joint pain may begin several months to up to 10 years before other symptoms appear. Additional symptoms involving the gastrointestinal system include steatorrhea (fatty stools), bloating, and gastrointestinal bleeding. The skin may become pigmented, taking on a gray-to-brown coloration. Symptoms such as fever, peripheral edema (swelling of the feet and hands), clubbing of the fingers, cough, pleuritic chest pain, and enlarged lymph glands (lymphadenopathy) also occur. The most common neurologic symptoms are mental status changes, confusion, and memory loss. Individuals with Whipple's disease may have abnormalities of the eye, such as ocular inflammation, vitreous opacities, and supranuclear ophthalmopegia. These conditions can affect the vision. Heart murmurs can also develop because of problems with the heart valves. Most individuals with Whipple's disease are anemic (have a low red blood cell count).

Treatment

The treatment of Whipple's disease often requires hospitalization. Prolonged antibiotic therapy with a drug that can treat central nervous system infections is used. These drugs include penicillin G, ampicillin, streptomycin, and trimethoprim-sulfamethoxazole. The reappearance of symptoms may indicate drug-resistant organisms, requiring a change of antibiotics. Occasionally corticosteroids can be used along with the antibiotics.

In addition, the nutritional deficiencies caused by the malabsorption must be treated. This is usually done with dietary supplements. The nutritional deficiencies may be severe enough that intravenous nutrition may have to be given.

The DOs

- Complete the prescribed antibiotic regimen to lessen the chances of relapse.
- The patient and family should watch for any neurologic changes such as mental status changes, memory loss, visual changes, headaches, or seizures.
- Maintain a proper diet.
- See your physician regularly for follow-up visits.

The DON'Ts

- Do not miss medication doses; Whipple's disease can relapse.
- Avoid alcohol.

When to Call Your Doctor

- If there is persistent abdominal pain and diarrhea.
- If you have a temperature of greater than 101°F.
- If being treated for Whipple's disease, call if symptoms worsen (or do not improve).
- If symptoms reappear or if new symptoms develop.

For More Information
National Digestive Diseases Information Clearinghouse
2 Information Way
Bethesda, MD 20892-3570
www.niddk.nih.gov
nddic@aerie.com

WOLFF-PARKINSON-WHITE SYNDROME

About Your Diagnosis

Wolff-Parkinson-White syndrome is commonly referred to as WPW. WPW is a condition in which the ventricles of the heart are electrically stimulated to contract out of sequence with the rest of the heart. The atria of the heart normally receive a signal to contract and force blood into the ventricle. The ventricle is properly filled before it contracts to send its blood out from the heart. If it is electrically excited out of order, the ventricle contracts before it has been completely filled with blood. This is an arrhythmia called *pre-excitation*. It can occur on either side of the heart. WPW is the most common type of pre-excitation syndrome. It causes the heart to beat too fast (tachycardia).

Living With Your Diagnosis

This condition is caused by an abnormal electrical pathway leading down to the ventricle from the atria. It can occur because of congenital abnormalities (problems present at birth), heart valve problems, hyperthyroidism, or hypertrophic cardiomyopathy (heart muscle disease). Persons with WPW often have no symptoms except those related to the medical condition that may have caused the WPW.

Sometimes symptoms of heart palpitations (irregular, pronounced, rapid beats) cause the heart to beat faster than usual for no apparent reason. You may have fainting or spells of lightheadedness. About half of persons with WPW never have symptoms. WPW is not rare, but because many persons with the condition never have symptoms, it is only found when you undergo an electrocardiogram (ECG) for another reason. The diagnosis of WPW is made on the basis of a characteristic pattern on an ECG.

Your diet does not generally affect this condition, but a healthy low-fat diet is generally recommended for anyone with a heart condition.

Treatment

Persons with this condition but no symptoms do not need treatment. They live as long as persons with normal hearts. Persons with symptoms should undergo an ECG while the symptoms are happening so that the physician can check the electrical pattern of the heart. Some patterns may necessitate hospitalization for intravenous medications to control the symptoms. Patients with symptoms not controlled with medications may need to undergo cardioversion (which means shock) or ablation (which means removal) of the electrical pathways.

Patients with symptoms of WPW frequently are able to stop the tachycardia by using one of several maneuvers. Straining (as if lifting something heavy) may slow the rapid heart rate. Gently massaging the carotid artery in the neck for a few seconds or applying a cold, wet towel to the face for a few minutes may slow the heart rate. These techniques should be tried as soon as symptoms are felt for best results.

Persons with frequent, recurrent symptoms may need medications. Medications for WPW are used either to manage the condition causing the arrhythmia or to control the response of the ventricle to the abnormal electrical pathway. Medications used to treat recurrent symptoms of WPW include atenolol, amiodarone, quinidine, procainamide, or propranolol.

The side effects of the medications should be monitored. Each of these medications can cause nausea, vomiting, or diarrhea. Each may lower the blood pressure and may cause additional arrhythmias. Atenolol and propranolol are beta-blockers and should be used with caution by persons with diabetes or asthma. They may decrease the ability to exercise because they prevent the heart from beating too fast. Quinidine may cause fever, rash, or cinchonism (ringing in the ears, dizziness, headache). Procainamide may cause a rash, fever, or joint pain.

The DOs

- Learn the maneuvers used to control tachycardia.
- Take your medications as prescribed.
- Stop smoking.
- Have a stress (exercise) test performed before starting any exercise program.

The DON'Ts

- Do not forget to take your medications on a regular schedule, that is, at the same time each day.

When to Call Your Doctor

- If you have new or worsening symptoms such as uncontrolled rapid heartbeat, fainting, shortness of breath or chest pain.
- If you have side effects of your medications.

For More Information
Contact the American Heart Association at 1-800-242-8721 and ask for the literature department.

Appendix 1

Breast Self-Examination (BSE)

Breast self-examination should be done once a month so that you become familiar with the usual appearance and feel of your breasts. Familiarity makes it easier to notice any changes in the breast from one month to another. Early discovery of a change from what is "normal" is the main idea behind BSE.

If you menstruate, the best time to do BSE is 2 or 3 days after your period ends, when your breasts are least likely to be tender or swollen. If you no longer menstruate, pick a day, such as the first day of the month, to remind yourself it is time to do BSE.

Here is how to do BSE:

1. Stand before a mirror. Inspect both breasts for anything unusual, such as any discharge from the nipples, puckering, dimpling, or scaling of the skin.

The next two steps are designed to emphasize any change in the shape or contour of your breasts. As you do them, you should be able to feel your chest muscles tighten.

2. Watching closely in the mirror, clasp your hands behind your head and press hands forward.
3. Next, press hands firmly on hips and bow slightly toward your mirror as you pull your shoulders and elbows forward.

Some women do the next part of the exam in the shower. Fingers glide over soapy skin, making it easy to concentrate on the texture underneath.

4. Raise your left arm. Use three or four fingers of your right hand to explore your left breast firmly, carefully, and thoroughly. Beginning at the outer edge, press the flat part of your fingers in small circles, moving the circles slowly around the breast. Gradually work toward the nipple. Be sure to cover the entire breast. Pay special attention to the area between the breast and the armpit, including the armpit itself. Feel for any unusual lump or mass under the skin.
5. Gently squeeze the nipple and look for a discharge. Repeat the exam on your right breast.
6. Steps 4 and 5 should be repeated lying down. Lie flat on your back, left arm over your head and a pillow or folded towel under your left shoulder. This position flattens the breast and makes it easier to examine. Use the same circular motion described earlier.

Repeat on your right breast.

[1]From US Department of Health and Human Services, National Institutes of Health, National Cancer Institute, US Public Health Service Pub. No 86-2000, 1986.

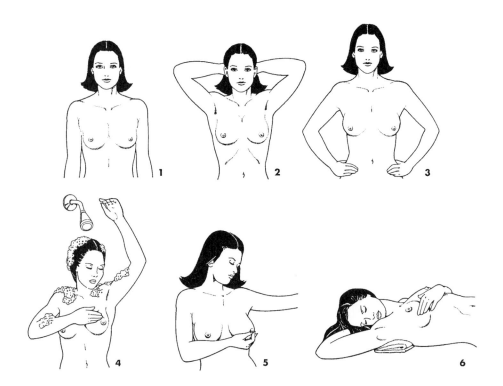

Appendix 2
Food Guide Pyramid

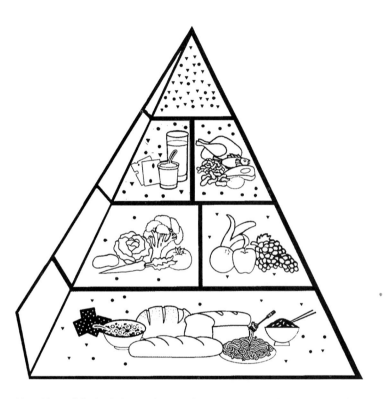

Food guide pyramid: guide to daily food choices. (From Nelson JK: Diet manual, a handbook of nutrition practices, US Department of Agriculture, US Department of Health and Human Services.)